HOLT

LEVEL RED

Decisions for Health

TEACHER EDITION

CONTENTS IN BRIEF

Teacher's Pages

Contents in Brief	T1
Program Overview	T2
Scope and Sequence	T4
Student Edition	T6
Teacher Edition	T8
Assessment Resources	T10
Teaching Resources	T12
Technology Resources	T14
Online Resources	T16
Activities	T18
Meeting Individual Needs	T20
Reading & Writing Skills	T22
Life Skills	T24
Cross-Disciplinary Skills	T25
Pacing Guide	T26
National Health Education Standards	T28
Sensitive Issues	T33

Student Edition
(recommended for 7th grade)

1	Health and Wellness	2
2	Successful Decisions and Goals	20
3	Building Self-Esteem	48
4	Physical Fitness	64
5	Nutrition and Your Health	92
6	A Healthy Body, a Healthy Weight	114
7	Mental and Emotional Health	132
8	Managing Stress	156
9	Encouraging Healthy Relationships	174
10	Conflict and Violence	196
11	Teens and Tobacco	218
12	Teens and Alcohol	244
13	Teens and Drugs	268
14	Infectious Diseases	298
15	Noninfectious Diseases and Disorders	320
16	Your Changing Body	346
17	Your Personal Safety	372
	Appendix	406
	Glossary	422

HOLT, RINEHART AND WINSTON
A Harcourt Education Company

Orlando • **Austin** • New York • San Diego • Toronto • London

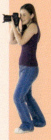

PROGRAM OVERVIEW

All the content you need with the flexibility you want!

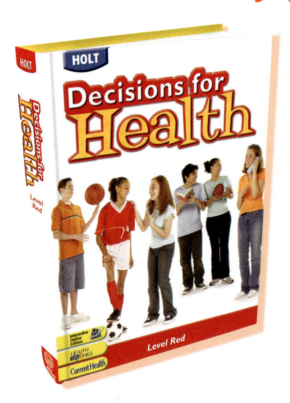

With its accessible two- to six-page lesson structure, **Decisions for Health** benefits both you and your students. Short, manageable lessons keep students focused on reading for understanding, while frequent assessment ensures comprehension. The flexible structure allows you to pick and choose what you want to teach.

A FOCUS ON LIFE SKILLS AND ACTIVITIES BOOSTS STUDENTS' UNDERSTANDING

- 9 **Life Skills** are developed and assessed throughout the program, with an added emphasis on decision-making and refusal skills.
- **Hands-On Activity** encourages active learning.
- Cross-disciplinary features throughout the program integrate language arts, math, science, and social studies skills into your core curriculum.
- Writing skills are developed through features such as **Start Off Write** and **Health Journal.**

REAL-LIFE FEATURES MAKE HEALTH RELEVANT TO STUDENTS

- The program incorporates feedback from a Teen Advisory Board.
- Realistic photos and graphics enhance lessons.
- Real-life examples like **Myth & Fact** keep students interested and dispel their misconceptions.

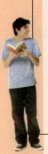

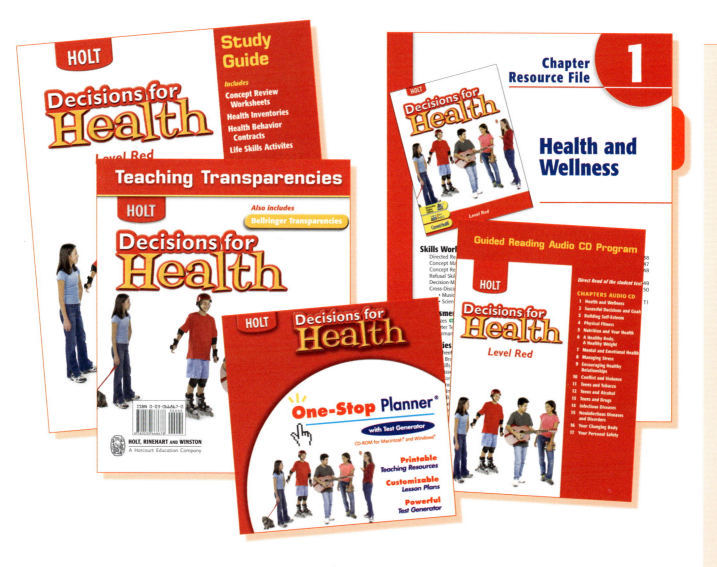

PROGRAM OVERVIEW

INTEGRATED TECHNOLOGY REINFORCES AND EXTENDS LEARNING

- Lighten the load with an interactive *Online Edition* or *CD-ROM Version* of the student text.

- **HealthLinks,** a Web service developed and maintained by NSTA, contains current and prescreened links to the best health-related Web sites available.

- *Current Health* online magazine articles and activities relate health to students' lives.

- All the resources you need are on the **One-Stop Planner® CD-ROM with Test Generator** with worksheets, customizable lesson plans, and the powerful **ExamView®** Test Generator.

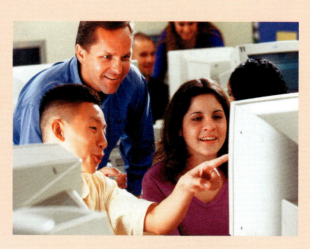

Health scope and sequence overview

Holt, Rinehart and Winston's health programs offer educators a complete health curriculum for grades 6-12. The Holt product development teams for both programs worked together to build a bridge between middle school and high school. Up-to-date health content, supported by a strong **Life Skills** emphasis (see page T24 for details) and effective activities, provide educators with two programs that help students make healthy lifestyle decisions.

Health educator research, state health curricula, and the National Health Education Standards were critical in determining overall program philosophies and content. Both programs offer a flexible format, easily customized to specific curriculum, to meet the needs of health educators and their students.

Decisions for Health for middle school uses a unique two- to six-page lesson organization. A **Health Handbook** at the end of *Lifetime Health* for high school contains, among other things, 37 **Express Lessons** of two to four pages each, giving teachers additional flexibility in presenting critical content.

Decisions for Health
MIDDLE SCHOOL

CH	LEVEL GREEN (recommended for 6th grade)	LEVEL RED (recommended for 7th grade)	LEVEL BLUE (recommended for 8th grade)
1	Health and Wellness	Health and Wellness	Health and Wellness
2	Making Good Decisions	Successful Decisions and Goals	Making Healthy Decisions
3	Self-Esteem	Building Self-Esteem	Stress Management
4	Body Image	Physical Fitness	Managing Mental and Emotional Health
5	Friends and Family	Nutrition and Your Health	Your Body Systems
6	Coping with Conflict and Stress	A Healthy Body, a Healthy Weight	Physical Fitness
7	Caring for Your Body	Mental and Emotional Health	Sports and Conditioning
8	Your Body Systems	Managing Stress	Eating Responsibly
9	Growth and Development	Encouraging Healthy Relationships	The Stages of Life
10	Controlling Disease	Conflict and Violence	Adolescent Growth and Development
11	Physical Fitness	Teens and Tobacco	Building Responsible Relationships
12	Nutrition	Teens and Alcohol	Conflict Management
13	Understanding Drugs	Teens and Drugs	Preventing Abuse and Violence
14	Tobacco and Alcohol	Infectious Diseases	Tobacco
15	Health and Your Safety	Noninfectious Diseases and Disorders	Alcohol
16		Your Changing Body	Medicine and Illegal Drugs
17		Your Personal Safety	Infectious Diseases
18			Noninfectious Diseases
19			Safety
20			Healthcare Consumer
21			Health and the Environment

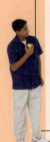

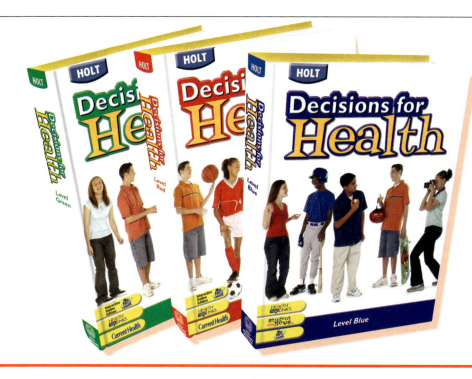
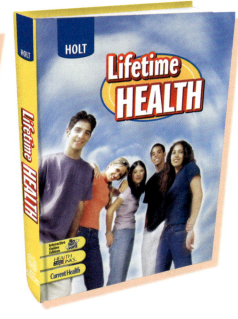

SCOPE AND SEQUENCE

Lifetime Health
HIGH SCHOOL

(recommended for grades 9-12)

- Leading a Healthy Life
- Skills for a Healthy Life
- Self-Esteem and Mental Health
- Managing Stress and Coping with Loss
- Preventing Violence and Abuse
- Physical Fitness for Life
- Nutrition for Life
- Weight Management and Eating Behaviors
- Understanding Drugs and Medicines
- Alcohol
- Tobacco
- Illegal Drugs
- Preventing Infectious Diseases
- Lifestyle Diseases
- Other Diseases and Disabilities
- Adolescence and Adulthood
- Marriage, Parenthood, and Families
- Reproduction, Pregnancy, and Development
- Building Responsible Relationships
- Risks of Adolescent Sexual Activity
- HIV and AIDS

Lifetime Health Express Lessons

How Your Body Works
- Nervous System
- Vision and Hearing
- Male Reproductive System
- Female Reproductive System
- Skeletal System
- Muscular System
- Circulatory System
- Respiratory System
- Digestive System
- Excretory System
- Immune System
- Endocrine System

What You Need to Know About…
- Environment and Your Health
- Public Health
- Selecting Healthcare Services
- Financing Your Healthcare
- Evaluating Healthcare Products
- Evaluating Health Web Sites
- Caring for Your Skin
- Caring for Your Hair and Nails
- Dental Care
- Protecting Your Hearing and Vision

First Aid and Safety
- Responding to a Medical Emergency
- Rescue Breathing
- CPR
- Choking
- Wounds and Bleeding
- Heat- and Cold-Related Emergencies
- Bone, Joint, and Muscle Injuries
- Burns
- Poisons
- Motor Vehicle Safety
- Bicycle Safety
- Home and Workplace Safety
- Gun Safety Awareness
- Safety in Severe Weather
- Recreational Safety

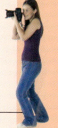

A Student Edition that builds understanding

Relevant graphics, tables, and photos enhance understanding with visual examples of concepts and topics.

The **Lessons** guide focuses reading with a preview of the chapter.

ENGAGING CONTENT GETS STUDENTS INVOLVED

What You'll Do lays out the objectives for each lesson, while **Terms to Learn** highlights new vocabulary.

Accessible navigation engages students with short, two- to six-page lessons, outline-style headings, content grouped into small chunks, and text that doesn't break between pages.

Links to **Current Health** online magazine articles offer articles that expand on content in meaningful ways.

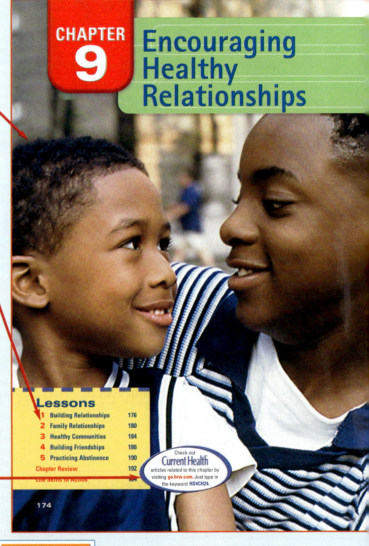

APPLYING HEALTH TO THE REAL WORLD

A variety of engaging features provoke thought and clear up misconceptions:

- **Myth & Fact** addresses common misunderstandings about health.
- **Teen Talk** answers real questions from real teens.
- **Warning!** calls attention to dangers to students' health.
- **Brain Food** motivates students with fun facts.

Myth & Fact

Myth: As soon as a drug's effects go away, the drug is out of your system.

Fact: The effects of a drug may stop after a few hours. However, the drug actually remains in your bloodstream for some time. Traces of some drugs can be found in the bloodstream for up to 2 months after the drug was taken.

Brain Food

A typical cigarette or a pinch of snuff can contain more than 10 milligrams of nicotine. Soaking this amount of tobacco in a few ounces of water overnight can make an effective insecticide.

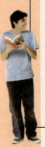

Relevant quotes from young people with whom your students can identify bring health issues home.

Health IQ prepares students for the subject ahead with pre-reading questions that test their existing knowledge.

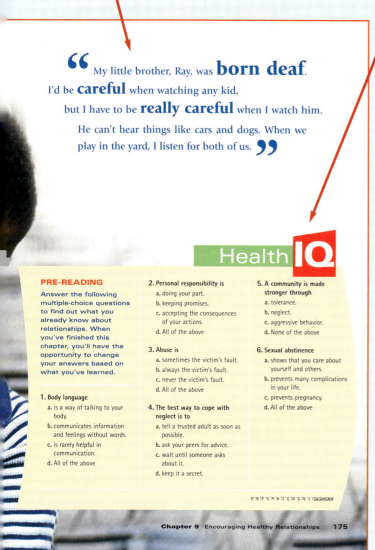

ACTIVITIES MOTIVATE STUDENTS

Hands-on Activity gives students a short hands-on experience to reinforce the concepts they're learning.

Life Skills Activity gets students thinking about **Life Skills** in real-life contexts and help build students' characters.

Life Skills in Action allows students to practice a **Life Skill** both in a guided and independent practice.

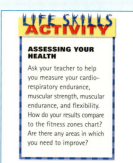

STUDY AND REVIEW SKILLS GET STUDENTS READY FOR TESTING

Lesson and **Chapter Reviews** check students' understanding of vocabulary and key concepts while developing critical-thinking and life skills.

Reading Check-Up finishes each chapter by prompting students to recall the **Health IQ** and reflect on what they've learned.

Study Tips for Better Reading gives students reading strategies to improve their comprehension, such as **Word Origins, Reading Effectively,** and **Compare and Contrast.**

CROSS-DISCIPLINARY CONNECTIONS MAKE CONTENT RELEVANT

Cross-disciplinary activities tie health issues with language arts, math, science, and social studies skills.

Students' writing skills are developed throughout the text. **Start Off Write** begins every section with a thought-provoking question about the lesson at hand, and **Health Journal** allows students to use their critical-thinking skills.

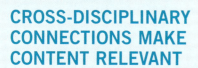

Using the six steps of decision making, explain how the founding fathers of the United States drew up the

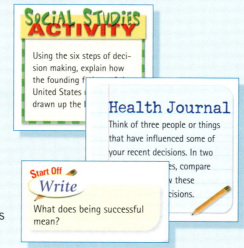

Health Journal
Think of three people or things that have influenced some of your recent decisions. In two compare these decisions.

Start Off Write
What does being successful mean?

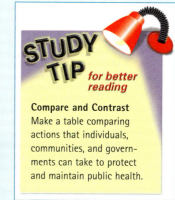

Compare and Contrast
Make a table comparing actions that individuals, communities, and governments can take to protect and maintain public health.

STUDENT EDITION

A Teacher Edition that makes planning easy

TEACHING RESOURCES DESIGNED FOR CONVENIENCE

The **Chapter Planning Guide** breaks each chapter into 45-minute blocks, and offers a full listing of activities and classroom resources available for that lesson and how to use them. Look for guidance on:

- Pacing
- Classroom Resources
- Activities and Demonstrations
- Skills Development Resources
- Review and Assessment
- Standards Correlation
- Chapter Review and Assessment Resources
- Online and Technology Resources
- Compression Guide

Background Information at the beginning of each chapter provides additional information on the upcoming lessons. Reproductions of the **Chapter Resources** available for each chapter are shown at the beginning of each chapter for easy reference.

A **Lesson Cycle** builds structure around every lesson:

- **Focus** uses the objectives to emphasize the up-coming content.

- **Motivate** uses demonstrations, discussions, and lively activities—such as **Role-Playing, Skit,** or **Poster Project**—to get students excited about the material.

- **Teach** presents various teaching techniques including **Debate, Life Skill Builder,** and more.

- Finally, **Close** with quiz questions ensures students understand the information covered and a **Reteaching** feature that helps students review concepts covered in the lesson.

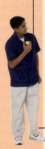

ACTIVITIES FOR EVERY LEARNING LEVEL

Activities are labeled to indicate ability level in the teacher's wrap—**Basic, General,** and **Advanced**—helping you choose the activities appropriate for each student. In addition, some are also labeled to identify activities that help with **Co-op Learning** or **English Language Learners.**

Learning styles—**Interpersonal, Intrapersonal, Auditory, Kinesthetic, Logical, Visual,** and **Verbal**—are addressed throughout so you can adapt material to different learning styles.

- An entire page of additional **Activities** is available at the beginning of each chapter.
- A **Bellringer** activity on a transparency begins each lesson with an activity designed to get students focused while you attend to administrative duties.
- **Activity** and **Group Activity** give you even more options for student interaction.
- Activities accompany each lesson of the **Teaching Sensitive Issues** section in the *Teacher Edition* to help you teach these difficult topics. See page T33 for the **Teaching Sensitive Issues** section.

Bellringer
Have students list the possible consequences for a teenager who was driving after drinking alcohol. (Answers will vary, but may include stories about the teenager being arrested, having a car wreck and damaging property, or killing himself or herself—or someone else—in the crash.)

Motivate
Activity — GENERAL
Drunk Drivers Have students design posters that warn young people about drunk driving or about accepting a ride with someone who is drunk. Hang completed posters in various locations around the school. You may wish to have a poster contest. Try to get a local grocery store, library, or video arcade to hang the winning poster in their establishment. **LS Visual**

CREATING RELEVANCE AND UNDERSTANDING

On almost every page you will find exciting features to help ignite class discussion and keep students thinking.

- Misconception Alert
- Using the Health IQ
- Attention Grabber
- Interdisciplinary Connections
- Real-Life Connection
- Reading Skill Builder
- Reteaching
- Sensitivity Alert
- Cultural Awareness

MATH CONNECTION — BASIC
Alcoholism's Cost Tell students that there are approximately 290 million people in the United States today. In 1998, alcoholism cost the United States $185 billion. Assuming the cost of alcoholism hasn't risen since 1998,

MUSIC CONNECTION — GENERAL
Communicating with Music Music has always been a method of communicating thoughts, feelings, and emotions. When students think about communicating with music, they might think of music with lyrics. Demonstrate that music can convey emotion without words by playing several examples of classical music for students. After each

Sensitivity ALERT
Discussing any family changes and problems can raise delicate issues. Avoid asking individual students questions in class about family finances, health problems, or any relationship problems they are having at home.

READING SKILL BUILDER — GENERAL
Anticipation Guide After students have read about the short-term responses to stress, ask them to anticipate the answers to the following questions:
1. What would happen if someone's fight-or-flight response were repeatedly stimulated by

Cultural Awareness
Laughter Therapy One way people in India deal with stress is by joining a laughter club. Large groups of people get together to laugh their way to good health. Research has shown that laughing lowers blood pressure, reduces stress hormones, and boosts the

MISCONCEPTION ALERT
Be sure students know that a certain amount of stress and change is normal. Every family goes through times of change and struggle. But when a change begins to have lasting, negative effects students should seek help from an adult family

INCLUSION STRATEGIES MAKE MATERIAL ACCESSIBLE TO ALL

Written by professionals in the field of special-needs education, two **Inclusion Strategies** in each chapter address the needs of students in your classroom. Each **Strategy** specifically identifies successful methods to assist you in meeting challenges you might face.

- Hearing Impaired
- Visually Impaired
- Learning Disabled
- Developmentally Delayed
- Attention Deficit Disorder
- Behavior Control Issues
- Gifted and Talented

INCLUSION Strategies — BASIC
- Developmentally Delayed
- Learning Disabled

Tell students that people are less likely to be influenced by TV shows if they can identify the pros and cons of a situation and relate their own values to what they see. For homework, have students watch (with their parents) a TV program about a family. Have students identify the positive and negative values illustrated in the shows. **LS Visual**

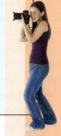

TEACHER EDITION

Assessment options help you track students' progress

PRE- AND POST-READING ASSESSMENT

- **Health IQ** is a pre-reading quiz to test students' prior knowledge.

- **Reading Checkup** at the end of each chapter refers students back to **Health IQ** questions so students can see how their understanding has changed.

Reading Checkup

Take a minute to review your answers to the Health IQ questions at the beginning of this chapter. How has reading this chapter improved your Health IQ?

Health IQ

PRE-READING
Answer the following true/false questions to find out what you already know about tobacco. When you've finished this chapter, you'll have the opportunity to change your answers based on what you've learned.

1. Smoking pipes or cigars can be as deadly as smoking cigarettes.
2. Nicotine is a drug.
3. Tobacco only affects a person after years of use.
4. Tobacco increases the risk of lung, mouth, throat, pancreatic, and bladder cancer.
5. It is against the law to sell any tobacco product to someone under the age of 18.
6. A person can easily quit smoking when he or she really wants to quit.
7. Young people do not become addicted to tobacco products as easily as adults do.
8. Sometimes, medicine can help a person quit using tobacco.
9. Positive peer pressure from friends can influence a teen to avoid tobacco.
10. Once a person has used tobacco, quitting the habit will not help him or her recover from the health effects.
11. Advertisements can encourage a false understanding of tobacco's effects.
12. Tobacco smoke can increase asthma symptoms in nonsmokers.

LESSON ASSESSMENT

- Comprehensive **Lesson Reviews** check students' understanding of vocabulary and key concepts while developing their critical-thinking skills.

- **Quiz**, found in the *Teacher Edition*, provides additional questions to assess student progress.

Lesson Review

Using Vocabulary
1. What is a carbohydrate, and how does your body use this nutrient?
2. What is a Calorie?

Understanding Concepts
3. Explain why a person should eat a variety of foods each day.

4. Explain why you must drink enough water every day.

Critical Thinking
5. **Making Inferences** Explain why you do not need to take vitamin pills if you have a healthy diet.

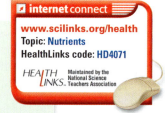

internet connect
www.scilinks.org/health
Topic: Nutrients
HealthLinks code: HD4071
HEALTH LINKS — Maintained by the National Science Teachers Association

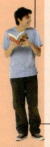

CHAPTER ASSESSMENT

- More extensive **Chapter Reviews** prepare students for testing by approaching the material from a variety of angles. Features include: **Using Vocabulary, Understanding Concepts, Critical Thinking,** and **Interpreting Graphics.**

- **Assignment Guide,** in the *Teacher Edition,* lets you see which questions correlate with a specific lesson so you can customize your review to the content you actually teach. This guide is a valuable resource for reteaching.

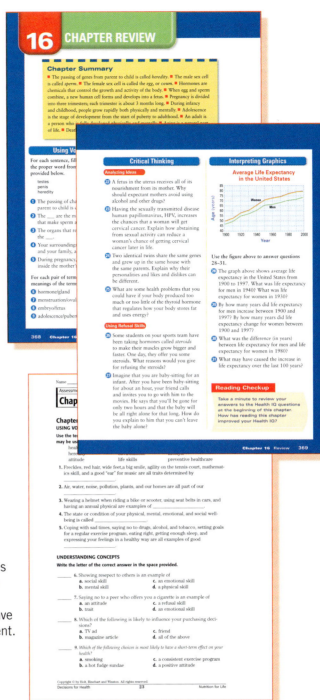

Assignment Guide

Lesson	Review Questions
1	2, 4, 6, 9, 10, 12, 15, 18, 19
2	14
3	16–17, 25–28
4	5, 8, 13, 22
5	19, 21, 23–24
6	3, 7, 8, 11, 20
2 and 4	1

- **Life Skills in Action** checks students' understanding of a specific life skill through guided and independent practice.

- Arranged by chapter, handy **Chapter Resource File** books assemble an invaluable collection of resources including a number of options for assessment. With **Performance-Based Assessments, Quizzes, Chapter Tests,** and **Test Item Listing** all in one place, you have fewer workbooks to juggle when preparing assessment.

- Review worksheets in the **Study Guide** help reinforce skills and concepts presented in the *Student Edition.*

CUSTOM ASSESSMENT

The *One-Stop Planner® CD-ROM with Test Generator* includes over a thousand test questions, allowing you to create customized assessment based on your teaching goals and the ability level of your class. See page T14 for more information.

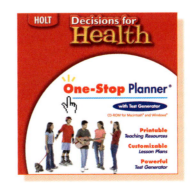

ASSESSMENT RESOURCES

TEACHING RESOURCES

Resources that make teaching easier

CHAPTER RESOURCE FILES— RESOURCES YOU NEED, LESS TO CARRY

A *Chapter Resource File* accompanies each chapter of *Decisions for Health*. Here you'll find everything you need to plan and manage your lessons in a convenient, time-saving format all organized into each chapter book. Also included is an introduction booklet, your guide to the resources found in each *Chapter Resource File*.

Includes:

Skills Worksheets
- Directed Reading
- Concept Mapping
- Concept Review
- Refusal Skills
- Decision-Making Skills
- Cross-Disciplinary

Assessments
- Quizzes
- Chapter Test
- Performance-Based Assessment
- Test Item Listing (for ExamView® Test Generator)

Activities
- Datasheets for In-Text Activities
- Life Skills
- Enrichment Activities
- Health Inventory
- Health Behavior Contract
- At-Home Activities (English and Spanish)

Teacher Resources
- Answer Keys
- Lesson Plans
- Parent Letter (English and Spanish)
- Teaching Transparency Preview

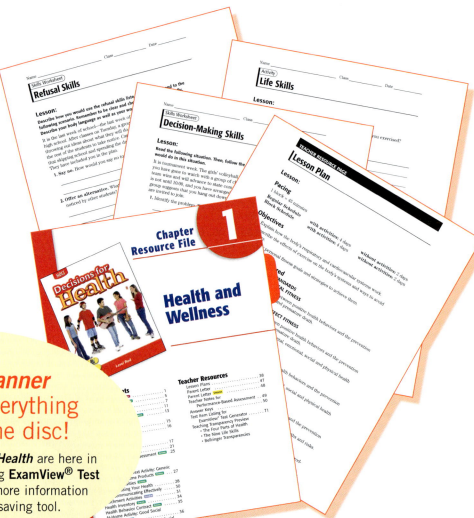

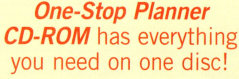

One-Stop Planner CD-ROM has everything you need on one disc!

All the resources for *Decisions for Health* are here in one place, along with the amazing **ExamView® Test Generator**. See page T14 for more information about this powerful time-saving tool.

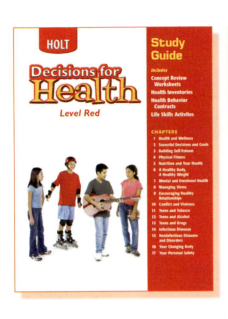
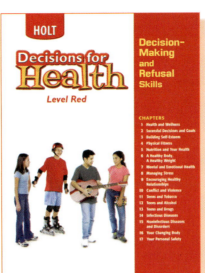
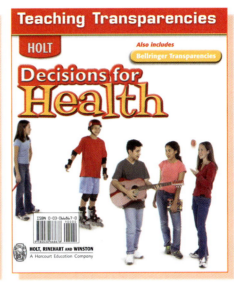

ADDITIONAL RESOURCES REINFORCE AND EXTEND LESSONS

- **Study Guide** contains review worksheets to reinforce the skills and concepts presented in the *Student Edition*.

- **Decision-Making and Refusal Skills Workbook** offers at least one worksheet per chapter that focuses on applying the key skills studied in the *Student Edition*.

- Over 80 full-color **Teaching Transparencies**, some utilizing graphics directly from the text, enhance classroom presentations. **Bellringer Transparencies** are also included to help you start off each lesson.

SPANISH RESOURCES

- A **Spanish Glossary** is right at students' fingertips in the *Student Edition*, following the **Glossary**. It shows the English term, its Spanish equivalent, and a definition in Spanish.

- **Study Guide** in Spanish contains review worksheets that reinforce the skills and concepts presented in the *Student Edition* that have been translated into Spanish.

- **Assessments** in Spanish include **Lesson Quizzes** and **Chapter Test**.

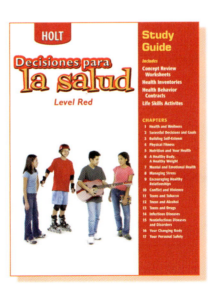
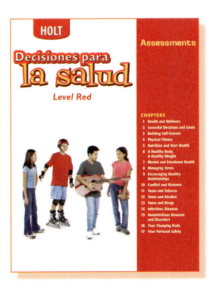

TEACHING RESOURCES

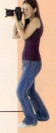

T13

TECHNOLOGY RESOURCES

Technology that enhances teaching

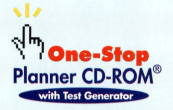
One-Stop Planner CD-ROM® with Test Generator

Planning and managing lessons has never been easier than with this convenient, all-in-one CD-ROM that includes a variety of timesaving features, including:

Printable resources and worksheets

The resources available for *Decisions for Health* are in one place, including skills development, concept practice, life skills practice, enrichment activities, Spanish materials, and transparency masters.

Customizable lesson plans

Tailor your lessons to your classroom's specific needs. Includes block-scheduling lesson plans in several word-processing formats.

Powerful ExamView® Test Generator

Contains test items organized by chapter, plus over a thousand editable questions, so you can put together your own tests and quizzes.

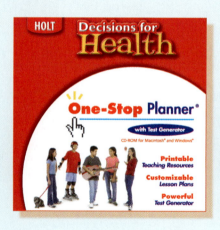

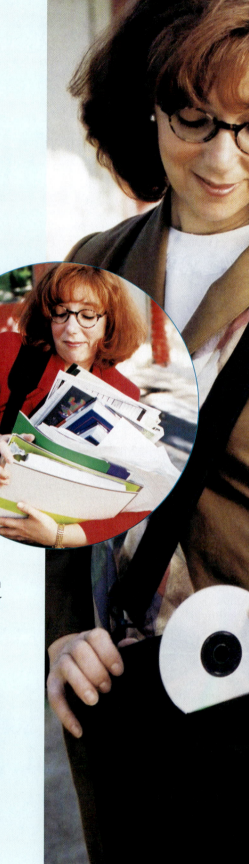

GUIDED READING AUDIO CD PROGRAM

This direct read of the textbook on audio CD makes content more accessible, especially for auditory learners and reluctant readers.

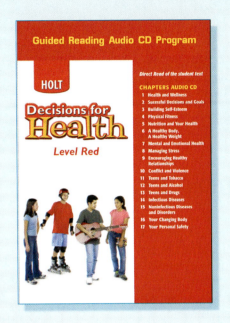

STUDENT EDITION, CD-ROM VERSION

Ideal for students who have limited access to the Internet, but who need to lighten the load of textbooks they carry home, the entire *Student Edition* is on one easy-to-navigate CD-ROM, page-for-page.

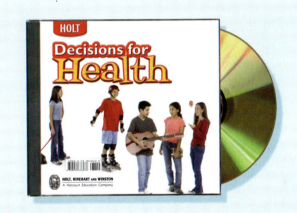

VIDEODISCOVERY® HEALTHSLEUTHS CD-ROMS

Get your students involved in a mystery with this intriguing 6-episode CD-ROM series, engaging students in critical thinking as they solve a fictitious mystery involving health concepts and human biology. Students use charts, graphs, photos, video interviews, and other tools to assist their sleuthing, then review what they have learned at the end with a test, recording everything in an online lab book for easy access.

VIDEO SELECT

Video Select gives you access to exciting and current videos for each chapter of *Decisions for Health.*

Look for **Video Select** boxes in the margin of the *Teacher Edition*, directing you to a Web site with information on recommended videos for each chapter.

Discover Films video and Holt have come together to bring you the best selection of motivating and educational health videos. Visit **go.hrw.com** to view a complete listing of available titles.

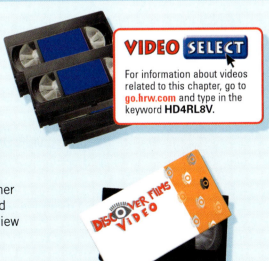

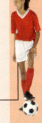

TECHNOLOGY RESOURCES

T15

ONLINE RESOURCES

Expand learning beyond the classroom

ONLINE EDITION—AN INTERACTIVE TEXTBOOK

Online textbooks from **Holt Online Learning** engage students in ways never before possible with traditional textbooks, providing interactivity and feedback with links to activities, homework help, and a host of other features. And since it's all online, it's available anytime, anywhere.

- Complete *Student Edition* online
- Interactive activities
- Immediate feedback
- Online study aids
- Additional homework

Contact your sales representative or call (800) HRW-9799 for more information.

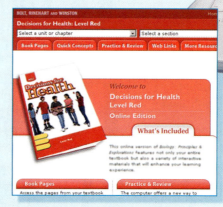

CURRENT HEALTH ONLINE ARTICLES EXTEND LEARNING

Current Health online articles and activities are correlated to the text and relate health to students' lives.

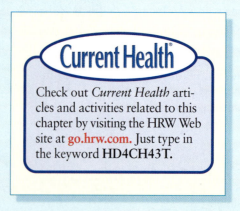

Check out *Current Health* articles and activities related to this chapter by visiting the HRW Web site at **go.hrw.com.** Just type in the keyword **HD4CH43T.**

student CNN News

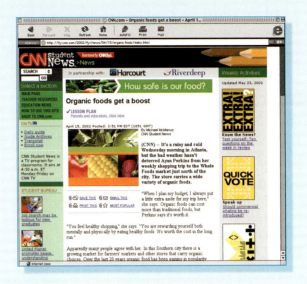

Go to **CNNStudentNews.com** for award-winning news and information for both teachers and students. You'll find a wealth of helpful information, including:
- News as it happens
- Classroom resources
- Student current events activities
- Lesson plans
- Projects and activities

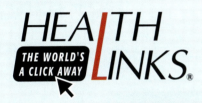

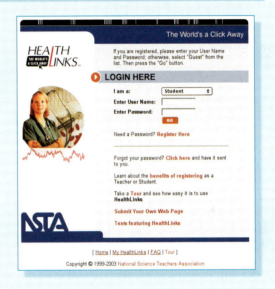

This Web service, developed and maintained by the National Science Teachers Association, contains links to up-to-date information and activities that relate directly to chapter topics, all prescreened so the content is safe and appropriate.

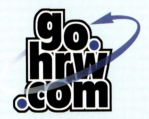

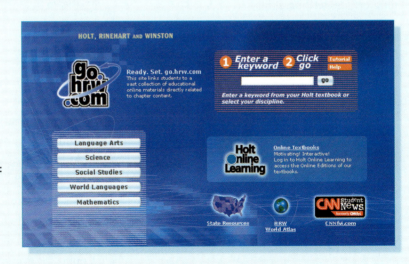

Holt, Rinehart and Winston's award-winning Web site, **go.hrw.com**, allows students to enrich their knowledge with Web links and activities. Here you'll find:
- Worksheets
- Activities
- Projects
- Research Articles and Ideas
- Interactive Quizzes
- Review Activities
- Teacher Resources

ONLINE RESOURCES

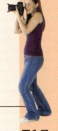

ACTIVITIES

Activities to engage every student

IN THE STUDENT EDITION

Health IQ offers pre-reading questions to assess students' prior knowledge and spark classroom discussion. Students reevaluate their answers in **Reading Checkup** at the end of the chapter.

Nine key **Life Skills** are supported throughout the program and developed in the following activities.

- **Life Skills Activity** gives students practice discussing and working with life skills in real-life contexts.

- **Life Skills in Action** is an opportunity to practice important life skills. Students role play in small groups in guided practice, then evaluate themselves and practice further on their own.

Hands-on Activity gives students a short, hands-on experience to reinforce the concepts they're learning.

Start Off Write begins every section with a thought-provoking question about the issue or subject students are about to explore, while building critical writing skills.

Writing skills are further developed as students are encouraged to keep a **Health Journal,** where they explore how health impacts their lives.

Cross-disciplinary Activities relate health concepts with language arts, math, science, and social studies skills.

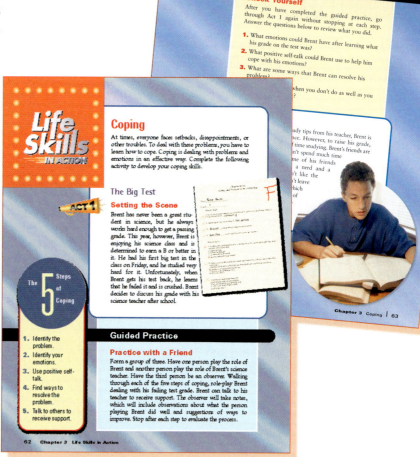

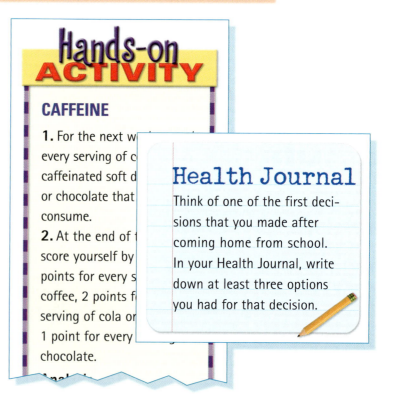

IN THE TEACHER EDITION

Additional activities found in the *Teacher Edition* also help illustrate health concepts. Look for:

- Activity
- Group Activity
- Bellringer
- Cross-Disciplinary Connections

Motivate
Activity — GENERAL

Drunk Drivers Have students design posters that warn young people about drunk driving or about accepting a ride with someone who is drunk. Hang completed posters in various locations around the school. You may wish to have a poster contest. Try to get a local grocery store, library, or video arcade to hang the winning poster in their establishment. **LS Visual**

Bellringer
Have students list the possible consequences for a teenager who was driving after drinking alcohol. (Answers will vary, but may include stories about the teenager being arrested, having a car wreck and damaging property, or killing himself or herself—or someone else—in the crash.)

CHAPTER RESOURCE FILES HAVE EVEN MORE ACTIVITIES

Look for a host of activity aids in our helpful *Chapter Resource Files*.

- Datasheets for In-text Activities
- Enrichment Activities
- Health Inventory
- Health Behavior Contract
- At-Home Activities (English and Spanish)

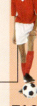

ACTIVITIES

T19

Meeting Individual Needs

Students have a wide range of abilities and learning exceptionalities. These pages show you how **Holt's Health Programs** provide resources and strategies to help you tailor your instruction to engage every student in your classroom.

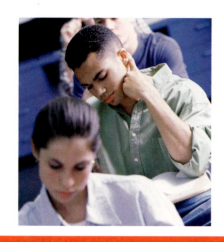

Learning exceptionality	Resources and strategies	
Learning Disabilities and Slow Learners Students who have dyslexia or dysgraphia, students reading below grade level, students having difficulty understanding abstract or complex concepts, and slow learners	• Inclusion Strategies labeled *Learning Disabled* • Activities and Alternative Assessments labeled *Basic* • *Reteaching* activities	• Activities labeled *Visual, Kinesthetic,* or *Auditory* • Hands-on activities or projects • Oral presentations instead of written tests or assignments
Developmental Delays Students who are functioning far below grade level because of mental retardation, autism, or brain injury; goals are to learn or retain basic concepts	• Inclusion Strategies labeled *Developmentally Delayed* • Activities and Alternative Assessments labeled *Basic*	• *Reteaching* activities • Project-based activities
Attention Deficit Disorders Students experiencing difficulty completing a task that has multiple steps, difficulty handling long assignments, or difficulty concentrating without sensory input from physical activity	• Inclusion Strategies labeled *Attention Deficit Disorder* • Activities and Alternative Assessments labeled *Basic* • *Reteaching* activities • Activities labeled *Co-op Learning*	• Activities labeled *Visual, Kinesthetic,* or *Auditory* • Concepts broken into small chunks • Oral presentations instead of written tests or assignments
English as a Second Language Students learning English	• Activities labeled *English-Language Learners* • Activities and Alternative Assessments labeled *Basic*	• *Reteaching* activities • Activities labeled *Visual*
Gifted and Talented Students who are performing above grade level and demonstrate aptitude in crosscurricular assignments	• Inclusion Strategies labeled *Gifted and Talented* • Activities and Alternative Assessments labeled *Advanced*	• *Connection* activities • Activities that involve multiple tasks, a strong degree of independence, and student initiative
Hearing Impairments Students who are deaf or who have difficulty hearing	• Inclusion Strategies labeled *Hearing Impaired* • Activities labeled *Visual*	• Activities labeled *Co-op Learning* • Assessments that use written presentations
Visual Impairments Students who are blind or who have difficulty seeing	• Inclusion strategies labeled *Visually Impaired* • Activities labeled *Auditory*	• Activities labeled *Co-Op Learning* • Assessments that use oral presentations
Behavior Control Issues Students learning to manage their behavior	• Inclusion Strategies labeled *Behavior Control Issues* • Activities labeled *Basic*	• Assignments that actively involve students and help students develop confidence and improved behaviors

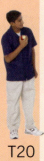

General Strategies The following strategies can help you modify instruction to help students who struggle with common classroom difficulties.

A student experiencing difficulty with...	May benefit if you...	
Beginning assignments	• Assign work in small amounts • Have the student use cooperative or paired learning • Provide varied and interesting activities	• Allow choice in assignments or projects • Reinforce participation • Seat the student closer to you
Following directions	• Gain the student's attention before giving directions • Break up the task into small steps • Give written directions rather than oral directions • Use short, simple phrases • Stand near the student when you are giving directions	• Have the student repeat directions to you • Prepare the student for changes in activity • Give visual cues by posting general routines • Reinforce improvement in or approximation of following directions
Keeping track of assignments	• Have the student use folders for assignments • Have the student use assignment notebooks	• Have the student keep a checklist of assignments and highlight assignments when they are turned in
Reading the textbook	• Provide outlines of the textbook content • Reduce the length of required reading • Allow extra time for reading • Have the students read aloud in small groups	• Have the student use peer or mentor readers • Have the student use books on tape or CD • Discuss the content of the textbook in class after reading
Staying on task	• Reduce distracting elements in the classroom • Provide a task-completion checklist • Seat the student near you	• Provide alternative ways to complete assignments, such as oral projects taped with a buddy
Behavioral or social skills	• Model the appropriate behaviors • Establish class rules, and reiterate them often • Reinforce positive behavior • Assign a mentor as a positive role model to the student • Contract with the student for expected behaviors • Reinforce the desired behaviors or any steps toward improvement	• Separate the student from any peer who stimulates the inappropriate behavior • Provide a "cooling off" period before talking with the student • Address academic/instructional problems that may contribute to disruptive behaviors • Include parents in the problem-solving process through conferences, home visits, and frequent communication
Attendance	• Recognize and reinforce attendance by giving incentives or verbal praise • Emphasize the importance of attendance by letting the student know that he or she was missed when he or she was absent	• Encourage the student's desire to be in school by planning activities that are likely to be enjoyable, giving the student a preferred responsibility to be performed in class, and involving the student in extracurricular activities • Schedule problem-solving meeting with parents, faculty, or both
Test-taking skills	• Prepare the student for testing by teaching ways to study in pairs, such as using flashcards, practice tests, and study guides, and by promoting adequate sleep, nourishment, and exercise • Decrease visual distraction by improving the visual design of the test through use of larger type, spacing, consistent layout, and shorter sentences	• During testing, allow the student to respond orally on tape or to respond using a computer; to use notes; to take breaks; to take the test in another location; to work without time constraints; or to take the test in several short sessions

MEETING INDIVIDUAL NEEDS

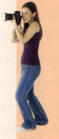

Build critical reading and writing skills

FEATURES HELP STUDENTS UNDERSTAND WHAT THEY READ

Health IQ offers multiple choice and true/false pre-reading questions at the start of each chapter that set the stage for reading the chapter. They assess students' prior knowledge and can be used to spark classroom discussion.

Reading Checkup refers students back to **Health IQ** to review what they've learned while reading the chapter.

Reading Checkup

Take a minute to review your answers to the Health IQ questions at the beginning of this chapter. How has reading this chapter improved your Health IQ?

Study Tip for Better Reading gives students reading strategies to improve their comprehension, including:
- Word Origins
- Reviewing and Taking Notes
- Organizing Information
- Reading Effectively
- Compare and Contrast
- Reviewing Information
- Interpreting Graphics

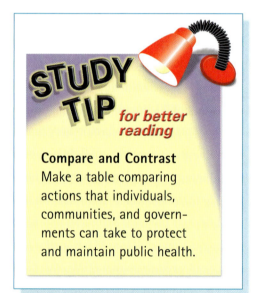

Compare and Contrast
Make a table comparing actions that individuals, communities, and governments can take to protect and maintain public health.

Reading skills are developed throughout the *Teacher Edition*. **Reading Skill Builder** offers reading strategies that help students' comprehension.

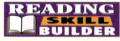 — GENERAL

Anticipation Guide After students have read about the short-term responses to stress, ask them to anticipate the answers to the following questions:

1. What would happen if someone's fight-or-flight response were repeatedly stimulated by a stressful situation but the person was helpless to flee or conquer? (If a stressor is not removed, a person's fight-or-flight response will lead to exhaustion.)

ADDITIONAL RESOURCES HELP IN READING COMPREHENSION

Directed Reading worksheets, found in the *Chapter Resource Files,* focus students' attention on key material and help them synthesize content.

Concept Review, found in the *Chapter Resource Files,* provides questions that help reinforce what students learned in each lesson.

Guided Reading Audio CD Program is a direct read of the *Student Edition* textbook on audio CD. This recording makes content more accessible, especially for auditory learners and reluctant readers.

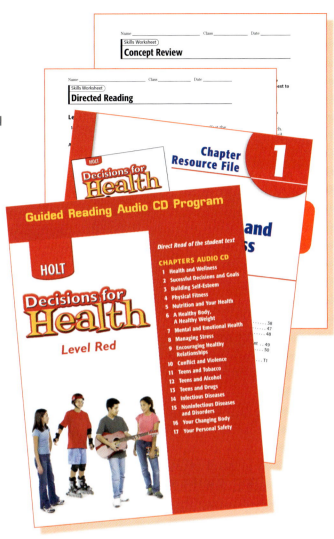

USEFUL FEATURES HELP BUILD WRITING SKILLS

Start Off Write begins every lesson with a thought-provoking question about the issue or subject students are about to explore, while building critical writing skills.

Writing and critical-thinking skills are further developed as students are encouraged to keep a **Health Journal,** where they explore how health issues impact their lives.

Look for **Writing** icons accompanying various activities in the teacher's wrap for more writing practice.

Start Off Write
What does being successful mean?

Health Journal
Think of three people or things that have influenced some of your recent decisions. In two or three sentences, compare and contrast how these affected your decisions.

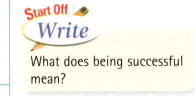
Communicating
Invite volunteers to skit that illustrates the fo scenario: "A classmate c leaves small gifts by your locker. The gestures are starting to make you feel uncomfortable. You decide to ask the individual to stop these

READING & WRITING SKILLS

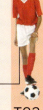

Life Skills

Nine key **Life Skills** are developed throughout the program with an emphasis on decision-making and refusal skills.

Life Skills
Making Good Decisions
Using Refusal Skills
Assessing Your Health
Evaluating Media Messages
Communicating Effectively
Setting Goals
Being a Wise Consumer
Practicing Wellness
Coping

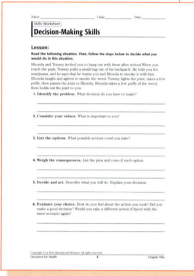
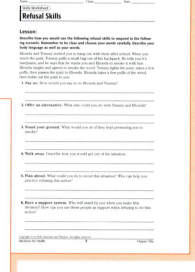

ACTIVITIES PROVIDE PRACTICE FOR LIFE SKILLS

- **Life Skills Activity** gives students practice discussing and working with **Life Skills** in real-life contexts.

- **Life Skills in Action** provides students with a step-by-step life skills practice. Students role play in small groups in guided practice, then evaluate themselves and practice further on their own.

- **Life Skill Builder** feature boxes in the *Teacher Edition* offer a number of different opportunities to practice all of the **Life Skills**.

- The **Chapter Review** reinforces **Making Good Decisions** and **Refusal Skills** in the **Critical Thinking** section of the review.

- The *Decision-Making and Refusal Skills Workbook* extends your resources with at least one worksheet per chapter that focuses on applying the key skills studied in the *Student Edition*.

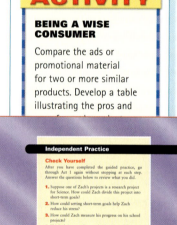
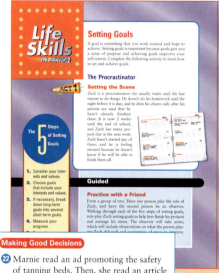
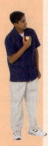

Skills are developed across other disciplines

CROSS-DISCIPLINARY ACTIVITIES

These activities call students' attention to connections between health and other disciplines like science, math, social studies, and language arts.

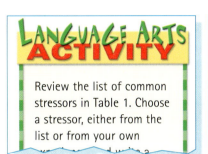

LANGUAGE ARTS ACTIVITY

Review the list of common stressors in Table 1. Choose a stressor, either from the list or from your own

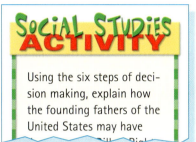

SOCIAL STUDIES ACTIVITY

Using the six steps of decision making, explain how the founding fathers of the United States may have

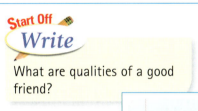

Start Off Write

What are qualities of a good friend?

Health Journal

Think of three people or things that have influenced some of your recent decisions. In two or three sentences, compare and contrast how these affected your decisions.

Numerous writing activities such as **Health Journal** and **Start Off Write** encourage written communication that will aid in all other subjects.

Using Vocabulary

❶ Use each of the following terms in a separate sentence: *positive stress, stress response, reframing,* and *prioritize.*

For each sentence, fill in the blank with the proper word from the word bank provided below.

stress	plan
stressor	defense mechanism
distress	stress management
positive stress	reframing
stress response	time management

THE TEACHER EDITION MAKES CONNECTIONS

The **Interdisciplinary Connection** feature in the *Teacher Edition* suggests activities and questions to draw students' attention to topics like math, biology, physical science, sports, art, language arts, and social studies, linking them back to health issues addressed in the text.

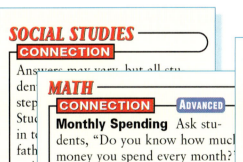

SOCIAL STUDIES CONNECTION

Answers may vary, but all students...

MATH CONNECTION — ADVANCED

Monthly Spending Ask students, "Do you know how much money you spend every month?" Have students keep track of every penny that they receive and every penny that they spend. Have them make a table, with categories

LANGUAGE ARTS CONNECTION — GENERAL

Point of View Students may think that all negative life events must cause distress. Remind students that it is not so much the events of life that are stressful, but how a person reacts to those events. Have students write a story about someone who at first perceives a stressor as negative, but then

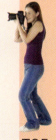

CROSS-DISCIPLINARY SKILLS

PACING GUIDE

Pacing and compression guidelines

The **Chapter Planning Guide** helps you organize your time and resources.

Pacing Each chapter is broken into several blocks. Each block consists of lessons that you can cover in approximately 45 minutes. The **Chapter Planning Guide** also lists activities, demonstrations, and worksheets that are available to accompany each lesson.

Assessment Each chapter includes enough assessment materials to fill two 45-minute blocks.

CHAPTER 16 Medicine and Illegal Drugs
Chapter Planning Guide

PACING	CLASSROOM RESOURCES	ACTIVITIES AND DEMONSTRATIONS
BLOCK 1 · 45 min pp. 394–397 **Chapter Opener**	CRF Health Inventory * GENERAL CRF Parent Letter *	SE Health IQ, p. 395 CRF At-Home Activity *
Lesson 1 What Are Drugs?	CRF Lesson Plan * TT Bellringer * TT How Drugs Enter the Body *	CRF Enrichment Activity * ADVANCED
BLOCK 2 · 45 min pp. 398–401 **Lesson 2** Using Drugs as Medicine	CRF Lesson Plan * TT Bellringer * TT Reading Prescription Medicine Labels *	TE Activity, pp. 398, 400 TE Demonstration Med-Alert Tags, p. 400 GENERAL CRF Life Skills Activity * GENERAL CRF Enrichment Activity * ADVANCED
BLOCK 3 · 45 min pp. 402–405 **Lesson 3** Drug Abuse and Addiction	CRF Lesson Plan * TT Bellringer *	TE Group Activity Skit, p. 404 GENERAL CRF Enrichment Activity * ADVANCED
BLOCK 4 · 45 min pp. 406–409 **Lesson 4** Stimulants and Depressants	CRF Lesson Plan * TT Bellringer *	SE Hands-on Activity, p. 407 CRF Datasheets for In-Text Activities * GENERAL TE Demonstration Modeling Euphoria, p. 407 GENERAL SE Science Activity, p. 408 CRF Enrichment Activity * ADVANCED
BLOCK 5 · 45 min pp. 410–413 **Lesson 5** Marijuana	CRF Lesson Plan * TT Bellringer *	TE Activities Modeling the Effects of Marijuana, p. 393F CRF Life Skills Activity * GENERAL CRF Enrichment Activity * ADVANCED
Lesson 6 Opiates	CRF Lesson Plan * TT Bellringer *	SE Social Studies Activity, p. 412 CRF Enrichment Activity * ADVANCED
BLOCK 6 · 45 min pp. 414–417 **Lesson 7** Hallucinogens and Inhalants	CRF Lesson Plan * TT Bellringer *	TE Activity Afterimages, p. 414 GENERAL TE Demonstration Fooling Your Senses, p. 415 GENERAL CRF Enrichment Activity * ADVANCED
Lesson 8 Designer Drugs	CRF Lesson Plan * TT Bellringer *	TE Group Activity Poster Project, p. 416 GENERAL CRF Enrichment Activity * ADVANCED
BLOCK 7 · 45 min pp. 418–423 **Lesson 9** Staying Drug Free	CRF Lesson Plan * TT Bellringer *	TE Activities Peer Pressure, p. 393F TE Group Activity Role-Playing, p. 418 GENERAL SE Life Skills in Action Using Refusal Skills, pp. 426–427 CRF Enrichment Activity * ADVANCED
Lesson 10 Getting Help	CRF Lesson Plan * TT Bellringer *	TE Group Activity Finding Help, p. 421 GENERAL TE Activity Skit, p. 421 ADVANCED CRF Enrichment Activity * ADVANCED
BLOCKS 8 & 9 · 90 min Chapter Review and Assessment Resources	SE Chapter Review, pp. 424–425 CRF Concept Review * GENERAL CRF Health Behavior Contract * GENERAL CRF Chapter Test * GENERAL CRF Performance-Based Assessment * GENERAL OSP Test Generator CRF Test Item Listing *	**Online Resources** go.hrw.com — Visit go.hrw.com for a variety of free resources related to this textbook. Enter the keyword HD4DR8. Holt Online Learning — Students can access interactive problem solving help and active visual concept development with the *Decisions for Health* Online Edition available at www.hrw.com. CNN Student News — cnnstudentnews.com Find the latest health news, lesson plans, and activities related to important scientific events.

393A Chapter 16 · Medicine and Illegal Drugs

Compression In many cases, a chapter will contain more material than you will have time to teach. The **Compression Guide** in each **Chapter Planning Guide** suggests lessons you can omit if you are short on time. The lessons suggested for omission often contain advanced material. You may also wish to consider using lessons omitted from class teaching as extension material for advanced students.

Compression guide:
To shorten your instruction because of time limitations, omit Lessons 4, 6, and 7.

KEY
- **TE** Teacher Edition
- **SE** Student Edition
- **OSP** One-Stop Planner
- **CRF** Chapter Resource File
- **TT** Teaching Transparency
- * Also on One-Stop Planner
- ■ Also Available in Spanish
- ♦ Requires Advance Prep

	SKILLS DEVELOPMENT RESOURCES	LESSON REVIEW AND ASSESSMENT	STANDARDS CORRELATION
			National Health Education Standards
	CRF Cross-Disciplinary * GENERAL CRF Directed Reading * BASIC	SE Lesson Review, p. 397 TE Reteaching, Quiz, p. 397 CRF Lesson Quiz * ■ GENERAL	
	SE Life Skills Activity Practicing Wellness, p. 399 TE Inclusion Strategies, p. 399 GENERAL TE Life Skill Builder Evaluating Media messages, p. 400 ADVANCED CRF Directed Reading * BASIC	SE Lesson Review, p. 401 TE Reteaching, Quiz, p. 401 CRF Concept Mapping * GENERAL CRF Lesson Quiz * ■ GENERAL	1.1, 1.7, 2.4, 2.6, 6.3
	SE Life Skills Activity, pp. 403, 405 CRF Cross-Disciplinary * GENERAL CRF Refusal Skills * GENERAL CRF Directed Reading * BASIC	SE Lesson Review, p. 405 TE Reteaching, Quiz, p. 405 CRF Concept Mapping * GENERAL CRF Lesson Quiz * ■ GENERAL	3.3, 6.3
	TE Reading Skill Builder Paired Summarizing, p. 407 BASIC SE Life Skills Activity Practicing Wellness, p. 408 TE Life Skill Builder Practicing Wellness, p. 408 BASIC CRF Directed Reading * BASIC	SE Lesson Review, p. 409 TE Reteaching, Quiz, p. 409 TE Alternative Assessment, p. 409 BASIC CRF Lesson Quiz * ■ GENERAL	3.2, 6.3
	TE Life Skill Builder Refusal Skills, p. 410 GENERAL CRF Directed Reading * BASIC	SE Lesson Review, p. 411 TE Reteaching, Quiz, p. 411 CRF Lesson Quiz * ■ GENERAL	6.3
	CRF Directed Reading * BASIC	SE Lesson Review, p. 413 TE Reteaching, Quiz, p. 413 CRF Lesson Quiz * ■ GENERAL	6.3
	TE Inclusion Strategies, p. 415 GENERAL CRF Decision-Making * GENERAL CRF Directed Reading * BASIC	SE Lesson Review, p. 415 TE Reteaching, Quiz, p. 415 CRF Lesson Quiz * ■ GENERAL	6.3
	TE Inclusion Strategies, p. 416 GENERAL TE Life Skill Builder Refusal Skills, p. 417 GENERAL CRF Directed Reading * BASIC	SE Lesson Review, p. 417 TE Reteaching, Quiz, p. 417 CRF Lesson Quiz * ■ GENERAL	6.3
	SE Life Skills Activity Using Refusal Skills, p. 419 TE Life Skill Builder Communicating Effectively, p. 419 GENERAL CRF Refusal Skills * GENERAL CRF Directed Reading * BASIC	SE Lesson Review, p. 419 TE Reteaching, Quiz, p. 419 CRF Lesson Quiz * ■ GENERAL	1.1, 1.4, 1.6, 3.1, 3.4, 3.6, 4.4, 5.1, 5.6, 6.3, 6.4, 7.1
	TE Life Skill Builder, pp. 421, 422, 422 GENERAL CRF Decision-Making * GENERAL CRF Directed Reading * BASIC	SE Lesson Review, p. 423 TE Reteaching, Quiz, p. 423 CRF Lesson Quiz * ■ GENERAL	1.4, 1.7, 2.2, 2.4, 2.6, 6.3, 7.4

HEALTH LINKS THE WORLD'S A CLICK AWAY
www.scilinks.org/health
Maintained by the National Science Teachers Association

Topic: Drugs
HealthLinks code: HD4030
Topic: Medicine Safety
HealthLinks code: HD4066
Topic: Drugs & Drug Abuse
HealthLinks code: HD4031

Technology Resources

One-Stop Planner All of your printable resources and the Test Generator are on this convenient CD-ROM.

Guided Reading Audio CDs

VIDEO SELECT For information about videos related to this chapter, go to go.hrw.com and type in the keyword **HD4DR8V**.

Chapter 16 • Chapter Planning Guide   **393B**

COMPRESSION GUIDELINES

National Health Education Standards

The following list shows the chapter correlation of *Decisions for Health* with the National Health Education Standards for grades 5–8. For further details, see the teacher's wrap of each chapter opener.

HEALTH EDUCATION STANDARD 1 — Students will comprehend concepts related to health promotion and disease prevention.

PERFORMANCE INDICATORS: As a result of health instruction in Grades 5–8, students will:

Standard	Correlation	
1. Explain the relationship between positive health behaviors and the prevention of injury, illness, disease, and premature death. Explain the relationship between positive health behaviors and the prevention of injury.	Chapter 1	1.3
	Chapter 4	4.2, 4.6, 4.8
	Chapter 5	5.1, 5.2
	Chapter 7	7.5
	Chapter 11	11.1, 11.6
	Chapter 12	12.1, 12.2, 12.3, 12.4, 12.5, 12.6, 12.7
	Chapter 15	15.1, 15.2, 15.3, 15.4, 15.5, 15.6, 15.7, 15.8, 15.9
	Chapter 16	16.2, 16.3
	Chapter 17	17.1, 17.2, 17.3, 17.4, 17.5, 17.6
	Chapter 20	20.5
2. Describe the interrelationship of mental, emotional, social and physical health during adolescence.	Chapter 1	1.1
	Chapter 3	3.1, 3.2, 3.3
	Chapter 7	7.1, 7.3
	Chapter 8	8.1, 8.2
	Chapter 16	16.6
3. Explain how health is influenced by the interaction of body systems.	Chapter 15	15.1, 15.2, 15.3, 15.4, 15.5, 15.6, 15.7, 15.8, 15.9
	Chapter 16	16.4
4. Describe how family and peers influence the health of adolescents.	Chapter 2	2.3, 2.4
	Chapter 3	3.1
	Chapter 5	5.1
	Chapter 7	7.5
	Chapter 9	9.1, 9.2, 9.3, 9.4, 9.5
	Chapter 11	11.5
	Chapter 12	12.1, 12.3, 12.5, 12.6, 12.7
	Chapter 14	14.4, 14.5
5. Analyze how environment and personal health are interrelated.	Chapter 1	1.2
	Chapter 7	7.4
	Chapter 15	15.4, 15.5, 15.6, 15.7
6. Describe ways to reduce risks related to adolescent health problems.	Chapter 1	1.3
	Chapter 2	2.2, 2.7
	Chapter 7	7.3, 7.5
	Chapter 9	9.1, 9.2, 9.4, 9.5
	Chapter 11	11.7
	Chapter 15	15.4, 15.6, 15.7
	Chapter 16	16.2, 16.3

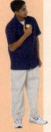

HEALTH EDUCATION STANDARD 1, continued

PERFORMANCE INDICATORS: As a result of health instruction in Grades 5–8, students will:

Standard	Correlation	
7. Explain how appropriate health care can prevent premature death and disability.	**Chapter 7** **Chapter 9** **Chapter 16** **Chapter 17**	7.4, 7.5 9.5 16.2, 16.3 17.7, 17.8
8. Describe how lifestyles, pathogens, family history, and other risk factors are related to the cause or prevention of disease and other health problems.	**Chapter 7** **Chapter 11** **Chapter 14** **Chapter 15**	7.4 11.2 14.1, 14.5 15.1, 15.2, 15.3, 15.4, 15.5, 15.6, 15.7, 15.8, 15.9

HEALTH EDUCATION STANDARD 2

Students will demonstrate the ability to access valid health information and health-promoting products and services.

PERFORMANCE INDICATORS: As a result of health instruction in Grades 5–8, students will:

Standard	Correlation	
1. Analyze the validity of health information, products, and services.	**Chapter 1** **Chapter 2**	1.4 2.3
2. Demonstrate the ability to utilize resources from home, school, and community that provide valid health information.	**Chapter 7**	7.5
3. Analyze how media influences the selection of health information and products.	**Chapter 1** **Chapter 2**	1.4 2.3
4. Demonstrate the ability to locate health products and services.	**Chapter 7** **Chapter 20**	7.5 20.4
5. Compare the costs and validity of health products.	**Chapter 1** **Chapter 14**	1.4 14.5
6. Describe situations requiring professional health services.	**Chapter 1** **Chapter 7** **Chapter 17** **Chapter 20**	1.3 7.4, 7.5 17.7, 17.8 20.4

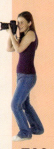

NATIONAL HEALTH EDUCATION STANDARDS

HEALTH EDUCATION STANDARD 3 — Students will demonstrate the ability to practice health-enhancing behaviors and reduce health risks.

PERFORMANCE INDICATORS: As a result of health instruction in Grades 5–8, students will:

Standard	Correlation		
1. Explain the importance of assuming responsibility for personal health behaviors.	Chapter 2 Chapter 9 Chapter 15 Chapter 20	2.1, 2.2, 2.4, 2.5, 2.7 9.1, 9.2, 9.3, 9.4, 9.5 15.4, 15.5, 15.6, 15.7 20.5	
2. Analyze a personal health assessment to determine health strengths and risks.	Chapter 1 Chapter 4	1.1 4.2	
3. Distinguish between safe and risky or harmful behaviors in relationships.	Chapter 2 Chapter 9 Chapter 14	2.3 9.2, 9.3, 9.4, 9.5 14.4	
4. Demonstrate strategies to improve or maintain personal and family health.	Chapter 1 1.1, 1.4 Chapter 2 2.2, 2.4, 2.5, 2.6, 2.7 Chapter 3 3.3 Chapter 4 4.2, 4.8 Chapter 5 5.3, 5.4 Chapter 6 6.2, 6.4	Chapter 7 7.2, 7.3, 7.4, 7.5 Chapter 9 9.1, 9.2, 9.3, 9.4, 9.5 Chapter 12 12.1, 12.2, 12.3, 12.4, 12.5, 12.6, 12.7 Chapter 17 17.1, 17.2, 17.3, 17.4, 17.5, 17.6	
5. Develop injury prevention and management strategies for personal and family health.	Chapter 4 Chapter 7 Chapter 14 Chapter 17	4.8 7.4, 7.5 14.5 17.1, 17.2, 17.3, 17.4, 17.5, 17.6, 17.7, 17.8	
6. Demonstrate ways to avoid and reduce threatening situations.	Chapter 2 Chapter 9 Chapter 10 Chapter 13 Chapter 17	2.7 9.1, 9.2, 9.4, 9.5 10.3, 10.4, 10.5 13.9 17.1	
7. Demonstrate strategies to manage stress.	Chapter 7 Chapter 8	7.3 8.2, 8.3, 8.4	

HEALTH EDUCATION STANDARD 4 — Students will analyze the influence of culture, media, technology, and other factors on health.

PERFORMANCE INDICATORS: As a result of health instruction in Grades 5–8, students will:

Standard	Correlation		
1. Describe the influence of cultural beliefs on health behaviors and the use of health services.	Chapter 2 Chapter 5	2.3 5.1	
2. Analyze how messages from media sources influence health behaviors.	Chapter 1 1.4 Chapter 2 2.3 Chapter 3 3.1	Chapter 6 6.2 Chapter 11 11.5 Chapter 12 12.3, 12.6, 12.7	
3. Analyze the influence of technology on personal health.	Chapter 4 Chapter 16	4.2 16.6	
4. Analyze how information from peers influences health.	Chapter 2 Chapter 9 Chapter 11 Chapter 12	2.3 9.1, 9.4, 9.5 11.5 12.1, 12.3	

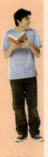

HEALTH EDUCATION STANDARD 5

Students will demonstrate the ability to use interpersonal communication skills to enhance health.

PERFORMANCE INDICATORS: As a result of health instruction in Grades 5–8, students will:

Standard	Correlation			
1. Demonstrate effective verbal and non-verbal communication skills to enhance health.	Chapter 6 Chapter 7 Chapter 8 Chapter 9 Chapter 10	6.7 7.2 8.3, 8.4 9.1, 9.2, 9.4, 9.5 10.2		
2. Describe how the behavior of family and peers affects interpersonal communication.	Chapter 1 Chapter 2 Chapter 7	1.1, 1.2, 1.3 2.3 7.5	Chapter 8 Chapter 9	8.2, 8.3, 8.4 9.1, 9.2, 9.3, 9.4, 9.5
3. Demonstrate healthy ways to express needs, wants, and feelings.	Chapter 2 Chapter 6 Chapter 7	2.7 6.3 7.2	Chapter 9 Chapter 10	9.1, 9.2, 9.3, 9.4, 9.5 10.2
4. Demonstrate ways to communicate care, consideration, and respect of self and others.	Chapter 2 Chapter 9	2.4 9.1, 9.2, 9.3, 9.4, 9.5		
5. Demonstrate communication skills to build and maintain healthy relationships.	Chapter 7 Chapter 9 Chapter 10	7.2 9.1, 9.2, 9.3, 9.4, 9.5 10.2		
6. Demonstrate refusal and negotiation skills to enhance health.	Chapter 2 Chapter 9 Chapter 10	2.7 9.4, 9.5 10.2	Chapter 11 Chapter 17	11.7 17.1
7. Analyze the possible causes of conflicts among youth in schools and communities.	Chapter 10 Chapter 17	10.1 17.1		
8. Demonstrate strategies to manage conflict in healthy ways.	Chapter 7 Chapter 10	7.1, 7.3 10.2, 10.3		

HEALTH EDUCATION STANDARD 6

Students will demonstrate the ability to use goal-setting and decision-making skills to enhance health.

PERFORMANCE INDICATORS: As a result of health instruction in Grades 5–8, students will:

Standard	Correlation			
1. Demonstrate the ability to apply a decision-making process to health issues and problems individually and collaboratively.	Chapter 2 Chapter 7	2.2 7.3, 7.5		
2. Analyze how health-related decisions are influenced by individual, family, and community values.	Chapter 2 Chapter 11 Chapter 12	2.3 11.5 12.3, 12.4, 12.5, 12.6, 12.7		
3. Predict how decisions regarding health behaviors have consequences for self and others.	Chapter 2 Chapter 9 Chapter 11 Chapter 12 Chapter 13	2.2 9.1, 9.2, 9.5 11.3 12.2, 12.3, 12.4, 12.5 13.5	Chapter 14 Chapter 15 Chapter 20	14.4 15.1, 15.2, 15.3, 15.4, 15.5, 15.6, 15.7, 15.8, 15.9 20.5

NATIONAL HEALTH EDUCATION STANDARDS

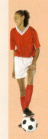

HEALTH EDUCATION STANDARD 6, continued

PERFORMANCE INDICATORS: As a result of health instruction in Grades 5–8, students will:

Standard	Correlation	
4. Apply strategies and skills needed to attain personal health goals.	Chapter 1 Chapter 2 Chapter 3 Chapter 4 Chapter 9	1.4 2.4, 2.5, 2.6, 2.7 3.3 4.2 9.5
5. Describe how personal health goals are influenced by changing information, abilities, priorities, and responsibilities.	Chapter 2	2.6
6. Develop a plan that addresses personal strengths, needs, and health risks.	Chapter 8 Chapter 12	8.4 12.6, 12.7

HEALTH EDUCATION STANDARD 7

Students will demonstrate the ability to advocate for personal, family, and community health.

PERFORMANCE INDICATORS: As a result of health instruction in Grades 5–8, students will:

Standard	Correlation	
1. Analyze various communication methods to accurately express health information and ideas.	Chapter 7	7.2
2. Express information and opinions about health issues.	Chapter 7	7.2
3. Identify barriers to effective communication of information, ideas, feelings, and opinions about health issues.	Chapter 8 Chapter 9	8.1, 8.2 9.2, 9.3, 9.4
4. Demonstrate the ability to influence others in making positive health choices.	Chapter 7 Chapter 9	7.5 9.1, 9.2, 9.3, 9.4, 9.5
5. Demonstrate the ability to work cooperatively when advocating for healthy individuals, families, and schools.	Chapter 9	9.1, 9.2, 9.3

Teaching Sensitive Issues

Contents

An Introduction to Teaching Sensitive Issues T34
Large-Scale Tragedy T40
Grief T42
Mental Illness T44
Suicide T46
Eating Disorders and Body Image T48
Cultural Tension and Stereotyping T50
Sexuality T52
Pregnancy T54
Sexually Transmitted Diseases T56
Gangs T58
Domestic Violence T60
Dating Violence T62

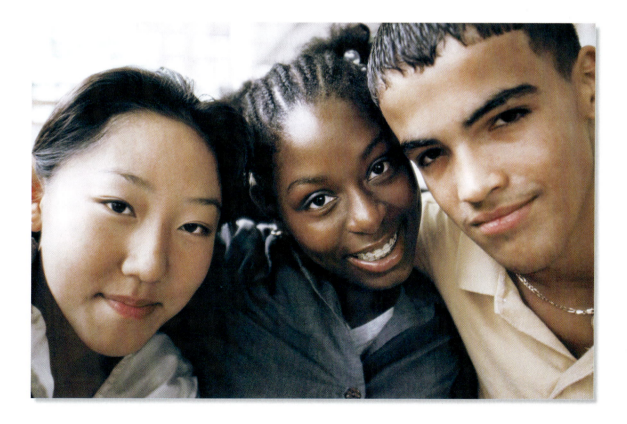

An Introduction to Teaching Sensitive Issues

Any issue that affects people personally or that can produce conflicting responses can be a sensitive issue. Helping students deal with a wide range of sensitive issues in adolescence will help them learn to cope with many of the difficult circumstances they will face throughout their lives. The purpose of this series is to help teachers develop strategies for addressing some of these issues.

Each issue addressed in this series is accompanied by activities for you to use either with individual students or with the class. Please review each set of activities to assess which activities are most appropriate for your students and which activities meet your district's policies.

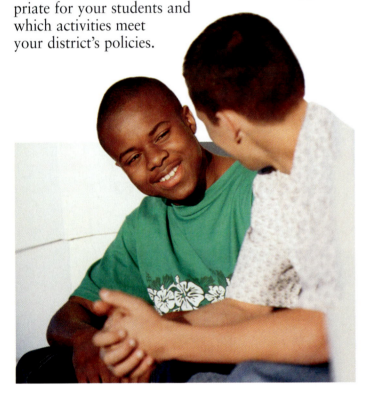

Why Sensitive Issues Arise

Sensitive issues arise for a number of reasons. Some sensitive issues, such as human development, may be part of a regular school curriculum and arise as a matter of course. Other sensitive issues arise when circumstances, such as the suicide of a young person in the community, a national tragedy, or the mental illness of a parent, require teachers or students to address these issues.

Sometimes, sensitive issues arise because of the physical and emotional transitions that occur during adolescence. During adolescence, teens begin experimenting with new and sometimes risky behaviors and peers take on new importance. Unless young teens have a strong sense of their own identity, standing up to peer pressure can be difficult. This pressure can lead to problems, such as depression and experimentation with drugs, alcohol, and sex, which are often difficult to discuss.

Sensitive issues affect people emotionally. No public consensus exists on how to deal with many sensitive issues, and attitudes about the issues can vary widely. Many sensitive issues are difficult to discuss without also discussing values and beliefs, and any public discussion of values and beliefs is likely to be controversial.

Why Sensitive Issues Need to Be Addressed

Although addressing sensitive issues can be controversial, avoiding them can cause larger problems. Teens often struggle to cope with problems such as cultural intolerance and domestic violence. And many teens make daily choices about issues such as pregnancy and gangs. Yet teens often do not feel comfortable speaking with their parents or other adults about these issues and few teens are able to provide their peers with well-informed support or direction. You can help by either directly addressing the issues that arise or by referring students to helpful resources.

Sometimes, a tragic event can overwhelm a school or other community. Students preoccupied with the effects of a tragic event often have trouble focusing on their schoolwork. Helping students cope with the effects of tragedy and respond in healthy ways can help them learn from the event and bring their focus back to their daily lives.

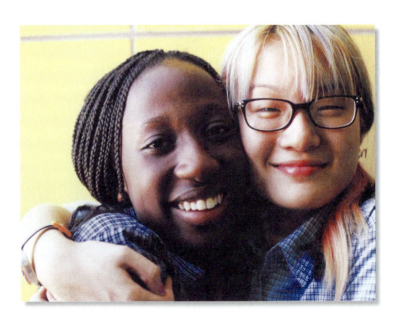

Working with Your District

Prior to teaching any of these issues, it is crucial for you to have a complete understanding of district and school philosophy and policies. The following tips may be helpful:

- Find out who is in charge of health programs for your district.
- Speak with district representatives, and set aside time to go to your district office to review policies, approved curriculum, and any other information that may be relevant.
- Determine which topics your district requires you to teach and which topics can and can not be discussed.
- Seek clarification for any policies that you do not understand.
- If possible, speak with another experienced health teacher and an administrator in your district to learn about specific sensitive issues and how the issues have been handled effectively in the past.
- Clearly state your objectives with your district and school administrator for final approval.
- For sensitive issues that relate to sex, sexuality, and pregnancy, find out whether parental consent is needed. Also, find out how much time must elapse between passing out consent forms and beginning a lesson.
- Find out what alternative arrangements must be made for the students of parents who do not consent.
- Find out what issues, facts, and information received from students must be reported, to whom you should report, and how you should report.
- If you have recently switched districts, do not assume the policies in the new district are the same as in the old.
- If district personnel change significantly, make sure you learn of any accompanying policy changes before teaching sensitive issues.
- Find out what referral resources are on site, such as a peer resource center, school nurse, or school psychologist, and which ones are available in your community.
- Find out which outside agencies are approved to serve as resources or guest presenters in the classroom, and review the agencies' curricula so that you are familiar with what will be presented in your classroom. When extending invitations, inform guest speakers of all district, school, and classroom guidelines that they must follow. If a speaker strays from the assigned topic, you must immediately decide if the new subject is appropriate to address at that time and, if necessary, stop the discussion. **Ultimately, you are responsible for what is discussed in the classroom, regardless of who introduces a subject.**
- You may wish to have a second adult present during some discussions, not only as an informational resource but also as a witness to the way material was addressed in your classroom.
- Do not read journals that students use in writing activities. Provide a written statement to your district and to students' parents or guardians that asserts you do not read student journals. If you do not state this policy in writing, you may be considered responsible for responding to the actions and behaviors students describe or even suggest in journal entries.

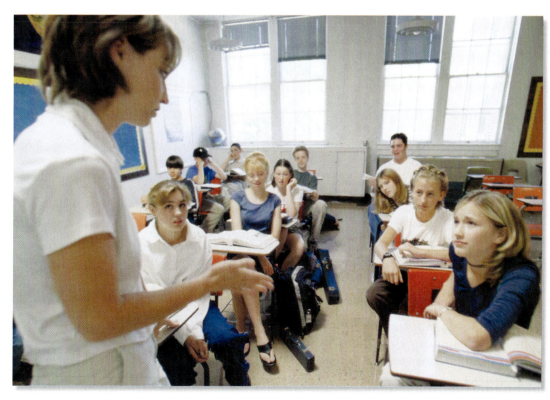

Working with Challenges

Sensitive issues can be difficult to address, but they provide teachers with important educational opportunities. Take full advantage of such "teaching moments" when they occur in your classroom. Sometimes, students will challenge you or their peers by deliberately initiating discussion about a sensitive issue, such as by insulting a group of people. Or a student could unknowingly approach an issue that you know many other students would find difficult to discuss. These moments can help begin discussion of important issues. For example, a student may frequently discuss his or her weight. Listen to these comments, and use them as an opportunity to teach.

You can also challenge teens to take personal responsibility. Provide teens information in an honest, nonjudgmental way to help them make sound, healthy decisions related to their own bodies, lifestyles, families, and communities. Encourage them to seek help from parents and other trusted adults.

To encourage students to ask questions, answer questions respectfully and thoughtfully. Remind students that there are no dumb questions. Remember that when students ask you questions, they are often looking for answers to more than the question they asked. For example, if a student asks about the risks of sexually transmitted diseases, he or she may also be asking about the risks of pregnancy or about the emotional risks and consequences of sexual activity. If you sense that a question has other questions behind it, you may want to find out which other concerns the student has. If a student asks a question about a sensitive issue, ask yourself, "Why is the student asking this question now? What larger issue might be helpful to address?" Don't be afraid to ask students questions, but avoid asking personal questions and stop asking if a student finds your questions upsetting. Keep your inquiries general. Be prepared to offer support, guidance, and referrals, as necessary. Most importantly, you should provide helpful, age-appropriate information and support within the guidelines set by your district.

Working with Parents

When dealing with sensitive issues, encourage teens to discuss these issues with their parents. Communicate to parents that you want what is best for their children. Keep in mind that parents are busy and that you are probably one of several teachers their child encounters each day. Your task will be to show parents that you care about each student and want each student to grow up healthy and well-educated. You and the parents can become partners and allies to help students navigate through the sensitive issues addressed in this series.

As children move into adolescence, parents often feel as if their children are pushing them away and are no longer interested in talking with them about tough issues. Some teens do pull away from their parents. However, if their parents will be open to their questions, many teens do want to talk to them about such issues.

Parents often underestimate their influence on their children's lives. In fact, as their children become teens, some parents may begin to pull away, often in frustration and fear. If both sides think there is no way to communicate and work together fairly, everybody loses.

As a teacher, you are in a position to help bridge the gap between students and parents. Encourage students to help their parents understand them. Always encourage students to go to their parents with problems and concerns. You may even help role-play how students might discuss sensitive issues with their parents.

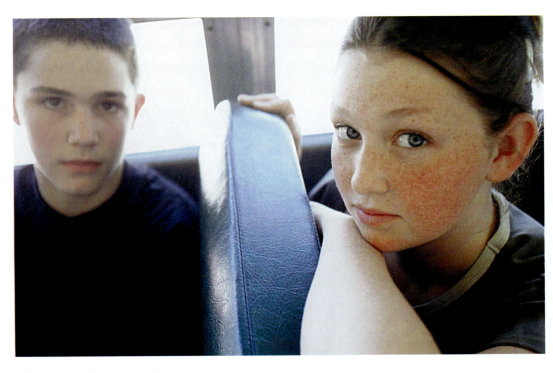

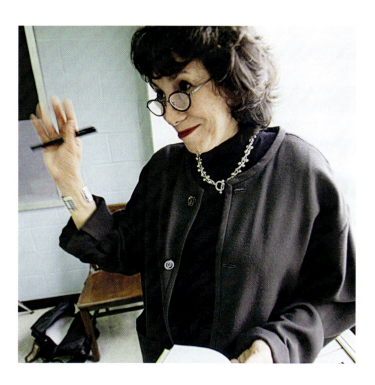

- If a teen is depressed, teachers and parents should talk with the teen about the depression, and should help him or her seek professional counseling.
- Unless teens are displaying dangerous or harmful behavior, teachers and parents should accept them as they are. Acceptance can be difficult at times. But acceptance is especially important while a teen is developing his or her identity.
- Many teens are not skilled at long-term thinking and planning about their lives. During difficult times, just getting through a day can seem like an accomplishment. Patience and compassion—along with appropriate discipline, boundaries, and structure—will go a long way in helping teens make it through this transitional time.

The Parent-Teacher Partnership

- Value parents. Recognize that you must become partners with them to help students work through many sensitive issues.
- Respect parents, and listen carefully to their concerns.
- Let parents know that you understand that, as a group, the parents of the students in your class may have diverse cultural beliefs and values and that you respect those beliefs and values.
- Let parents know you appreciate and share many of their concerns regarding adolescent behavior.
- Although many adults feel that some students are too young to hear about sex, gangs, and other sensitive issues, most students have already heard something about these issues and will learn additional information about these subjects from peers, TV, and the Internet. Parents and teachers can work together to provide children with reliable, helpful information.
- If a student has begun to participate in a pattern of risky behaviors, these behaviors will not change overnight. Help parents understand that it may take time for the teen to learn to make healthier decisions.

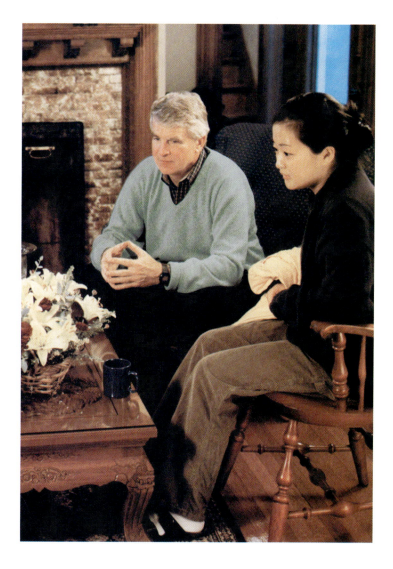

Teen Needs

When developing a partnership with parents, consider the following developmental needs of middle school students:

- Middle school students identify with their peers, want to belong, and need opportunities to form positive relationships with other teens. However, they also need caring relationships with adults who love them, respect them, and provide structure and discipline.
- Many young teens are very critical of themselves. Adults can help teens appreciate their uniqueness and differences while being clear about limits, boundaries, and expectations. Clearly defining limits helps young teens feel more secure.
- During puberty, many teens experience rapid and uneven growth that can make them feel very uncomfortable about their bodies.
- Creative expression is important for teens to learn more about who they are and to let the world know what is unique about them. They need to discover their strengths to help them feel less self-conscious and self-critical. Teachers and parents can encourage exploration of a variety of activities, including volunteering, to help the teens discover healthy activities of interest to them. For example, volunteering at an animal shelter or zoo or tutoring younger children can help a sad or bored teen gain a new sense of involvement in the larger community. Community service also helps foster a sense of compassion and responsibility for others.
- Encourage parents to help teens develop social skills by encouraging their teens to share their ideas about the world. While doing this, parents can model good listening skills, such as asking for clarification when ideas are not clear and respectfully sharing thoughts and opinions about those ideas.

Teens and Risk-Taking

It is important for teens to learn to discern healthy risks from bad risks. Show teens how to weigh the dangers and benefits of a particular situation and to know how his or her own strengths and weaknesses may affect the consequences. When teens learn the power of their own choices, they can gain self-confidence. Any risk involving the possibility of teens hurting themselves or others is a bad risk and should be discouraged.

Many parents have difficulty addressing risk-taking behaviors with teens. On one hand they want to protect teens, while on the other hand they recognize that teens have to be able to make their own mistakes. Striking a balance between the teen's safety and his or her autonomy can be one of the most difficult challenges parents face. Parents may find it helpful to think back to their own childhood and remember various risks they took, to realize they gradually modified their behavior as they went along, and to remember that they got through that period relatively unharmed.

Some degree of risk-taking is part of adolescence. Risk-taking is one way teens develop their identity. Much of adolescent risk-taking is actually healthy and helps teens grow by allowing them to try new things and test themselves and their abilities. However, dangerous behavior requires an immediate response. If a parent thinks a teen may be in danger, refer the parent to professionals who can help.

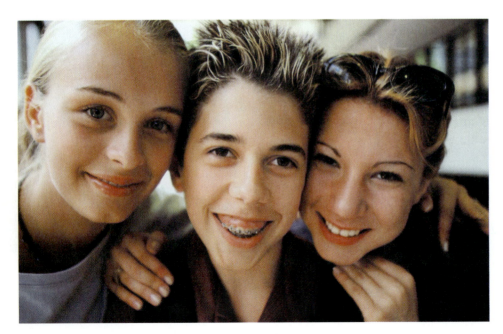

Tips for Success

- In class, be aware of your responses to questions and comments about sensitive issues. Teens will observe your body language, tone of voice, attitudes, and confidence. They will perceive your level of comfort. If you feel uncomfortable, want to avoid discussing an issue, or think that a behavior is wrong, students will know. Your response may also determine which questions students think they can ask about the issue. So, honesty is very important. Do not bluff or offer disingenuous answers. It is OK to let students know that you are uncomfortable discussing an issue or that you do not know the answer to a question. You can also research the topic and report back to the students. Encourage students to discuss the topics with their parents or other trusted adults.

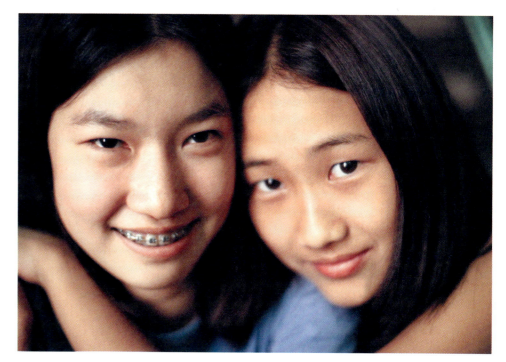

- Be aware of your own biases and values. Are you the best person to teach a particular issue? A teen's life experience may be such that you will alienate him or her if your bias enters the presentation or discussion. If there is an issue that needs to be addressed but that you feel you can not present in a neutral way, try to find another teacher or speaker to teach that issue.

- Set and enforce boundaries. Have clear expectations of student behavior.

- Encourage students to speak freely, but make sure they understand what information you are legally required to report.

- Do not share your opinions or personal life with students.

- Whenever possible, enlist the support of administrators and parents. Parental support is of particular value. Get parents involved as often as possible when you are discussing sensitive subjects.

- Create a classroom environment that is nonjudgmental and respectful and that celebrates differences in people. No matter how homogeneous your class may seem, your class is made of individuals.

- As part of your classroom environment, include posters and resource numbers for places students may contact, such as mental health hotlines, suicide prevention centers, and child abuse prevention organizations. Make sure that you provide only resources that your district has approved.

- Some issues, such as issues involving sexuality, may be inappropriate for students in your district to research. But when student investigation is appropriate, ask students—either individually or in teams—to research an issue and report back to the class what they have found. You can follow up their presentation with an activity from this series. Learning about some issues may inspire students to take action. For example, students learning about violence may want to learn to become peer mediators.

- At all times, you must realize you are a teacher, not a trained counselor or therapist. This series is intended to assist you by providing background information about sensitive issues that you may encounter and by offering activities to help students better understand those issues. If a student needs help with these issues you should identify local resources, both at school and within the community, that can accept your referrals. Listening, showing that you care, and assisting in locating appropriate referrals are the most effective ways you can help.

- Provide an anonymous question box that you check regularly. Be sure to follow district rules when answering questions.

Large-Scale Tragedy

Introduction

Although we would like to protect children from tragedy, it is impossible to isolate them from many of the major traumas and disasters of the world. These traumas and disasters include natural phenomena, such as earthquakes, hurricanes, and tornadoes, and human-made tragedies, such as terrorism, suicides, and shootings. Some tragic events happen locally, while others happen far away. Local traumatic events directly affect students, and media coverage makes national tragedies significant for students living thousands of miles away from the incident.

People respond to traumatic incidents in many ways. Physical reactions may include rapid heartbeat, fatigue, nightmares, insomnia, hyperactivity, exhaustion, lack of activity, headaches, stomach problems, and appetite changes. Cognitive reactions may include difficulty concentrating, making decisions, and solving problems; memory problems; and an inability to attach importance to anything other than the incident. Emotional reactions may include fear, anxiety, guilt, depression, emotional numbness, feelings of helplessness, oversensitivity, anger, violent fantasies, or sadness.

An intense reaction to trauma is often referred to as post-traumatic stress disorder (PTSD). Symptoms of PTSD include mood swings, dramatic behavioral changes, poor concentration, hyperactivity, nightmares, or flashbacks. These symptoms may persist for a month or more or may not occur until several months after the trauma. If you see symptoms of PTSD, immediately refer the student to a trained health professional.

Teen Concerns

- Traumatic events change the way people see themselves and their world. Teens may feel helpless and unsettled during a crisis, and they need accurate and timely information to prevent rumors and false information from causing further anxiety.
- Students will have different reactions to a tragedy as well as different abilities to cope with it. Teens need to be reassured that there can be a variety of responses to the same event and that there is no such thing as a correct response. They also need to know that the amount of time it takes to heal varies from person to person. Having the time and opportunity to work through feelings about tragedies is essential.

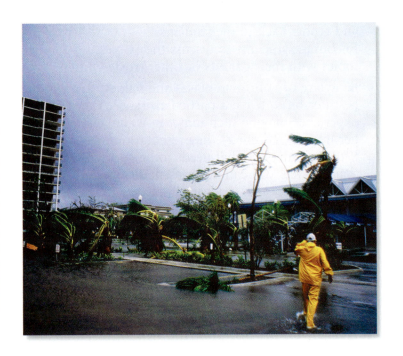

What You Can Do

- Know your school's and your district's crisis and disaster response plan and your role in the plan.
- Take care of yourself physically and emotionally so that you are able to help your students.
- If your classroom was directly affected by the tragedy, remove from your classroom-related signs of the tragedy. For example, remove items broken by an earthquake.
- For a while, plan shorter lessons taught at a slower pace and give less homework.
- Pay attention to your students so that you have a sense of how they are coping. Set aside time to discuss the event and its effects. Encourage students to express their feelings either aloud or in writing.
- Acknowledge that traumatic events often lead to strong feelings, such as intense anger or fear.

- Set aside time over the next few months to discuss practical issues related to recovery.
- Help students learn what they need to do to be safe.
- Identify all available resources, such as university programs, volunteer agencies, and local health and mental health agencies.
- Recognize reactions to trauma and disaster. Students may act out in response to an event.
- Be clear about your behavioral expectations, especially if students behave inappropriately. Help students understand and manage their anger.
- Recognize that traumatized adolescents are at risk for reckless behavior that can lead to injury, including drug and alcohol use. Discuss these risks and the need to be especially careful in the weeks and months ahead.
- Encourage students to limit their time watching news coverage about the event, especially if the event is being covered on an ongoing basis. Help students process what they have seen on TV.
- Encourage students to alternate between periods of inactivity and exercise to help cope with the physical effects of distress.
- Encourage students to participate in extracurricular activities.
- Be aware of students who seem to assume too much responsibility for what has happened. These students may be struggling with PTSD.
- If a student has become withdrawn or excessively quiet, talk to him or her. Provide new opportunities for him or her to participate in class. If the behavior continues, refer the student to people who can help.
- Help students develop a school or neighborhood improvement project to help others in the community.

ACTIVITIES

Group Activity
Responding to Tragedy

After a tragic event occurs, ask students to share the feelings, thoughts, and questions that they had when they first heard about or witnessed the event. On the board, make three lists: one for feelings, one for thoughts, and one for questions. (Possible feelings include confusion, anger, fear, sadness, disorientation, and numbness. Possible thoughts include, "This should not have happened. I want to run away. I want to help." Possible questions include, "How will this affect me? How will this affect my family? Why did it happen? Am I in danger?") Point out the variety of thoughts and feelings that can result from one crisis. If the event was far away, ask students, "Why are we moved by events that occur far away from us? What connects us to events that occur throughout the country and the world? How large is our community?" Conclude by reviewing some of the primary thoughts and feelings, and acknowledge the universality and individuality of reactions to traumatic events.

Writing Activity
Chronicling a Response

Ask students to create a notebook or journal in which they can freely express their feelings. Ask students to bring in a magazine or newspaper article about the tragedy. Have students paste this article to the front of their notebook. During the weeks following the tragedy, allow time for students to write reflective journal entries and drawings. Questions to prompt students include the following:

- What do you understand about what happened?
- What questions do you want answered?
- How do you feel about what happened?
- Whom have you been speaking to about the event?
- How can we support the people who were directly affected by this tragedy?

(**Caution:** You may be held responsible for information in the journals unless you have a written policy stating that you will not read journal entries and you follow that policy.) Have students write in their journals periodically, because their emotions will change over time.

Extension Activity
Identifying Resources

Ask students, "To whom can we turn in times of community or national tragedy?" Write volunteer's responses on the board. Give students a list of local people and organizations that your school and district have identified as resources to address crises.

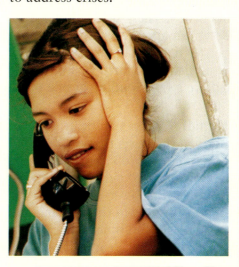

Grief

Introduction

Grieving a death or another significant loss is often very difficult. Losing someone or something important can be emotionally disorienting, troubling, or even devastating. Furthermore, a death in a family sometimes poses practical concerns. For example, if the family member had provided financial support, losing that support may result in lifestyle changes.

While the death of a loved one is often the most significant loss a person can face, other significant losses are also common. These losses include a best friend moving, a close friend changing schools, parents divorcing, a pet running away or dying, or personally experiencing a change in physical ability, such as becoming a paraplegic.

Teaching about grief can raise sensitive issues about personal experiences, beliefs, and values. Respecting people's privacy, beliefs, and values is the first step in helping people understand grief.

Teen Concerns

- While experiencing grief at any age is challenging, it can be particularly difficult for teens. Adolescence is a time when people look to the future and to the possibilities of what they will do with their lives and what they will contribute to the world. It is a time when many people feel invincible. When young people are faced with the death of a loved one, they may think that their world has been shaken. The teen not only has lost someone but may also suddenly feel vulnerable to death, perhaps for the first time.
- Teens in grief may fear living without the person they lost. Some teens suddenly fear their own death or the death of another close relative or friend. For example, after the death of a classmate's parent, teens may fear that their own parents or caregivers will soon die.

Stages of Grief

You can introduce the issue of death or loss to your class by discussing the main stages of grief, which are listed below. These stages do not always occur in the order given and they simplify a very complex process. A person may remain in one stage for a long time or may go back and forth between stages. But the stages listed are a basic outline of one theory about how people grieve.

- **Denial** After a significant loss, a person often feels nothing or insists that no change has occurred because of the loss. For example, some children sincerely hope and believe that their parents will get back together, even after a divorce. This stage is an important time in the grieving process because it allows a person time to organize feelings and responses to the death or loss. A person in this stage needs understanding and time.
- **Anger** After a person experiences a significant loss, his or her world has changed, and he or she may feel angry about that change. In teens, anger can show itself in the form of disruptive or aggressive behavior, diminished academic performance, and sleep disturbances. It is important to help teens express anger in positive and healthy ways.
- **Bargaining** People who have lost someone or something sometimes try to bargain physically, psychologically, or spiritually to restore what they have lost. For example, a man in grief over a divorce may promise his ex-wife that he will correct every problematic behavior he has if she will return to the marriage. People at this stage are usually beginning to face the hard truth that a permanent change has occurred.

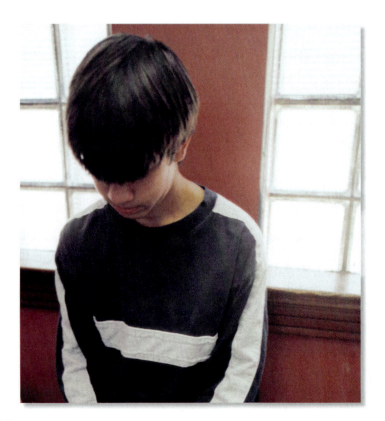

- **Despair** When people feel loss, they may feel helpless. They may cry frequently, withdraw from activities, or become lethargic. They may avoid doing things they enjoyed in the past. If a person is experiencing too much emotional distress, withdrawing can be a healthy, self-protective response. Teens at this stage need to be reassured that others understand their grief and that their feelings of sadness will decrease over time. If a teen exhibits a deeply depressed or irritable mood or persistent feelings of worthlessness, guilt, or hopelessness, he or she should be referred to professional help. Anyone depressed to the point of having suicidal thoughts should receive professional counseling as soon as possible.
- **Acceptance** Eventually, a grieving person begins to feel more hopeful and comes to accept the loss. Many people approaching this stage appreciate encouragement to begin the return to a balanced, active life.

What You Can Do

- If a student chooses to tell you about grief that he or she is feeling, listen to the student. Be sympathetic, respond authentically, give the student permission to be sad, and refer the student for help if his or her grief appears to be resulting in depression.
- If a student, teacher, or other significant member of the school or community dies, obtain accurate information about the death and determine what information is appropriate to share.
- Help students identify the feelings they may experience after losing someone or something important: sadness, anger, regret, a feeling of missing or longing for the deceased, worry, fear of being alone, disorientation, numbness, confusion, or guilt. These feelings may vary from day to day depending on who or what was lost, and all of these feelings can be part of a healthy response.
- Educate students about manifestations of grief, such as poor concentration, nightmares, headaches, forgetfulness, lack of appetite, and sleep difficulties. People may dream about the person who has died or may suddenly think they see the person in a familiar place.
- Help students identify what they can do to feel better. Let them know that strong emotions and thoughts related to death and loss eventually fade or change over time. The strong feelings may return on significant dates, such as birthdays, or at significant events, such as graduations. In time, students will be able to move through their sad feelings.
- Advise students that during the grieving process, taking good physical care of oneself—by eating well, sleeping, and exercising—is important and helpful.
- Advise students to reach out to others, such as family, friends, teachers, counselors, and members of their religious or spiritual communities.

ACTIVITIES

Discussion
How Do People Grieve?
People respond to loss in many ways. Begin a discussion by asking students, "How do people respond when they lose something or someone important to them?" *(Sample answers: People can feel sad, lonely, angry, guilty, frustrated, confused, numb, or relieved.)*

Writing Activity
A Letter
If a student asks you how he or she can respond to a death, you may invite the student to write a letter to the person the student has lost. The letter can express feelings of gratitude for time spent together and feelings associated with the loss. If appropriate, encourage the student to write a letter to the family of the person who died. This letter may include what the person who died meant to the student and may describe memorable times. The student may choose to keep the letter or to send the letter to family members of the person who died. Afterward, ask students to write down what they learned by writing the letter.

Extension Activity
Cultural Awareness
Ask students to research the ways in which communities from various countries honor those who have died. For example, in Mexico, the deceased are honored during an annual ritual held in November. This ritual is called *El Dia de Los Muertos* (The Day of the Dead). Students can use the Internet or school library to conduct their research. Have students present their findings to the class.

Mental Illness

Introduction

A mental illness is any disorder that affects behavior, thoughts, or emotions. Mental illnesses are not rare. Mental health professionals estimate that in any given year, more than 54 million Americans have a mental illness, although fewer than 8 million seek treatment. The two most common types of mental illnesses are depression and anxiety disorders, and each type of these illnesses affects 19 million American adults annually.

Causes of mental health problems vary but can include one or a combination of any of the following: excessive stress from a particular situation or series of events, environmental stress, genetic factors, or biochemical imbalances. Symptoms of the more common disorders may include changes in mood, personality, and personal habits as well as social withdrawal. Many people can learn to cope with or treat a mental illness if they receive proper care.

Care for mental illnesses is not always easy to get. Medically underserved communities frequently lack resources to care adequately for mentally ill people. Sometimes, care is not sought. Cultural barriers often keep people from disclosing symptoms of a mental illness, even to medical professionals.

Learning that a loved one has a mental illness can be both physically and emotionally difficult. Often, the members of the family do not discuss the matter with people outside the family for personal reasons. Keeping the matter private can lead children to think that the problem is a secret and a source of shame or fear.

Teen Concerns

- One in five children has a diagnosable mental illness or an emotional or behavioral disorder.
- An estimated two-thirds of young people with mental health problems are not receiving the help they need.
- If parents have an anxiety disorder, studies suggest it is more likely that their children have that disorder, as well.
- As many as one in eight adolescents may have depression.
- Schizophrenia occurs in approximately three out of every 1,000 adolescents.
- Children of parents addicted to alcohol or other drugs are up to four times more likely to develop substance abuse and mental health problems than other children are.
- Twenty percent of incarcerated youths have a serious emotional disturbance, and most (about 70 percent) have mental health problems.
- Children whose parents have an untreated mental illness are at risk of developing social, emotional, and behavioral problems. Children may take on inappropriate levels of responsibility in caring for themselves and managing the household. They may blame themselves for their parent's illness and become isolated from their peers and others. They may also be at increased risk for problems with schoolwork, alcohol and other drugs, and relationships. On the other hand, many children of parents with untreated mental illness are resilient and able to thrive, in spite of environmental and genetic vulnerability.

Some Signs of Mental Illness in Teens

The warning signs and symptoms of mental illness in youth include

- substance abuse
- an inability to cope with problems and daily activities
- a prolonged negative mood, often accompanied by poor appetite or thoughts of death
- frequent complaints of physical ailments
- defiance of authority
- an intense fear of weight gain
- a change in sleeping or eating habits
- frequent outbursts of anger
- episodes of truancy, theft, or vandalism

What You Can Do

- Teach students about various mental illnesses that generally affect teens and their families.
- Let students know there is both help and hope for successful treatment of a mental or emotional problem.
- Seek help from a school counselor for any student you suspect may be suffering from a mental illness.
- Know about resources available for students or their families, including school counselors, local health departments' mental health division, other mental health organizations, family physicians, family services agencies, religious leaders, emergency rooms, and crisis centers.
- If a student has a parent whose mental illness keeps the parent from being supportive, help the student develop healthy coping tools. Those tools include positive self-esteem, interest in and success at school, positive peer relationships, healthy engagement with adults outside the home, and the ability to articulate feelings.
- Be aware that a student with an untreated mental illness is at increased risk for drug abuse, suicide, eating disorders, gang involvement, and sexual activity.

ACTIVITIES

Writing Activity
Mental Health

Instruct students to write about what they know about mental health. Ask students, "What does it mean to be mentally healthy?" (Sample answers: feeling good, strong, confident, and enthusiastic about life) Ask, "What does it mean to have a mental illness?" (Note: Be careful not to put students on the spot. A student with a mentally ill family member may not wish to discuss the issue at all. However, this activity may encourage students who might have family members that are struggling with a mental illness to discuss the problem with you privately.) This activity provides you the opportunity to clarify myths students may hold about people who have a mental illness.

Discussion
Helping Yourself

Ask students, "How do we contribute to our own mental health?" Write student responses on the board. (Sample answers: get enough sleep, eat properly, exercise, express feelings, avoid using drugs, become involved in meaningful activities, spend time with supportive friends and family members, spend time reflecting, laugh, sing) Ask students, "How much sleep is enough sleep? Do you get enough sleep? Do you get too much sleep? What is a well-balanced diet? Do you eat a well-balanced diet? Do you let people know when you feel very sad or anxious?" Encourage students to look critically at their habits and modify them if necessary. Share your healthy habits, such as routine exercising or healthy eating habits, with students. Let them know the benefits of such habits, especially over time.

Extension Activity
Interview

Have students interview mental health professionals. Students may ask their interviewees to describe what they do and the kinds of problems they treat. They may also ask the mental health professionals to describe some healthful activities many people can do to stay mentally healthy. The interviewees may describe the mental and physical benefits people can get from these activities. Students can make posters illustrating what the mental health professional does and the suggestions he or she has for helping people stay mentally healthy.

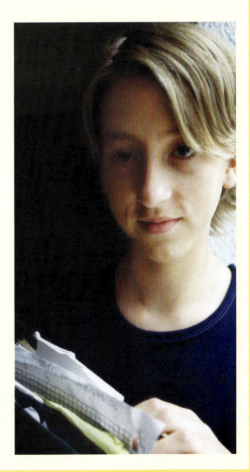

Suicide

Introduction

Suicide is the eighth leading cause of death in the United States, regardless of age, sex, or race. Problems, such as stressful events, substance abuse, and mental illness (including depression, anorexia nervosa, and anxiety) can increase the risk of suicide. Most people who attempt suicide do not want to kill themselves but are looking for a way to end the deep, emotional pain they are experiencing.

Teen Concerns

- Suicides among teenagers in the United States have increased dramatically in recent years. Suicide is now the third leading cause of death for young people aged 15 to 24 and is the fourth leading cause of death for people ages 10 to 14. Males are four to five times more likely than females to succeed at committing suicide.
- Teens often experience confusion, self-doubt, stress, and fear. Some of these feelings may seem overwhelming to a teen and can lead to depression and suicidal feelings. For some teens, issues related to their family structure, including divorce, moving, and the formation of a new family with stepparents and stepsiblings, can be very unsettling and can intensify self-doubts.
- Some teens respond in unhealthy ways to the intense pressure to succeed in school and in sports. While some young people may appear to be excelling, they may actually be very self-critical and feeling inadequate.
- Children exposed to violence, life-threatening events, or traumatic losses are at increased risk for alcohol and substance abuse, depression, and suicide.
- People intent on killing themselves are difficult to stop. However, many people attempting suicide are trying to solve a problem, not trying to die. In such cases, suicide can often be prevented with proper intervention.

Warning Signs of Teen Suicide

Never ignore signs that a student may be considering suicide. Examples of signs include

- suicide notes
- a plan or method
- threats (Direct threats include, "I am going to kill myself," and "I want to die." Indirect threats include, "The world would be better off without me," and "Nothing matters." The indirect signs may be seen or heard in jokes, in continued references to death, or in suicidal themes in school assignments.)
- previous attempts at suicide
- depression, which is a mental illness in which a person feels extremely sad and hopeless for long periods of time
- masked depression, which includes risk-taking behaviors, such as gunplay, alcohol or substance abuse, or acts of aggression
- self-mutilating behavior
- frequent complaints about physical symptoms that often relate to emotions, such as headaches, fatigue, or stomachaches
- making final arrangements, such as giving away valued possessions
- inability to think rationally or to concentrate
- feeling persistent boredom, which may be apparent through classroom behavior, academic performance, or conversation
- changes in physical appearance and habits, such as sudden weight gain or loss, disinterest in hygiene or appearance, and sleeping in class
- sudden changes in friends, behaviors, and personality, such as withdrawing from normal relationships, having increased absenteeism, running away, lacking involvement in regular interests and activities, and isolation

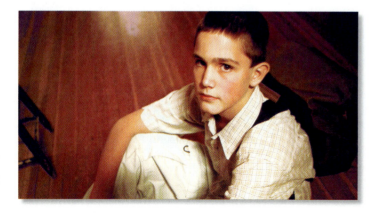

What You Can Do

- You may wish to have another adult witness any discussion you have with students about suicide.
- Know your district and school policy on reporting students at risk for suicide, and adhere to the guidelines of that policy.
- If you have no guidelines, inform both a school counselor or administrator and a parent or caregiver if a student raises the issue of suicide. Encourage your school district to develop guidelines for handling this issue.
- Never minimize the thoughts a suicidal person expresses or describe them as foolish, and never use logic to try to convince a suicidal person that he or she has many reasons to live.
- If you are worried about a student, let him or her know. Do not be afraid to ask questions about suicide. (Direct questions include, "Are you thinking about killing yourself?" "Do you have a plan?" and "Have you ever considered suicide before?") You will not initiate thoughts about it just by asking. In fact, asking will provide the student with assurance that somebody cares and will give the student a chance to talk about problems.
- If a student answers affirmatively to any of the questions in the point above, he or she is at risk. Do not leave a student alone if you have determined he or she is at risk for committing suicide. Do not send suicidal students to a counselor alone. Escort them yourself to an appropriate adult who will help.
- Let students know that you care and want to know if they or someone they know is considering suicide.
- Encourage students to tell an adult if they know someone who is thinking about commiting suicide.
- Know your local suicide prevention hotline number, and make this number available to students.
- Be aware of suicide contagion. If a suicide is successful in your school or area, some people may now be at higher risk of considering suicide themselves. These people include any student who assisted a person in committing suicide. For example, they may have helped write a note, provided the means for the suicide, or been involved in a suicide pact. Other people at risk include a student who knew of the suicide plans but did not divulge them to an adult; best friends; siblings or other relatives; students with a history of suicidal threats or attempts; students who identify closely with the situation of the person who committed suicide; a student who was committed to trying to keep the student alive; and any other students who are feeling desperate for any reason and see suicide as an option.
- Be an advocate for a teen if other adults are minimizing risk factors and warning signs. Continue your advocacy until you are sure the student is safe.

ACTIVITIES

Discussion
Misconception Quiz

Have students indicate which of the following statements are true and which are false:

1. If a person jokes about committing suicide that means he or she will not really do it.
2. Suicide is the third leading cause of death for people ages 15 to 24.
3. If you are worried that someone you know is thinking about committing suicide, you should ask him or her questions about how he or she feels.
4. People who threaten to commit suicide want to die.
5. Sometimes, people who are depressed do risky things, such as drink alcohol or play with weapons.

(Answers: 1. false; 2. true; 3. true; 4. false; 5. true)

Ask students if the answers to the quiz surprised them. Allow students to express their surprise, confusion, and fear. (Sample answers: "I thought if someone were going to commit suicide, he or she would keep it quiet—you know, not tell anyone. I think it would be hard to talk to someone who seems really depressed. I mean, what would I say? I always thought depressed people were silent and alone. I didn't know they could be right here being loud.")

Explain that depression can manifest itself in many ways, such as risk-taking behaviors; frequent complaints about headaches, fatigue, or stomachaches; persistent boredom; and sudden changes in friends, behaviors, and personality. Stress that if he or she thinks a friend is depressed or contemplating suicide, it is important to seek appropriate adult help for that friend.

Writing Activity
Trusted Adults

Students should list at least two adults who could help them if they needed to talk about a problem or ask for advice. Remind students to contact these people whenever they think they are in danger or need to talk.

Decisions for Health • Teaching Sensitive Issues

Eating Disorders and Body Image

Introduction

No single factor can explain an eating disorder. A need for control, biochemical changes, and societal pressures can all contribute to eating disorders in teens. But body image is frequently a factor. If teens think they are fat, they can develop unhealthy eating habits. These unhealthy habits can lead to eating disorders. The most common eating disorders are anorexia nervosa, bulimia, and binge eating.

In spite of tremendous emphasis on being thin in today's society, eating disorders are rarely just about weight; frequently they are accompanied by symptoms of low self-esteem and illustrate feelings of helplessness. Controlling eating behavior may be the only area where people with eating disorders think they have power or control in their life. An eating disorder can develop as a way of handling stress and anxiety. People can have a combination of more than one eating disorder, which increases health risks. Approximately half of patients with anorexia also develop bulimia. The majority of people with anorexia have clinical depression as well.

Teen Concerns

- Teens' body image is often an inaccurate picture of what they look like. Often, when teens look in the mirror, they are not just looking at themselves. They are comparing themselves to people they find attractive or peers who have bodies they prefer to their own. These comparisons influence the development of eating disorders.
- Weight is often tied to a teen's self-esteem. This may be especially true for girls. Dieting can become a way of life from a very young age and, along with anorexia nervosa and bulimia, can be dangerous to a growing body.
- Anorexic and bulimic girls often have irregular menstrual periods. Anorexia nervosa typically shows up in early to mid adolescence. Frequently, teens with anorexia try hard to please others. Anorexia is one of the most common psychiatric diagnoses in young women and has one of the highest death rates of any mental health condition.
- Some teen athletes can also be susceptible to weight issues. Many teens feel pressure to lose weight in unhealthy ways so that they can participate in sports. For example, wrestlers often feel pressure to maintain a particular weight. Wrestlers may drop 5 to 15 pounds so that they can wrestle in a particular weight class. They may fast, throw up, or try to sweat or spit off fluids to "make weight." These practices can lead to dehydration and poor performance and contribute to a loss of muscle mass over time. Some wrestlers' weight fluctuates as much as fifteen pounds in a week's time. Young dancers and gymnasts also often experience tremendous pressure to maintain a specific body weight and may develop eating disorders.

Common Eating Disorders

- **Anorexia nervosa** is very serious and potentially life threatening. Its characteristics are self-starvation and excessive weight loss. A person with anorexia nervosa usually refuses to maintain a healthy body weight for their body type, age, and activity level; has an intense fear of gaining weight or being overweight; feels overweight even after dramatic weight loss; and is extremely concerned about body weight and body shape.
- **Bulimia nervosa** is also very serious and potentially life threatening. It is characterized by a cycle of bingeing and purging. The bulimic person typically eats large quantities of food in short periods of time, often eats secretly, and eats to a point of feeling out of control. After the binge, a bulimic person induces vomiting, abuses a laxative or diuretics, or exercises obsessively or compulsively.
- **Binge eating disorder** is primary characteristic is frequent episodes of uncontrolled eating of large quantities of food in short periods of time. The person with the disorder often eats secretly. The person usually feels out of control when bingeing and later feels shame, disgust, or guilt.

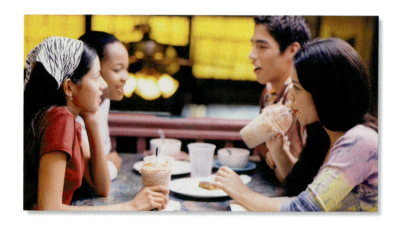

What You Can Do

- Help students differentiate between healthy eating and emotional eating. Share information about eating disorders and their dangers.
- Help students see how images in the media often distort the true diversity of healthy human body types and shapes.
- Help students build healthy self-esteem.
- Help students understand the role of genetics in body type and shape.
- Help students make a connection between respecting diversity in shape and weight and respecting diversity in gender and race.
- Encourage students to be active and to appreciate the abilities of their bodies.
- Let students know that people are much more than their appearance.
- If you suspect a student has an eating disorder, talk with the student's family and encourage the student to seek professional help.

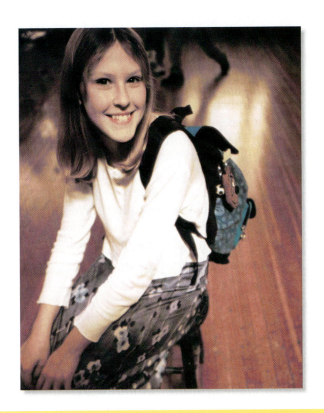

ACTIVITIES

Writing Activity
Poem

Have students fill in the blanks in the following poem template with positive words.

I am a _____ (boy/girl)

with _____, _____ hair (color) (texture)

that says I'm _____. (adjective)

I am a _____ (boy/girl)

with _____, _____ eyes (color) (adjective)

that say I'm _____. (adjective)

I am a _____ with _____, (boy/girl) (adjective)

_____ arms that (adjective)

can _____ and (verb)

_____. (verb)

I am a _____ with _____, (boy/girl) (adjective)

_____ legs that (adjective)

can _____ and (verb)

_____. (verb)

I am a _____ with a heart that (boy/girl)

sings _____ (words from a song)

and a mind that can _____, (verb)

_____ and _____. (verb) (verb)

I am _____, _____ (adjective) (adjective)

and_____. (adjective)

Ask for volunteers to share their poems.

Writing Activity
TV Types

For homework, ask students to watch TV for 30 minutes and to make a chart or table describing the types of bodies they see. Students may chart this information for a single show, including commercials, or they may choose to flip through the channels and chart this information for a number of shows. Ask students to note patterns. (Sample answer: Most of the women and men are tall. Many of the women are very thin. I saw very few Asian American people on TV.) Ask students to write answers to the following questions: "Do you compare yourself with the people you see on TV? How did you respond when you noticed the characteristics of the people on the shows? Why? Do the people in your life—your parents, neighbors, and teachers—look like the people on TV? What are some similarities and differences? What did this exercise teach you about media body images?"

Decisions for Health • Teaching Sensitive Issues

Cultural Tension and Stereotyping

Introduction

Many people suffer mistreatment because of assumptions made about them as individuals based on their race, ethnicity, beliefs, or associations. Some of these tensions are exacerbated by widely held, pervasive, and negative stereotypes. People who are not part of a mainstream culture because of race, language, ethnicity, or religious differences often feel marginalized. Often they do not see themselves represented well in the media, in historical reports, or in positions of authority.

Discussing race and identity in the United States is complicated. For example, the national census conducted in the year 2000 counted over 280 million Americans. Many respondents identified with 1 of 16 racial categories provided. And over 15 million people chose the category "some other race." More than 6 million people described themselves as belonging to two or more races. The United States is a diverse country. Helping students understand the strengths of that diversity can help them develop their social health.

Teen Concerns

- Schools provide the opportunity for young people to encounter people who are unlike them, and in the future, schools in the United States will be even more diverse. Students often share classes, sports teams, and extracurricular clubs with people of different ethnicities, cultures, and religions. Thus, they are in a good position to learn about the various populations that make up the United States.

- With guidance, intolerant students can learn to overcome feelings of fear and mistrust of people they perceive to be different. If a teacher creates a classroom environment that promotes tolerance, students can begin to listen to and respect each other, establish friendships, and build tolerant communities.

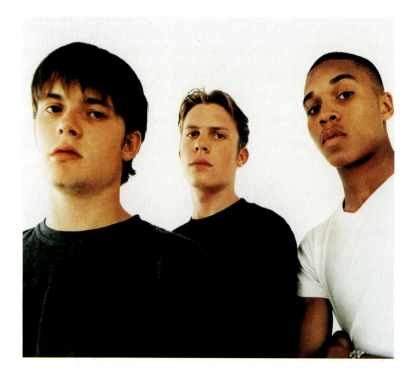

What You Can Do

- Treat all students with respect, and provide opportunities for all students to succeed in the classroom.
- Before you begin talking about issues of race and ethnicity, help students develop a list of ground rules phrased as "I" statements, such as "I will not use derogatory language" and "I will listen when someone is speaking." Post the list, and enforce these ground rules.
- Acknowledge that race and ethnicity are important components of identity to some people and that these components should be respected in all people.
- Routinely talk about issues of tolerance and fairness.
- Point out stereotypes in the print and electronic media when they arise in class.

- Point out that some stereotypes are based on gender, age, and interests.
- Point out that stereotypes that seem to promote positive behavior or values can be problematic. For example, if someone claims that all people of a group are good at math or are great musicians, individuals in that group are not being judged as individuals who have their own ideas, talents, and preferences.
- Be aware of how race and ethnicity affect the students in your class, but do not single out any student, especially if that student is the only individual of a particular race or ethnicity. Do not assume any one person can or will represent the views of all people of that ethnicity.
- Provide students with the opportunity to talk to each other about a variety of topics not specific to race or ethnicity. Students from different ethnic or racial groups may share similar values, lifestyles, and experiences. Discovering common characteristics helps promote tolerance.
- If you encounter a situation involving race or ethnicity that you feel unqualified to address effectively, refer the problem to a colleague who is qualified.

ACTIVITIES

Writing Activity
Stereotypes

Tell students to write about a time they were stereotyped, they stereotyped someone, they saw someone being stereotyped, or they felt different or out of place.

Instruct students to do the following:
1. Describe what happened.
2. Explain how you felt.
3. Explain what could have been done differently.

Encourage students to use descriptive language and dialogue.

Group Activity
Poster Project

Have students use discarded magazines to explore how advertisements target specific groups. Have students investigate how the ads use stereotypes to promote products. Encourage all students to empathize with the members of groups stereotyped in the ads. Students can create posters from ads they find in the magazines. Have students write on the posters comments about the stereotypes they see promoted in the ads.

Extension Activity
Identifying Stereotypes in Our Society

Challenge students to be conscious of the stereotypes they encounter daily. Ask them to keep a log of the stereotypes they see and hear. Students can get their data from school hallways, the bus, music, TV, and movies. After students have collected their data, ask, "How common were acts of stereotyping? Who tried to stop the stereotyping? What stops stereotyping? Do you respond to stereotyping differently now than before you began the lesson?"

Discussion
Harmful Stereotypes

Ask the class to come up with a class definition of *stereotype,* and write the definition on the board. (Sample answers: the belief that all people from a certain race or ethnicity are the same; to think something bad about someone because of his or her race or ethnicity; to judge someone by the way he or she looks before you get to know him or her.) Ask students why stereotypes are harmful. (Sample answer: Many stereotypes are based on incorrect assumptions. And people are individuals who should not be judged by how other people behave.)

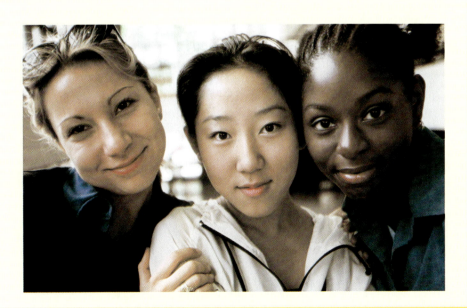

Decisions for Health • Teaching Sensitive Issues

Sexuality

Introduction

We express our sexuality through our actions, mannerisms, dress, speech, and feelings toward other people. Sexuality can involve feelings about one's body, desire for physical closeness to others, and a desire for emotional intimacy. In other words, sexuality includes everything that makes a person a sexual being. *Sexual harassment* is any unwanted remark, behavior, or touch that has sexual content. Both males and females can be victims of sexual harassment. Sexual harassment is always wrong.

Sexual identity refers to an individual's predominant attraction toward other people. People who have sexual desire for people of the opposite gender are called *heterosexual*. (A slang term for *heterosexual* is *straight*.) People who have sexual desire for people of either gender are called *bisexual*. People who have sexual desire for people of their own gender are called *homosexual*. (Another term for *homosexual* is *gay*.) Homosexual women are also called *lesbians*. Surveys indicate that 3 to 10 percent of the population is gay. No one knows for sure why some people are straight, some are bisexual, and others are gay.

Teen Concerns

- Teens may associate sexuality with sexual activity or other forms of physical intimacy. Teens are surrounded by media images that encourage specific physical expressions of male and female sexual behavior. Some of the behaviors are risky. These media images can create unreasonable or even dangerous expectations about how teens should or should not express their sexuality. Sexual expression in real life is subtle and complicated. Teen sexuality involves all of the expressions of how teens sense themselves as males and females and all of the human attractions they feel. Teen sexuality is not limited to physical appearance or expression. For example, teens may express their sexuality through bravado, athletic prowess, humor, maturity, or daring.
- Media messages aimed at teens frequently equate sexual activity with love, and teens easily confuse sexual activity with intimacy. Teens will sometimes bypass the stage of getting to know someone and assume that love will naturally follow if they become sexually involved. So, both boys and girls need to be given the tools to deal respectfully with their sexuality and feelings of attraction. Teens need to be reminded that expressing sexuality requires healthy respect for themselves and others, that responsible actions need to be in line with their values, and that actions have consequences. Teens also need careful guidance in understanding that they are valuable as people and are not mere objects to be decorated, displayed, and coveted.

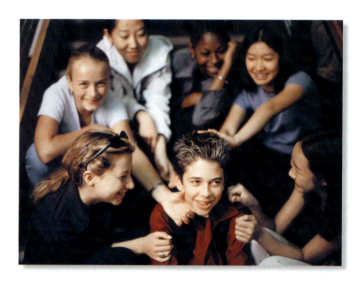

What You Can Do

- Be aware of your school's policies and guidelines about discussing sex and sexuality with students. Follow these policies and guidelines.
- Tell students that sexuality is part of being alive. During adolescence, the way that teens express themselves may change, and desires for sexual activity can become stronger.
- Tell students that they should always be themselves. Tell them not to pretend to be someone they are not. Being themselves helps teens develop relationships with people who like them and respect them for who they really are.
- Remind students that sexual activity is not a game. Sex involves the risk of being hurt—or hurting someone else—physically and emotionally.
- Remind students that sexual abstinence is the only sure way to protect themselves from the risks of sexual activity, including pregnancy and infection by sexually transmitted diseases.

- Remind students that they can say no to sexual activity even if they have already been sexually active.
- Explain to students some healthy ways that young teens can show each other affection. Examples include spending time together, helping each other with projects, complimenting each other, and holding hands.
- Help students learn about healthy relationships, and encourage relationships based on respect, trust, honesty, fairness, equality, responsibility, and good communication. People in healthy relationships care enough about each other to protect each other from unintended pregnancy and sexually transmitted infections. They never use pressure, guilt, or force to have sex.
- Help students understand that sexuality develops at its own pace. Tell students that it is OK if they are not attracted to either boys or girls.
- Help teens understand the need to always insist that other people respect them.
- If you discuss the issue of homosexuality in class, discuss it respectfully. Be aware that someone in your class may be homosexual or related to someone who is homosexual, or have a friend who is homosexual.
- Remind students that sexual harassment is always wrong. Students who are harassed by their peers because of their sexual identity may develop feelings of isolation. Students who feel isolated may be at great risk for engaging in high-risk behaviors.
- Help students understand that sexual intimacy will not guarantee that their partner will be committed to them.
- Help students understand that some people whom they find attractive will not find them attractive in return. If a person gives attention to someone who asks him or her to stop, the person giving the attention should stop immediately. Giving unwanted attention is harassment.

ACTIVITIES

Writing Activity
Attraction

Propose the following scenario: "Paul likes to show off in front of Emily. He especially likes her smile and her laugh. When Emily is around, Paul tells jokes loudly to try to make her laugh more. Emily likes Paul, too. She likes the way he cares for his cat, Elmo, which has a broken leg. But she doesn't think Paul's jokes are very funny." Then ask students, "What are some of the ways Paul and Emily are attracted to each other?" (Sample answer: He likes her laugh. She likes his caring.) "Does Paul know what Emily finds attractive about him?" (no) "If Paul and Emily could talk about what they find attractive in each other, what do you think they would say?" (Sample answer: Emily might say that she likes Paul because he is caring and that he doesn't need to try to make her laugh so much. Paul might say that he likes Emily and tells the jokes only because he likes to hear her laugh.) Remind students that all of the things Paul and Emily find attractive in each other are expressions of their sexuality. They cannot control what the other person finds attractive.

Group Activity
Role-Playing

Have interested students role-play the following scenarios:
- Brenda would like Neil to stop following her and putting notes in her locker.
- Kevin would like Monica to stop following him and putting notes in his locker.
- John keeps sending Katie love letters. Katie's friend, Ann, knows and is bothered that John is harassing Katie.
- Cody doesn't play tennis but really likes Lucy, who is good at tennis.

Have students discuss the scenarios and identify healthy and unhealthy behaviors.

Discussion
Sex

If appropriate for your class, ask students, "What are some reasons teens have sex?" Write student responses on the board. (Sample answers: they think they are in love, loneliness, curiosity, peer pressure, to feel close with someone, to get or keep a boyfriend or girlfriend, boredom, rebellion, to get experience, they are drunk or on drugs and so have impaired judgment) Then ask, "What can happen when two people have sex for different reasons?" (Sample answers: If one person is having sex out of curiosity and another is doing it because he or she feels in love with the other person, the person in love may feel used. If one person wants to feel close to someone and the other person is curious, the one wanting to feel close may get his or her feelings hurt.) Refer to the list on the board. Ask students, "Which of these reasons are inappropriate reasons for having sex? Why?"

Decisions for Health • Teaching Sensitive Issues

Pregnancy

Introduction

The decision for teens to engage in sexual activity is based on many variables. These variables may include curiosity, peer pressure—especially if teens think everybody else is having sex, a desire for affection, physical desire, a desire to feel close to someone, revenge, an inability to refuse, a desire for acceptance, to please a boyfriend or girlfriend, or a belief that engaging in sexual intercourse proves one's independence or adulthood. Some teens have sexual intercourse against their better judgment. Some have sex under the influence of alcohol or other drugs. Few young people fully understand the emotional ramifications of having sex or the possible physical consequences of having sex. Many teens do not realize that having vaginal intercourse, even once and for the first time, can cause pregnancy.

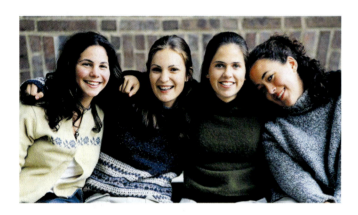

Teen Concerns

- Four out of 10 girls in the United States become pregnant at least once by age 20.
- One million teenage girls get pregnant every year in the United States.
- Teens are vulnerable to fleeting feelings of affection and peer pressure. During this time of experimentation, many teenagers make short-term decisions that have long-term consequences.
- Many girls today have rapidly maturing bodies. By the time they reach middle school, many girls have bodies that have already reached physical maturity. These girls may receive attention from boys or men who are much older than they are. This attention may seem flattering, but it can also be confusing and extremely dangerous. An older boy or man may try to take advantage of teen girls.
- The idea of having a baby can seem very romantic to some teens. Some mistakenly think that having a baby will bring them closer to their partner. For a young person who does not receive sufficient love and attention, having a baby can seem like a way to have someone to love and someone who can provide love.

Facts About Pregnancy

Know the facts about pregnancy, and share these facts with your students. For example, a female can get pregnant

- during her first sexual experience
- when she is having her period
- if she does not have an orgasm
- if she rarely has vaginal intercourse
- if she urinates, showers, or douches right after having vaginal intercourse
- if the male pulls his penis out of her vagina before he ejaculates
- if she has not had her first period
- if she is not yet a teenager

Pregnancy can be dangerous for teens. For example, the teen mother's pelvis may not be large enough for a full-grown fetus to pass through. Many teens have babies who have a low birth weight, which is a risk to the baby's health and well-being.

What You Can Do

- Be aware of your district's policies about advising students who are pregnant or have other medical problems. Follow those policies.
- Have a school nurse, counselor, or other adult witness discussions about sexuality or pregnancy.
- Emphasize that abstinence is the only sure way to avoid pregnancy.
- Be aware that you may have a student in your class who is a parent, knows a teen parent, or was born to a teen parent. Discuss teen pregnancy respectfully and carefully.
- Talk to students about the responsibility and consequences of having sex. Make sure that both boys

Decisions for Health • Teaching Sensitive Issues

and girls understand the emotional and physical ramifications.

- Understand the reasons that young people may want to have sex. Help students identify more-appropriate behavior for teens.
- Emphasize that even though intimate relationships between young teens and older people may be enticing and flattering, these relationships are often physically and emotionally risky.
- If a pregnant teen wants to talk, listen carefully and without judging. Assure the teen that you care and that you want her to be safe and healthy.
- Encourage students who are concerned about pregnancy to talk with their families and trusted community members. Provide students with names and contact information for district-approved community resources from which they can obtain more help.

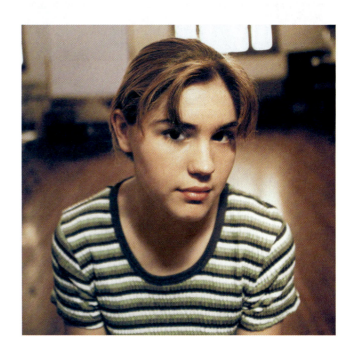

ACTIVITIES

Discussion
Parental Responsibilities
Ask students, "What are some responsibilities that parents have for babies?" (Sample answers: changing diapers, feeding and bathing the baby and buying food and clothes) Write student responses on the board. Ask students, "On average, how much does it cost to support a child for the first year of life?" Have each student write his or her estimate on a small piece of paper. (Sample answer: On average, it costs families $8,400 to $9,600 to support a child in the first year of life.) Discuss the difficulty of attending school and earning enough money to support a family.

Group Activity
Poster Project
Instruct students to create a collage that uses words and images to express their understanding of positive, healthy relationships and appropriate nonsexual expressions of love and care. (Images may include pictures of two people holding hands, looking at each other affectionately, playing together, doing chores, eating together, and raising a family together. Words may express support, understanding, compassion, hugging, laughing, honesty, and trust.) Students may draw these images or cut them out of magazines. Ask students to write about why they included certain images and words, paste their reasons to the back of their collages, and display the collages around the classroom.

Writing Activity
Interview
Instruct students to think of five open-ended interview questions to ask parents. Next, ask students to interview a parent whom they know. The parent should not be one of their own parents. (Sample questions: What was the hardest part about raising your child? How did your life change once you had a child? As a parent, what do you wish you had done differently? What qualities do you think a person has to have to be a good parent? What challenges did you face by having a child at the age you were?) Ask the students to use the answers to their interview questions and information from class discussion to write a reflective essay in response to the question "What does it take to raise a child?" (Sample answer: It takes patience, love, and a stable home to raise a child. Parents have to be thoughtful, organized, and prepared to give up a lot of things that many teens take for granted, such as free time.)

Extension Activity
Time Spent Parenting
Have students explore the following questions: "On average, how much time does a parent spend changing diapers? On average, how many hours a night does a new mother sleep? On average, how many pounds of supplies and equipment must a mother carry when taking an infant to the doctor, grocery store, or home of another family member?" Have students write their thoughts on these questions in their notebook or journal. Let them know that you do not have exact answers to the questions but that being aware of the various parenting responsibilities is important.

Decisions for Health • Teaching Sensitive Issues

Sexually Transmitted Diseases

Introduction

Sexually transmitted diseases (STDs) are diseases or infections passed from one person to another during sexual contact. The most dangerous STD is HIV (human immunodeficiency virus), which often leads to AIDS (acquired immune deficiency syndrome). While medications to manage HIV are available, AIDS is fatal. HIV is most often transmitted through vaginal, anal, or oral sexual contact or through shared needles, but it can also be passed from mother to child during pregnancy, birth, or breast-feeding. Symptoms of AIDS include chronic fatigue, fever, chills or night sweats, unexplained weight loss more than 10 pounds, swollen lymph glands, purple blotches on the skin, constant diarrhea, persistent white spots in the mouth, dry cough, and shortness of breath. A blood test to detect the antibody to HIV is the most accurate way to know if one is infected.

Hepatitis B is a virus transmitted the same way that HIV is transmitted. However, hepatitis B is easier to get than HIV because hepatitis B can also be passed through shared toothbrushes, razors, and similar objects. Symptoms of Hepatitis B include nausea, fever, loss of appetite, dark urine, abdominal pain, and yellow eyes and skin. No cure for Hepatitis B exists. But symptoms can be treated, and a vaccine is available. Hepatitis B can cause serious liver damage and can lead to death.

Some STDs are caused by bacteria. These diseases include chlamydia, gonorrhea, and syphilis. These infections can be treated with antibiotics, but if left untreated, they may cause permanent harm, and death.

Pubic lice, also called *crabs,* are parasites that live in the pubic hair. Scabies are mites that burrow under the skin, most often in the genital area. Pubic lice and scabies can be passed through sexual contact, through close physical contact with another person, and by sharing towels, clothing, and bedding with an infected person. The main symptom of pubic lice and scabies is severe itching. Both can be treated by using prescribed lotions or shampoos and by washing all clothing and bedding in hot water.

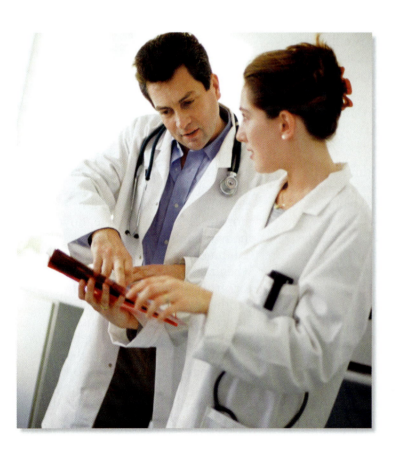

Teen Concerns

- An estimated 15 million new cases of STDs occur annually in the United States. Four million of these cases are among teens. About 25 percent of sexually active teens are infected with an STD every year. Half of new HIV infections occur in people under 25. AIDS is the sixth leading cause of death among people aged 15 to 24.
- In a 1998 survey, 82 percent of teens said they knew a lot or a fair amount about STDs, but 74 percent did not know that chlamydia is curable, and 54 percent did not know that herpes in not curable.
- Of sexually experienced teens in the 1998 survey, 67 percent did not perceive themselves to be at risk for contracting an STD even though 43 percent did not regularly use condoms, 70 percent had never gotten tested for STDs, 55 percent had not discussed STDs with any sexual partner, and 57 percent had never discussed STDs with a medical provider.

What You Can Do

- Encourage sexual abstinence among teens.
- Help teens understand that if they have sex just once with only one partner, they can be at risk for STD infection.
- Help teens realize that people may not always be truthful when discussing topics such as sex, the number of partners they have had, and any STDs they may have had. People infected with an STD may not have any symptoms and may not know they are infected.
- If a student approaches you with concern for his or her health, follow the guidelines of your school, district, and state. You may need to report the problem. You may wish to have another adult present to witness any conversations you have with a student about STDs.
- In a neutral, nonjudgmental way, create a dialog with the student to help determine risk. Find out what he or she might be doing that could put him or her at risk for contracting an STD.
- Help the student understand that he or she can take responsibility for being tested and changing high-risk behaviors.
- Offer options about what he or she might do or where he or she can get tested or get counseling. Encourage the student to choose a positive next step rather than telling him or her what to do.

ACTIVITIES

Writing Activity
Misconception Quiz

Have students indicate whether they think each of the following statements is true or false.

1. You can tell if a person has an STD just by looking at him or her.
2. All STDs can be cured.
3. Some STDs go undetected because infected people have no symptoms.
4. Drug and alcohol use and abuse can influence a person's risk behaviors.
5. There is no cure for HIV.

(1. false; 2. false; 3. true; 4. true; 5. true)

Discussion
STDs

After the quiz, allow students to ask questions and express opinions about some of the facts associated with STDs. Provide accurate information about STDs. Ask students, "How can a person protect himself or herself from contracting an STD?" (Sample answer: not having sexual intercourse) Inform students about the dangers of having sex. Point out that they may be more likely to be talked into having sex if they are intoxicated. In fact, some people don't even remember what they did while they were intoxicated. Make available to students local STD referral numbers that your district approves.

Extension Activity
101 Ways to Express Affection

Challenge your students to come up with a list of 101 healthy ways to express care and affection for another person. (Sample answers: by holding hands, hugging, writing a poem, giving a gift, making a meal, listening, laughing at his or her jokes, playing basketball together, and supporting him or her while he or she plays sports) Instruct students to choose 10 activities from their list and create an illustrated pamphlet. The pamphlet should include drawings and magazine photographs that depict the activity and should explain why the activity is an expression of caring and affection and how receiving or giving this expression of care and love feels. (The pamphlet may include the following: "When you listen to me, you show that you care about what I think and feel. When I know you care, I feel special and important.")

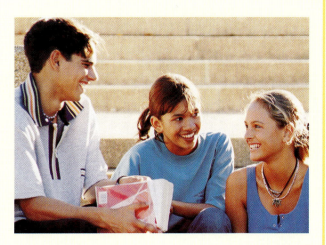

Gangs

Introduction

Most public schools in the United States are safe places for teaching and learning. But in many schools, serious problems with gangs disrupt teaching and learning, threaten the safety of students, and create an environment of fear. Gangs are organized groups of violent youths. Gangs have played a significant role in the increase in school violence over the past 3 decades.

If gangs and gang activity threaten students' safety in school, schools, communities, and families must cooperate to make students' environment safe. The presence of gangs on school property is not the school's fault, and the elimination of gangs is not solely the school's responsibility. The elimination of gangs is everybody's responsibility.

There are many theories to explain why youths join gangs. Some studies indicate that youths join gangs because they seek protection or because they feel coerced into doing so. Associating with known gang members, having gangs in the neighborhood, having a relative in a gang, failing in school, having a delinquency record, and abusing drugs all increase the likelihood that a teen will join a gang. A lack of access to resources, training, and education also seem to contribute to gang involvement. Gangs provide their members with material incentives, financial security, and physical protection, but they often do so illegally, dangerously, and at the expense of the autonomy of their members.

Teen Concerns
- The violence prevalent in society makes its way into the schools. If students feel unsafe and are not grounded in meaningful activities, they are at increased risk of joining gangs. Once joined, gangs are very difficult to leave.
- Statistics about gangs are never exact, but the following is information collected by the National Youth Gang Center's sixth annual Gang Survey, for the year 2000:
  - More than 24,500 gangs were active in the United States in 2000.
  - There were 772,500 active gang members in the United States in 2000.

The Characteristics of Gangs
- Gangs often develop along racial and ethnic lines.
- Gangs express their culture through unique colors, signs, clothes, language, and graffiti.
- Gangs stake out their own territory.
- Gangs operate as an organization.

What You Can Do
- Recognize why youths are drawn to gangs, identify what gangs offer to young people in your area, and create a thoughtful, comprehensive and community-based approach to gang prevention.
- Work with students to improve their academic performance, and instill positive attitudes about school.
- Assist students in finding meaningful activities, clubs, and interests.
- Integrate conflict resolution and peer mediation throughout the curriculum. Students need to be taught appropriate behavior for settling disputes.
- Become informed about the level and types of gang activity in your school district.
- Pay attention to your students. If you think a student is a member of a gang or may be tempted to join a gang, refer him or her to community personnel or to organizations that work specifically with gang issues.

- Communicate your concerns about specific students to school counselors, community agencies, and parents. All community members need to participate in the elimination of gangs.
- Listen to students involved with gangs, and gently encourage them to seek support to get out of gangs.
- Help students get into mentoring programs in which adults provide support, guidance, and assistance to youths, such as Big Brothers Big Sisters. It is best if the needs and interests of youths drive the mentoring relationship. Benefits of mentoring youths include increased focus, motivation, and positive attitudes; improved trust and communication with parents; enhanced learning skills; increased self-esteem and self-control; emotional support; decreased drug and alcohol use; and decreased absences from school.
- If a student engages in inappropriate behavior, follow your school's disciplinary policies.

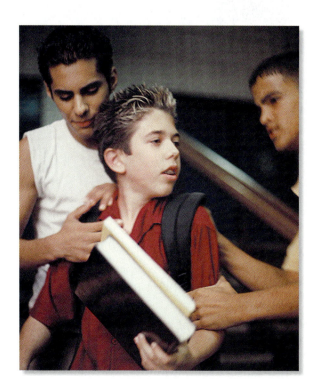

ACTIVITIES

Discussion
Analyzing Conflict

One of the attractions that some teens see in gangs is the perceived ability of gangs to protect them in conflicts. Working on conflict management skills can help teens see alternatives to gang involvement. Ask students, "What causes conflict between students?" (Sample answers: feeling disrespected, gossip, and misunderstandings) Write student responses on the board. Then ask, "What causes conflict between children and their parents?" (Sample answers: differing perspectives and miscommunication) Write student responses on the board. Instruct students to describe in writing a conflict they had with someone. Have students include how the conflict started, who said what to whom, how the conflict ended, how they felt, how they think the other person felt, and what could have been done differently. Ask volunteers to share what they have written.

Writing Activity
Perspective

Instruct students to write about a conflict they had, from the point of view of the other person in the conflict. Students should write in the first person. (Sample answers: I heard she was talking about me, so I went up to her. She was standing there with her friends, looking scared; I had another fight with my son. I wish he would just talk to me instead of always running out or hiding in his room.) Ask students how difficult it was to write about the situation from the other person's point of view. Ask students if doing this exercise helped them better understand the other person's perspective. Encourage students to try to understand another person's viewpoint when they encounter future conflicts.

Writing Activity
Keeping Safe

Ask students, "How can you be safe from gangs? What can you do if you come in contact with gang members who bother or threaten you?" (Sample answer: I can talk to a trusted adult as soon as possible, make sure that the adult knows that the threat is real and serious, and notify the police.)

Group Activity
Role-Play

Remind students that when someone offers them incentives to join a gang, those incentives have a price. Gangs are very dangerous. Remind students to use their refusal skills: avoid dangerous situations; say no; stick to the issue; remember your values; and walk away. Encourage students to use these skills if they are ever invited to participate in gang activity. Have students role-play using these refusal skills in the following scenario: "Someone offers money, drugs, clothing, jewelry, clothes, or power in exchange for your involvement in a gang."

Decisions for Health • Teaching Sensitive Issues

Domestic Violence

Introduction

Domestic violence is violence that occurs in the home, usually when one person tries to gain power and control over another person through physical, emotional, or sexual abuse.

Forms of abuse

- Physical abuse is physical mistreatment of another person that causes bodily harm. Physical abuse is also called *battering*.
- Emotional abuse is the repeated use of actions and words that imply a person is worthless or powerless.
- Verbal abuse is the use of hurtful words to intimidate, manipulate, hurt, or dominate another person.
- Sexual abuse is unwanted sexual activity with an adult or any sexual contact with a child.

Facts about Domestic Violence

- Battering is the most common violent crime in the United States and is a significant health problem.
- Domestic violence against women occurs once every 15 seconds.
- More than one-third of the women murdered every year are victims of domestic violence.
- Domestic violence caused the deaths of more than 1,200 women in 1999.

Batterers come from all social classes and ethnicities and from both genders. However, males commit 95 percent of the reported incidents of assaults in relationships, and 95 percent of the victims of battering are female.

People remain in abusive relationships for a variety of reasons, including fear, guilt, shame, economic reliance, loss of self-confidence, failure to recognize the behavior as abuse, confusion, a commitment to reforming the abuser, a belief that abuse is a sign of love or passion, a lack of a support system or a safe place to go, a belief that the children somehow benefit if the relationship is kept intact, and a lack of knowledge about legal rights.

A violent relationship often gets worse over time unless something changes. Specifically, the person who is violent needs to take active steps to become nonviolent or the victim needs to leave the relationship completely.

Teen Concerns

- It is estimated that between 3 million and 4 million children in the United States witness physical abuse of one parent by another each year.
- Approximately half of the men who assault their wives also abuse their children.
- Domestic violence is a learned behavior. Many children who have witnessed domestic violence in their homes have become involved in a violent relationship. Male children who witness a father beating a mother are 700 times more likely to abuse their adult female partner.
- Exposure to violence in the home can also result in diminished academic performance, substance abuse, teen pregnancy, and suicidal behavior.

Signs of Child Abuse

Know the signs of child abuse, and enforce child abuse-reporting policies in your school, district, and state. The following list describes some of the symptoms of children who suffer abuse or who frequently witness abuse. They may

- fear adults
- show physical evidence of abuse
- abuse alcohol or other drugs
- break things on purpose or by accident
- engage in aggressive behavior
- easily become angry
- be abnormally shy
- think or talk about killing themselves or others
- avoid going home (For example, victims may spend a lot of time at school helping others.)
- run away from home

What You Can Do

- Give students clear messages that violence is wrong and should never be tolerated.
- Give students clear messages that it is not OK for anyone to abuse them in any way.
- If a student tells you he or she is being abused, believe him or her and offer to help seek professional assistance.

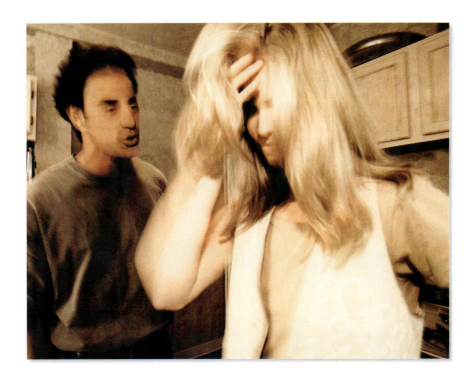

ACTIVITIES

Writing Activity
Misconception Quiz

Have students indicate which of the following statements are true and which are false.

1. Battering is the most common violent crime in the United States.
2. Domestic violence against women occurs once every 15 minutes in the United States.
3. A batterer can be from any place or social class.
4. A violent relationship will get worse over time unless the person who is violent takes active steps to change his or her behavior.
5. A person can easily leave a relationship in which there is domestic violence.
6. Domestic violence is a learned behavior.

(1. true; 2. false; 3. true; 4. true; 5. false; 6. true)

Discussion
Domestic Violence

Use the writing activity to initiate a class discussion. Provide the facts, where appropriate, for the false statements.

Stress that domestic violence is learned and that anyone living in a home where violence occurs is at much higher risk for later becoming involved in a violent relationship. Conclude the discussion by emphasizing that help is available for anyone in an abusive relationship, whether that person is an intimate partner of the abuser or a child of the abuser. Share with students the approved, local resource numbers that anyone can use to get help.

Discussion
Abuse

Explain to students the various types of abuse. Tell students that no one deserves to be abused and that abuse is always wrong. Ask students why children who are being abused at home may have difficulty seeking help. (Sample answer: Children love their parents, are afraid of retaliation, and are afraid that their families will break up.) Explain that the best hope a child has to end the abuse is for an adult who cares about the child to step in and help stop the abuse. Ask students to list those adults who might be able to help. (Sample answers: other adult family members, neighbors, coaches, teachers, activity leaders, and the parents of friends) Ask students what these adults have in common. (Sample answer: They care about the children and are in a position to help.) Explain that after these trusted adults know about the problem they can help stop the abuse. Ask how these adults might learn about the problem. (Sample answer: An abused child could tell them.) Ask how a victim of abuse might start a difficult conversation about his or her abuse. (Sample answer: The victim could say to a trusted adult, "I need to talk to someone." Most adults can help guide the conversation from there.)

Decisions for Health • Teaching Sensitive Issues

Dating Violence

Introduction

Dating violence is the physical, sexual, emotional, or verbal abuse of one partner by the other in a dating relationship. Unfortunately, dating violence is very common. Either gender can suffer abuse in a relationship, but females are more likely than males to be the victims of violence in a relationship. Dating violence can be very damaging and even deadly.

Dating violence often occurs in cycles. The abuse often gets worse with each cycle. The first stage of the cycle is when one person demoralizes and begins controlling another person. The second stage is characterized by an increase in tension. This stage can last minutes, months, or years. Things feel very strained for the victim suffering the abuse. The victim may think that he or she must do everything perfectly and fears what might happen if he or she does not. The third stage is the explosion. Often, this stage is the most dramatic and visible one of the abuse cycle. The fourth stage is called *the honeymoon* and is the stage in which the abuser realizes the relationship is in danger and is nice to the victim. The abuser becomes apologetic and promises that the violence will never happen again. The abuser may give gifts to the victim. Or the abuser may blame the abuse on the victim. Because the victim's self-esteem is low, he or she often believes the abuser, which leads the couple back to the tension-building stage.

Date or acquaintance rape is sexual activity by force or threat by someone known to the victim. Rape is a physical assault, but it also challenges people's basic beliefs in their own safety and the predictability of their environment, their trust and mutual respect in relationships, and their self-confidence and autonomy or control. Many rape victims struggle with feelings of personal responsibility or self-blame. Self-blame can stem from a need to find a reason for the assault. Finding a reason is a way to try to regain control. As a victim tries to make sense of a rape, helping the victim see that the rapist is at fault is important.

Teen Concerns

- Dating is a new experience for teens, so they need to learn what is normal and healthy in a dating relationship. Because of a lack of experience or lack of healthy role models, many teens who experience dating violence are not aware their relationships are unhealthy. Without positive role models, teens may not realize it is not permissible for a boyfriend or girlfriend to hurt them, try to hurt them, force them to have sex, threaten them, harass them, stalk them, or destroy things that belong to them.
- Approximately one out of every 10 teenagers experiences physical violence in a dating relationship. Approximately 70 to 90 percent of rapes are by an acquaintance. The majority of victims are aged 16 to 24. Teen relationship abuse puts young people at risk for adult relationship abuse. Many teens are vulnerable. Teens who do not feel close to their parents or other adults may look to a dating relationship—even an unhealthy one—to meet their needs for closeness and intimacy. They may think that they need to handle a violent relationship themselves to appear mature.

Signs of an Abusive Relationship

Help students understand the signs of an abusive relationship. These signs include a boyfriend or girlfriend who

- hits, pushes, or slaps
- becomes jealous or possessive
- intimidates
- pressures the partner to be sexually active
- abuses alcohol or other drugs
- touches in ways that the partner does not like
- likes to play-fight in ways that are upsetting
- calls the partner disrespectful names or puts him or her down
- does not care how the partner feels or what he or she thinks
- blames the partner for problems the partner does not control
- tries to control the partner
- tries to keep the partner away from friends and family

Signs of a Teen at Risk
Be aware of signs that indicate a teen may be in a violent relationship. These signs include the following:
- bruises or other signs of physical injury or damaged property
- a boyfriend or girlfriend who is extremely possessive
- secretive behavior or evidence of shame, hostility, or isolation

What You Can Do
- Tell teens that dating abuse and violence is wrong.
- Tell teens that *no* means "no." And even if a partner has voluntarily participated in some amount of sexual activity before, he or she can always refuse to participate in sexual activity.
- Tell students that harassment and sexual harassment are dangerous and always wrong. Harassment can also lead to violence. Tell students that if anyone harasses them or anyone they know in order to begin, continue, or renew an unwanted or unhealthy relationship, the students should use assertive behavior and their refusal skills to end the harassment. Tell the students that if the harassment continues after they have tried to end it, they should tell a trusted adult as soon as possible.
- Teach your students about gender roles and stereotypes. Help students see the stereotypes reinforced by many forms of children's play and entertainment. Help teens understand that referring to people of either gender by derogatory terms is unacceptable.
- Teach students how to build healthy, respectful relationships. Help them appreciate healthy family patterns in which people are supportive. Teach students that people in healthy relationships respect the expression of feelings and opinions; the freedom to question a partner and explore problems; time alone and with friends; individual beliefs and goals; and the right to one's own body.
- If students are in an abusive relationship, tell them to take the problem seriously, plan for their safety, and seek help. If anyone they know is being abused, students should encourage the person to talk about the abuse and to get help. They can remind the victim that without help, abuse usually doesn't go away, and in fact, usually gets worse.
- Tell students to communicate clearly and to let a partner know they will not tolerate any abuse.
- If you learn that someone has been physically or sexually assaulted, assist him or her in getting help. Adhere to the reporting policies in your district. Refer the person for emotional support and counseling, if possible.
- Let students know that abuse is never the victim's fault. Tell students to avoid, resolve, or end any relationship that causes fear or problems.
- Inquire about successful teen programs in your community including peer education, support groups, safety planning, and other services.
- Be prepared to handle a situation in which a student says, "I would like to tell you something, but you cannot tell anyone else." You cannot make that promise. Make sure students know what you must report and to whom you must report it.

Tips for Avoiding Dating Violence
Tell teens the following tips for avoiding dating violence:
- Make sure your parents or guardians know where you are going and who will be with you.
- Always have a way to get home.
- Carry enough change to use a pay phone.
- Know your limits or boundaries before a situation arises and communicate those limits clearly.
- Avoid being alone with a new aquaintance.
- Never put another's feelings ahead of your own safety.
- Avoid alcohol and other drugs.
- Trust your instincts about any concerns you may have about a potential date.
- Get to know the person before going out alone with that person or go out in a group.
- Never allow another person to control you, which includes not allowing anyone to tell you how to dress and who to have as friends.

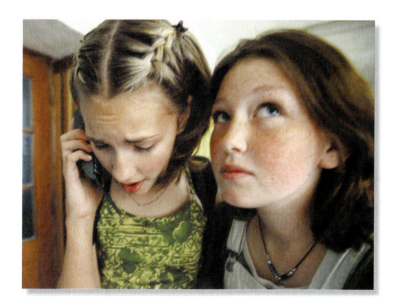

ACTIVITIES

Discussion
Dating Behaviors

- On the board, write "Appropriate Dating Behaviors," and write student responses under this heading. (Be clear that you are not asking about sexual activity, and offer examples of the behaviors you are studying. Students should offer examples acceptable for a classroom discussion.) (Sample answers: I want my boyfriend to hold my hand. I want my date to tell me that I am good at basketball, bowling, or dancing. I want my date to laugh at my jokes. I want my boyfriend to listen to me when I talk. I want my girlfriend to ask questions when I tell her something. I want my date to be happy.) If students offer responses that are inappropriate, tell them that their responses will be listed elsewhere on the board. After completing the next activity, you and the class will decide whether to put that behavior on the "appropriate" or "inappropriate" list.

- On the board, write "Inappropriate Dating Behaviors," and write student responses under this heading. (Sample answers: I don't want my date to tell me I look bad. I don't want my date to try to make me go somewhere I don't want to go. I don't want my boyfriend to demand to know where I have been and with whom I was talking. I don't want my girlfriend to tell me whom I should be friends with. I don't want my boyfriend to try to make me do something I don't want to do. I don't want my date to try to make me do something that would break my parents' rules. I don't want to do anything that I'd find embarrassing.)

- Explain to students that when they are on a date, they never have to do anything that they don't want to do. Stress that if a student feels uncomfortable or unsafe he or she has the responsibility to express his or her concerns or end the date or relationship.

Group Activity
Role-Playing

Ask for three pairs of students to volunteer to role-play appropriate and inappropriate dating behaviors in front of the class.

- **Pair 1** Have one student demonstrate two inappropriate dating behaviors, and have the other student not resist or express concern. Ask the class, "How do you think the victim of the inappropriate behavior felt? Why didn't he or she express concern or leave? What could the victim have done to make himself or herself more comfortable or safe in that situation?"

- **Pair 2** Have one student demonstrate two inappropriate dating behaviors, and have the other student voice concern, resist, or leave. Ask the class, "What did the victim of the inappropriate dating behavior do well? Why do you think the victim acted like that? Do you think he or she should go out with this person again?"

- **Pair 3** Have both students demonstrate two appropriate dating behaviors. Ask the class, "How do you think the two people on this date felt? Should they go out with each other again?"

Explain to students that they have the right to be treated well, that real affection is respectful, and that no one has the right to force them to do something unwelcome or unsafe. Stress that they should practice strategies for expressing their concern and removing themselves from uncomfortable or unsafe dating situations.

Conclude the lesson by letting students know that violence is never appropriate in relationships.

Photo Credits for Teaching Sensitive Issues

T33, Digital Image copyright © 2004 Artville; T34 (tl), Digital Image copyright © 2004 PhotoDisc, Inc.; (br), Digital Image copyright © 2004 Artville; T35, T36, Digital Image copyright © 2004 Artville; T37 (tl), Digital Image copyright © 2004 Artville; (br), CORBIS Images/HRW; T38, T39, Digital Image copyright © 2004 Artville; T40, CORBIS Images/HRW; T41, © Digital Vision; T42, T45, T46, Digital Image copyright © 2004 Artville; T48, Digital Image copyright © 2004 PhotoDisc, Inc.; T49, Digital Image copyright © 2004 Artville; T50, © Digital Vision; T51, T52, Digital Image copyright © 2004 Artville; T54, CORBIS Images/HRW; T55, Digital Image copyright © 2004 Artville; T56, © Brand X Pictures; T57, © Digital Vision; T58, John Langford/HRW; T59, Digital Image copyright © 2004 Artville; T61, CORBIS Images/HRW; T63, Digital Image copyright © 2004 Artville.

HOLT
Decisions for Health

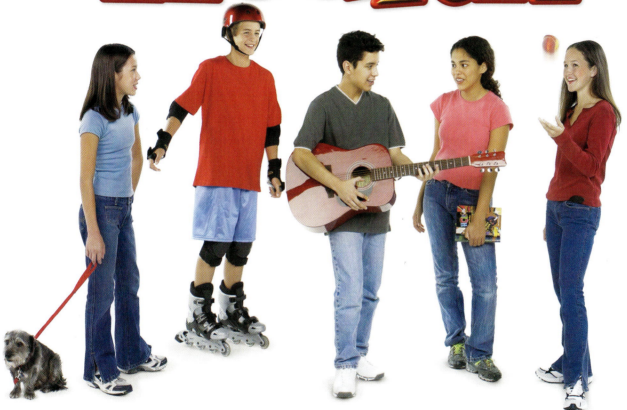

Teacher Edition

HOLT, RINEHART AND WINSTON
A Harcourt Education Company

Orlando • **Austin** • New York • San Diego • Toronto • London

Acknowledgments

Contributing Authors

Katy Z. Allen
Science Writer and Former Science Teacher
Wayland, Massachusetts

Balu H. Athreya, M.D.
Staff Physician
Alfred I. duPont Hospital for Children
Wilmington, Delaware

Kate Cronan, M.D.
Chief, Division of Emergency Medicine
Alfred I. duPont Hospital for Children
Wilmington, Delaware

Sharon Deutschlander
Department of Health and Physical Education
Indiana University of Pennsylvania
Indiana, Pennsylvania

Efrain Garza Fuentes, Ed.D.
Director, Patient and Family Services
Childrens Hospital Los Angeles
Los Angeles, California

Keith S. García, M.D., Ph.D.
Instructor of Psychiatry
Washington University School of Medicine
St. Louis, Missouri

Patricia J. Harned, Ph.D.
Director of Character Development and Research
Ethics Resource Center
Washington, D.C.

Craig P. Henderson, LCSW, MDIV
Therapist
Youth Services of Tulsa
Tulsa, Oklahoma
Trainer
National Resource Center for Youth Services
Norman, Oklahoma

Jack E. Henningfield, Ph.D.
Associate Professor of Behavioral Biology
The Johns Hopkins University School of Medicine
Baltimore, Maryland

Peter Katona, M.D., FACP
Associate Professor of Clinical Medicine, Infectious Disease Division, Department of Medicine
UCLA School of Medicine
Los Angeles, California

Linda Klingaman, Ph.D.
Professor
Indiana University of Pennsylvania
Indiana, Pennsylvania

Joe S. McIlhaney, Jr., M.D.
President
The Medical Institute for Sexual Health
Austin, Texas

Kweethai Chin Neill, Ph.D., C.H.E.S., FASHA
Assistant Professor, Department of Kinesiology, Health Promotion, and Recreation
University of North Texas
Denton, Texas

Christine Rose, M.S.
Project Director, Innovators Combating Substance Abuse
Robert Wood Johnson Foundation
Pinney Associates
Bethesda, Maryland

Stephen E. Stork, Ed.D., C.H.E.S.
Assistant Professor
Department of Kinesiology, Health Promotion, and Recreation
University of North Texas
Denton, Texas

Richard Yoast, Ph.D.
Director, American Medical Association Office of Alcohol and Other Drug Abuse
Director, Robert Wood Johnson Foundation National Alcohol Program Offices
American Medical Association
Chicago, Illinois

Copyright © 2004 by Holt, Rinehart and Winston

All rights reserved. No part of this publication may be reproduced or transmitted in any form or by any means, electronic or mechanical, including photocopy, recording, or any information storage and retrieval system, without permission in writing from the publisher.

Requests for permission to make copies of any part of the work should be mailed to the following address: Permissions Department, Holt, Rinehart and Winston, 10801 N. MoPac Expressway, Building 3, Austin, Texas 78759.

ONE-STOP PLANNER is a trademark licensed to Holt, Rinehart and Winston, registered in the United States of America and/or other jurisdictions.

CNN and CNN Student News are trademarks of Cable News Network LP, LLLP. An AOL Time Warner Company.

HealthLinks is a service mark owned and provided by the National Science Teachers Association. All rights reserved.

Current Health is a registered trademark of Weekly Reader Corporation.

ExamView is a registered trademark of FSCreations, Inc.

Printed in the United States of America

ISBN 0-03-066816-6

1 2 3 4 5 6 7 048 08 07 06 05 04 03

Contributing Writers

Presentation Series Development

Carol Badran, M.P.H.
Health Educator
San Francisco Department
  of Public Health
San Francisco, California

Pirette McKamey
Teacher
Thurgood Marshall Academic
  High School
San Francisco, California

Inclusion Specialists

Ellen McPeek Glisan
Special Needs Consultant
San Antonio, Texas

Joan A. Solorio
Special Education Director
Austin Independent
  School District
Austin, Texas

Feature Development

Katy Z. Allen
Wayland, Massachusetts

Angela Berenstein
Princeton, New Jersey

Marilyn S. Chakroff
Christiansted, Virgin Islands

Mickey Coakley
Pennington, New Jersey

Allen Cobb
La Grange, Texas

Theresa Flynn-Nason
Voorhees, New Jersey

Chris Hess
Boise, Idaho

Charlotte W. Luongo
Austin, Texas

Eileen Nehme, M.P.H.
Austin, Texas

Clementina S. Randall
Quincy, Massachusetts

Answer Checking

Helen Schiller
Taylor, South Carolina

Medical Reviewers

David Ho, M.D.
Professor and Scientific Director
Aaron Diamond AIDS
  Research Center
The Rockefeller University
New York, New York

Ichiro Kawachi, Ph.D., M.D.
*Associate Professor of Health
  and Social Behavior*
School of Public Health
Harvard University
Boston, Massachusetts

Leland Lim, M.D., Ph.D.
Year II Resident
Department of Neurology
  and Neurological Sciences
Stanford University School
  of Medicine
Palo Alto, California

Iris F. Litt, M.D.
Professor
Department of Pediatrics
  and Adolescent Medicine
School of Biomedical
  and Biological Sciences
Stanford University
Palo Alto, California

Ronald Munson, M.D., F.A.A.S.P.
*Assistant Clinical Professor,
  Family Practice*
Health Sciences Center
The University of Texas
San Antonio, Texas

Alexander V. Prokhorov, M.D., Ph.D.
*Associate Professor of
  Behavioral Science*
M.D. Anderson Cancer Center
The University of Texas
Houston, Texas

Gregory A. Schmale, M.D.
Assistant Professor
Pediatrics and Adolescent
  Sports Medicine
University of Washington
Seattle, Washington

Hans Steiner, M.D.
*Professor of Psychiatry and
  Director of Training*
Division of Child Psychiatry
  and Child Development
Department of Psychiatry
  and Behavioral Sciences
Stanford University School
  of Medicine
Palo Alto, California

Professional Reviewers

Nancy Daley, Ph.D., L.P.C., C.P.M.
Psychologist
Austin, Texas

Linda Gaul, Ph.D.
Epidemiologist
Texas Department of Health
Austin, Texas

Linda Jones, M.S.P.H.
*Manager of Systems
  Development Unit*
Children with Special
  Healthcare Needs Division
Texas Department of Health
Austin, Texas

William Joy
President
The Joy Group
Wheaton, Illinois

Edie Leonard, R.D., L.D.
Nutrition Educator
Portland, Oregon

JoAnn Cope Powell, Ph.D.
*Learning Specialist
  and Licensed Psychologist*
Counseling, Learning and
  Career Services
University of Texas
  Learning Center
The University of Texas
Austin, Texas

Hal Resides
Safety Manager
Corpus Christi Naval Base
Corpus Christi, Texas

Professional Reviewers
(continued)

Eric Tiemann, E.M.T.
Emergency Medical Services
Hazardous Waste Division
Travis County Emergency
  Medical Services
Austin, Texas

Lynne E. Whitt
Director
National Center for Health
  Education
New York, New York

Academic Reviewers

Nigel Atkinson, Ph.D.
*Associate Professor of
  Neurobiology*
Institute For Neuroscience
Institute for Cellular and
  Molecular Biology
Waggoner Center for Alcohol
  and Addiction Research
The University of Texas
Austin, Texas

John Caprio, Ph.D.
George C. Kent Professor
Department of Biological
  Sciences
Louisiana State University
Baton Rouge, Louisiana

Joe Crim, Ph.D.
*Professor and Head, Biological
  Sciences Department*
University of Georgia
Athens, Georgia

Susan B. Dickey, Ph.D., R.N.
*Associate Professor, Pediatric
  Nursing*
College of Allied Health
  Professionals
Temple University
Philadelphia, Pennsylvania

Stephen Dion
Associate Professor
Sport Fitness
Salem College
Salem, Massachusetts

Ronald Feldman, Ph.D.
*Ruth Harris Ottman Centennial
  Professor for the
  Advancement
  of Social Work Education
Director, Center for the
  Study of Social Work Practice*
Columbia University
New York, New York

William Guggino, Ph.D.
Professor of Physiology
The Johns Hopkins University
  School of Medicine
Baltimore, Maryland

Kathryn Hilgenkamp, Ed.D., C.H.E.S.
*Assistant Professor, Community
  Health and Nutrition*
University of Northern
  Colorado
Greeley, Colorado

Cynthia Kuhn, Ph.D.
*Professor of Pharmacology and
  Cancer Biology*
Duke University Medical Center
Duke University
Durham, North Carolina

John B. Lowe, M.P.H., Dr. P.H., F.A.H.P.A.
Professor and Head
Department of Community and
  Behavioral Health
College of Public Health
The University of Iowa
Iowa City, Iowa

Leslie Mayrand, Ph.D., R.N., C.N.S.
Professor of Nursing
Pediatrics and Adolescent
  Medicine
Angelo State University
San Angelo, Texas

Karen E. McConnell, Ph.D.
Assistant Professor
School of Physical Education
Pacific Lutheran University
Tacoma, Washington

Clyde B. McCoy, Ph.D.
Professor and Chair
Department of Epidemiology
  and Public Health
University of Miami School of
  Medicine
Miami, Florida

Hal Pickett, Psy.D.
*Assistant Professor of
  Psychiatry*
Department of Psychiatry
University of Minnesota
  Medical School
Minneapolis, Minnesota

Philip Posner, Ph.D.
*Professor and Scholar in
  Physiology*
College of Medicine
Florida State University
Tallahassee, Florida

John Rohwer, Ph.D.
Professor
Department of Health Sciences
Bethel College
St. Paul, Minnesota

Susan R. Schmidt, Ph.D.
Postdoctoral Psychology Fellow
Center on Child Abuse and
  Neglect
The University of Oklahoma
  Health Sciences Center
Oklahoma City, Oklahoma

Stephen B. Springer, Ed.D., L.P.C., C.P.M.
*Director of Occupational
  Education*
Southwest Texas State
  University
San Marcos, Texas

Richard Storey, Ph.D.
Professor of Biology
Colorado College
Colorado Springs, Colorado

Acknowledgments continued on page 455.

Contents in Brief

Chapters

1	Health and Wellness	2
2	Successful Decisions and Goals	20
3	Building Self-Esteem	48
4	Physical Fitness	64
5	Nutrition and Your Health	92
6	A Healthy Body, a Healthy Weight	114
7	Mental and Emotional Health	132
8	Managing Stress	156
9	Encouraging Healthy Relationships	174
10	Conflict and Violence	196
11	Teens and Tobacco	218
12	Teens and Alcohol	244
13	Teens and Drugs	268
14	Infectious Diseases	298
15	Noninfectious Diseases and Disorders	320
16	Your Changing Body	346
17	Your Personal Safety	372

Contents

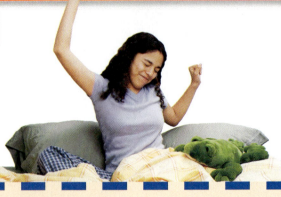

CHAPTER 1 — Health and Wellness 2

Lessons

1. **Being Healthy and Well** 4
   - Health Journal 5
   - Life Skills Activity: Making Good Decisions 6
2. **Influences on Your Health** 8
   - Myth and Fact 9
3. **Making Good Health Choices** 10
   - Life Skills Activity: Assessing Your Health 11
4. **Nine Life Skills for Better Health** 12
   - Hands-on Activity: Generic Versus Brand-Name Products 13
   - Cross-Discipline Activity: Language Arts 13
   - Life Skills Activity: Practicing Wellness 14

Chapter Review 16
Life Skills in Action: Setting Goals: Lonely Logan 18

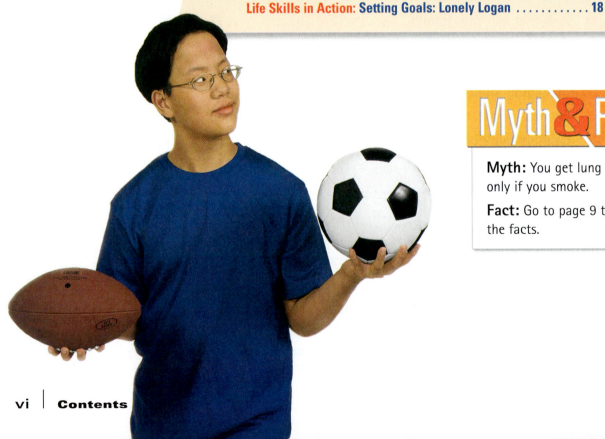

Myth & Fact

Myth: You get lung cancer only if you smoke.

Fact: Go to page 9 to get the facts.

CHAPTER 2 Successful Decisions and Goals 20

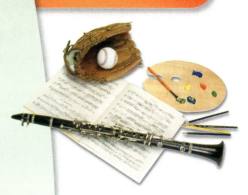

Lessons
1. Decisions and Consequences 22
2. Six Steps to Making Good Decisions 24
   - Health Journal 25
   - Life Skills Activity: Making Good Decisions 27
3. Influences on Your Decisions 28
   - Life Skills Activity: Being a Wise Consumer 30
4. Setting Healthy Goals 32
   - Health Journal 33
   - Cross-Discipline Activity: Social Studies 34
5. How to Reach Your Goals 36
6. Changing Your Goals 38
7. Skills for Success 40
   - Hands-on Activity: Listening Lab 41
   - Health Journal 42

Chapter Review 44

Life Skills in Action: Using Refusal Skills:
Reanna's Refusal 46

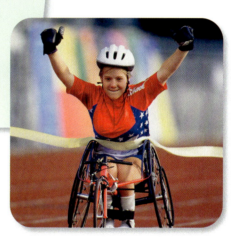

CHAPTER 3 Building Self-Esteem 48

Lessons
1. Self-Esteem and Your Life 50
   - Hands-on Activity: Self-Esteem Booster 52
   - Health Journal 53
2. Your Self-Concept 54
3. Keys to Healthy Self-Esteem 56
   - Cross-Discipline Activity: Language Arts 57
   - Life Skills Activity: Using Refusal Skills 58

Chapter Review 60

Life Skills in Action: Coping: The Big Test 62

Contents | vii

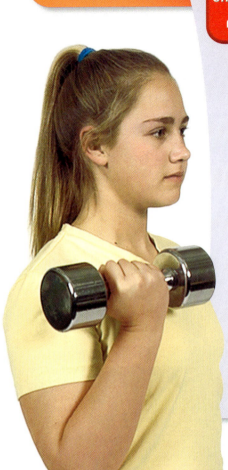

CHAPTER 4 Physical Fitness 64

Lessons
1 The Parts of Fitness 66
2 Your Fitness Program 68
    Life Skills Activity: Practicing Wellness 70
3 Energy for Exercise 72
    Health Journal 73
4 Sports and Competition 74
5 Weight Training 76
    Cross-Discipline Activity: Science 77
6 Injury 80
    Health Journal 80
7 Common Injuries 82
8 Eight Ways to Avoid Injury 84
    Life Skills Activity: Evaluating Media Messages 86

Chapter Review 88

Life Skills in Action: Assessing Your Health:
    Swim Team Tryouts 90

CHAPTER 5 Nutrition and Your Health 92

Lessons
1 Nutrition and Diet 94
    Life Skills Activity: Communicating Effectively 96
    Cross-Discipline Activity: Social Studies 96
    Health Journal 97
2 The Six Essential Nutrients 98
    Hands-on Activity: Brown Bag Test 100
3 Balancing Your Diet 102
4 Building Healthful Eating Habits 106
    Life Skills Activity: Practicing Wellness 107
    Life Skills Activity: Making Good Decisions 108
    Health Journal 109

Chapter Review 110

Life Skills in Action: Making Good Decisions:
    What's for Lunch? 112

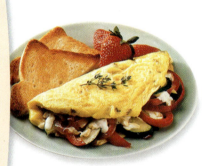

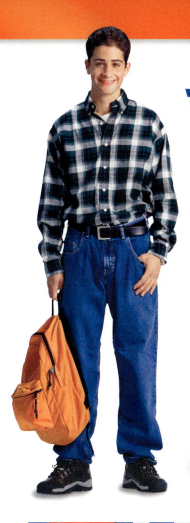

CHAPTER 6
A Healthy Body, a Healthy Weight 114

Lessons
1. **What Is Body Image?** 116
   - Health Journal 117
2. **Building a Healthy Body Image** 118
   - Life Skills Activity: Evaluating Media Messages 119
3. **Eating Disorders** 120
   - Life Skills Activity: Making Good Decisions 123
4. **Managing Your Weight** 124
   - Health Journal 126
   - Cross-Discipline Activity: Math 127

Chapter Review 128

Life Skills in Action: Practicing Wellness:
   The Junk Food Junkie 130

CHAPTER 7
Mental and Emotional Health 132

Lessons
1. **Kinds of Emotions** 134
   - Cross-Discipline Activity: Social Studies 135
2. **Expressing Emotions** 138
   - Life Skills Activity: Communicating Effectively 139
3. **Managing Your Emotions** 140
   - Life Skills Activity: Coping 141
   - Hands-on Activity: Using Positive Self-Talk 142
4. **Mental Illness** 144
5. **Getting Help** 148
   - Health Journal 149
   - Life Skills Activity: Making Good Decisions 151

Chapter Review 152

Life Skills in Action: Communicating Effectively:
   Sean's Sadness 154

Myth & Fact

Myth: A person can tell if he or she is going to like or dislike another person the first time they meet.

Fact: Go to page 136 to get the facts.

Contents | ix

CHAPTER 8 Managing Stress 156

Lessons

1 **Stress Is Only Natural** 158
   - Life Skills Activity: Assessing Your Health 160
   - Health Journal 161
2 **The Effects of Stress** 162
   - Cross-Discipline Activity: Science 163
3 **Defense Mechanisms** 164
   - Hands-on Activity: Stressors 165
4 **Managing Distress** 166
   - Hands-on Activity: Stress Management 167
   - Life Skills Activity: Coping 168

Chapter Review 170

Life Skills in Action: Setting Goals:
   The Procrastinator 172

Myth & Fact

Myth: All stress is bad.
Fact: Go to page 159 to get the facts.

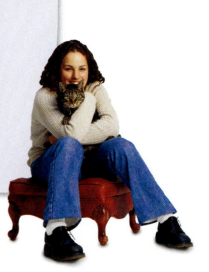

CHAPTER 9 Encouraging Healthy Relationships 174

Lessons

1 **Building Relationships** 176
   - Cross-Discipline Activity: Language Arts 178
2 **Family Relationships** 180
   - Life Skills Activity: Coping 182
   - Health Journal 183
3 **Healthy Communities** 184
4 **Building Friendships** 186
   - Life Skills Activity: Making Good Decisions 187
   - Health Journal 188
5 **Practicing Abstinence** 190
   - Health Journal 191

Chapter Review 192

Life Skills in Action: Evaluating Media Messages:
   Happy Family? 194

x | Contents

CHAPTER 10 Conflict and Violence 196

Lessons

1 What Is Conflict? 198
    Health Journal 200
2 Communicating During Conflicts 202
    Hands-on Activity: Body Language on TV 203
    Life Skills Activity: Communicating Effectively 204
3 Getting Help for Conflicts 206
    Health Journal 206
    Cross-Discipline Activity: Language Arts 207
4 Violence: When Conflict Becomes Dangerous 208
    Life Skills Activity: Making Good Decisions 210
    Health Journal 211
5 Preventing Violence 212

Chapter Review 214

Life Skills in Action: Communicating Effectively:
    The Threat 216

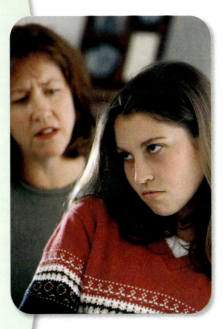

CHAPTER 11 Teens and Tobacco 218

Lessons

1 Tobacco: Dangerous from the Start 220
2 Tobacco Products, Disease, and Death 224
    Hands-on Activity: How Much Tar? 225
3 Social and Emotional Effects of Tobacco 228
    Life Skills Activity: Assessing Your Health 229
4 Forming a Tobacco Addiction 230
5 Why People Use Tobacco 232
    Health Journal 233
6 Quitting 234
    Life Skills Activity: Using Refusal Skills 236
    Health Journal 237
    Cross-Discipline Activity: Math 237
7 Choosing Not to Use Tobacco 238
    Health Journal 239

Chapter Review 240

Life Skills in Action: Making Good Decisions:
    Tobacco Troubles 242

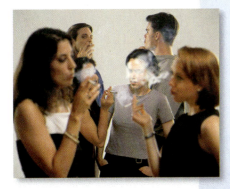

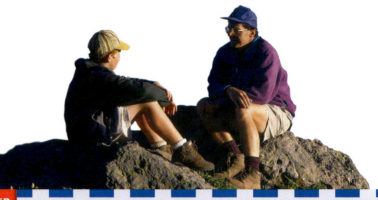

CHAPTER 12 Teens and Alcohol 244

Lessons

1. Understanding Teens and Alcohol 246
2. Alcohol and Your Body 248
   - Hands-on Activity: Delayed Reaction Time 250
3. Alcohol, You, and Other People 252
4. Drunk Driving 256
5. Alcoholism 258
   - Teen Talk 259
6. Resisting the Pressure to Drink 260
   - Health Journal 261
7. Alternatives to Alcohol 262
   - Life Skills Activity: Practicing Wellness 263

Chapter Review 264

Life Skills in Action: Using Refusal Skills:
   Sophie and the Secret Alcohol 266

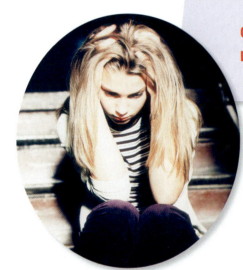

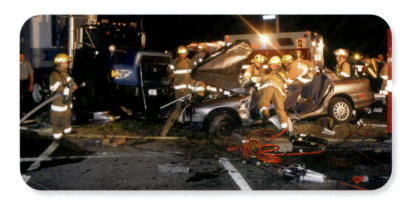

Myth & Fact

Myth: Using tobacco in the form of chewing tobacco or snuff is much safer than smoking.

Fact: Go to page 272 to get the facts.

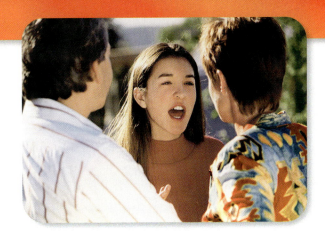

CHAPTER 13 Teens and Drugs 268

Lessons

1	Using Drugs	270
2	The Use of Drugs as Medicine	274
	Health Journal	275
3	Drug Misuse and Abuse	276
	Life Skills Activity: Practicing Wellness	277
4	Drug Addiction	278
5	The Consequences of Drug Abuse	280
	Life Skills Activity: Making Good Decisions	281
	Cross-Discipline Activity: Science	282
6	Stimulants and Depressants	284
7	Marijuana	286
8	Hallucinogens and Inhalants	288
9	Staying Drug Free	290
	Hands-on Activity: Why Stay Drug Free?	291
	Health Journal	293

Chapter Review 294

Life Skills in Action: Coping: The Drug Problem 296

Contents | xiii

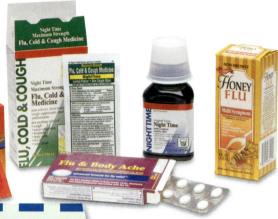

CHAPTER 14 Infectious Diseases 298

Lessons

1. **What Is an Infectious Disease?** 300
   - Hands-on Activity: Infectious Handshake 301
2. **Bacterial Infections** 302
3. **Viral Infections** 306
   - Health Journal 307
   - Cross-Discipline Activity: Science 308
   - Life Skills Activity: Practicing Wellness 309
4. **Sexually Transmitted Diseases** 310
5. **Preventing the Spread of Infectious Diseases** 314

Chapter Review 316

Life Skills in Action: Making Good Decisions:
   Juan's Illness 318

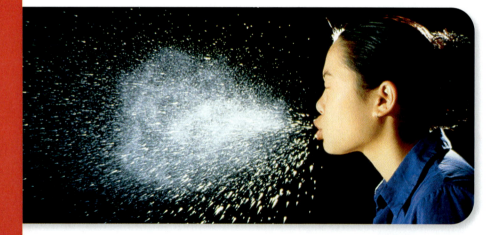

Myth & Fact

Myth: You catch a cold when you are out in cold or wet weather.

Fact: Go to page 307 to get the facts.

xiv | Contents

CHAPTER 15 Noninfectious Diseases and Disorders 320

Lessons

1. Noninfectious Diseases and Body Systems 322
2. Circulatory System 324
   - Teen Talk 325
   - Hands-on Activity: Heartbeats 326
3. Respiratory System 328
   - Life Skills Activity: Making Good Decisions 329
4. Nervous System 330
5. Endocrine System 332
   - Life Skills Activity: Being a Wise Consumer 333
6. Digestive System 334
7. Urinary System 336
8. Skin, Bones, and Muscles 338
   - Hands-on Activity: How Much Skin Do You Have? ... 339
9. Eyes and Ears 340
   - Health Journal 341

Chapter Review 342

Life Skills in Action: Coping: Derek's Depression 344

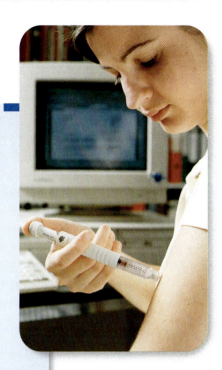

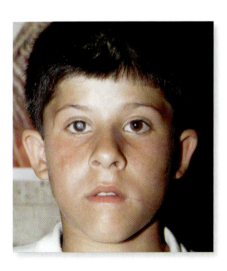

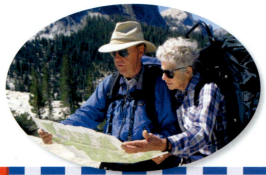

CHAPTER 16 Your Changing Body 346

Lessons

1	**What Makes You You** 348
	Hands-on Activity: The Eyes Have It 349
2	**The Male Reproductive System** 350
	Life Skills Activity: Assessing Your Health 353
3	**The Female Reproductive System** 354
	Teen Talk 357
4	**The Endocrine System** 358
5	**Growing Up** 360
	Health Journal 362
	Cross-Discipline Activity: Language Arts 363
6	**Becoming an Adult** 364
	Life Skills Activity: Making Good Decisions 365
	Health Journal 366

Chapter Review 368

Life Skills in Action: Assessing Your Health:
  Puberty Blues 370

> **Myth & Fact**
>
> **Myth:** Ovulation always happens on the fourteenth day of the menstrual cycle.
>
> **Fact:** Go to page 355 to get the facts.

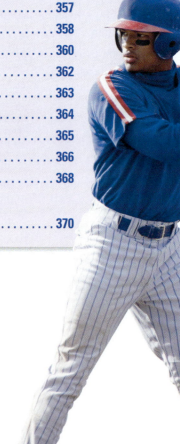

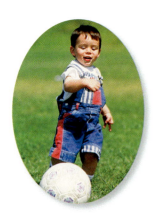

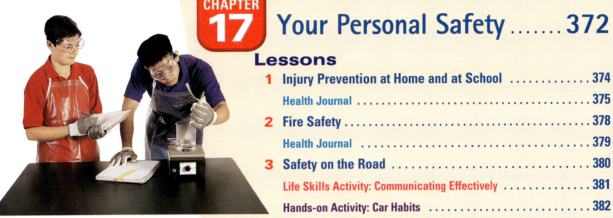

CHAPTER 17 Your Personal Safety 372

Lessons

1 Injury Prevention at Home and at School 374
  Health Journal 375
2 Fire Safety 378
  Health Journal 379
3 Safety on the Road 380
  Life Skills Activity: Communicating Effectively 381
  Hands-on Activity: Car Habits 382
4 Safety Outdoors 384
5 Natural Disasters 388
  Life Skills Activity: Communicating Effectively 390
6 Deciding to Give First Aid 392
  Life Skills Activity: Practicing Wellness 393
7 Abdominal Thrusts and Rescue Breathing 394
8 First Aid for Injuries 398
  Cross-Discipline Activity: Science 400

Chapter Review 402

Life Skills in Action: Being a Wise Consumer:
  The Best Baby Seat 404

Myth & Fact

Myth: You should slap a choking person on the back.

Fact: Go to page 395 to get the facts.

Appendix

The Food Guide Pyramid 406
Alternative Food Guide Pyramids 407
Calorie and Nutrient Content of Common Foods 408
Food Safety Tips 410
The Physical Activity Pyramid 411
Water Safety 412
Staying Home Alone 413
Emergency Kit 414
Internet Safety 415
Baby Sitter Safety 416
The Body Systems 418

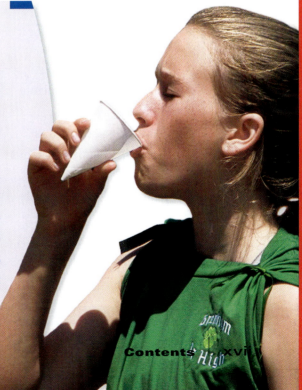

Activities

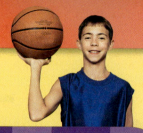

Hands-on ACTIVITY

Generic Versus Brand-Name Products ... 13	How Much Tar? ... 225
Listening Lab ... 41	Delayed Reaction Time ... 250
Self-Esteem Booster ... 52	Why Stay Drug Free? ... 291
Brown Bag Test ... 100	Infectious Handshake ... 301
Using Positive Self-Talk ... 142	Heartbeats ... 326
Stressors ... 165	How Much Skin Do You Have? ... 339
Stress Management ... 167	The Eyes Have It ... 349
Body Language on TV ... 203	Car Habits ... 382

LIFE SKILLS ACTIVITY

Making Good Decisions ... 6	Coping ... 182
Assessing Your Health ... 11	Making Good Decisions ... 187
Practicing Wellness ... 14	Communicating Effectively ... 204
Making Good Decisions ... 27	Making Good Decisions ... 210
Being a Wise Consumer ... 30	Assessing Your Health ... 229
Using Refusal Skills ... 58	Using Refusal Skills ... 236
Practicing Wellness ... 70	Practicing Wellness ... 263
Evaluating Media Messages ... 86	Practicing Wellness ... 277
Communicating Effectively ... 96	Making Good Decisions ... 281
Practicing Wellness ... 107	Practicing Wellness ... 309
Making Good Decisions ... 108	Making Good Decisions ... 329
Evaluating Media Messages ... 119	Being a Wise Consumer ... 333
Making Good Decisions ... 123	Assessing Your Health ... 353
Communicating Effectively ... 139	Making Good Decisions ... 365
Coping ... 141	Communicating Effectively ... 381
Making Good Decisions ... 151	Communicating Effectively ... 390
Assessing Your Health ... 160	Practicing Wellness ... 393
Coping ... 168	

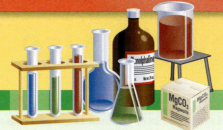

Cross-Discipline ACTIVITY

Language Arts 13	Language Arts 178
Social Studies 34	Language Arts 207
Language Arts 57	Math 237
Science 77	Science 282
Social Studies 96	Science 308
Math 127	Language Arts 363
Social Studies 135	Science 400
Science 163	

Life Skills IN ACTION

Setting Goals 18	Making Good Decisions 318
Using Refusal Skills 46	Coping 344
Coping 62	Assessing Your Health 370
Assessing Your Health 90	Being a Wise Consumer 404
Making Good Decisions 112	
Practicing Wellness 130	
Communicating Effectively 154	
Setting Goals 172	
Evaluating Media Messages 194	
Communicating Effectively 216	
Making Good Decisions 242	
Using Refusal Skills 266	
Coping 296	

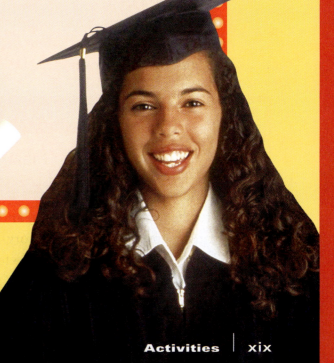

How to Use Your Textbook

Your Roadmap for Success with *Decisions for Health*

Read the Objectives

The objectives, which are listed under the **What You'll Do** head, tell you what you'll need to know.

STUDY TIP Reread the objectives when studying for a test to be sure you know the material.

Study the Key Terms

Key Terms are listed for each lesson under the **Terms to Learn** head. Learn the definitions of these terms because you will most likely be tested on them. Use the glossary to locate definitions quickly.

STUDY TIP If you don't understand a definition, reread the page where the term is introduced. The surrounding text should help make the definition easier to understand.

Start Off Write

Start Off Write questions, which appear at the beginning of each lesson, help you to begin thinking about the topic covered in the lesson.

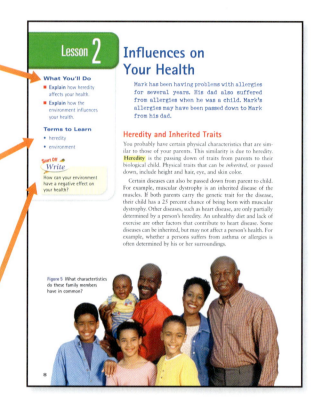

Take Notes and Get Organized

Keep a health notebook so that you are ready to take notes when your teacher reviews the material in class. Keep your assignments in this notebook so that you can review them when studying for the chapter test.

↗ Be Resourceful, Use the Web

Internet Connect boxes in your textbook take you to resources that you can use for health projects, reports, and research papers. Go to **scilinks.org/health** and type in the HealthLinks code to get information on a topic.

Visit go.hrw.com
Find worksheets, *Current Health* magazine articles online, and other materials that go with your textbook at **go.hrw.com**. Click on the textbook icon and the table of contents to see all of the resources for each chapter.

Use the Illustrations and Photos

Art shows complex ideas and processes. Learn to analyze the art so that you better understand the material you read in the text.

Tables and graphs display important information in an organized way to help you see relationships.

A picture is worth a thousand words. Look at the photographs to see relevant examples of health concepts you are reading about.

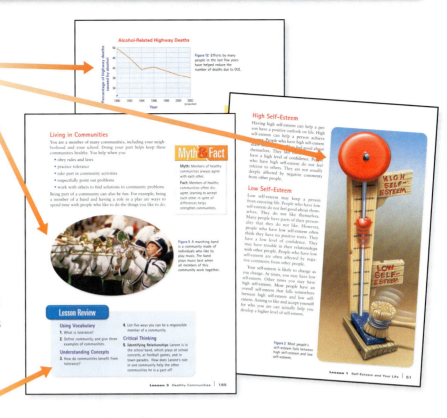

Answer the Lesson Reviews

Lesson Reviews test your knowledge over the main points of the lesson. Critical Thinking items challenge you to think about the material in greater depth and to find connections that you infer from the text.

STUDY TIP When you can't answer a question, reread the lesson. The answer is usually there.

Do Your Homework

Your teacher will assign Study Guide worksheets to help you understand and remember the material in the chapter.

STUDY TIP Answering the items in the Chapter Review will prepare you for the chapter test. Don't try to answer the questions without reading the text and reviewing your class notes. A little preparation up front will make your homework assignments a lot easier.

Visit Holt Online Learning
If your teacher gives you a special password to log onto the **Holt Online Learning** site, you'll find your complete textbook on the Web. In addition, you'll find some great learning tools and practice quizzes. You'll be able to see how well you know the material from your textbook.

Holt Online Learning
For more information go to:
www.hrw.com

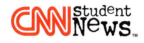

Visit CNN Student News
You'll find up-to-date events in science at cnnstudentnews.com.

How to Use Your Textbook | xxi

CHAPTER 1

Health and Wellness
Chapter Planning Guide

PACING	CLASSROOM RESOURCES	ACTIVITIES AND DEMONSTRATIONS
BLOCK 1 • 45 min pp. 2–7 **Chapter Opener**	CRF Health Inventory * ■ GENERAL CRF Parent Letter * ■	SE Health IQ, p. 3 CRF At-Home Activity * ■
Lesson 1 Being Healthy and Well	CRF Lesson Plan * TT Bellringer * TT The Four Parts of Health *	TE Activities Wellness Collage Box, p. 1F TE Demonstration Breaking Habits, p. 5 GENERAL TE Activity Poster Project, p. 6 BASIC TE Group Activity Popularity, p. 6 GENERAL CRF Life Skills Activity * ■ GENERAL CRF Enrichment Activity * ADVANCED
BLOCK 2 • 45 min pp. 8–11 **Lesson 2** Influences on Your Health	CRF Lesson Plan * TT Bellringer *	TE Activities Wellness in Your Community, p. 1F TE Activities Sports and Health, p. 1F CRF Enrichment Activity * ADVANCED
Lesson 3 Making Good Health Choices	CRF Lesson Plan * TT Bellringer *	TE Group Activity Lifestyle Choices, p. 10 GENERAL TE Activity Lifestyles of a Student, p. 11 GENERAL CRF Enrichment Activity * ADVANCED
BLOCK 3 • 45 min pp. 12–15 **Lesson 4** Nine Life Skills for Better Health	CRF Lesson Plan * TT Bellringer * TT The Nine Life Skills *	SE Language Arts Activity, p. 13 SE Hands-on Activity, p. 13 CRF Datasheets for In-Text Activities * GENERAL TE Activity Role-Playing, p. 13 GENERAL TE Group Activity Life Skill Charades, p. 13 GENERAL TE Activity Difficult Situations, p. 14 GENERAL SE Life Skills in Action Setting Goals, pp. 18–19 CRF Life Skills Activity * ■ GENERAL CRF Enrichment Activity * ADVANCED

BLOCKS 4 & 5 • 90 min Chapter Review and Assessment Resources

- SE Chapter Review, pp. 16–17
- CRF Concept Review * ■ GENERAL
- CRF Health Behavior Contract * ■ GENERAL
- CRF Chapter Test * ■ GENERAL
- CRF Performance-Based Assessment * GENERAL
- OSP Test Generator
- CRF Test Item Listing *

Online Resources

Visit **go.hrw.com** for a variety of free resources related to this textbook. Enter the keyword **HD4HW7**.

Students can access interactive problem solving help and active visual concept development with the *Decisions for Health* Online Edition available at **www.hrw.com**.

CNN student News
cnnstudentnews.com
Find the latest health news, lesson plans, and activities related to important scientific events.

Compression guide:
To shorten your instruction because of time limitations, omit Lesson 3.

KEY

TE Teacher Edition	**CRF** Chapter Resource File	***** Also on One-Stop Planner
SE Student Edition	**TT** Teaching Transparency	■ Also Available in Spanish
OSP One-Stop Planner		◆ Requires Advance Prep

SKILLS DEVELOPMENT RESOURCES	LESSON REVIEW AND ASSESSMENT	STANDARDS CORRELATION
		National Health Education Standards
TE Life Skill Builder Setting Goals, p. 4 `GENERAL` TE Inclusion Strategies, p. 5 `BASIC` SE Life Skills Activity Making Good Decisions, p. 6 CRF Cross-Disciplinary * `GENERAL` CRF Directed Reading * `BASIC`	SE Lesson Review, p. 7 TE Reteaching Quiz, p. 7 TE Alternative Assessment, p. 7 `GENERAL` CRF Concept Mapping * `GENERAL` CRF Lesson Quiz * ■ `GENERAL`	1.2, 3.2, 3.4
TE Inclusion Strategies, p. 10 `GENERAL` CRF Cross-Disciplinary * `GENERAL` CRF Refusal Skills * `GENERAL` CRF Directed Reading * `BASIC`	SE Lesson Review, p. 9 TE Reteaching, Quiz, p. 9 CRF Lesson Quiz * ■ `GENERAL`	1.3, 1.5
SE Life Skills Activity Assessing Your Health, p. 11 CRF Decision-Making * `GENERAL` CRF Refusal Skills * `GENERAL` CRF Directed Reading * `BASIC`	SE Lesson Review, p. 11 TE Reteaching, Quiz, p. 11 CRF Lesson Quiz * ■ `GENERAL`	1.1, 1.6, 2.6
SE Life Skills Activity Practicing Wellness, p. 14 CRF Decision-Making * `GENERAL` CRF Directed Reading * `BASIC`	SE Lesson Review, p. 15 TE Reteaching, Quiz, p. 15 TE Alternative Assessment, p. 15 `GENERAL` CRF Concept Mapping * `GENERAL` CRF Lesson Quiz * ■ `GENERAL`	2.1, 2.3, 2.5, 3.4, 4.2, 6.4

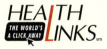

www.scilinks.org/health

Maintained by the **National Science Teachers Association**

Topic: Depression
HealthLinks code: HD4026

Topic: Genes and Traits
HealthLinks code: HD4045

Topic: Physical Fitness
HealthLinks code: HD4076

Technology Resources

 One-Stop Planner
All of your printable resources and the Test Generator are on this convenient CD-ROM.

 Guided Reading Audio CDs

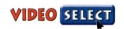
For information about videos related to this chapter, go to **go.hrw.com** and type in the keyword **HD4HW7V**.

Chapter 1 • Chapter Planning Guide **1B**

Chapter 1: Health and Wellness
Chapter Resources

Teacher Resources

TEACHING TRANSPARENCIES
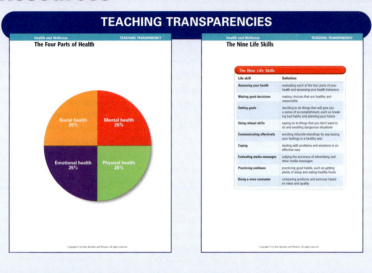

BELLRINGER TRANSPARENCIES
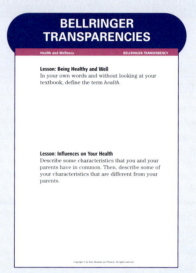

LESSON PLANS
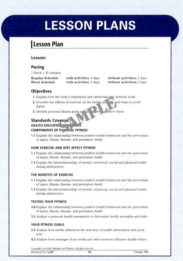

PARENT LETTER
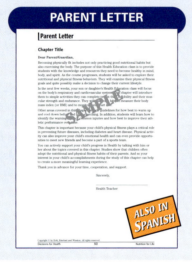

TEST ITEM LISTING
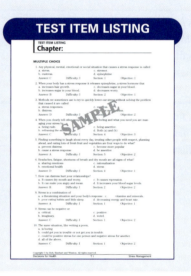

Meeting Individual Needs

DIRECTED READING
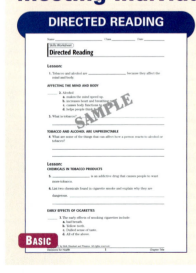

CONCEPT MAPPING
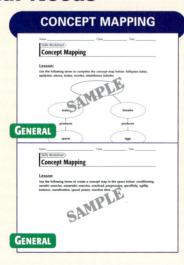

CONCEPT REVIEW
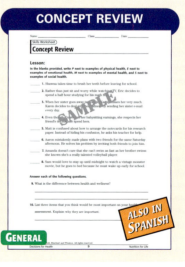

ENRICHMENT ACTIVITIES
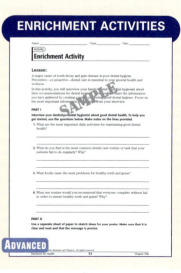

Resources

These worksheet pages can be found in the Chapter Resource File and the One-Stop Planner. The transparencies can be found in the Teaching Transparencies binder and on the One-Stop Planner.

Activities

LIFE SKILLS ACTIVITIES
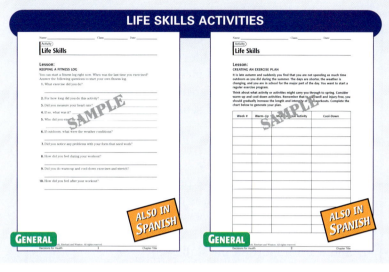

AT-HOME ACTIVITY
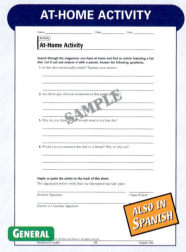

DATASHEETS FOR IN-TEXT ACTIVITIES
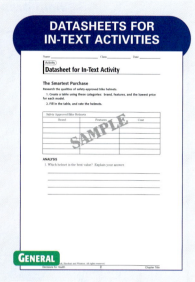

Applications

DECISION-MAKING
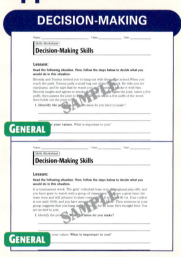

REFUSAL SKILLS
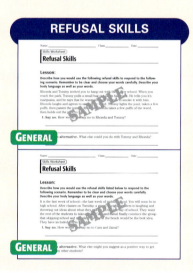

CROSS-DISCIPLINARY
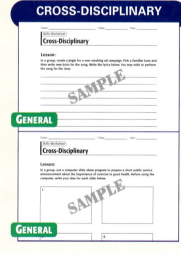

HEALTH BEHAVIOR CONTRACT
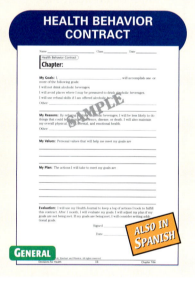

Assessments

HEALTH INVENTORY
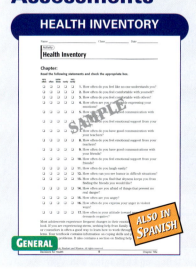

LESSON QUIZZES
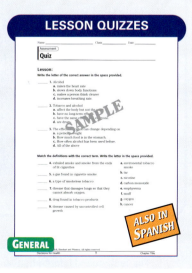

CHAPTER TEST
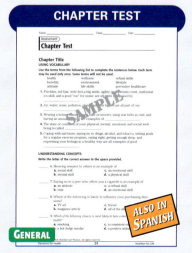

PERFORMANCE-BASED ASSESSMENT
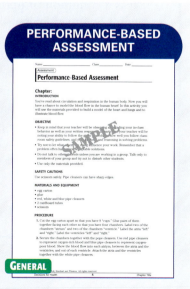

Chapter 1 • Chapter Resources and Worksheets   **1D**

Chapter 1: Background Information

The following information focuses on the concept of wellness and discusses how the four parts of health are interrelated. This material will help prepare you for teaching the concepts in this chapter.

What Is Wellness?

- The concept of wellness is difficult to define, but generally wellness is the balance of the many parts of health. Achieving wellness requires active pursuit of all four parts of health—physical, emotional, mental, and social. While it helps to think of physical, emotional, mental, and social health as separate entities, it is important to realize that these four parts of health are interrelated. Being aware of the connections among the different parts of health can help a person choose behaviors that will promote the different parts of his or her health, and therefore contribute substantially to their overall wellness. To better understand the concept of wellness, the following definitions from leaders of the wellness movement have been included.

  - Wellness is a state of complete physical, mental, and social well-being and not merely the absence of disease or infirmity. (World Health Organization)

  - Wellness is much more than simply not being sick. It is a condition of optimal physical, mental, and emotional well-being. Wellness is a preventive way of living that reduces—sometimes even eliminates—the need for remedies. Wellness emphasizes personal responsibility for making the life style choices and self-care decisions that will improve the quality of your life. One crucial belief is that preventing illness is even more important than treating it, especially since many chronic diseases are incurable. (Berkeley Wellness Letter)

  - Wellness is a positive, day-to-day approach to a long, healthful, active life. It includes both highly scientific and practical medicine—from the latest research and most advanced tests to reliable home remedies and common sense. (Berkeley Wellness Letter)

Sports and Wellness

- One activity that can have positive effects on many parts of a person's health is playing sports. Playing sports can help a young person improve his or her physical health, develop a strong social network, and learn important life skills.

- Studies have even shown that students who participate in sports are less likely to be regular tobacco users, and girls who play sports have a more positive body image and lower levels of depression than girls who do not play sports.

- Sports participation reduces the risk of premature death, as well as reduces the risk of heart disease, hypertension, colon cancer, and diabetes mellitus. Physical activity is important for the health of muscles, bones, and joints.

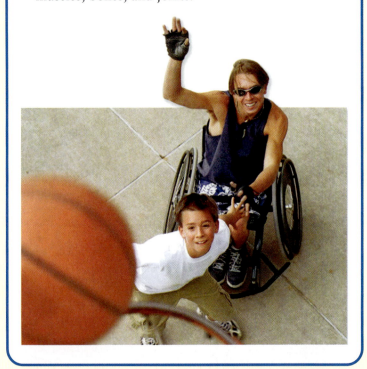

For background information about teaching strategies and issues, refer to the Professional Reference for Teachers.

ACTIVITIES

CHAPTER 1

Consider using the activities on this page as students explore the lessons of this chapter. Look for other activities throughout the Student Edition chapter.

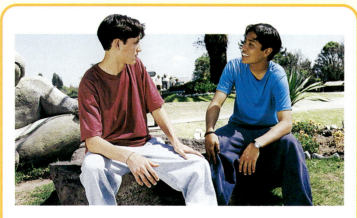

Wellness Collage Box

Procedure Making a wellness collage box will help students explore the private and public aspects of their personal wellness. Each student will need a shoebox. Provide a variety of magazines, markers, colored pencils, paper, and glue sticks. Have students begin by making two lists. One list should be things they do publicly for their wellness, such as playing sports, socializing with friends, and wearing their seat belt and protective sports gear. The other list should be things students do that are private, such as personal hygiene practices, a journal, and practicing relaxation exercises. Let students know that it is their decision as to what they consider to be public or private. Then, have the students decorate the outside of their shoebox with images or words that represent things from their public list. Have students decorate the inside of their shoebox with images and words that represent things from their private list. Students may volunteer to share their collages with the class.

Analysis Ask students the following questions after they have completed their collage boxes.

- Which part of the collage was more difficult for you to represent, the public or the private things that you do for your wellness? (Answers may vary depending on the student.)

- Which part of your health was the most represented in your collage? (Answers may vary. At this time, students will probably have more items that represent their physical or social health.)

- Which part of your health was the least represented in your collage? (Answers may vary.)

Sports and Health

This exercise is designed to help students explore how the four parts of health are interrelated. Lead students in a discussion by asking the following questions related to sports or substitute another activity.

- In what ways could playing sports help or hurt the physical part of your health? the emotional part of your health? the mental part of your health? the social part of your health?

- How might heredity affect your ability to play sports?

- How might your environment affect your ability to play sports?

- What kinds of preventive measures are important when playing sports?

- What life skills does playing sports help teach?

Promoting Wellness in Your Community

Many local and state health departments have wellness campaigns targeting specific health issues. Have students contact their local health departments to learn about issues in their communities and how they can help contribute to the wellness efforts.

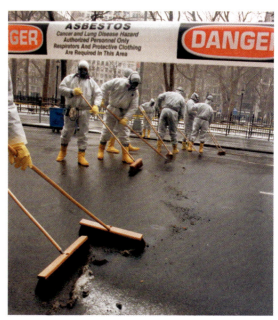

Chapter 1 • Activities **1F**

CHAPTER 1

Overview

Tell students that this chapter will help them learn about the four parts of their health and what wellness means. Students will also learn about the different influences on their health, about the importance of making good choices about health, and about the life skills that will help them be healthy.

Question Box

Students may feel more comfortable asking questions if you set up a Question Box to collect their questions. Have students write and anonymously submit their questions about their health, wellness, and influences on their health. Address these questions during class, or use these questions to introduce lessons that cover related topics.

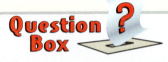

Check out *Current Health* articles and activities related to this chapter by visiting the HRW Web site at **go.hrw.com.** Just type in the keyword **HD4CH16T.**

Chapter Resource File

- Directed Reading BASIC
- Health Inventory GENERAL
- Parent Letter

CHAPTER 1 Health and Wellness

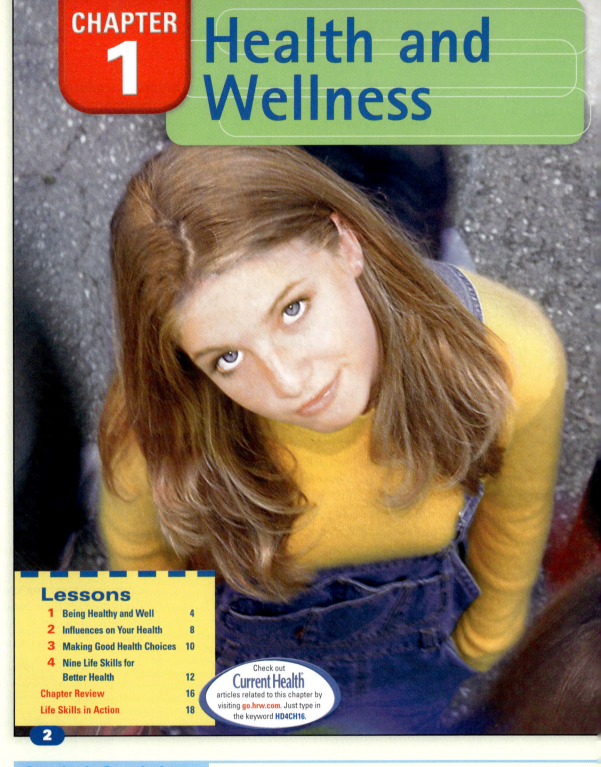

Lessons

1	Being Healthy and Well	4
2	Influences on Your Health	8
3	Making Good Health Choices	10
4	Nine Life Skills for Better Health	12

Chapter Review 16
Life Skills in Action 18

Check out *Current Health* articles related to this chapter by visiting go.hrw.com. Just type in the keyword **HD4CH16.**

Standards Correlations

National Health Education Standards

1.1 (partial) Explain the relationship between positive health behaviors and the prevention of injury, illness, disease, and premature death. (Lesson 3)

1.2 Describe the interrelationship of mental, emotional, social, and physical health during adolescence. (Lesson 1)

1.3 Describe how family and peers influence the health of adolescents. (Lesson 2)

1.5 Analyze how environment and personal health are interrelated. (Lesson 2)

1.6 Describe ways to reduce risks related to adolescent health problems. (Lesson 3)

2.1 Analyze the validity of health information, products, and services. (Lesson 4)

2.3 Analyze how media influences the selection of health information and products. (Lesson 4)

2.5 Compare the costs and validity of health products. (Lesson 4)

2.6 Describe situations requiring professional health services. (Lesson 3)

> "I belong to a lot of **school** groups, and I'm making pretty good **grades**. I have a lot of **friends**, too. I really like where I am **in my life** right now."

Using the Health IQ

Misconception Alert
Answers to the Health IQ questions may help you identify students' misconceptions.

Question 1: Students may know that many physical traits, such as hair and eye color, height, and curly hair, are traits that are passed down from their parents but may not realize that certain diseases can also be inherited.

Question 3: Students may associate the word *hygiene* with things like using deodorant or brushing their teeth. But students may not realize that hygiene includes the simple act of washing their hands before they eat and after they use the bathroom.

Question 4: Students may not have heard the term *social health* and may think of it simply as a measure of how popular they are. In reality, social health really has little to do with the number of friends a person has but is more about a person's ability to interact with others in a positive, mutually respectful way.

Answers
1. d
2. d
3. c
4. b
5. a
6. a

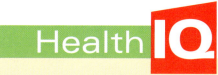

PRE-READING
Answer the following multiple-choice questions to find out what you already know about health and wellness. When you've finished this chapter, you'll have the opportunity to change your answers based on what you've learned.

1. Which of the following characteristics is NOT hereditary?
   a. the tendency to get certain diseases or conditions
   b. height
   c. eye color
   d. taste in music

2. Brushing and flossing your teeth regularly is an example of
   a. a healthy lifestyle.
   b. preventive healthcare.
   c. good hygiene.
   d. All of the above

3. Which of the following behaviors is an example of good hygiene?
   a. eating a balanced diet
   b. avoiding harmful substances
   c. washing your hands
   d. getting plenty of exercise

4. Your social health is made up of all of the following EXCEPT
   a. being a team player.
   b. exercising.
   c. sharing your true feelings with your friends.
   d. being considerate of others.

5. Telling someone that you do not want to do something is an example of
   a. using refusal skills.
   b. practicing wellness.
   c. coping.
   d. making good decisions.

6. Being able to express yourself clearly to avoid misunderstandings describes which of the following skills?
   a. communicating effectively
   b. practicing wellness
   c. coping
   d. emotional health

ANSWERS: 1. d; 2. d; 3. c; 4. b; 5. a; 6. a

3.2 Analyze a personal health assessment to determine health strengths and risks. (Lesson 1)

3.4 (partial) Demonstrate strategies to improve or maintain personal and family health. (Lessons 1 and 4)

4.2 Analyze how messages from media and other sources influence health behaviors. (Lesson 4)

6.4 Apply strategies and skills needed to attain personal health goals. (Lesson 4)

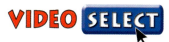

For information about videos related to this chapter, go to **go.hrw.com** and type in the keyword **HD4HW7V**.

Lesson 1

Focus

Overview
Before beginning this lesson, review with your students the objectives listed under the What You'll Do head in the Student Edition. Tell students that this lesson will help them learn about the four parts of health. Tell students they will also learn the difference between health and wellness.

🔔 Bellringer
Ask students to write a definition of health without looking at their book.

Answer to Start Off Write
Sample answer: I can eat nutritious foods, get plenty of rest, and exercise regularly.

Motivate

Discussion — GENERAL

Overall Health Once students have written their own definition of health, ask them the following questions:

- Did anyone's definition address any aspects of health other than the physical aspect?
- Does anyone think that health is more than just physical? What else might health include?

LS Interpersonal

Sensitivity ALERT
Be aware that some students may not have the opportunity or financial resources to get to the doctor or dentist as often as they should, which is suggested in the last bullet.

Lesson 1 — Being Healthy and Well

What You'll Do
- Identify the four parts of health.
- Explain the difference between health and wellness.

Terms to Learn
- health
- wellness

Start Off Write
Write down three things that you can do daily to improve your physical health.

Mary and Chris have been helping to plan the seventh-grade dance. They have been juggling these duties with their schoolwork and responsibilities at home. Now both girls are feeling tense and tired. And they miss seeing their other friends.

Mary and Chris have a lot going on in their lives. The stress of their many activities is affecting their overall health. **Health** is the condition of physical, emotional, mental, and social well-being. To be healthy, you need to balance your physical, emotional, mental, and social health. In this lesson, you will learn ways that you can maintain each part of your health to stay healthy.

Physical Health

The part of health that deals with the body is *physical health*. The following are habits you should practice to have good physical health:

- Eat a balanced diet.
- Get plenty of exercise.
- Get 8 hours of sleep every night.
- Avoid drugs, alcohol, and tobacco.
- Practice safety by wearing protective sports gear and selt belts whenever you are in a moving vehicle.
- Practice good hygiene. *Hygiene* is the practice of keeping clean to prevent the spread of disease.
- Visit your doctor and dentist regularly.

Remember that today's choices will affect your physical health for years to come. And the choices you make now are going to be tomorrow's habits. So, make them good habits!

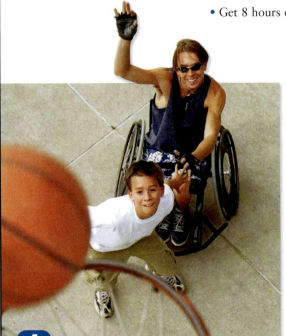

Figure 1 Playing sports is not only fun, but it is a good way to keep yourself physically fit.

Life SKILL BUILDER — GENERAL

Setting Goals Ask students to copy the bulleted list of good physical health habits on this page in their textbook. Have students identify each habit as being something that they do often, sometimes, rarely, or never. Ask students to choose one thing that they either do rarely or never, and encourage them to try to make this a new health habit. Ask students to volunteer their answers. **LS Verbal**

Chapter Resource File
- Directed Reading BASIC
- Lesson Plan
- Lesson Quiz GENERAL

Transparencies
TT Bellringer
TT The Four Parts of Health

4 Chapter 1 • Health and Wellness

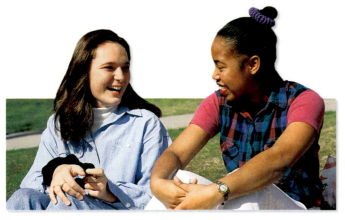

Figure 2 It's great to have friends you can talk to about your problems.

Emotional Health

Your emotional health can affect how you feel about yourself and how you treat other people. *Emotional health* is the way you recognize and deal with your feelings. An emotionally healthy person has the ability to

- express emotions in calm and healthy ways
- deal with sadness and get help for depression
- accept his or her strengths and weaknesses

During adolescence, you experience some major life changes. Your body is changing and you also have more responsibilities both at home and at school. As a result, you may become more emotional than you once were. Although having emotional ups and downs isn't pleasant, this experience is a normal part of growing up. Talk to your parents if you have concerns about controlling your emotions or if you are worried about being depressed.

Mental Health

Being able to easily adjust to change is a sign of good mental health. *Mental health* is the way that you cope with the demands of daily life. Having good mental health means that you can

- solve problems with little trouble
- deal with stress effectively
- accept new ideas

Your mental health can be affected by many of the same things that affect your physical health. For example, lack of sleep hurts your mental alertness and your ability to deal with stress. Good judgment comes more easily after a good night's sleep.

Health Journal
Write a few lines in your Health Journal about a time when one of your friends helped you work through a difficult problem.

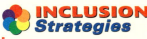

INCLUSION Strategies — BASIC

- Hearing Impaired • Attention Deficit Disorder

Students often benefit from concrete examples. Give the following examples of what sharing one's feelings is and is not. Sharing feelings is NOT: 1. I hate school, 2. I don't like cabbage. 3. My teacher Mr. Miller is dumb. Sharing feelings IS: 1. Spring is my favorite season because the new growth lifts my spirits. 2. I feel very peaceful when I have the family room to myself. 3. I feel jealous of students who easily get good grades.

Discuss that sharing feelings is a way to reach out to others and to share your inner self.

Teach

Demonstration — GENERAL

Breaking Habits This activity is designed to help students understand the concept of a habit. Bring to class about ten pencils or sticks that can easily be broken. Give one of the pencils to a student and ask him or her to break it. Have the student report on how difficult it was to break the pencil. (It should be quite easy.) Then give the same student three pencils and ask him or her to break them at the same time. If the student is able to break the three pencils, ask him or her how hard it was compared with breaking just one. (It should have been much harder.) Give the student five pencils in a bundle and ask him or her to break all five at the same time. (The student will not be able to break them.) Let the students know that each pencil represents a behavior, such as flossing your teeth or smoking a cigarette. The bundle of pencils represents a habit. Help students understand that a behavior contributes to the development of a habit. **LS Kinesthetic/Visual**

Discussion — GENERAL

Emotional Health Have students define *emotional health*. Ask students how their emotional health might affect the following:

- their relationships with friends and family
- their success in school

LS Interpersonal

Answer to Health Journal
Answers may vary. This Health Journal can be used to begin a class discussion on emotions. Remember that some students may be uncomfortable sharing personal information.

Lesson 1 • Being Healthy and Well 5

Teach, continued

Activity —— BASIC
Poster Project This activity will allow students to make a visual representation of wellness. Have students write definitions for each part of health based on what that part of health means to them, or what goals they may have related to that part of their health. Provide students with poster boards, construction paper, magazines, markers, scissors, and glue. Tell students they can use different colors of construction paper to represent each part of health. Tell students to place words or images from magazines on each piece of paper to represent that part of health. Encourage students to hang their creations around the room.
LS Kinesthetic

Group Activity —— GENERAL
Popularity To generate a discussion about the relationship between social health and popularity, ask students to list three characteristics of someone who they think is socially healthy. Then, have the students list three characteristics of someone who they consider to be popular. After students have completed their lists, ask students the following questions:

- Do you think that social health always means being popular?
- In what ways might the desire for popularity get in the way of achieving social health?

Help students understand that it is the quality, not the quantity, of relationships that contributes to a person's social health.
LS Interpersonal

Career —— GENERAL
Sociologists A sociologist is a person who studies human societies. This person researches the origin and development of a society, which includes how the society is organized and how it functions as a group. Sociologists look at the way people in a society interact with each other, and how they interact with people in different societies. **LS Verbal**

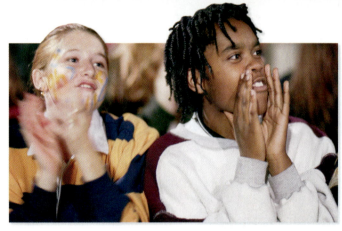

Figure 3 Spending time with your friends is important for your social health.

Social Health

Good social skills help you get along better with people. The way you interact with other people describes your *social health*. You can build good social skills in the following ways:

- Be considerate of other people. Treat others the way that you would like to be treated.
- Show respect for other people.
- Share your true feelings with your friends.
- Be dependable.
- Volunteer to do things for your community.
- Be supportive of your friends when they make the right choice.

Having friends and being close to your family give you a sense of belonging. You know that these people care about you. And when you know that your friends and family care about you and want the best for you, you feel even better about yourself. As a result, you want to be a better person and do things for your friends and family.

LIFE SKILLS ACTIVITY

MAKING GOOD DECISIONS

A new student has joined your class. Some of the popular students in the class are making fun of her when the teacher's back is turned. What will you do? Will you join these students so you can be part of their crowd? If not, what are some things that you could do to let these students know that you don't approve of their actions? How do you think you would feel if you were this new student?

LIFE SKILLS ACTIVITY

Answer
Answers may vary. Sample answer: I would give the other students a look of disapproval, and later, I would tell them that their actions were very rude and hurtful to the new student. I would ask them to put themselves in her place.

6 Chapter 1 • Health and Wellness

Wellness

Your overall wellness is affected by each of the four parts of your health. **Wellness** is a state of good health that is achieved by balancing your physical, emotional, mental, and social health. For example, if you are physically, emotionally, and mentally healthy but have ignored the social part of your health, you can't achieve total wellness.

If you are not sure of your level of wellness, take a health assessment. A *health assessment* is a set of questions that rates your overall health. The following are examples of questions that you should ask yourself:

- Do I get at least 8 hours of sleep each night?
- Do I eat balanced meals?
- Is talking openly with my friends an important part of my day?
- Do I have a trusted adult, such as a parent, who is a main source of support for me?
- Do I deal well with stress?

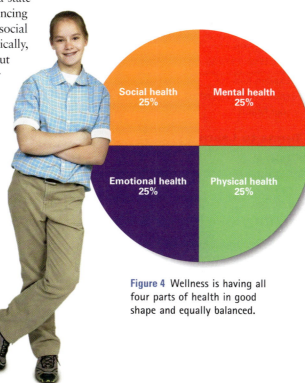

Figure 4 Wellness is having all four parts of health in good shape and equally balanced.

Lesson Review

Using Vocabulary
1. Distinguish between health and wellness.

Understanding Concepts
2. Identify the four parts of health. Write a sentence describing each part.
3. Explain why you must balance all four parts of health to achieve wellness.
4. Why is hygiene important for good physical health?
5. Explain what a health assessment is and how it can help you rate your overall health.

Critical Thinking
6. **Analyzing Ideas** Your friend is sad because she thinks none of her friends care about her. What part of her health is out of balance? Explain.

internet connect
www.scilinks.org/health
Topic: Depression
HealthLinks code: HD4026
HEALTH LINKS. Maintained by the National Science Teachers Association

Close

Reteaching — BASIC

Defining Health Have students work in groups of four. One student in each group will choose one of the four parts of health and will become the "expert" on that part of health. Allow the students to spend 15 minutes reading and writing questions about their topic. Each expert will explain his or her area of health to the other members of the group. After all students have completed their turn, ask students from each group to volunteer to ask their questions to the class. The questions should be representative of the four parts of health. **LS Verbal**

Quiz — GENERAL

1. Good hygiene is an important aspect of which part of health? (Good hygiene is an important part of physical health.)
2. Being dependable is an important element of which part of health? (Being dependable is an important part of social health.)
3. What is one way to measure your overall health? (You can take a health assessment to measure your overall health.)

Alternative Assessment — GENERAL

Assessing Your Health Organize students in small groups and ask them to read the bulleted questions on this page. Ask students to make a Health Assessment Quiz. Students may use the questions on this page or they may think of other questions. Suggest that the students give points for answers. For example, an answer of "Always" gets 5 points, "Sometimes" will earn 4 points, "Rarely" gets 2 points, and "Never" has a value of 0 points. Have the student groups exchange quizzes with other groups. **LS Verbal**

Answers to Lesson Review

1. Health is the state of good physical, emotional, mental, and social well-being. Wellness is a state of good health that is achieved by having these four parts of health balanced.
2. The four parts of health are physical, emotional, mental, and social. Sample answer: Physical health has to do with taking care of your body. Emotional health is the way that you express your feelings. Mental health is how you cope with everyday problems. Social health is how you interact with other people.
3. If any part of your health isn't as good as it should be, then your health is not balanced, and you have not achieved wellness.
4. Hygiene is important because it helps to prevent the spread of diseases.
5. A health assessment is a set of questions that allows you to rate each part of your health. A low score on any part of the assessment means that part of your health needs improvement.
6. Sample answer: My friend's sadness means that her emotional health is out of balance.

Lesson 1 • Being Healthy and Well

Lesson 2

Focus

Overview
Before beginning this lesson, review with your students the objectives listed under the What You'll Do head in the Student Edition. In this lesson, students will learn how heredity and the environment can influence a person's health and wellness.

🔔 Bellringer
Ask students to describe some traits that they have in common with their parents and some traits that are different from their parents.

Answer to Start Off Write
Sample answer: If I breathe polluted air, the environment is affecting my health adversely.

Motivate

Discussion — GENERAL
Twins Have students imagine that they have an identical twin who went to live with another family at birth. Ask students to identify ways that their twin may be like them, and ways that their twin may be different. Ask students to explain their answers. (Explain to students that their twin would have similar physical characteristics because of their common heredity, but some characteristics may be different due to different environments.)
LS Interpersonal

Sensitivity ALERT
Be aware that students who are adopted may be sensitive about issues of heredity.

Lesson 2 — Influences on Your Health

Mark has been having problems with allergies for several years. His dad also suffered from allergies when he was a child. Mark's allergies may have been passed down to Mark from his dad.

What You'll Do
- Explain how heredity affects your health.
- Explain how the environment influences your health.

Terms to Learn
- heredity
- environment

Start Off Write
How can your environment have a negative effect on your health?

Heredity and Inherited Traits

You probably have certain physical characteristics that are similar to those of your parents. This similarity is due to heredity. **Heredity** is the passing down of traits from parents to their biological child. Physical traits that can be *inherited*, or passed down, include height and hair, eye, and skin color.

Certain diseases can also be passed down from parent to child. For example, muscular dystrophy is an inherited disease of the muscles. If both parents carry the genetic trait for the disease, their child has a 25 percent chance of being born with muscular dystrophy. Other diseases, such as heart disease, are only partially determined by a person's heredity. An unhealthy diet and lack of exercise are other factors that contribute to heart disease. Some diseases can be inherited, but may not always affect a person's health. For example, whether a persons suffers from asthma or allergies is often determined by his or her surroundings.

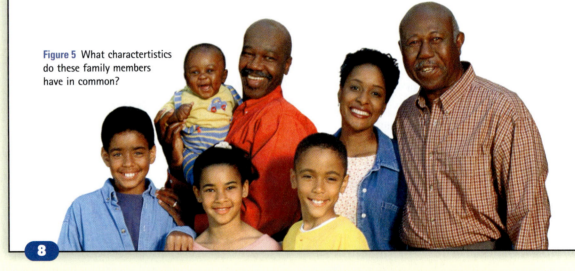

Figure 5 What charactertistics do these family members have in common?

REAL-LIFE CONNECTION — GENERAL
Family Traits Ask the students to make two columns on a piece of paper. Title the first column "Characteristic" and title the second column "Family member." Under the first column, students should write a characteristic about themselves, such as height, sense of humor, or specific talents. Under the second column, have students identify which family member has that similar trait. **LS** Verbal

Chapter Resource File
- Directed Reading BASIC
- Lesson Plan
- Lesson Quiz GENERAL

Transparencies
TT Bellringer

---

8 Chapter 1 • Health and Wellness

Your Environment

Some disease can be triggered by your environment. Your **environment** includes all of the living and nonliving things around you. Asthma attacks are one such example of the way in which the environment can affect your health. Environmental factors that may bring on an asthma attack include things such as air pollution, tobacco smoke, and pollen. Emotional stress has also been known to trigger asthma attacks.

Your environment can affect more than just your physical health. For example, your emotional and mental health can suffer from noise pollution around your home or school. Loud or constant noise disturbs your ability to concentrate, thereby causing you stress. Your emotional health can even be affected by the amount of daylight you receive. Seasonal affective disorder, or SAD, causes depression in some people if they do not get enough sunlight. Most of the time, people suffer from SAD during the winter months, when there are fewer daylight hours. SAD is treated by having the patient sit in front of a light box for a certain period of time.

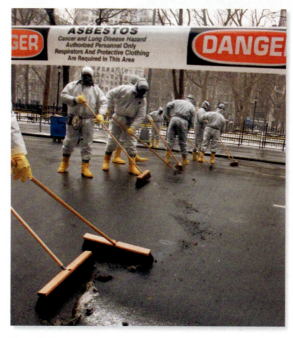

Figure 6 Years ago, asbestos was used as fireproof insulation in buildings. Today, we know that asbestos is an environmental hazard because it damages your lungs.

Myth & Fact

Myth: You get lung cancer only if you smoke.

Fact: It is possible to get lung cancer from second-hand smoke as well as other kinds of air pollutants.

Lesson Review

Using Vocabulary
1. Define the term *heredity*.

Understanding Concepts
2. Explain how heredity influences your health.
3. What are ways that the environment can affect your health?

Critical Thinking
4. **Making Inferences** What can you do to reduce health hazards such as air and water pollution?
5. **Identifying Relationships** Poor air quality is an environmental factor that can trigger asthma attacks. What kind of environment would be healthy for a person with asthma? Explain your answer.

internet connect
www.scilinks.org/health
Topic: Genes and Traits
HealthLinks code: HD4045
HEALTH LINKS. Maintained by the National Science Teachers Association

Lesson 3 Focus

Overview
Before beginning this lesson, review with your students the objectives listed under the What You'll Do head in the Student Edition. This lesson helps students understand how their lifestyle and attitude affects their health. Students will also learn some ways they can take responsibility for their health.

Bellringer
Ask students to describe the characteristics of a person with a good attitude.

Answer to Start Off Write
Accept all reasonable answers. Sample answer: To have a healthier lifestyle, I should avoid harmful substances such as tobacco and alcohol, and I should eat a balanced diet.

Motivate

Group Activity —— GENERAL
Lifestyle Choices Ask students to work in pairs and discuss healthy and unhealthy lifestyles. Ask students to write a description of a healthy lifestyle. Then, ask students to write a description of an unhealthy lifestyle. When students have completed their lists, ask volunteers to write their ideas on the board. Afterwards, have students place a checkmark by the lifestyle choices that they have control over. Help students understand that their lifestyle is the result of choices they make and that their lifestyle affects their health. Students fluent in another language can write their descriptions in both English and their other language. **LS Verbal** — English Language Learners

---

Lesson 3 — Making Good Health Choices

What You'll Do
- **Describe** the relationship between your lifestyle and your health.
- **Identify** four things that you can do to have a healthy lifestyle.
- **Explain** how your attitude affects your health.
- **Explain** what you can do to take responsibility for your healthcare.

Terms to Learn
- lifestyle
- attitude
- preventive healthcare

Start Off Write
Describe ways that you can have a healthier lifestyle.

Taitia was entering a new school and decided that this was a good time to make some changes. Taitia wanted to learn how to make better choices about things that influence her health and life.

At some point, you may decide to make some major changes in your life just as Taitia did. In this lesson, you'll learn how you can take responsibility for your health by making good choices.

Living Healthily

Every day, you make choices that influence your health. For example, you choose what to eat for lunch, when to study, what to do for fun, and whom to have as your friends. These choices determine your lifestyle. A **lifestyle** is a set of behaviors that you live by. To maintain a healthy lifestyle, you will want to develop a good attitude about your health. Your **attitude** is a way of acting, thinking, or feeling that causes you to make one choice over another. A good attitude will allow you to listen to advice about healthy living. It will also help you avoid things that will harm you, such as tobacco, alcohol, and drugs. A good attitude puts you in charge of your health.

Taking Control of Your Health

How can you take charge of your health? Like Taitia, you must first decide to improve your lifestyle. Next, you should decide which part of health you want to work on. For example, you may want to focus on your physical health by starting an exercise routine. But don't forget your emotional, mental, and social health, too. If you are not exactly sure how to improve a certain part of your health, talk to your parents or another trusted adult.

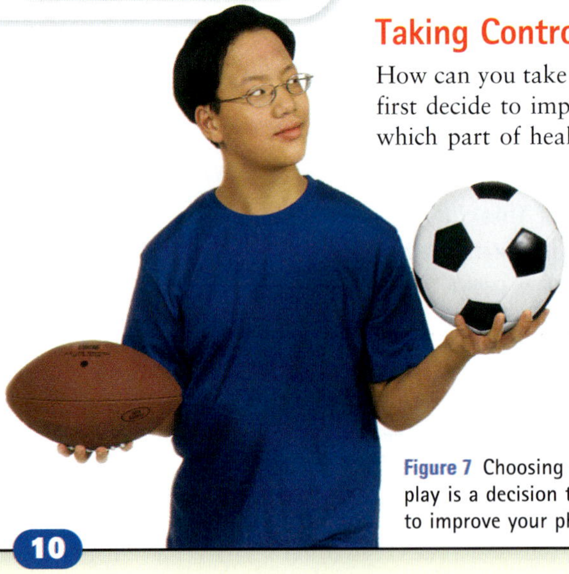

Figure 7 Choosing which sport to play is a decision that you can make to improve your physical health.

INCLUSION Strategies — GENERAL
- Behavior Control Issues • Developmentally Delayed

These students often do not recognize that they make many daily choices. Ask each student to list 10 choices they have made today. Create a running list of choices on the board by having one student start the list and then having others add to the list. Some possible choices include the following: what to eat for breakfast, which shampoo to use, and what to wear to school.

Chapter Resource File
- Directed Reading **BASIC**
- Lesson Plan
- Lesson Quiz **GENERAL**

Transparencies
- TT Bellringer

---

10 Chapter 1 • Health and Wellness

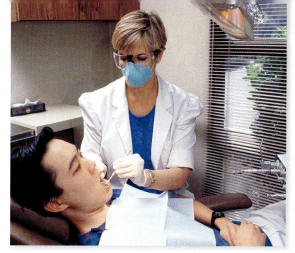

Figure 8 Having a dental exam every year is a good way to find and fill cavities before they get very large.

Healthcare and Personal Responsibility

What responsibilities do you have? You may answer that you are responsible for cleaning your room and feeding your dog. But what is your responsibility for your healthcare. How often do you

- brush and floss your teeth?
- eat healthy food, exercise, and sleep for 8 hours every night?
- wear safety equipment when you play sports?
- buckle your seat belt?
- avoid behavior that will get you in trouble?

If you do these things regularly, you are being responsible for your health by practicing preventive healthcare. **Preventive healthcare** is taking steps to help prevent illness and accidents. These steps include regular visits to your doctors and dentist as well as regular vaccinations. Finding health problems early can prevent serious illness.

LIFE SKILLS ACTIVITY

ASSESSING YOUR HEALTH

Work in a group so that you can share ideas. Draw two columns on a piece of paper. In the first column, write the ways that you already practice preventive healthcare. In the other column, write things that you could start doing to prevent illness or accidents.

Lesson Review

Using Vocabulary

1. Define the term *lifestyle*.
2. Identify three ways to practice preventive healthcare.

Understanding Concepts

3. List four health choices that you make every day.
4. How does your attitude influence the decisions that you make about your health?

Critical Thinking

5. **Identifying Relationships** How can breaking bad habits improve your lifestyle?

internet connect
www.scilinks.org/health
Topic: Physical Fitness
HealthLinks code: HD4076
HEALTH LINKS. Maintained by the National Science Teachers Association

---

Answers to Lesson Review

1. A lifestyle is a set of behaviors by which you live.
2. Preventive healthcare can be practiced by regularly visiting the dentist, wearing a seatbelt in the car, and wearing a bicycle helmet.
3. Sample answer: I can choose to exercise, eat healthy foods, get eight hours of sleep, and avoid harmful substances every day.
4. Having a good attitude allows you to listen to advice about all parts of your health. You will want to make good choices about things that will affect you and your health.
5. Sample answer: Breaking bad habits, such as skipping breakfast or eating too many unhealthy snacks can improve your lifestyle because you will be changing your behavior to improve your health.

Teach

Activity — GENERAL

Writing **Lifestyles of a Student**
Ask students to write a brief description of their personal lifestyle. Then, have students answer the following questions:

- What things do I do that have a positive effect on my physical, mental, social and emotional health?
- What things do I do that have a negative effect on my physical, mental, social and emotional health?
- What is one thing I could start doing or stop doing that would help me have a healthier lifestyle?

LS Verbal

Close

Reteaching — BASIC

Attitudes Ask students to think about a time when they had a bad attitude about something and a time when they had a good attitude about something. Ask them how their different attitudes affected their decisions and behaviors. Help students see how their attitude affects the choices and behaviors that make up their lifestyle. **LS** Auditory

Quiz — GENERAL

1. What is one lifestyle choice that will have a long-term effect on your health? (Sample answer: choosing not to smoke)
2. Regular checkups are examples of what kinds of healthcare? (preventive)
3. What is a proactive approach to health? (A proactive approach is purposefully doing something to improve your health.)

Lesson 3 • Making Good Health Choices

Lesson 4

Focus

Overview
Before beginning this lesson, review with your students the objectives listed under the What You'll Do head in the Student Edition. In this lesson, students will learn about different life skills. Students will also learn how to assess their progress in learning these life skills, and understand how using these skills can improve their health and wellness.

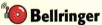**Bellringer**

Ask students to write a definition for the term *refusal skills*.

Answer to Start Off Write
Accept all reasonable answers. Sample answer: Life skills are skills that will help you deal with difficult situations.

Motivate

Discussion — GENERAL

Tough Situations Ask students to write a few paragraphs about one of the following situations:

- having a misunderstanding with a friend or family member
- making a difficult decision
- dealing with a challenge such as moving

Let students know that each of us will face these types of situations throughout our lives. Therefore, it is important to develop the skills needed to handle these situations.

LS Intrapersonal

Lesson 4 — Nine Life Skills for Better Health

What You'll Do
- **Identify** the nine life skills that can improve your life and health.
- **Describe** how practicing the life skills can help you master them.
- **Explain** how you can assess your progress in learning the life skills.
- **Describe** why the life skills should be a part of your daily life.

Terms to Learn
- life skills

Start Off Write
What are life skills?

Stephanie and her sister, Shannon, are always arguing about things that seem unimportant. They both want to get along better with each other, but they are not sure what to do to improve their relationship.

Stephanie and Shannon probably just need to learn how to communicate better. Good communication is one of the nine life skills you will learn about in this lesson. **Life skills** are skills that will help you deal with the many kinds of situations that you will face throughout your life.

The Nine Life Skills

Using life skills can help you maintain a healthy lifestyle. They can help you solve both simple problems and more complicated health problems. Table 1, on the next page, lists and briefly explains each life skill. As you read through this textbook, you will become more familiar with these life skills. In each chapter, you will have several opportunities to practice using the life skills.

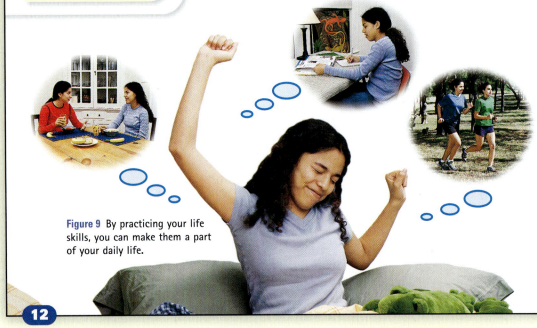

Figure 9 By practicing your life skills, you can make them a part of your daily life.

 Life SKILL BUILDER — GENERAL

Making Good Decisions Have students work in groups of four. Tell students to think of a problem that requires a difficult decision. Have two of the students role-play a good solution to the problem, and have the other two students role-play a bad solution.

Chapter Resource File
- Directed Reading BASIC
- Lesson Plan
- Datasheets for In-Text Activities
- Lesson Quiz GENERAL

Transparencies
- TT Bellringer
- TT The Nine Life Skills

12 Chapter 1 • Health and Wellness

TABLE 1 The Nine Life Skills

Life skill	Definition
Assessing your health	evaluating each of the four parts of your health and assessing your health behaviors
Making good decisions	making choices that are healthy and responsible
Setting goals	deciding to do things that will give you a sense of accomplishment, such as breaking bad habits and planning your future
Using refusal skills	saying no to things that you don't want to do and avoiding dangerous situations
Communicating effectively	avoiding misunderstandings by expressing your feelings in a healthy way
Coping	dealing with problems and emotions in an effective way
Evaluating media messages	judging the accuracy of advertising and other media messages
Practicing wellness	practicing good habits, such as getting plenty of sleep and eating healthy foods
Being a wise consumer	comparing products and services based on value and quality

LANGUAGE ARTS ACTIVITY

Select three life skills from the table on this page, and write a story about a student who improved his or her lifestyle by using these three life skills.

Hands-on ACTIVITY

GENERIC VERSUS BRAND-NAME PRODUCTS

1. Your teacher will provide you with at least two items that are the same type of product but different brands. One item will be a generic, or store brand, and the other item will be a brand-name product. You will compare these products.
2. Look at the items' packaging. Note which package is more attractive.
3. Compare the price of each item.
4. Compare the ingredients on the label of each item.
5. With your teacher's permission, test both the generic and brand-name products.

Analysis

1. Make a chart that has two rows. In each of the rows, write the name of one of the items. Make five columns, and title the columns "Packaging," "Price," "Ingredients," "Quality," and "Overall rating."

2. Fill in each column with an analysis of your findings. You may analyze your findings by answering the following questions:
   - Would you buy one product instead of the other based on the appearance of the package?
   - What is the difference in the prices of the two items?
   - Is there a difference in the kinds of ingredients?
   - Did you notice any difference in the quality of the products?

3. Summarize your findings by writing a paragraph about whether brand-name products are worth the extra money.

Teach

Group Activity —— GENERAL

Life Skill Charades Organize students into two teams. Write each of the life skills on separate pieces of paper. Put all the pieces into a container, and flip a coin to see which team goes first. Have someone from the first team draw a slip of paper, read the life skill, and return the paper to the container. Then have that person act out (without using words) the life skill for the rest of his or her team. Give the team three minutes to guess the life skill. Have the teams take turns until everyone has gotten a chance to act out a life skill, or until an appropriate stopping point is reached. **LS Kinesthetic/Visual**

Activity —— GENERAL

Role-Playing Have students select and role-play one of the following scenarios:
- you and your best friend argued and aren't speaking to each other
- your pet is missing
- your family is being transferred by your father's employer to another state

After each role-play, ask the class for suggestions on how the situation could have been handled differently. **LS Kinesthetic/Visual**

READING SKILL BUILDER —— BASIC

Discussion Have students work in pairs. Tell the students to take turns reading each life skill aloud. After the students have read all of the life skills, instruct them to think of a situation in which each life skill could be used. **LS Verbal**

Answer to Language Arts Activity
Answers may vary, but the stories should include any three of the nine life skills.

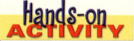

Answer
It is suggested for this activity that at least two types of products are provided for the students to compare. One type of product should be a generic brand, and the other type should be a brand-name product. For example, have students compare the store brand of shampoo to a brand-name shampoo. Other suggestions are paper towels, canned food, toothpaste, and cleaning supplies.

Lesson 4 • Life Skills for Better Health

Teach, continued

Activity — GENERAL

Difficult Situations Have students write about a time when they needed to use one of the nine life skills described in this lesson, but they found it difficult to do so. To guide their writing, have students answer the following questions:

- What made the situation difficult?
- Do you usually avoid using this life skill? Explain your answer.
- What situations do you anticipate facing in the future that will require using this same skill?
- What are some ways that you could practice the life skill to make it easier to use next time you need it?

LS Intrapersonal/Verbal

Cultural Awareness — ADVANCED

Physical Fitness Across the World Have students explore different sports that students from other cultures play with their friends. Start by asking students to list some of their favorite sports. Then have students use the Internet or library to research other sports played in different parts of the world. If possible, have students learn the rules and explain these rules to the class. Ask students which life skills they use when playing sports. **LS** Verbal

LIFE SKILLS ACTIVITY

PRACTICING WELLNESS

Work in groups of two or three students. With your teacher's help, choose one of the life skills to role-play. If you like, you can also role-play your life skill in front of the class.

LANGUAGE ARTS CONNECTION

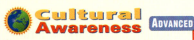

Everyday Skills Have students select a scientist with whom they are familiar. Have students write an imaginary scenario about this scientist and how he or she may have used life skills in his or her research. The stories can be humorous, but still must accurately describe the life skill, as well as the scientist's work. Ask for volunteers to read their stories out loud to the class if appropriate.

Practice Makes Perfect

You may find that using certain life skills is difficult or awkward at first. But that is true of any new skill that you are trying to learn. Remember that the best way to master any skill is to practice it. Try practicing one of the life skills that you think you may have trouble with. First, think of a situation in which you may need this skill and play out the situation in your mind. For example, what would you do if you said no to a friend but that person wouldn't take no for an answer? Would you stand your ground or give in to your friend? Remember that if you prepare yourself for these kinds of situations, you will have less trouble when you face the real thing. Practice these skills, and you will soon find them easier to use.

Assessing Your Progress

You may already be familiar with some of the life skills, while other life skills may be new to you. But, you will want to assess the progress that you are making in using all of these skills. To assess your progress, ask yourself questions such as the following:

- Which skills do I use most often?
- Which skills do I rarely use but should use more often?
- Are there skills that I don't feel comfortable using?
- Am I having problems with a specific skill?
- How can I improve my use of life skills?

Some skills are more difficult to master than others are. So, spend time practicing the skills that you have trouble with. It may help to role-play a life skill with a friend or family member. And remember that you can always talk to your parents or another trusted adult to get advice on how best to use certain life skills.

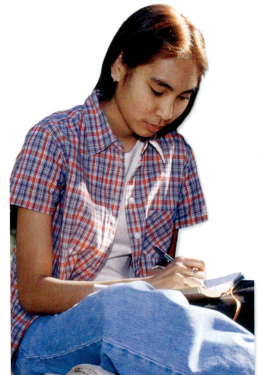

Figure 10 Keep a record of daily events in your life. This record will show you how well you are using the life skills.

LIFE SKILLS ACTIVITY

Answer
Students will choose various scenarios to role-play. Make sure that each scenario accurately represents the life skill that the students are role-playing.

Maintaining a Healthy Lifestyle

Life skills will help you make good choices both now and in the future. Remember that you want to maintain the four parts of your health to achieve wellness. The following examples describe ways that you can keep your health balanced:

- Spending quality time with parents and friends can improve your social health.
- Talking openly about problems and expressing yourself in healthy ways can improve your emotional health.
- Opening your mind to new ideas and new ways of doing things can improve your mental health.
- Eating properly, getting rest, and exercising regularly can improve your physical health.

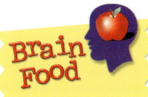

Brain Food

The risk of cancer can be reduced by eating at least five servings of fruits and vegetables every day and by decreasing the fat in your diet.

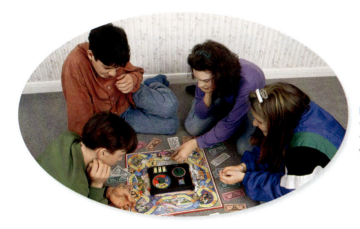

Figure 11 What life skills would you possibly use when playing a game with your friends?

Lesson Review

Using Vocabulary

1. Define the term *life skill*, and briefly describe each life skill.

Understanding Concepts

2. Explain how you can assess your progress in using the life skills.
3. Describe why life skills should be a part of your everyday life.
4. How does practicing the life skills help you master them?

Critical Thinking

5. **Making Inferences** Which life skill would you use in each of the following situations?
   - You and your brother argued, and now you aren't talking to each other.
   - Two brands of shampoo are advertised as being the best.
   - Your friend wants to copy your homework.

Answers to Lesson Review

1. Life skills are skills that help you deal with situations that can affect your health. Students should list and describe the nine skills in the table on the second page of this lesson.
2. You can assess your progress in using the life skills by asking yourself which skills you use most and which skills you use least. You can think about which skills you are having trouble with and how you can improve your use of those skills.
3. Using life skills every day can help you maintain a healthy lifestyle and can help you solve problems when they arise.
4. You will become more familiar and more comfortable using the life skills when you practice them regularly.
5. Sample answer: I would use the following skills: communicating effectively, being a wise consumer, and using refusal skills.

Close

Reteaching — BASIC

Using Life Skills Have students choose one or two life skills that they want to improve. Instruct the students to write the skill or skills on a piece of paper. Then, have students write a plan explaining how they will improve the skill or skills. Tell the students to keep a journal to detail their progress over the next two weeks. At the end of the two weeks, have students volunteer to tell the class about their experience. **LS Verbal**

Quiz — GENERAL

1. Explain the meaning of the term *coping*. (Coping is dealing with problems and emotions in an effective way.)
2. Why is it important to be a wise consumer? (Being a wise consumer helps you get the best value and quality for your money.)
3. Why would it be useful to role-play different life skills? (Role-playing helps you practice the life skills so you will be prepared to use them when you need them.)

Alternative Assessment — GENERAL

Summarizing Have students write on a piece of paper the title of each of the four heads in this lesson. Have students write a summary of the material under each head. When students have completed their assignment, tell them to read the lesson objectives and make sure their summaries have covered this material.

Lesson 4 • Life Skills for Better Health

CHAPTER 1 REVIEW

Assignment Guide

Lesson	Review Questions
1	5, 7–10, 18
2	1, 4, 11–12, 19
3	2–3, 6, 13–14, 17
4	15–16, 20–22

ANSWERS

Using Vocabulary
1. heredity
2. preventive healthcare
3. lifestyle
4. environment
5. hygiene
6. attitude
7. wellness

Understanding Concepts
8. The four parts of health are physical, emotional, mental and social.
9. Health is a condition of physical, emotional, mental, and social well-being. Wellness occurs when all of these parts of health are optimal and balanced.
10. Seven things that you can do for good physical health are: eating healthy foods, exercising, getting plenty of sleep, avoiding harmful substances, practicing good hygiene, wearing protective sports gear and seat belts, and avoiding behaviors that could be dangerous.
11. Certain diseases can be passed down from parents to their biological children.
12. The environment can affect your health if you have to breathe smog-filled air or pollutants that can cause allergies and asthma attacks.
13. You can choose to spend time with family and friends, talk openly about your problems to a caring friend or family member, be open to new ideas, and take care of your physical health.
14. Five things that you can do to practice preventive healthcare are to avoid behavior that will get you into trouble, practice good hygiene, eat nutritious foods, wear safety equipment when playing sports, and buckle your seat belt.
15. The nine life skills are: assessing your health, making good decisions, setting goals, using refusal skills, communicating effectively, coping, evaluating media messages, practicing wellness, and being a wise consumer.
16. To assess your life skills, you can ask yourself these questions: "Which skills do I use most often? Am I having problems with a specific skill? How can I improve my use of life skills? Which skills should I be using more often? Do I feel comfortable using all of the skills?"

CHAPTER 1 REVIEW

Chapter Summary
- The four parts of your health are physical, emotional, social, and mental health.
- A balanced diet, exercise, and 8 hours of sleep each night are needed for good physical health.
- Expressing your feelings in a healthy way is a sign of good emotional health.
- Having good mental health helps you deal with problems effectively.
- Getting along well with other people is a sign of good social health.
- Wellness is having all parts of your health balanced.
- Your heredity and environment can influence your health.
- Your lifestyle and attitude affect your health.
- Life skills help you deal with problems that can affect your health, and these skills should be used in your everyday life.

Using Vocabulary

For each sentence, fill in the blank with the proper word from the word bank provided below.

hygiene	heredity
environment	life skills
preventive healthcare	health
lifestyle	attitude
health assessment	wellness

1. The passing of traits from a parent to his or her offspring is ___.
2. Taking care of yourself before you have an accident or get an illness is ___.
3. The set of behaviors by which you live is your ___.
4. The ___ is everything around you, including the air.
5. Someone who is always clean and well groomed is said to have good ___.
6. Your ___ includes a state of mind that affects the decisions you make.
7. Your ___ is based on balanced physical, mental, emotional, and social well-being.

Understanding Concepts

8. Name the four parts of your health.
9. How does the term *wellness* differ from the term *health*?
10. What seven things can you do to contribute to good physical health?
11. How does heredity influence your health?
12. How can the environment affect your health?
13. What four choices can you make to ensure a healthy lifestyle?
14. What are five things you can do to practice preventive healthcare?
15. List the nine life skills.
16. What five questions can you ask yourself to assess your life skills?
17. What is the relationship between having a good attitude and living a healthy lifestyle?

Critical Thinking

Applying Concepts

18. You've had infectious mononucleosis for a month, and your physical health isn't as good as is should be. Does your poor physical health have any effect on the other parts of your health? Explain your answer.

19. Your friend has learned that her father has an inherited medical condition. She is afraid that she may get it, too. How can your friend become informed about this medical condition? What information could you give her that would help her?

Making Good Decisions

20. Your friend told you that he has not been feeling well and doesn't have the energy to do anything. He said that some of his other friends suggested taking over-the-counter pills that would help him stay awake. Do you think that these pills are safe because they are sold over the counter? What could you say to your friend to help him?

21. Your friend's grandfather died a few months ago. Your friend has been quiet and doesn't want to hang out with anyone anymore. He finally tells you that he feels guilty because during his grandfather's illness, he spent more time with his friends than with his grandfather. What can you tell your friend to help him with his feelings?

22. Your friend has not been making good grades lately. She says that she prefers doing other things to studying. What life skills would you suggest to your friend to improve her grades?

Interpreting Graphics

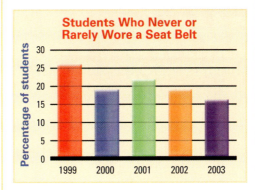

Use the figure above to answer questions 23–27.

23. What percentage of students never or rarely wore seat belts in 1999? in 2003?
24. According to this graph, what is the trend in the number of students who wear seat belts?
25. What percentage of students never or rarely wore seat belts in 2001?
26. What greater percentage of students wore seat belts in 2003 than in 2001?
27. What is one reason that you can give to explain why students are being more responsible in later years?

Reading Checkup

Take a minute to review your answers to the Health IQ questions at the beginning of this chapter. How has reading this chapter improved your Health IQ?

Model

Introduce this activity by reminding students that using this Life Skill will help them take personal responsibility for their behavior. Then, review the scenario with the class.

Prepare students for this activity by modeling each of the steps of the skill. Make sure students understand each step before you move on to the next one.

Guided Practice: Practice with a Friend

Guided Practice is the stage in which you and the students analyze their approach to solving the problem given in the scenario and analyze their ability to set goals. Have students read Act 1. Discuss with the class the situation described and the way students are to act it out. Organize the class into groups of three. In each group, one person plays the role of Logan, another person plays Amy, and the third person is the observer.

Proper pacing during the Guided Practice is important. The suggestions listed below will help you control the pace.

1. Stop after completing each step of setting goals.
2. Discuss with each group the observer's comments.
3. Ask the other members of each group to listen to the observer's suggestions and to suggest ways to improve their ability to set goals.
4. Instruct students to repeat the steps that need improvement and to include their modifications.

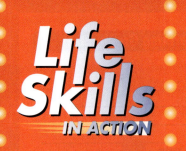

Life Skills IN ACTION

Setting Goals

A goal is something that you work toward and hope to achieve. Setting goals is important because goals give you a sense of purpose and achieving goals improves your self-esteem. Complete the following activity to learn how to set and achieve goals.

Lonely Logan

ACT 1

Setting the Scene

Logan's family moved to a new city over the summer. He started 7th grade in his new school a few weeks ago. Since then, Logan has met a lot of people but doesn't feel like he has any friends. Logan's older sister, Amy, isn't having any problems making new friends. Logan doesn't want to feel lonely forever, so he asks Amy for advice.

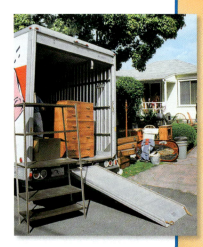

The 5 Steps of Setting Goals

1. Consider your interests and values.
2. Choose goals that include your interests and values.
3. If necessary, break down long-term goals into several short-term goals.
4. Measure your progress.
5. Reward your success.

Guided Practice

Practice with a Friend

Form a group of three. Have one person play the role of Logan and another person play the role of Amy. Have the third person be an observer. Walking through each of the five steps of setting goals, role-play Logan setting and working toward his goal of making new friends. Amy may give him advice and support when necessary. The observer will take notes, which will include observations about what the person playing Logan did well and suggestions of ways to improve. Stop after each step to evaluate the process.

5. Check to make sure that students understand each step before they move on to the next step.
6. If time permits, repeat the exercise three times, switching roles each time. Each student should have the opportunity to play each role. `Co-op Learning`

18 Chapter 1 • Life Skills in Action

Independent Practice

Check Yourself

After you have completed the guided practice, go through Act 1 again without stopping at each step. Answer the questions below to review what you did.

1. What interests and values could Logan consider before setting his goal?
2. Logan's long-term goal is to make new friends. What short-term goals could help him to meet his long-term goal?
3. How does Logan's goal relate to the four parts of his health?
4. What is one of your long-term goals? On which part of your health does your goal focus?

On Your Own

After several weeks, Logan has made many new friends. Two of his friends are reporters for the school newspaper. Logan thinks it would be fun to be a reporter and knows that working on the newspaper will allow him to spend more time with his friends. His friends tell him that he has to apply for a position as a reporter and write a sample newspaper article. Make a poster that shows how Logan could use the five steps of setting goals to work toward his goal of being a reporter.

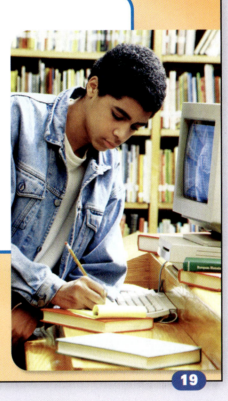

Independent Practice: Check Yourself

Instruct students to repeat Act 1 without stopping at each step. Remind students to apply what they learned in the Guided Practice to the Independent Practice.

Encourage students to use the Check Yourself questions as a starting point for reviewing and analyzing their Independent Practice. Remind students that as they change roles, the answers to these questions may change for each actor. Encourage students to create additional questions for checking their ability to set goals. When students have finished the Independent Practice, have them answer the Check Yourself questions in writing. Use their answers to assess their understanding of the steps of setting goals and to assess their use of the steps.

Check Yourself Answers

1. Sample answer: Logan should consider his interests in sports and other extracurricular activities and consider values such as being nice to other people and being a good friend.
2. Sample answer: Logan can set a short-term goal to speak to a new person every day or can set a goal to join a school sports team or club.
3. Sample answer: Logan's goal of making new friends will positively affect his social health. His goal will also improve his emotional health by making him happier. If Logan's emotional health improves, his mental health will also improve. If Logan decides to achieve his goal by joining a sports team, it will improve his physical health.
4. Sample answer: I have a long-term goal of going to college. This goal focuses on my mental health.

Act 2: On Your Own

This additional scenario gives students an opportunity to apply what they have learned in both the Guided Practice and the Independent Practice to a new situation.

Suggest to students that they use the Check Yourself questions as a starting point for setting goals in the new situation. Encourage students to be creative and to think of ways to improve their ability to set goals.

Assessment

Review the posters that students have created as part of the On Your Own activity. The posters should show that the students followed the steps of setting goals in a realistic and effective manner. Display the posters around the room. If time permits, discuss some of the posters with the class.

CHAPTER 2

Successful Decisions and Goals
Chapter Planning Guide

PACING	CLASSROOM RESOURCES	ACTIVITIES AND DEMONSTRATIONS
BLOCK 1 • 45 min pp. 20–23 **Chapter Opener**	**CRF** Health Inventory * ■ GENERAL **CRF** Parent Letter * ■	**SE** Health IQ, p. 21 **CRF** At-Home Activity * ■
Lesson 1 Decisions and Consequences	**CRF** Lesson Plan * **TT** Bellringer *	**TE** Activities Truth or Consequences, p. 19F **CRF** Enrichment Activity * ADVANCED
BLOCK 2 • 45 min pp. 24–27 **Lesson 2** Six Steps to Making Good Decisions	**CRF** Lesson Plan * **TT** Bellringer * **TT** Steps to Making Good Decisions *	**TE** Activities Mock Trial, p. 19F **TE** Group Activity Brainstorming, p. 25 ◆ BASIC **TE** Activity Options, p. 25 GENERAL **CRF** Enrichment Activity * ADVANCED
BLOCK 3 • 45 min pp. 28–31 **Lesson 3** Influences on Your Decisions	**CRF** Lesson Plan * **TT** Bellringer *	**TE** Activity Identifying Pressure, p. 29 GENERAL **TE** Group Activity Skit, p. 30 GENERAL **TE** Activity Ins and Outs, p. 30 GENERAL **CRF** Enrichment Activity * ADVANCED
BLOCK 4 • 45 min pp. 32–37 **Lesson 4** Setting Healthy Goals	**CRF** Lesson Plan * **TT** Bellringer *	**TE** Activity, pp. 32, 33 GENERAL **TE** Group Activity Role-Playing, p. 33 BASIC **SE** Social Studies Activity, p. 34 **TE** Activity Dream College, p. 34 ◆ BASIC **CRF** Life Skills Activity * ■ GENERAL **CRF** Enrichment Activity * ADVANCED
Lesson 5 How to Reach Your Goals	**CRF** Lesson Plan * **TT** Bellringer *	**TE** Activity Skit, p. 37 BASIC **CRF** Enrichment Activity * ADVANCED
BLOCK 5 • 45 min pp. 38–43 **Lesson 6** Changing Your Goals	**CRF** Lesson Plan * **TT** Bellringer *	**TE** Group Activity Road Map Detours, p. 38 ◆ GENERAL **CRF** Enrichment Activity * ADVANCED
Lesson 7 Skills for Success	**CRF** Lesson Plan * **TT** Bellringer * **TT** Using Refusal Skills 1 * **TT** Using Refusal Skills 2 *	**TE** Demonstration Communicating Emotions, p. 40 GENERAL **SE** Hands-on Activity, p. 41 **CRF** Datasheets for In-Text Activities * GENERAL **TE** Group Activity, pp. 41, 42 **TE** Activity Refusal Skills, p. 42 BASIC **SE** Life Skills in Action Using Refusal Skills, pp. 46–47 **CRF** Life Skills Activity * ■ GENERAL **CRF** Enrichment Activity * ADVANCED

BLOCKS 6 & 7 • 90 min — Chapter Review and Assessment Resources

- **SE** Chapter Review, pp. 44–45
- **CRF** Concept Review * ■ GENERAL
- **CRF** Health Behavior Contract * ■ GENERAL
- **CRF** Chapter Test * ■ GENERAL
- **CRF** Performance-Based Assessment * GENERAL
- **OSP** Test Generator
- **CRF** Test Item Listing *

Online Resources

Visit **go.hrw.com** for a variety of free resources related to this textbook. Enter the keyword **HD4DE7**.

Students can access interactive problem solving help and active visual concept development with the *Decisions for Health* Online Edition available at **www.hrw.com**.

CNN Student News
cnnstudentnews.com
Find the latest health news, lesson plans, and activities related to important scientific events.

Chapter 2 • Successful Decisions and Goals

Compression guide:
To shorten your instruction because of time limitations, omit Lessons 3 and 6.

KEY

- **TE** Teacher Edition
- **SE** Student Edition
- **OSP** One-Stop Planner
- **CRF** Chapter Resource File
- **TT** Teaching Transparency
- ✱ Also on One-Stop Planner
- ■ Also Available in Spanish
- ♦ Requires Advance Prep

SKILLS DEVELOPMENT RESOURCES	LESSON REVIEW AND ASSESSMENT	STANDARDS CORRELATION
		National Health Education Standards
TE Life Skill Builder Evaluating Media Messages, p. 23 ♦ GENERAL **CRF** Directed Reading * BASIC	**SE** Lesson Review, p. 23 **TE** Reteaching, Quiz, p. 23 **CRF** Lesson Quiz * ■ GENERAL	3.1
TE Life Skill Builder, pp. 24, 26 GENERAL **SE** Life Skills Activity Making Good Decisions, p. 27 **CRF** Cross-Disciplinary * GENERAL **CRF** Decision-Making * GENERAL **CRF** Directed Reading * BASIC	**SE** Lesson Review, p. 27 **TE** Reteaching, Quiz, p. 27 **TE** Alternative Assessment, p. 27 ADVANCED **CRF** Lesson Quiz * ■ GENERAL	1.6, 3.1, 3.4, 6.1, 6.3
TE Life Skill Builder Evaluating Media Messages, p. 28 ♦ GENERAL **SE** Study Tip Reading Effectively, p. 29 **TE** Reading Skill Builder Anticipation Guide, p. 29 BASIC **SE** Life Skills Activity Being a Wise Consumer, p. 30 **TE** Life Skill Builder Being a Wise Consumer, p. 30 ADVANCED **CRF** Decision-Making * GENERAL **CRF** Directed Reading * BASIC	**SE** Lesson Review, p. 31 **TE** Reteaching, Quiz, p. 31 **TE** Alternative Assessment, p. 31 ♦ BASIC **CRF** Lesson Quiz * ■ GENERAL	1.4, 2.1, 2.3, 3.3, 4.1, 4.2, 4.4, 5.2, 6.2
TE Life Skill Builder Setting Goals, p. 33 GENERAL **TE** Life Skill Builder Setting Goals, p. 34 GENERAL **CRF** Directed Reading * BASIC	**SE** Lesson Review, p. 35 **TE** Reteaching, Quiz, p. 35 **TE** Alternative Assessment, p. 35 ADVANCED **CRF** Concept Mapping * GENERAL **CRF** Lesson Quiz * ■ GENERAL	1.4, 3.1, 3.4, 5.4, 6.4
TE Life Skill Builder Evaluating Media Messages, p. 36 GENERAL **TE** Inclusion Strategies, p. 36 BASIC **CRF** Refusal Skills * GENERAL **CRF** Directed Reading * BASIC	**SE** Lesson Review, p. 37 **TE** Reteaching, Quiz, p. 37 **CRF** Lesson Quiz * ■ GENERAL	3.1, 3.4, 6.4
CRF Refusal Skills * GENERAL **CRF** Directed Reading * BASIC	**SE** Lesson Review, p. 39 **TE** Reteaching, Quiz, p. 39 **CRF** Lesson Quiz * ■ GENERAL	3.4, 6.4, 6.5
TE Inclusion Strategies, p. 41 GENERAL **TE** Life Skill Builder Using Refusal Skills, p. 42 GENERAL **CRF** Cross-Disciplinary * GENERAL **CRF** Directed Reading * BASIC	**SE** Lesson Review, p. 43 **TE** Reteaching, Quiz, p. 43 **TE** Alternative Assessment, p. 43 ADVANCED **CRF** Concept Mapping * GENERAL **CRF** Lesson Quiz * ■ GENERAL	1.6, 3.1, 3.4, 3.6, 5.3, 5.6, 6.4

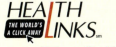

www.scilinks.org/health

Maintained by the **National Science Teachers Association**

Topic: Smoking and Health
HealthLinks code: HD4090

Topic: Truth in Advertising
HealthLinks code: HD4103

Topic: Building a Healthy Self-Esteem
HealthLinks code: HD4020

Topic: Communication Skills
HealthLinks code: HD4022

Technology Resources

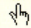 **One-Stop Planner**
All of your printable resources and the Test Generator are on this convenient CD-ROM.

 Guided Reading Audio CDs

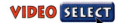

For information about videos related to this chapter, go to **go.hrw.com** and type in the keyword **HD4DE7V**.

Chapter 2 • Chapter Planning Guide   19B

CHAPTER 2
Successful Decisions and Goals
Chapter Resources

Teacher Resources

TEACHING TRANSPARENCIES

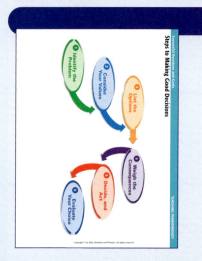
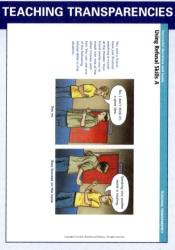
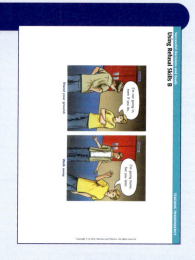

BELLRINGER TRANSPARENCIES

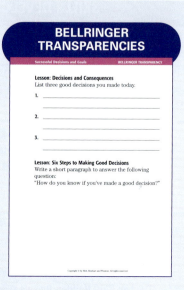

LESSON PLANS

PARENT LETTER

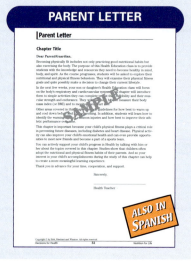

TEST ITEM LISTING

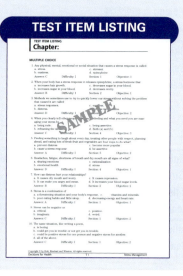

Meeting Individual Needs

DIRECTED READING
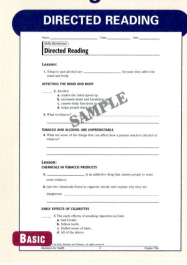
BASIC

CONCEPT MAPPING
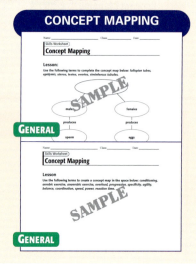
GENERAL

CONCEPT REVIEW
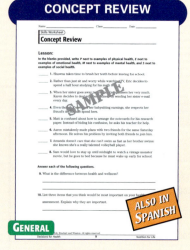
GENERAL

ENRICHMENT ACTIVITIES
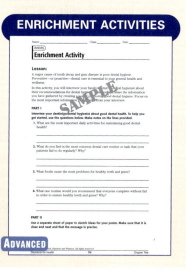
ADVANCED

Resources

These worksheet pages can be found in the Chapter Resource File and the One-Stop Planner. The transparencies can be found in the Teaching Transparencies binder and on the One-Stop Planner.

Activities

LIFE SKILLS ACTIVITIES   **AT-HOME ACTIVITY**   **DATASHEETS FOR IN-TEXT ACTIVITIES**

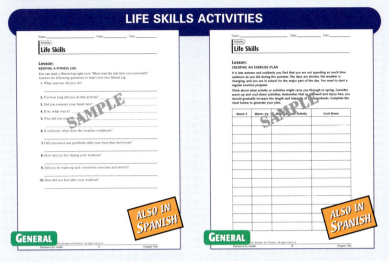
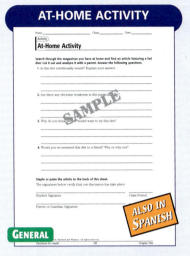
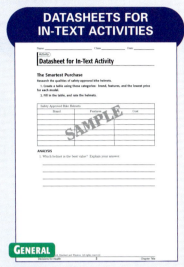

Applications

DECISION-MAKING   **REFUSAL SKILLS**   **CROSS-DISCIPLINARY**   **HEALTH BEHAVIOR CONTRACT**

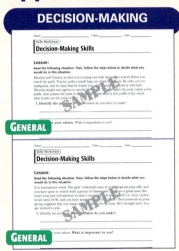
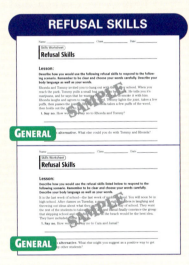
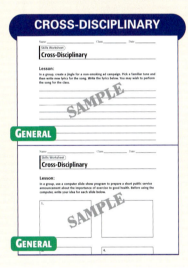
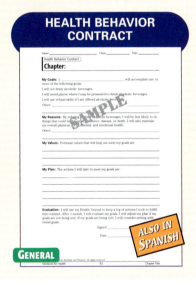

Assessments

HEALTH INVENTORY   **LESSON QUIZZES**   **CHAPTER TEST**   **PERFORMANCE-BASED ASSESSMENT**

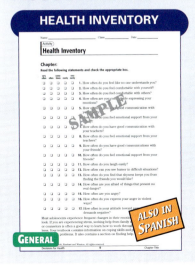
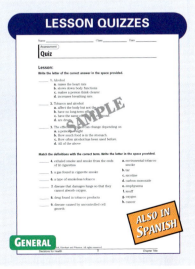
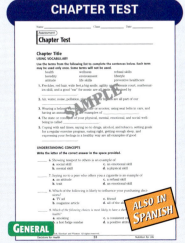
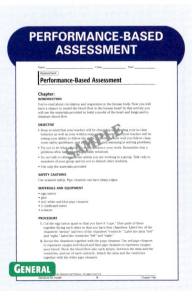

Chapter 2 • Chapter Resources and Worksheets   **19D**

Background Information

CHAPTER 2

The following information focuses on identifying interests and reaching goals. This material will help prepare you for teaching the concepts in this chapter.

Identifying Interests

- People who are the happiest are those who do what interests them most. However, sometimes it is difficult to pinpoint what a person's interests are. Below are a few activities that can help a person identify his or her interests.

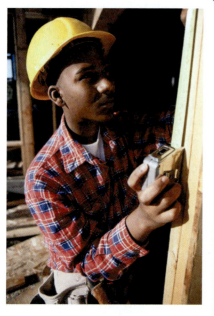

- **Nurture Yourself** Practicing good health behaviors—such as getting plenty of exercise and sleep, and eating nutritious foods—helps one hear his or her inner voice. A 20-minute walk in the park (without a radio) is a wonderful way to clear one's mind and to get in touch with oneself.

- **Become Aware** Things that excite, motivate, and touch a person emotionally are indicative of a person's interests. What does a person daydream about? These images are a great way for someone to become aware of his or her interests and desires.

- **Without Regret** One way to identify interests is to ask the question, "What would I do if I wanted to live my life without regrets?"

Tips on Reaching Goals

- **Work on One Goal at a Time** Some people overwhelm themselves by working on too many things at the same time. Sometimes, it helps to choose to work on only one thing at a time. Doing this will make it is easier to stay focused and to become successful.

- **Brainstorm** Brainstorming is an excellent way to come up with options and different ways to meet a goal.

- **Encourage Friends** A little encouragement goes a long way, and it can help motivate a person when a task seems daunting, or when he or she feels discouraged. If you give your friends encouragement, they will encourage you as you work toward your goals.

- **Take Action** Taking action may sometimes mean taking risks. But, taking risks sometimes yields the greatest rewards.

Removing Obstacles

- The most common obstacles to reaching goals are the lack of time, the lack of money, and fear. Below are some tips on how to overcome these obstacles.

  - **Time** A person can find the time to pursue a goal by doing a few simple things, such as turning off the television 2 to 3 hours per week, getting up one hour earlier once a week, and setting aside one hour every weekend. Doing this will provide up to 20 hours a month to pursue a goal.

  - **Money** Community centers provide many free programs that can help someone pursue his or her goals. Furthermore, libraries have information and books on grants, scholarships, fellowships, and contests.

  - **Fear** One way you can get over being afraid of trying something new is to ask others for advice or participate in a brainstorming session. Often, others will bring up options that you may not have previously considered.

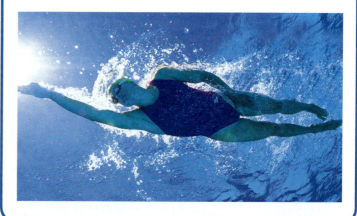

For background information about teaching strategies and issues, refer to the Professional Reference for Teachers.

ACTIVITIES

CHAPTER 2

Consider using the activities on this page as students explore the lessons of this chapter. Look for other activities throughout the Student Edition chapter.

Mock Trial

Explain to students that judges and juries make important decisions every day. They must decide the guilt or innocence of accused criminals and they must assign responsibility for problems. Tell students that they are going to stage a mock trial and compare the proceedings to the decision-making process in this chapter. However, instead of hearing a criminal case, they will put a controversial issue on trial.

Procedure Have the class pick an issue to put on trial. Form two groups with 3 to 5 students in each group. One group is the prosecution team (argues against the issue) and the other is the defense team (argues in favor of the issue). The rest of the class will be the jury. You will be the judge, but the jury will make the final decision.

Have students research the positive and negative consequences surrounding the issue and develop a case with the information they found. Conduct a mock trial by allowing a 5-minute presentation from each side, an opportunity for the jury to ask both sides questions, and a 2-minute rebuttal from each side. The jury should deliberate and vote on the issue.

Analysis Ask students the following questions:

- Which step of the six-step decision-making process did the trial most resemble? (The trial most resembled step four: weigh the consequences.)

- Why is it important for the prosecution and defense to research and present good information and facts? (Sample answer: The jury needs the information in order to make the right decision.)

- How is a trial different from your own decision making? How is it similar? (Sample answers: It is different because you don't have a jury—you have to make the decision yourself. It is similar because the jury weighs evidence just as you weigh consequences when making decisions.)

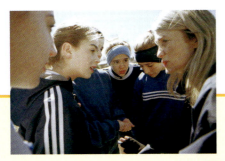

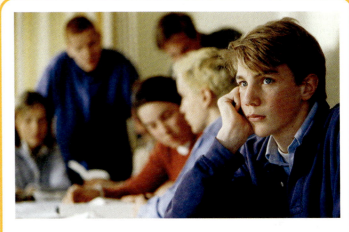

Truth or Consequences

Hands on

Procedure Have students work in groups to create a board game called *Truth or Consequences*. Students must develop rules, board design, and game pieces. Student must also write the Decision Cards and the Consequence Cards described below. All board games must adhere to the following criteria:

- The object of the game is to be the first person to reach a spot on the board called "Honesty."

- If a player lands on a "Decisions" square, he must draw a Decision Card. Each Decision Card describes a decision the player has to make. After making his or her decision, the player must then draw a Consequence Card. Consequence Cards may have positive consequences or negative consequences. For example, a player may be instructed to move forward, move backward, or to lose a turn.

Analysis Give students a chance to play their games and ask the following questions:

- How were the decisions you made while playing your game different from the decisions you make in real life? (Sample answer: In this game, I didn't worry about making bad decisions because the consequences were not real.)

- How were the decisions you made while playing your game similar to the decisions you make in real life? (Sample answer: Like in real life, all the decisions I made led to a consequence.)

Chapter 2 • Activities   19F

CHAPTER 2

Overview

In this chapter students learn that their decisions have consequences that affect themselves and others. Students learn to make good decisions using a six-step process. Students also learn how their values, their family, their friends, and the media influence their decisions. This chapter explains the importance of setting goals, explains how goals build healthy relationships, and relates achieving goals to success. Finally, students learn the importance of using good communication skills and refusal skills.

Question Box

Students may feel more comfortable asking questions if you set up a Question Box to collect their questions. Have students write and anonymously submit their questions about decision making and goal setting. Address these questions during class, or use these questions to introduce lessons that cover related topics.

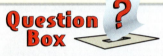

Check out *Current Health* articles and activities related to this chapter by visiting the HRW Web site at **go.hrw.com**. Just type in the keyword **HD4CH17T**.

Chapter Resource File
- Directed Reading BASIC
- Health Inventory GENERAL
- Parent Letter

CHAPTER 2 Successful Decisions and Goals

Lessons
1. Decisions and Consequences — 22
2. Six Steps to Making Good Decisions — 24
3. Influences on Your Decisions — 28
4. Setting Healthy Goals — 32
5. How to Reach Your Goals — 36
6. Changing Your Goals — 38
7. Skills for Success — 40

Chapter Review — 44
Life Skills in Action — 46

Check out *Current Health* articles related to this chapter by visiting **go.hrw.com**. Just type in the keyword **HD4CH17**.

Standards Correlations

National Health Education Standards

2.3 (partial) Analyze how media influences the selection of health information and products. (Lesson 3)

3.1 Explain the importance of assuming responsibility for personal health behaviors. (Lesson 1)

4.1 (partial) Describe the influence of cultural beliefs on health behaviors and the use of health services. (Lesson 3)

4.2 Analyze how messages from media and other sources influence health behaviors. (Lesson 3)

4.4 Analyze how information from peers influences health. (Lesson 3)

5.1 Demonstrate effective verbal and nonverbal communication skills to enhance health. (Lesson 7)

5.3 Demonstrate healthy ways to express needs, wants, and feelings. (Lesson 7)

5.5 Demonstrate communication skills to build and maintain healthy relationships. (Lesson 7)

5.6 (partial) Demonstrate refusal and negotiation skills to enhance health. (Lesson 7)

6.1 (partial) Demonstrate the ability to apply a decision-making process to health issues and problems individually and collaboratively. (Lesson 2)

> **"My friends** kept **bugging** me to go to this **party.** I didn't know **anyone** that was going to be there, so I **didn't want to go.** But my friends just kept pushing me. Finally, I had to put my foot down and tell them to quit bothering me. I must have gotten through to them, because after that they left me alone.**"**

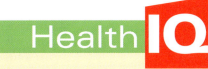

PRE-READING

Answer the following multiple-choice questions to find out what you already know about making decisions. When you've finished this chapter, you'll have the opportunity to change your answers based on what you've learned.

1. Which of the following is an example of peer pressure?
   a. You have power over your actions.
   b. An adult has power over your actions.
   c. Your friend has power over your actions.
   d. The media has power over your actions.

2. Choose the correct statement about values.
   a. Values are beliefs that are important to you.
   b. Values change as goals change.
   c. Values change depending on your situation.
   d. Values are the beliefs you get from your friends.

3. Which of the following statements about interests is true?
   a. Interests never change.
   b. Interests change easily.
   c. Interests are steps to reaching your goal.
   d. Interests always lead to a career.

4. Success can best be defined by
   a. making good decisions.
   b. defining your values.
   c. becoming famous.
   d. reaching your goals.

5. What may cause you to change your action plan?
   a. a change in interests
   b. a change in goals
   c. a setback
   d. all of the above

6. When you make a good decision, you
   a. do what other people tell you to do.
   b. make a lot of money.
   c. carefully consider your options.
   d. make others happy.

ANSWERS: 1. c; 2. a; 3. b; 4. d; 5. d; 6. c

Using the Health IQ

Misconception Alert
Answers to the Health IQ questions may help you identify students' misconceptions.

Question 4: Some students may think that success is defined by how much money a person has or by how famous a person is. Point out that money and fame are only true measures of success if obtaining them was a person's goal in the first place.

Question 6: Some students may be surprised to learn that making others happy does not determine whether a decision is good or bad. Explain to students that they should not aim to please other people. Instead, they should focus on their values and carefully consider all of their options before making a decision.

Answers
1. c
2. a
3. b
4. d
5. d
6. c

VIDEO SELECT
For information about videos related to this chapter, go to **go.hrw.com** and type in the keyword **HD4DE7V**.

6.2 Analyze how health-related decisions are influenced by individuals, family, and community values. (Lessons 2–3)

6.3 Predict how decisions regarding health behaviors have consequences for self and others. (Lesson 1)

6.4 Apply strategies and skills needed to attain personal health goals. (Lesson 5)

6.5 (partial) Describe how personal health goals are influenced by changing information, abilities, priorities, and responsibilities. (Lesson 6)

Chapter 2 • Successful Decisions and Goals

Lesson 1

Focus

Overview
Before beginning this lesson, review with your students the objectives listed under the What You'll Do head in the Student Edition. In this lesson, students learn that a good decision is a responsible decision. Students also learn that decisions have consequences and learn that there are different types of consequences.

Bellringer
Ask students to list three good decisions they made this morning. (Sample answer: Getting ready for school, eating a healthy breakfast, and selecting warm clothes to wear.) **LS** Verbal

Answer to Start Off Write
Accept all reasonable answers. Sample answer: A consequence of deciding to go bowling was that I had fun with my friends.

Motivate

Discussion ——— GENERAL
Bad Decisions Ask students to describe a decision that they made that resulted in negative consequences. What were the consequences? If they could make the same decision again, what would they do differently? What do they predict the consequences of the new decision to be? **LS** Verbal

Lesson 1 — Decisions and Consequences

What You'll Do
- **Explain** how a good decision is a responsible decision.
- **Explain** the different types of consequences that decisions have.

Terms to Learn
- good decision
- consequence

Start Off Write
What was the consequence of the last decision that you made?

What are three decisions you've made since you woke up this morning? You make decisions every day, from what clothes to wear to what lunch to eat. You control what happens to you. And each day is shaped by your decisions.

Most teenagers think they don't have much control over their life. But you probably have more control than you realize! In this lesson, you'll learn more about what you can control and how your decisions affect you.

You Are in Control

Being in control means that you can make your own choices. You make choices every day. You don't have to do what your friends tell you to do. You make choices about how you will act, what you will do, and who your friends are. A *decision* is a choice that you make and act upon. But how do you know if you are making a good decision? A **good decision** is a decision in which you have carefully considered the outcome of each choice. A good decision is a responsible decision. To be responsible, you must think through each decision to select the best choice possible. A responsible person knows right from wrong and makes wise choices.

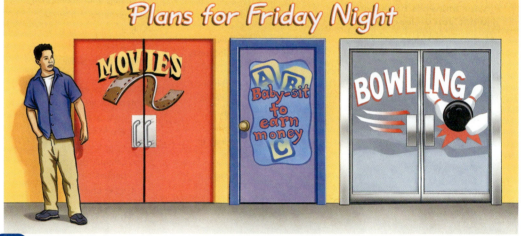

Figure 1 Even decisions about what to do on a Friday night can be difficult to make.

22

MISCONCEPTION ALERT

Consequences Some students may think that a decision not to do something does not have any consequences. Tell students the following may help them understand that such decisions do have consequences: "If you decide not to buy a pair of shoes, you will not have new shoes, the salesperson will not receive credit for a sale, and another person will have a chance to buy the shoes."

Chapter Resource File
- Directed Reading BASIC
- Lesson Plan
- Lesson Quiz GENERAL

Transparencies
TT Bellringer

22   Chapter 2 • Successful Decisions and Goals

Your Decisions Have Consequences

Whenever you make a decision, something happens. For example, if you decide to turn on a light, the room you are in fills with light. Your decision to turn on a light had a consequence. A ==consequence== is the result of a decision. Every decision has consequences. Even a decision to do nothing has consequences. For example, if it's time to sign up for electives at school and you do nothing, what happens? You won't get the classes you want, and you may have to take a class you don't want to take.

Consequences of your decisions not only affect you but also affect the people around you. There are three types of consequences:

- *Positive consequences* help you or others.
- *Negative consequences* do harm to you or to others.
- *Neutral consequences* are neither helpful nor harmful.

What consequences occur if a player on the soccer team shown in Figure 2 decides to quit? A positive consequence is that the player will have more free time. A negative consequence is that the team will lose an experienced player. The player's decision affects her and the people around her.

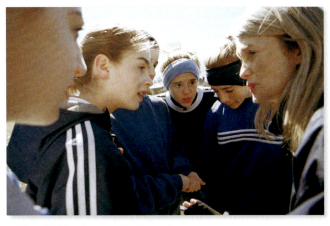

Figure 2 If a player quits, the entire team will suffer the consequences!

Lesson Review

Using Vocabulary
1. Use an example to explain what a good decision is.
2. What is a consequence?

Understanding Concepts
3. What is the difference between positive, negative, and neutral consequences?
4. How does a responsible person make good decisions?

Critical Thinking
5. **Making Predictions** What consequences would your decision to join the track team have for your family? for your friends?

Teach

Life SKILL BUILDER — GENERAL

Evaluating Media Messages
Have students sort through newspapers to find three current events in which a person made a decision that resulted in a consequence. Students should find an example for each type of consequence—positive, negative, and neutral. Ask students to identify the decisions made and the consequences of each decision. Invite volunteers to summarize their articles in front of the class. **LS Verbal**

Close

Reteaching — BASIC

Distinguishing Consequences
Pair each student with a partner. Have one student give an example of a good decision he or she made that had a positive consequence. Have the same student describe a decision that he or she made that had negative consequences and then describe a decision that had neutral consequences. Students should switch roles and repeat the activity. **LS Intrapersonal**

Quiz — GENERAL

Decide if the situations listed below have mostly positive consequences, negative consequences, or neutral consequences.

1. sleeping eight hours each night (positive consequences)
2. turning your homework in two days late (negative consequences)
3. planting a garden (positive consequences)
4. waiting until the second ring before you pick up the telephone (neutral consequences)
5. talking while you wait in line at the cafeteria (neutral consequences)

Answers to Lesson Review

1. Answers may vary but each answer should be an example of a decision in which a person has carefully considered the outcome of each choice.
2. A consequence is the result of a decision.
3. Positive consequences help you or others, negative consequences harm you or others, and neutral consequences are neither helpful nor harmful.
4. A responsible person thinks through each decision to select the best choice possible.
5. Answers may vary. Sample answer: My family would enjoy watching me compete at track meets and would have to take me to and from practice. I would not be able to see my friends as much after school while I am training.

Lesson 1 • Decisions and Consequences

Lesson 2

Focus

Overview
Before beginning this lesson, review with your students the objectives listed under the What You'll Do head in the Student Edition. This lesson explains the six steps to making good decisions and describes how values influence a person's decisions. Students will learn the importance of evaluating decisions by looking at the benefits and risks of all options.

 Bellringer
Have students write a short paragraph to answer to the question: "How do you know if you made a good decision?" **LS Verbal**

Answer to Start Off Write
Accept all reasonable answers. Sample answer: Weighing the consequences of each option will help you make the best choice possible.

Motivate

Life SKILL BUILDER — GENERAL

Assessing Your Health Have students identify three bad habits they would like to change. Ask students to think about each of these habits and try to decide what causes the habits. For example, a student might bite her nails when she is nervous. Once students have identified the causes of their bad habits, they can start to devise a plan to change their behaviors using the six steps outlined in this lesson. **LS Intrapersonal**

Lesson 2 — Six Steps to Making Good Decisions

What You'll Do
- **List** the six steps to making good decisions.
- **Describe** how your values influence your decisions.
- **Explain** the importance of looking at the benefits and risks of your options.
- **Explain** why you should evaluate your decisions.

Terms to Learn
- values
- option
- brainstorming

 Start Off Write
Why should you weigh the consequences before you make a decision?

Emma really isn't sure what to do. Elizabeth, her friend, asked her to go to the movies on the same night that Bobby asked her to his party. She doesn't want to hurt anyone's feelings. How can she decide what to do?

Whether you're choosing what you will do Friday night or what career you want to have someday, making decisions is tough! In this lesson, you'll learn six steps that you can follow to make good decisions. You'll see how your values influence your choices. You will also learn how to make the best choices possible.

Identify the Problem

The first step in making a decision is to identify the problem. For example, what would you do if your friends dared you to cut class with them? At first, you may think that the problem is taking the dare. You might take the dare just because they asked you to. However, the real problem is to decide if missing class is okay. If you thought about that problem, your decision might be very different. Problems can be hard to identify. Asking a parent or trusted friend for advice may help you.

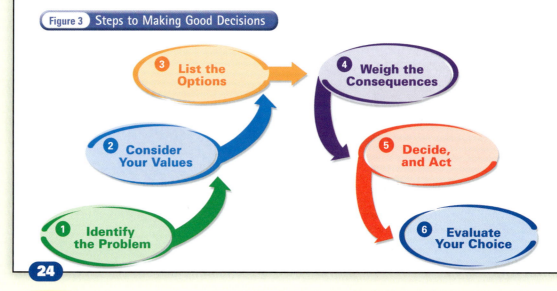

Figure 3 Steps to Making Good Decisions

Career

Emergency Room Doctor Tell students that emergency room doctors must make fast decisions. Because the consequences of their decisions can vary greatly, their decisions must also be very reliable. Emergency room doctors may go through a similar decision-making process like the one described in this lesson, but they do so very quickly.

Chapter Resource File
- Directed Reading **BASIC**
- Lesson Plan
- Lesson Quiz **GENERAL**

 Transparencies
TT Bellringer
TT Steps to Making Good Decisions

24 Chapter 2 • Successful Decisions and Goals

Consider Your Values

Knowing your values will help you make good decisions. **Values** are the beliefs that you consider to be of great importance. Some good values are honesty, kindness, and generosity. It's important to know your values before you face problems. Your values influence your decisions by guiding you when problems arise. For example, if you value being responsible, you won't skip class. How do you determine your values? Think about what kind of person you want to be. In other words, think about your character. *Character* is the way a person thinks, feels, and acts. Your character is a reflection of your values. Character based on good values will help you make good decisions.

Health Journal
List four values that are very important to you. Describe why making a decision that goes against these four values would be difficult.

List the Options

After you consider your values, the next step is to list your options. **Options** are different choices that you can make. The best way to identify your options is by brainstorming with several other people. **Brainstorming** is thinking of all the possible ways to carry out your decision. If possible, you should write down your ideas. A written list will allow you to quickly compare your options. For example, when you are deciding if you will cut class, one option is to tell your friends no. A second option is to agree with your friends' idea and cut class together. Another possibility is to suggest that you all go to class but do something fun after school. There is always more than one option for you to choose from.

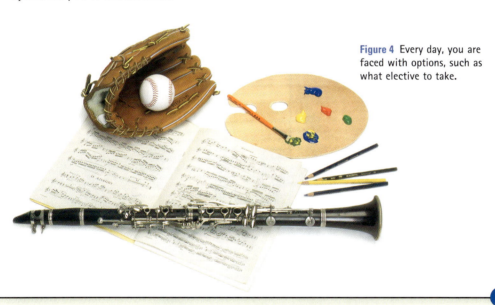

Figure 4 Every day, you are faced with options, such as what elective to take.

Cultural Awareness — BASIC

Comparing Values Tell students that showing respect for parents and elders is a common value across cultures. Invite students from different cultures and backgrounds to describe some of the ways they show respect for elders. Ask the rest of the class to compare the actions described with the signs of respect they use. Also ask students to identify some signs of respect they think could be used in their own cultures. **LS Interpersonal**

Answer to Health Journal
Answers may vary. This Health Journal can be used to begin a class discussion on values and decision making. Remember that some students may be uncomfortable sharing personal information.

Teach

Discussion — GENERAL

Identifying Values To help students identify their values, ask them the following questions:

- What values have your parents tried to instill in you? (Sample answers: Get an education and respect others.)
- What values are reflected in laws? (Sample answer: Do not kill or harm anyone or take or destroy another person's possessions.)
- What values have you learned from the media? (Sample answer: Be tolerant of other people who come from different backgrounds.)

Finally, have students list some of their values. Remind students that their values influence the decisions they make. **LS Verbal**

Group Activity — BASIC

Brainstorming Distribute crayons, paper, 2 triangles, and 1 circle to each group. Ask groups to create as many pictures as they can in 5 minutes according to these rules:

- Use only the 3 shapes given to them. Dots, lines, and curves are allowed, but they cannot be used to make other shapes.
- Trace around each shape, but do not change its size.

Explain to students that this is a brainstorming process and that brainstorming can be used to solve many types of problems. **LS Visual** **English Language Learners**

Activity — GENERAL

Options Tell students the following: "You are responsible for the household budget and need to cut expenses. List ways that you could save money." (Sample answers: cancel magazine subscriptions, turn off lights, and rent movies less frequently) **LS Logical**

Lesson 2 • Six Steps to Making Good Decisions

Teach, continued

Discussion — BASIC

Transportation Ask students to brainstorm the benefits and risks of riding a bicycle to school. (Sample answers: Benefits include exercise, getting fresh air, and having independence. Risks include problems with safety, arriving late because you are going slower, and having trouble carrying several things.) Ask students to describe things a person can do to reduce the risks listed. (Sample answers: Following bicycle safety rules and wearing safety equipment can reduce the safety risk. Leaving earlier would get a person to school on time. Storing some equipment in a school locker would reduce one's load.) **LS** Verbal

Life SKILL BUILDER — GENERAL

Making Good Decisions Tell students that they sometimes will have to make decisions to do something despite the risks involved. In order for the students to make good decisions in such situations, they must determine if the benefits outweigh the risks. For example, a student might decide to join the school football team although he knows that there is a risk that he might be injured. However, joining the team will teach him discipline, will provide him with exercise, and will help him make new friends. Explain that people should not always avoid risks, but they should carefully consider whether certain risks are worth taking. Have students describe a time in which they made a decision that involved taking risks. **LS** Intrapersonal

Myth & Fact

Myth: If you change your mind about a decision you made, you will look like a person who can't stick with a decision.

Fact: Making a decision that is right for you is more important than worrying about what other people think.

Weigh the Consequences

When you weigh the consequences of a possible decision, you compare the benefits and risks of your options. Every option will have risks and benefits to consider. Start by making two columns. Label one column "Benefits" and the other column "Risks." Consider the example of cutting class again. One benefit of deciding to skip class is that your friends wouldn't be angry with you. Another benefit is not having to sit through your least favorite class. But what are the risks? First, cutting class would get you in serious trouble with the school. Second, you would miss the lesson and get behind, which could cause your grade to suffer. Another, more serious risk is that your parents might lose trust in you. Now, look at your list. Do the benefits outweigh the risks? Whenever you have to make a decision, weigh the benefits and risks of each option very carefully. Doing so will help you make good decisions.

Decide, and Act

You have done your best to think about your options. Now you are ready to act on your decision. Think hard. Some decisions can be made only once. When you make your choice, take action! For example, you decide that getting in trouble with your parents and the school is not worth cutting class. In this case, the risks of cutting class certainly outweigh the benefits. So, you decide to tell your friends that you aren't cutting class with them. When they try to change your mind, you stay firm. You make a decision, and you follow through with it. Making a choice and acting on your decision are important in decision making.

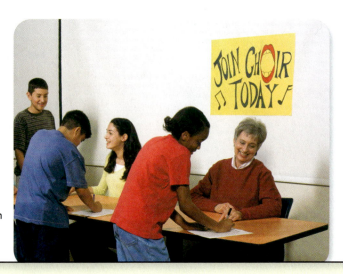

Figure 5 These teens have decided to join choir. By signing up for choir, they are following through with their decision.

SOCIAL STUDIES CONNECTION — ADVANCED

The Bill of Rights Remind students that after the United States declared its independence from England, the U.S. debated which rights and values to uphold for all citizens. Have students investigate the debates over the Bill of Rights. Students should list the benefits and risks of one item in the Bill of Rights. Students should also summarize how some of these rights changed over time and describe how these changes took place. **LS** Verbal

26 Chapter 2 • Successful Decisions and Goals

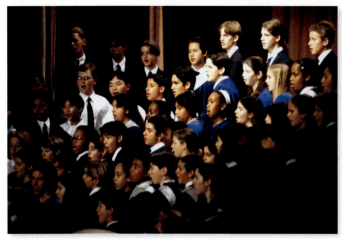

Figure 6 These teens appear happy with their decision to join the choir.

Evaluate Your Choice

You made your decision, and you carried it out. But you aren't finished yet. You may face this problem again, so it is important to look back at your decision. If you answer yes to one or more of the following questions, you may want to choose a different option in the future.

- Did your decision harm anyone?
- Were you unhappy with the result?
- Would another option have had a better consequence?

By evaluating your choices, you learn which options work for you and which don't. Using this procedure takes practice. But the more you use it, the easier it gets!

LIFE SKILLS ACTIVITY

MAKING GOOD DECISIONS

In a small group, think of a situation in which a decision is needed. Write your scenario on a card, and swap cards with another group. In your group, brainstorm ways to solve the problem. Remember to use the six-step method for making decisions. What was your group's decision? Each group will evaluate the other group's decision.

Lesson Review

Using Vocabulary

1. Define the term *values* in your own words. How do your values influence your decisions?
2. What is an option?
3. Explain what you do when you brainstorm.

Understanding Concepts

4. Why should you weigh the risks and benefits of your options?

5. Why is it important to evaluate your choices?

Critical Thinking

6. **Making Good Decisions** Imagine a situation in which you are having trouble making a decision. Write down each of the six decision-making steps. Then apply each step to the situation that you imagined.

internet connect
www.scilinks.org/health
Topic: Smoking and Health
HealthLinks code: HD4090
HEALTH LINKS. Maintained by the National Science Teachers Association

---

Answers to Lesson Review

1. Values are beliefs you consider to be of great importance. Values guide you when you are making decisions.
2. Options are different choices that you can make.
3. When you brainstorm, you think of as many options as you can and write them down.
4. Weighing the risks and benefits of your options will help you make good decisions.
5. It is important to evaluate your choices because you learn which options work for you and which options do not work. If you face the same problem again, you will be better prepared for it.
6. Answers may vary, but all answers should describe an application of the six steps outlined in this lesson.

Close

Reteaching — BASIC

Mnemonic Device Write the following terms on the blackboard: *problem, values, options, consequences, action,* and *evaluation*. Have students make a sentence using the first letters in each term to help them remember the six steps to making good decisions. (Sample sentence: Please vacuum over carpets and everywhere.) Have them use their sentence to summarize this lesson with a partner.
LS Verbal

Quiz — GENERAL

1. What are three things you could ask yourself when evaluating your decisions? (Sample answer: You should ask if the decision was harmful, if it made you happy, and if you could have made a better choice.)
2. How does a written list help a person who is brainstorming? (A written list allows you to quickly compare your options.)
3. Does a person experience consequences if they decide against doing something? Explain with an example. (Sample answer: yes; If you don't join the school choir, you will not be able to sing in the choir concert.)

Alternative Assessment — ADVANCED

Historical Decisions Encourage interested students to research and write a report about a courageous historical figure who acted on his or her values in spite of the possible consequences of his or her decision. In their report, students should explain how the decisions of these people changed the course of history. **LS Verbal**

Lesson 3

Focus

Overview
Before beginning this lesson, review with your students the objectives listed under the What You'll Do head in the Student Edition. This lesson describes several influences on decision making.

Bellringer
Have students list the names of five people they know who influence their decisions. After each name, students should describe how the person influences them.
LS Interpersonal

Answer to Start Off Write
Accept all reasonable answers. Sample answer: My mother influences my decisions because she cares about me and I respect her opinions.

Motivate

Discussion — GENERAL
Influences Start a discussion with your students about the influences in their lives by asking the following questions:

- How do your parents or caregivers influence the decisions you make? (Sample answer: My parents expect me to get good grades, so I study very hard.)
- How do your friends influence your decisions? (Sample answer: I want my friends to like me, so I do things that they like to do.)
- Describe a time that you wanted something after seeing a commercial for it. (Answers may vary.)

LS Intrapersonal

Lesson 3 — Influences on Your Decisions

What You'll Do
- **Describe** how family and cultural traditions influence your decisions.
- **Explain** how peer pressure affects the decisions that you make.
- **Identify** the media as a major influence in your decision making.
- **Explain** how your decisions change based on new information.

Terms to Learn
- peer pressure

Start Off Write
Who influences most of your major decisions? Why is this person so influential?

Marcus is trying to decide what CD to buy. His friend is telling him to get the newest rock release. But he really wants to buy a new rap CD. At the same time, he knows that his parents would like him to develop an interest in classical music.

Like Marcus's choices, many of your choices are influenced by other people. Your family, friends, other people, and things around you all have an influence on your decisions.

Your Family

Your family is the most important influence in your life. Every family has values, cultural beliefs, and traditions. How often you have to help out at home reflects your family value of responsibility. What your parents say about dating reflects their cultural beliefs. What your family does on holidays reflects your family's traditions. These values, beliefs, and traditions are a part of your character. You are aware of them whenever you make decisions. Therefore, they influence your decisions.

Your family also affects your decisions about your health practices. Decisions you make about how much you exercise, what food you eat, and how you react to stress probably reflect your family's habits.

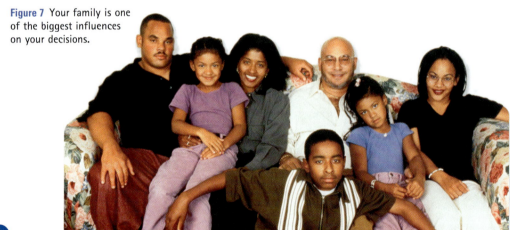

Figure 7 Your family is one of the biggest influences on your decisions.

 — GENERAL

Evaluating Media Messages Show students a videotape of an episode of a family sitcom. Ask students to analyze how the members of the family influence each other. Ask students to explain how the influences shown are similar to or different from the influences in their families. Finally, ask students to describe how the television show does or does not accurately depict reality. **Note:** You may need to obtain the permission of your school's administration before showing the video. **LS Verbal**

Chapter Resource File
- Directed Reading **BASIC**
- Lesson Plan
- Lesson Quiz **GENERAL**

Transparencies
TT Bellringer

---

28 Chapter 2 • Successful Decisions and Goals

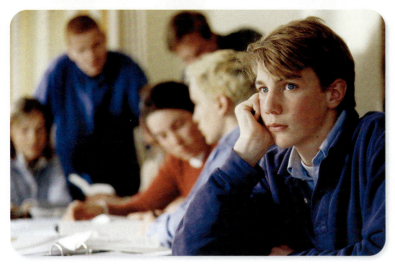

Figure 8 Convincing your friends to ask the new student to join your group is an example of positive peer pressure.

Peer Pressure

Your peers are another important influence in your life. A *peer* is someone who is about the same age as you are and with whom you interact. Sometimes, you get pressure from your peers to do something. This pressure is called peer pressure. Peer pressure is a feeling that you should do something that your friends want you to do. Peer pressure can come from one friend or from a group of friends. Groups can have a powerful influence on teens. A group expects certain behaviors from its members. Think about a certain group at your school. Do the members of the group dress alike? Do they enjoy most of the same activities? Peer pressure from a group can be particularly powerful. It is hard to say no to a group of people who are your friends.

Most teens face peer pressure related to drinking alcohol, smoking, cheating, or gossiping. In these situations, your friends may tell you that everyone else is doing these things. By telling you that, your friends put pressure on you to go along with them. But everyone else is probably not doing the things that your friends are suggesting. This kind of peer pressure is negative. *Negative peer pressure* is pressure to do things that could harm you or others. But not all peer pressure is negative. *Positive peer pressure* influences you to do something that will benefit you or someone else. For example, if your friends are studying together for a big math test, you may join in and study, too. This kind of peer pressure makes you feel good about yourself and your friends.

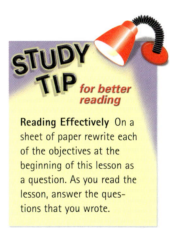

Study Tip for better reading

Reading Effectively On a sheet of paper rewrite each of the objectives at the beginning of this lesson as a question. As you read the lesson, answer the questions that you wrote.

Teach

READING SKILL BUILDER — BASIC

Anticipation Guide Before students read this lesson, have them answer the following true/false questions. Give students a chance to revise their answers after reading the lesson.

- All peer pressure is bad. (false)
- TV, music, magazines, and the Internet are all part of the media. (true)
- People are the only influence on your decision making. (false)

LS Verbal

MISCONCEPTION ALERT

Nonverbal Peer Pressure Some students may think that peer pressure is always manifested as verbal communication—such as when a peer says, "Everybody's doing it." Tell students that peer pressure can also be very subtle. For example, if many people are smoking at a party, a teen may feel pressure to smoke in order to fit in.

Activity — GENERAL

Identifying Pressure Encourage students to remember a time when they did something that conflicted with their values because of negative peer pressure. How did they feel? (Sample answer: I felt bad. I felt as if I was breaking the law.) Have students write down what a peer said or did to influence their decision. Students should draw a one-picture cartoon of a "peer-pressure monster" using the information they wrote down. **English Language Learners**

LS Visual

REAL-LIFE CONNECTION — ADVANCED

Family Documentary Have interested students make a family profile using photographs or a video camera. The focus of the documentary is to reflect on their family's values, cultural beliefs, traditions, health practices, and exercise routines. **LS** Visual

Attention Grabber

Tell students the following statistics to illustrate the prevalence of peer pressure:

One out of every five teens reports feeling peer pressure to consume alcoholic drinks and one out of every twelve teens reports feeling peer pressure to use drugs.

Lesson 3 • Influences on Your Decisions   **29**

Teach, continued

Life SKILL BUILDER — ADVANCED

Being a Wise Consumer Have students design and conduct an experiment to test the validity of a television commercial's claim. (Sample experiment: Hold a blind "taste-test" of fruit juices to see how many people prefer the taste of one brand over another.) Ask students to evaluate the accuracy of the commercial. Have students write a letter to the manufacturer of the product describing their experiment, their results, and their conclusions. **LS Logical**

Group Activity — BASIC

Skit Have students work in small groups to write and perform a skit of a television commercial that targets teens. Students should identify a product in which teens might be interested and think of things to say about the product that will convince teens to buy the product. If students want more of a challenge, they should pick a product that does not appeal to teens. **LS Kinesthetic**

Activity — GENERAL

Ins and Outs Have students brainstorm lists of things that they consider to be "in" and things that they think are "out." Students can list fashion trends, hairstyles, music, and activities. After students finish their lists, ask students to pick one item from their "in" list and analyze why it is popular. Have students identify things on their "out" list that used to be popular and ask them to explain why it is no longer popular. **LS Verbal**

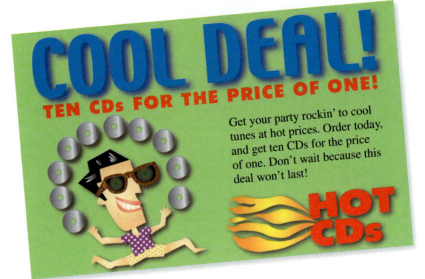

Figure 9 How are you influenced by ads like the one shown above?

LIFE SKILLS ACTIVITY

BEING A WISE CONSUMER

Think of three commercials that you heard on TV or on the radio. Which of these ads do you think are truthful? Which of these ads do you think may contain false claims? Explain your answers.

Other Influences in Your Life

Your family and friends are not the only influences in your life. Some of the most powerful messages that you hear come from the media. The media includes TV, radio, the Internet, movies, magazines, music, and news reports. The media tells you what is going on in the world. The media gives you messages about what is important, what is good, and what is bad. But not all of the information you receive is correct. Commercials can be an example of misinformation.

Some of the products advertised on TV don't do what advertisers claim. Advertisers want you to identify with their products. So, they try to make you believe that you will become more popular or feel better about yourself if you use the products. But most products won't make you be popular or feel better about yourself. Yet it is hard not to believe the messages, at least a little. You want to believe that you can feel better, have more friends, and change things that you don't like about yourself. As a result, you might decide to buy some of the products after hearing these messages from the media.

Learn the truth about advertising. There are many good sources of information. Seek out accurate information about products. Talk with your parents. You will discover how much the media really influences you.

TECHNOLOGY CONNECTION — ADVANCED

V Chip The V Chip is a computer chip placed in some television sets that can be used to block the viewing of certain shows. For example, a parent can use a V Chip to prevent their child from watching a show that contains adult language. Have interested students research the V Chip and write a persuasive essay either appraising or criticizing its use. **LS Verbal**

LIFE SKILLS ACTIVITY

Answer
Accept all reasonable answers.

Extension: Ask students to explain why some advertisers might use false claims in their commercials.

When Things Change

New information causes people to change their minds and to make new decisions. For example, from the 1950s to the 1970s, cigarette ads on TV made smoking seem cool. The ads influenced many people to start smoking. At that time, nobody knew that smoking was harmful. Scientific studies later showed that cigarettes are dangerous and addictive and can cause lung diseases. Studies also found that smoking affects not only smokers but also the people around the smoking. Some health organizations started to make commercials explaining the dangers of smoking. People started to quit after learning that smoking was a dangerous habit.

When you receive new information, stop and think. First, make sure you can trust the information to be true. Then, think about how the information affects you. You may have to make new decisions based on the information. You also may have to rethink decisions you made in the past. If you do, remember to follow the six steps to making good decisions!

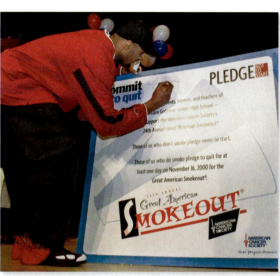

Figure 10 The Great American Smokeout is one of many campaigns against smoking.

Lesson Review

Using Vocabulary
1. What is peer pressure?

Understanding Concepts
2. Describe how your family influences your decisions.
3. Explain how peer pressure affects the decisions that you make.
4. What is the media? How does it influence your choices?

Critical Thinking
5. **Analyzing Ideas** Describe a time when you had to rethink a decision because something changed.
6. **Applying Concepts** You see a commercial that says a product will make you lose weight without dieting or exercising. Should you believe this claim? Explain.

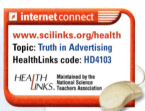

internet connect
www.scilinks.org/health
Topic: Truth in Advertising
HealthLinks code: HD4103
HEALTH LINKS. Maintained by the National Science Teachers Association

Lesson 4

Focus

Overview
Before beginning this lesson, review with your students the objectives listed under the What You'll Do head in the Student Edition. This lesson explains why goals are important, describes how values and interests influence your goals, and compares short-term goals and long-term goals.

🔔 Bellringer
Have students list three goals that they have. Once students have written their goals, ask them to estimate how long it will take them to achieve these goals.
LS Intrapersonal

Answer to Start Off Write
Accept all reasonable answers. Sample answer: A goal is something you work toward and hope to achieve.

Motivate

Activity — GENERAL
Building Self-Esteem Encourage students to remember a time when they achieved an important goal. Ask them to write a description of the situation or draw a picture illustrating their accomplishment. Encourage students to post their description or drawing in their bedroom where they will see it every day.
English Language Learners
LS Intrapersonal

Lesson 4

What You'll Do
- **Explain** why goals are important.
- **Identify** two influences on your goals.
- **Compare** short-term goals and long-term goals.
- **Describe** how goals can help build healthy relationships.

Terms to Learn
- goal
- self-esteem
- interest

Start Off Write
What is a goal?

Setting Healthy Goals

Jim and Parag are good friends and have known each other since they were 4 years old. Jim has always wanted to become a great judge. Parag wants to be a famous surgeon when he grows up.

Jim and Parag are good friends. But like most friends, they don't always like the same things. They also have different goals. A **goal** is something that you work toward and hope to achieve. In this lesson, you will learn why goals are important. You will also learn how to set goals.

Why Are Goals Important?
Goals are an important part of growing up. They give you a sense of purpose and direction. As you accomplish your goals, your self-esteem grows. **Self-esteem** is the way you value, respect, and feel confident about yourself. For example, suppose you set a goal of earning an A in math. You study and do your homework every day. Many days, you see a tutor. When you get your report card and see that you earned an A, you are very proud of yourself. When you set and reach goals, you always feel good about your achievement and yourself.

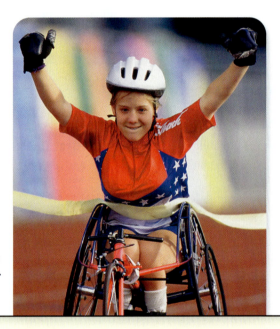

Figure 11 Accomplishing goals builds self-esteem.

32

MISCONCEPTION ALERT
Self-Esteem Some students may confuse self-esteem with being boastful or proud. Tell students that some boastful people have high self-esteem, but others do not. Explain that sometimes people brag about their abilities because they have low self-esteem and are trying to make themselves feel better by looking for recognition. Also tell students that some people with high self-esteem are very humble.

Chapter Resource File
- Directed Reading **BASIC**
- Lesson Plan
- Lesson Quiz **GENERAL**

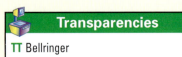
Transparencies
TT Bellringer

TABLE 1 The Relationship Between Values, Interests, and Goals

Value	Interest	Possible goal
Self-expression	public speaking	to act in a play
Helping others	woodworking	to help elderly people with household projects
Self-discipline	running	to run a 10-kilometer race
Honesty	current events	to join the newspaper staff

Examining Your Values

Your values influence the goals that you set. Remember that a value is an important belief. It is a reflection of the kind of person you want to be. Think about your values when you set goals. You are more likely to reach goals that are based on your values. In the example at the beginning of the lesson, both Jim and Parag value helping other people. But Jim wants to become a judge, while Parag wants to become a surgeon.

Your personal values develop over time and are based on your experiences. Not everyone has the same values, although there are certain values that most people believe in. For example, most people believe in honesty and responsibility. When you know your values, setting goals for yourself is easier.

Health Journal
Using Table 1 as an example, write down one thing that you value and one thing that interests you. How would you combine your value and your interest to set a possible goal?

Defining Your Interests

You also have interests. An 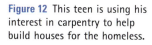 interest is something that you enjoy and want to learn more about. You can have an interest in things such as art, athletics, music, or science. Like your values, your interests influence your goals. But unlike values, which develop over a long period of time, interests can start quickly and can end just as fast. You may have an interest in tennis for several months. But soon you may find that your interest has changed to basketball. Values usually do not change this rapidly. If you value honesty now, you will probably value it later in life, too. Your values reflect your character. Your interests reflect your personality and tastes.

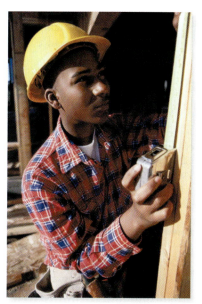

Figure 12 This teen is using his interest in carpentry to help build houses for the homeless.

Teach

Discussion — ADVANCED
Childhood Traits Have students list four traits that they liked in themselves as a young child. (Sample answers: being straightforward and honest, not being stressed out, not caring what other people think about them, and being carefree) Ask students how these childhood traits are reflected in their current values. (Sample answer: I am straightforward when I talk to others and I always tell the truth because I value honesty.)
LS Intrapersonal

Answer to Health Journal
Answers may vary. This Health Journal may be a good introduction to the lesson. You may want to assign this writing exercise the day before you teach the lesson. After teaching the lesson, ask students if they would change what they wrote in their Health Journal.

Activity — GENERAL
Identifying Values Have students list five people—either living or dead—that they admire. Ask students: "What traits do the people on your list have that you would like to see in yourself?" (Sample answers: self-discipline, honesty, responsibility, and helping others)
LS Intrapersonal

Group Activity — BASIC
Role-Playing Have students work in pairs to role-play a scene in which a student talks with his or her guidance counselor about setting goals. The student playing the role of the counselor should ask the other student questions that lead him or her to identify his or her values and interests. The counselor should then help the student develop a goal based on the values and interests named.
LS Kinesthetic   Co-op Learning

Life SKILL BUILDER — GENERAL
Setting Goals Ask students to list five hobbies, classes, or skills that interest them right now. Have students brainstorm jobs that involve one or more of their current interests. Finally, have students research the training or education they would need to begin a career with one of the jobs on their list. **LS Verbal**

Teach, continued

Activity — BASIC

Dream Collage Ask students to finish this sentence with five different answers: "If I could do anything, I would try ___." After they finish their sentences, have students look for images in magazines, newspapers, or the Internet that illustrate their sentences. Students should cut these images out, and paste them on a poster board as a collage. Students can also draw their own images for the collage. Have students present their collages to the class or display them around the classroom. **LS Visual**

PHYSICAL SCIENCE CONNECTION — ADVANCED

Architectural Engineering Tell students that architects design bridges in stages. The long-term goal of a bridge designer is to build a bridge that will withstand strong winds and heavy loads without falling into the water. The short-term goals of a designer include building the main structure, stabilizing it, and testing it. Have student work in small groups to design and build a bridge out of toothpicks and glue. The bridge should span two desks that are 1 foot apart. Test the stability of these bridges by hanging weights from the center until the bridge breaks or begins to sag. If students are interested, hold a contest to see which group can build the strongest bridge. **LS Logical**

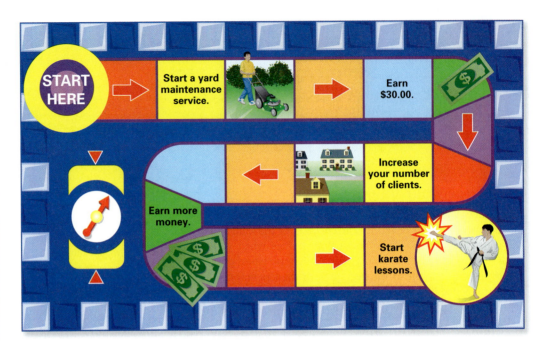

Figure 13 For Jeff to reach his long-term goal of taking karate lessons, he must first accomplish several short-term goals.

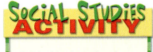

Political leaders often have goals they wish to achieve while in office. Research the goals set and achieved by former Presidents of the United States.

Short-Term Goals and Long-Term Goals

After you have determined your values and interests, you are ready to identify your goals. There are two kinds of goals: short-term goals and long-term goals. *Short-term goals* are tasks that you can accomplish in hours, days, or weeks. For example, making a good grade on a test is a short-term goal. Finishing your chores in time to watch a TV show is a short-term goal.

Long-term goals may take months or even years to reach. Usually, long-term goals are made up of several short-term goals and even other long-term goals. For example, suppose you set a long-term goal of going to college. What goals would help you reach your final goal? One goal would be to make good grades in your classes so that you can graduate. Another might be to save money to help pay for your tuition. Getting accepted into college is another goal. Each goal builds on the other to help you reach your long-term goal. The key to reaching a long-term goal is to identify all of the other goals that make up that goal. Then, you must work through all of your goals. If you don't accomplish one goal along the way, don't give up! Think about what you can do to get back on track. You may need to change one of your short-term goals. Or you may need to add a goal to your plans. There is more than one way to reach your final goal.

Life SKILL BUILDER — GENERAL

Setting Goals Ask students to list ten things that they could have as short-term goals for this week. (Sample answers: organize my room, complete all of my homework, exercise for twenty minutes every day, and write a letter to friend or relative) Encourage students to pick three things on their list and do them. After a week passes, poll students to find out who accomplished their goals. **LS Verbal**

Answer to Social Studies Activity
Accept all reasonable answers.

Extension: Ask students why they think that Presidents set goals for themselves and for the country.

Goals Build Healthy Relationships

Goals not only help you in your activities and at school but also can help you build healthy relationships. A healthy relationship begins when you and a friend or family member work toward goals together. For example, many people around you can help you reach your goal of going to college. Your parents help by giving you support every day. They may also teach you how to save money and may work with you to fill out college applications. Your friends help you reach your goal by studying with you so that you will earn good grades. Your teachers also help you reach your goal. Teachers can help you choose classes that will prepare you for college and can teach you good study habits. Working with others to reach a goal strengthens your relationships with them.

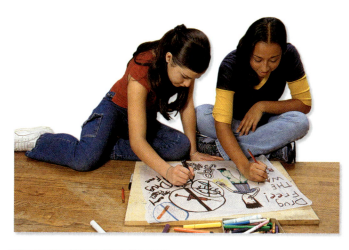

Figure 14 Working with others to achieve a goal helps build healthy relationships.

Lesson Review

Using Vocabulary
1. Define the term *interest*.
2. What is the relationship between having self-esteem and achieving goals?

Understanding Concepts
3. Explain the importance of interests and values in setting your goals.
4. How do short-term goals and long-term goals differ?
5. How do goals build healthy relationships?

Critical Thinking
6. **Making Inferences** Alan enjoyed fishing a few years ago. Now, he prefers to go hiking. Did his interests change, his values change, or did both change? Explain.

Answers to Lesson Review
1. An interest is something that you enjoy and want to learn more about.
2. When you reach your goals, you feel good about your achievements and your self-esteem grows.
3. You are more likely to achieve goals that reflect your interests and values.
4. Short-term goals are tasks that you can accomplish in hours, days, or weeks. Long-term goals may take months or years to reach.
5. Working with others to reach a goal strengthens your relationships with them.
6. Answers may vary. Sample answer: Alan's interests changed. He used to like fishing, but now he likes hiking. Alan's values did not change. He still values spending time outdoors and enjoying nature.

Close

Reteaching — BASIC
Goals Have pairs of students distinguish between their short-term and long-term goals by specifying what they plan to do today, this week, this month, and this year. Ask students what they hope to accomplish five years and ten years from now. Explain to students that the goals they wish to accomplish in less than a month are short-term goals. Further explain that long-term goals may take months or years to accomplish. **LS Verbal**

Quiz — GENERAL
1. Define the term *self-esteem*. (Self-esteem is the way you value, respect, and feel confident about yourself.)
2. Explain the difference between the development of interests and the development of values. (Interests can develop quickly and change just as quickly, whereas values take a long time to develop and usually do not change very easily.)
3. What is the key to reaching a long-term goal? (The key to reaching a long-term goal is to identify all of the other goals that make up that goal.)

Alternative Assessment — ADVANCED
Writing — Letter to the Mayor Encourage students to write a letter to the mayor of your city about the goals he or she is trying to reach during his or her term in office. **LS Verbal**

Lesson 4 • Setting Healthy Goals   35

Lesson 5 Focus

Overview
Before beginning this lesson, review with your students the objectives listed under the What You'll Do head in the Student Edition. In this lesson, the students will learn the relationship between goals and success. Students also read about the importance of learning from their mistakes.

🔔 Bellringer
Have students write a brief paragraph about what success means to them. Invite volunteers to read their paragraphs to the class.
LS Verbal

Answer to Start Off Write
Accept all reasonable answers. Sample answer: If you learn from your mistakes, you won't make the same mistakes again when trying to reach your goal.

Motivate

 — GENERAL

Evaluating Media Messages
Have students describe a movie in which a character used persistence to reach his or her goal. What obstacles did the character overcome to reach the goal? What setbacks did he or she encounter and how did this character overcome these setbacks? Be sure the students do not discuss R-rated movies.
LS Verbal

Lesson 5 — How to Reach Your Goals

What You'll Do
- **Explain** the relationship between goals and success.
- **Describe** how you can learn from your mistakes.

Terms to Learn
- success
- persistence

Start Off Write
Why must you learn from your mistakes to reach your goals?

Elena daydreams about making the winning basket for her team. She practices shooting baskets every day. Elena's goal is to become a professional basketball player.

No matter what your goal is, you will need to make many decisions along the way. In this lesson, you will learn how to use the six steps to making good decisions to reach your goals.

Reaching Your Goals

Success is the achievement of your goals. You can follow the six steps to making good decisions to reach goals. For example, let's say you set a goal to get in shape.

- **Identify the problem.** How do you get in shape?
- **Consider your values.** You value being physically fit.
- **List the options.** Your options are to ride a stationary bike or jog.
- **Weigh the consequences.** If the weather is bad, you won't be able to run. The bike is indoors.
- **Decide, and act.** You decide to ride the bike.
- **Evaluate your choice.** You ride for an hour every day. You are getting in shape! You reached your goal.

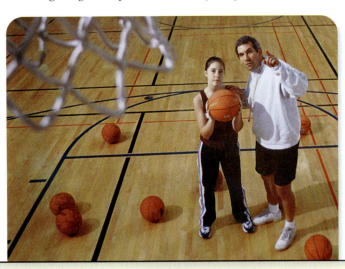

Figure 15 Many goals require a lot of practice.

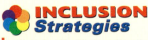 BASIC

• Learning Disabled • Attention Deficit Disorder

Give students a chance to get out of their seats and to gain a concrete understanding of persistence. Organize students into two teams. Tell students they are not to talk, run, nor touch anyone during this activity. Team 1 members are to cross from one side of the room to the other. Team 2 members should try to stop Team 1 members. Discuss signs of persistence that were displayed.
LS Kinesthetic

Chapter Resource File
- Directed Reading **BASIC**
- Lesson Plan
- Lesson Quiz **GENERAL**

Transparencies
TT Bellringer

---

36 Chapter 2 • Successful Decisions and Goals

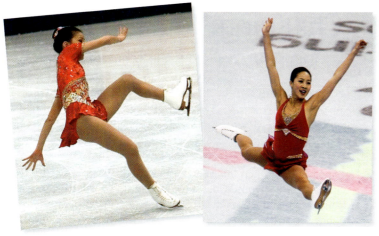

Figure 16 Mistakes can be valuable learning tools. They make you think about how you can improve.

Learning from Your Mistakes

The most important thing to remember about goals is that it takes time, energy, and determination to reach them. Success rarely comes easily, so persistence is important. Persistence is the commitment to keep working toward your goal even when things that make you want to quit happen. Sometimes, it will be hard to stay focused. And you will make mistakes along the way. Everyone who sets goals sometimes makes a bad decision when trying to reach his or her goal. To be successful, you must learn from your mistakes. Take time to think about what you did. What can you do differently next time? Making a mistake might have gotten you off track temporarily, but do not let it stop you from reaching your goal. You can get back on track again. Tell yourself that making a mistake is OK. You must convince yourself to stay positive and keep going.

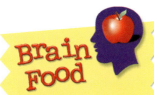

Brain Food

The greatest challenge Thomas Edison faced while inventing the light bulb was to find a material that would glow without burning. Edison tried more than 1,600 materials before he found the right one.

Lesson Review

Using Vocabulary

1. In your own words, define success.
2. What is persistence?

Understanding Concepts

3. Explain the relationship between goals and success.

4. Explain how a mistake can be a valuable learning tool.

Critical Thinking

5. **Applying Concepts** Using the six steps to making decisions, outline a plan for reaching one of your goals.

Lesson 6

Focus

Overview
Before beginning this lesson, review with your students the objectives listed under the What You'll Do head in the Student Edition. In this lesson, students learn the importance of measuring their progress when pursuing a goal. Students also learn why changing their plans is sometimes a part of reaching their goals.

🔔 Bellringer
Have students list things or activities that can be measured. (Sample answers: counting how many sit-ups you can do and taking a test)
LS Logical

Answer to Start Off Write
Accept all reasonable answers. Sample answer: I measure my progress toward my goal of earning a good grade in history class by writing down my grades on my daily assignments.

Motivate

Group Activity — GENERAL
Road Map Detours Organize the class into groups of four. Give each group a road map and the names of two cities. The groups should plan which roads to take from one city to another and write down their plan. After each group has their plan, tell students that one of the roads they chose is closed for construction. Have groups redesign their travel plan with the new information. Tell students that people sometimes have to take detours while working toward a goal. **LS Visual**

Lesson 6

What You'll Do
- **Explain** the importance of measuring your progress when pursuing a goal.
- **Explain** why changing your plans is sometimes part of reaching your goals.

Terms to Learn
- coping

Start Off Write
How do you measure your progress when reaching a goal?

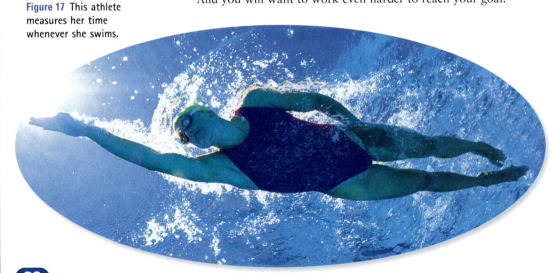

Figure 17 This athlete measures her time whenever she swims.

SOCIAL STUDIES CONNECTION — ADVANCED
✏️ **Pioneers** Briefly discuss how the western part of the United States became settled by people traveling in covered wagons. Have the students research and write a paper about some of the problems that the settlers faced as they traveled into new territory. In their papers, students should suggest ways that these people may have coped with the obstacles that they faced.
LS Verbal

Changing Your Goals

Manuel did not make the tennis team the first time he tried out. At first, he wasn't sure whether to try out for the team again or to try something new. Manuel decided that being on the tennis team was important enough to him to try out again.

Like Manuel, when things don't go as planned, you may be disappointed, but you do not have to give up on your dreams. In this lesson, you'll look at ways to measure your progress as you work toward a goal. You will also see how to make changes to meet your goal.

Measuring Your Progress

Your goal is to run the mile faster and to break your old record. After a month, how can you tell if you are running faster? You can time yourself. When you are trying to reach a goal, it is important to measure your progress. By measuring your progress, you can see if you are on the right track. And the only way to be sure that you have progressed is to check your results. Scores, grades, and measurements are ways that you can track your progress. You can also make charts or keep a journal. Reviewing results is just as important as working on the goal itself. When you see how far you've come, you will feel great. And you will want to work even harder to reach your goal.

Chapter Resource File
- Directed Reading **BASIC**
- Lesson Plan
- Lesson Quiz **GENERAL**

Transparencies
TT Bellringer

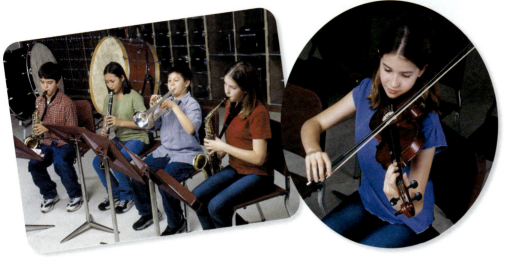

Figure 18 Goals sometimes change because our interests change.

Changing Your Plan

Sailors chart a course on a map to show where they want to go. Even with the best boat and the best skills, they still have to change course sometimes. You face the same situation when you try to reach a goal. You may have all of the desire and skill in the world, but sometimes you will have to change your direction. You will occasionally have to cope with setbacks. **Coping** is dealing with problems in an effective way. When things don't go as planned, try a different path. You may find new energy to keep working toward your original goal. You might even find that your new direction inspires you to work toward a new goal. Remember that goals worth achieving are not easy to reach. Such goals are rarely reached on the first try.

Lesson Review

Using Vocabulary

1. Define the term *coping*.

Understanding Concepts

2. Why is it important to measure your progress as you work toward a goal?

3. Explain why changes must sometimes be made when you work toward a goal.

Critical Thinking

4. **Applying Concepts** Why is it important to learn to cope with disappointments at an early age? How do you think your ability to cope with disappointments will help you as you get older?

5. **Making Inferences** Identify three reasons why a plan for reaching a goal may need to be changed.

Lesson 7

Focus

Overview
Before beginning this lesson, review with your students the objectives listed under the What You'll Do head in the Student Edition. This lesson explains why communication and refusal skills are important for achieving success.

 Bellringer
Have students list characteristics of a good listener. *(Sample answers: Good listeners don't interrupt other people, they maintain eye-contact, and they pay attention when other people are speaking.)* **LS Interpersonal**

Answer to Start Off Write
Accept all reasonable answers. Sample answer: I look at them when they are talking and I ask questions about what they have said to me.

Motivate

Demonstration — **GENERAL**

Communicating Emotions Ask two students to volunteer for this demonstration. Tell students that there are several ways that a person can communicate their emotions to other people. Challenge the two volunteers to demonstrate four or more ways to communicate happiness and sadness. *(Sample answers: telling a person that they are happy or sad, smiling or frowning, laughing or crying, and drawing a smiley face or a frowning face)* **LS Kinesthetic**

Lesson 7

What You'll Do
- **Explain** why communication is important.
- **Identify** four skills that you need to be a good listener.
- **Identify** five refusal skills.

Terms to Learn
- communication
- refusal skill

Start Off Write
What do you do to let people know that you are listening to them?

REAL-LIFE CONNECTION — **ADVANCED**

Sign Language Encourage interested students to take a course in sign language. Tell students that they can practice using their new communication skills with people in the community who have hearing impairments. **LS Kinesthetic**

Skills for Success

```
Keesha hates it when her friend Maren
doesn't listen to her. Sometimes, Keesha
will be talking about something really
important when she realizes that Maren
hasn't heard a word that she has said.
```

Keesha wishes that Maren had better listening skills. In this lesson, you'll learn how to communicate so that people will listen to you. You will also learn listening skills.

Communication

Sometimes, it is difficult to get your ideas across. To do so, you need to be able to communicate. **Communication** is the ability to exchange information and the ability to express your thoughts and feelings clearly. The ability to communicate is an important skill, especially when you are trying to reach a goal. This skill allows you to let others know exactly what you want or expect so that no misunderstandings take place. Someone can offer good advice to you only if he or she knows your intentions. When you express your ideas, be open, but choose your words carefully. Good communication can mean the difference between getting the information you need to reach a goal or not.

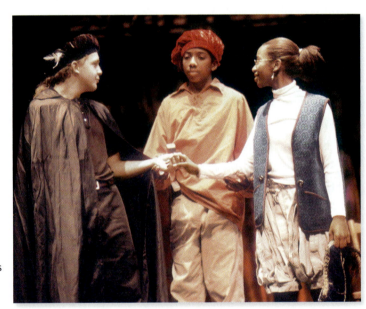

Figure 19 Good communication skills are important here as well as in everyday life.

Chapter Resource File
- Directed Reading **BASIC**
- Lesson Plan
- Lesson Quiz **GENERAL**

Transparencies
TT Bellringer
TT Using Refusal Skills 1
TT Using Refusal Skills 2

40 Chapter 2 • Successful Decisions and Goals

Listening Skills

Having good listening skills is as important to reaching your goal as communicating clearly is. To develop good listening skills, follow these suggestions:

- **Pay attention to the person who is speaking.** Facing a person shows that you are interested in what the person is saying.
- **Make eye contact.** Looking around makes people think that you are not listening to them.
- **Nod when you understand.**
- **Ask questions when you don't understand.** Try to ask open-ended questions. *Open-ended questions* call for an answer other than yes or no. Ask questions such as, "What do you think about that?"

How do good listening skills help you reach your goals? Very few people reach their goals without help from others. To get this help, you need to listen to the person who is giving you advice. People can point you in the right direction and can give you tips to save you time and energy. But you must listen!

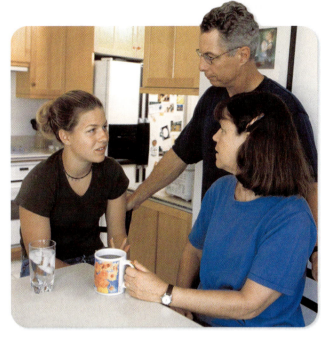

Figure 20 What listening skills are this teen's parents exhibiting?

Hands-on ACTIVITY

LISTENING LAB

1. Go to a place where students spend time talking together.
2. Find a place where you can observe some people without disturbing them. Be sure to take a pencil and a piece of paper with you.
3. What do you observe about the way that students talk and listen to each other?

Note the following things in your observations:
- body position
- facial expressions
- tone of voice
- hand movements
- eye contact

Analysis

1. Describe your observations. For example, could you tell if the people were friends or if they were casual acquaintances? Were they happy, sad, or angry with each other? Explain.

Teach, continued

Using the Figure — GENERAL
At the Movies Have students study the figure shown at the top of this page and the top of the next page of the Student Edition. Ask students the following questions:

- Which refusal skill will not work in the situation shown? Explain. (Avoiding dangerous situations will not work because the teen is already at the movie theater.)
- Which refusal skill do you think is the most effective? Explain. (Sample answer: Walking away is most effective because the teen won't feel any pressure after he leaves.)
- What would you do if you were in this situation? (Answers may vary.)

LS Verbal

Group Activity — ADVANCED
Reworked Stories Have students work in small groups to rewrite a children's story and change the plot such that the main character uses refusal skills to avoid trouble. For example, Little Red Riding Hood can use refusal skills to tell the Big Bad Wolf that she will not stray from the path to her grandmother's house. Invite volunteers to read their story aloud to the class. **LS** Verbal

Activity — BASIC
Refusal Skills Have students list scenarios in which they would use refusal skills. (Sample answers: refusing to drink at a party, refusing to take drugs or use tobacco, and refusing to commit a crime) **LS** Verbal

---

Figure 21 Using Refusal Skills

You and a friend have just finished watching a movie at the theater. Your friend wants you to sneak into one of the other movies with him. You can use any of the following refusal skills in this situation.

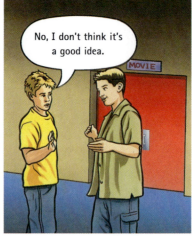

Say no.

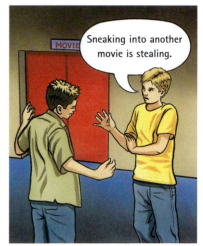

Stay focused on the issue.

Refusal Skills

Sometimes, saying no when you are faced with peer pressure is difficult. But remembering your values and goals will give you the strength to say no. How do you say no? You use refusal skills. **Refusal skills** are strategies to avoid doing something you don't want to do. There are five ways to deal with negative peer pressure.

- **Avoid dangerous situations.** You won't have to say no if you avoid situations that you know will be a problem.
- **Say, "No."** Use a tone of voice that shows that you mean no.
- **Stay focused on the problem.** Picture what is wrong with the situation. Point out the problem if your friends argue with you.
- **Stand your ground.** Don't give in when your friends give you a hard time.
- **Walk away.** If your friends won't accept a simple no, walking away may be the best thing to do.

Using refusal skills will help you stay focused on your goals. Friends may use negative peer pressure to try to get you to do things that are not good for you. These kinds of things never help you reach your goals. They distract you and get you off track. Using refusal skills help you throughout your life. Begin practicing these skills now to keep your goals in sight.

Health Journal
Write a journal entry about a time when you were faced with negative peer pressure. Describe how you handled the situation.

Background
Refusal Skill Success A recent study showed that inner-city students who participated in a Life Skills Training program were less likely to use tobacco, alcohol, and drugs than students who did not participate were. This training program involved more than 3,600 New York City seventh graders and taught the students to use refusal skills, social skills, and self-management skills.

Life SKILL BUILDER — GENERAL
Using Refusal Skills Have students use their refusal skills as they role-play the following scenario: "You are babysitting for your neighbor's two young children. After the children go to bed, your two best friends call and say that they want to come over to watch movies on your neighbor's new big-screen TV. You don't think it is a good idea. What should you do?" **LS** Kinesthetic

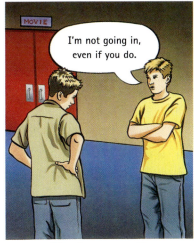
Stand your ground.

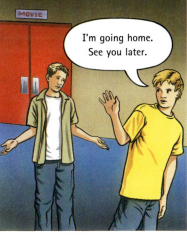
Walk away.

Putting It All Together

Suppose you are helping your dad build a room onto your house. When you need a certain tool, you reach into the toolbox and pull out the tool that is best suited for the job. Think of the skills in this lesson as tools in a toolbox. Each skill is a tool that you can use to solve a certain problem. If you need information to reach a goal, use good communication to express what you want to know. When getting advice, use your listening skills to get the information you need. If you find yourself in a situation in which you need to say no, use one or more of your refusal skills. These skills can help you in everyday life as well as in problem situations. Remember these skills, and use them often!

Lesson Review

Using Vocabulary
1. Define the term *communication*.
2. What are refusal skills?

Understanding Concepts
3. Why are communication and listening skills important? What four things make you a good listener?

Critical Thinking
4. **Analyzing Ideas** List the five refusal skills. Which refusal skill do you use the most? Which skill is the most difficult for you to use? Explain why.

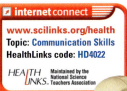

internet connect
www.scilinks.org/health
Topic: Communication Skills
HealthLinks code: HD4022
HEALTH LINKS. Maintained by the National Science Teachers Association

Close

Reteaching — BASIC

Comprehension Check Write the headings and subheadings of this lesson on the chalkboard. Have students work in pairs to summarize the material below each heading without looking at the textbook. If a pair is having trouble, have one student in the pair reread the difficult parts and explain them to his or her partner. **LS** Verbal

Quiz — GENERAL

1. How is communication related to goals? (Good communication can mean the difference between getting the information you need to reach a goal or not.)
2. What are open-ended questions? (Open-ended questions are questions that call for an answer other than yes or no.)
3. How do refusal skills help you reach your goals? (Refusal skills help you stay focused on your goals. You can use refusal skills when faced with negative peer pressure that might distract you from your goals.)

Alternative Assessment — ADVANCED

Analyzing Literature Interested students could analyze a short story by indicating which parts of the story illustrate good communication and good listening skills. In addition, students can explain how a character could have used refusal skills to avoid trouble. **LS** Verbal

Answers to Lesson Review

1. Communication is the ability to exchange information and the ability to express your thoughts and feelings clearly.
2. Refusal skills are strategies to avoid doing something you don't want to do.
3. Communication is important because it allows you to let others know exactly what you want or expect. Listening skills are important because they help you avoid misunderstandings. Four things that make a person a good listener are paying attention to the person speaking, making eye contact, nodding when you understand, and asking open-ended questions.
4. Five refusal skills are avoiding dangerous situations, saying "no," staying focused on the problem, standing your ground, and walking away. Sample answer: Walking away is most difficult for me because I don't want to look like a coward.

Chapter 2 Review

Assignment Guide

Lesson	Review Questions
1	6, 16
2	1, 4, 10
3	11, 18, 22–25
4	2, 5, 7, 12
5	13
6	8
7	3, 9, 14–15, 17, 19–20
1 and 7	21

ANSWERS

Using Vocabulary

1. options
2. goal
3. refusal skills
4. values
5. interest
6. good decision
7. self-esteem
8. coping

Understanding Concepts

9. Four skills of being a good listener are paying attention to the person speaking, making eye contact, nodding when you understand, and asking open-ended questions.
10. The six steps to making good decisions are identify the problem, consider your values, list the options, weigh the consequences, decide, and act, and evaluate your choice.
11. Sometimes, you have to make new decisions or rethink decisions you made in the past based on new information.
12. Goals are important because they give you a sense of purpose and direction.
13. Making mistakes contributes to success if you learn from your mistakes.
14. You should ask open-ended questions if you don't understand what someone is saying.
15. Five ways to refuse are avoiding dangerous situations, saying no, staying focused on the problem, standing your ground, and walking away.
16. Answers may vary. Sample answer: A positive consequence of studying for a test all weekend is that you will earn a good grade. A negative consequence is that you will not able to spend time with your friends.

CHAPTER 2 REVIEW

Chapter Summary

- A good decision has a positive outcome. ■ A consequence is the result of a decision. ■ There are six steps to making good decisions. ■ Values are beliefs that you consider to be of great importance. ■ Brainstorming can help you identify options when making a decision. ■ Your decisions are influenced by your family, your friends, and the media. ■ Peer pressure can be negative or positive. ■ Your values and interests influence your goals. ■ There are short-term goals and long-term goals. ■ Success is the achievement of your goals. ■ You should measure your progress and be persistent when working toward a goal. ■ Communication and listening skills are important when working toward a goal. ■ Refusal skills are ways to avoid doing something that you don't want to do.

Using Vocabulary

For each sentence, fill in the blank with the proper word from the word bank provided below.

brainstorming	goal
refusal skills	persistence
interest	self-esteem
values	consequence
options	coping
good decision	

1. When making a decision, ___ are the possible choices you can make.
2. Planning to save $100 to buy something you want is called a(n) ___.
3. Actions that mean "no" are called ___.
4. Your ___ are made up of all of the beliefs that you consider important.
5. Wanting to know more about stamp collecting would be a(n) ___.
6. A(n) ___ is one that is responsible.
7. If you value and respect yourself you have high ___.
8. Sometimes, plans do not go as expected, but ___ is the ability to move beyond the problems.

Understanding Concepts

9. What are the four skills of being a good listener?
10. What are the six steps to making good decisions?
11. How do your decisions change based on new information?
12. Why are goals important?
13. How does making mistakes contribute to success?
14. What should you do if you don't understand someone?
15. List five different strategies that indicate refusal.
16. Give an example of a positive consequence and an example of a negative consequence.

Critical Thinking

Analyzing Ideas

17. You are trying to tell a friend about a problem that you have. He doesn't seem to be listening to you. What nonverbal communication clues might tell you that he isn't listening? What could you tell your friend about good listening skills?

18. You see a commercial on television that shows athletes wearing a certain kind of shoe. Do you think that you need those shoes to be an athlete? Why do you think that advertisers use sports heroes to sell their products? Explain your answer.

Using Refusal Skills

19. You are taking a test in class, and you see one of your friends cheating. When she sees that you realize what is going on, she asks you if you want the answers, too. What refusal skills would you use in this situation?

20. Imagine that all your friends have started wearing a certain type of shirt. They are all telling you that you need to wear the same type of shirt as them. You don't like the style of the shirt. What refusal skills would you use?

21. A friend dares you to shoplift an item from a store. Your friend says that you are a coward if you don't do it. You think about it. List some of the consequences of not shoplifting the item. Describe how you can use refusal skills in this situation.

Interpreting Graphics

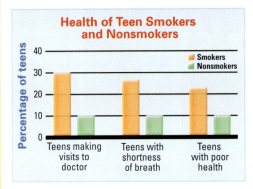

Use the figure above to answer questions 22–25.

22. Overall, do you think smokers or nonsmokers are healthier? Explain your answer.

23. The number of smokers who visit the doctor is greater than the number of students who report poor health. Why do you think this happens?

24. Athletes depend on being healthy and being able to breathe easily while exercising. Do you think many athletes smoke? Explain.

25. If your friend wanted to start smoking, how would you use the chart above to convince him otherwise?

Reading Checkup

Take a minute to review your answers to the Health IQ questions at the beginning of this chapter. How has reading this chapter improved your Health IQ?

Chapter Resource File

- Concept Review GENERAL
- Concept Mapping GENERAL
- Performance Based Assessment GENERAL
- Chapter Test GENERAL

Critical Thinking

Analyzing Ideas

17. Sample answer: Your friend may not be listening if he is looking away and not facing you. You could tell him that good listening skills are important to avoid misunderstandings.

18. No, you do not need that shoe to be an athlete. Advertisers use athletes to make us believe that we might perform like sports stars if we buy their products.

Using Refusal Skills

19. Sample answer: I would say "no" by shaking my head and keeping my eyes on my own test so that the teacher doesn't think that I'm cheating, too.

20. Sample answer: I would stand my ground by telling my friend that I don't want a new shirt.

21. Sample answer: Some negative consequences of not shoplifting are that my friend will call me a coward and might stop liking me. Some positive consequences are that I will not get in trouble with the law or my parents, and that I will be upholding my values. I would stay focused on the problem and explain why shoplifting is wrong.

Interpreting Graphics

22. Nonsmokers are healthier than smokers are. Fewer nonsmokers have poor health.

23. Sample answer: Teens who go to the doctor tend to be healthier than teens who don't go to the doctor.

24. no; Smoking makes it difficult for an athlete to perform well because it interferes with breathing. The percentage of smokers that report shortness of breath is about 26 percent.

25. Sample answer: I could show my friend the chart to prove how bad smoking is for a person's health.

Model

Introduce this activity by reminding students that using this Life Skill will help them take personal responsibility for their behavior. Then, review the scenario with the class.

Prepare students for this activity by modeling each of the steps of the skill. Make sure students understand each step before you move on to the next one.

Guided Practice: Practice with a Friend

Guided Practice is the stage in which you and the students analyze their approach to solving the problem given in the scenario and analyze their use of refusal skills. Have students read Act 1. Discuss with the class the situation described and the way students are to act it out. Organize the class into groups of three. In each group, one person plays the role of Reanna, another person plays Kelsey, and the third person is the observer.

Proper pacing during the Guided Practice is important. The suggestions listed below will help you control the pace.

1. Stop after completing each step of using refusal skills.
2. Discuss with each group the observer's comments.
3. Ask the other members of each group to listen to the observer's suggestions and to suggest ways to improve their refusal skills.
4. Instruct students to repeat the steps that need improvement and to include their modifications.
5. Check to make sure that students understand each step before they move on to the next step.
6. If time permits, repeat the exercise three times, switching roles each time. Each student should have the opportunity to play each role. Co-op Learning

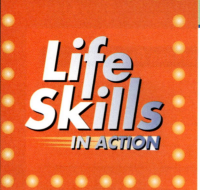

Life Skills IN ACTION

Using Refusal Skills

Using refusal skills is saying no to things you don't want to do. You can also use refusal skills to avoid dangerous situations. Complete the following activity to develop your refusal skills.

Reanna's Refusal

ACT 1

Setting the Scene

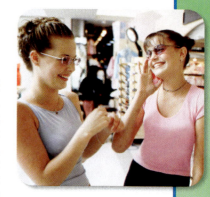

Reanna and her best friend Kelsey are shopping at the mall. Near the end of their shopping trip, Reanna sees a bracelet that she likes a lot. Unfortunately, she cannot buy the bracelet because she has already spent all of her money. Kelsey tells Reanna that she should just take the bracelet. "It's small," Kelsey says, "No one will ever notice that it is missing."

The 5 Steps of Using Refusal Skills

1. Avoid dangerous situations.
2. Say "No."
3. Stand your ground.
4. Stay focused on the issue.
5. Walk away.

Guided Practice

Practice with a Friend

Form a group of three. Have one person play the role of Reanna and another person play the role of Kelsey. Have the third person be an observer. Walking through each of the five steps of using refusal skills, role-play Reanna responding to Kelsey. Kelsey should try to convince Reanna to shoplift the bracelet. The observer will take notes, which will include observations about what the person playing Reanna did well and suggestions of ways to improve. Stop after each step to evaluate the process.

46   Chapter 2 • Life Skills in Action

Independent Practice

Check Yourself

After you have completed the guided practice, go through Act 1 again without stopping at each step. Answer the questions below to review what you did.

1. To stand her ground, what could Reanna say to Kelsey?
2. What could Reanna say to convince Kelsey that shoplifting is wrong?
3. How could Reanna avoid dangerous situations similar to this one in the future?
4. Think about a time when you had to say no to a good friend. Why was it difficult to say no?

On Your Own

At school the next day, Kelsey hands Reanna a present. Reanna opens it and finds the bracelet that Kelsey tried to convince her to steal. Reanna asks Kelsey if she paid for the bracelet. Kelsey admits that she didn't and tells Reanna not to say anything about it. Reanna tries to give the bracelet back to Kelsey, but Kelsey insists that she keep it. Draw a comic strip that shows how Reanna could use the five steps of using refusal skills in this situation.

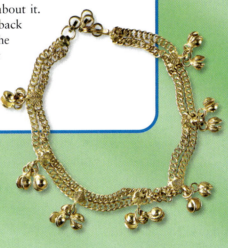

Independent Practice: Check Yourself

Instruct students to repeat Act 1 without stopping at each step. Remind students to apply what they learned in the Guided Practice to the Independent Practice. Students do not have to use every step to refuse successfully.

Encourage students to use the Check Yourself questions as a starting point for reviewing and analyzing their Independent Practice. Remind students that as they change roles, the answers to these questions may change for each actor. Encourage students to create additional questions for checking their use of refusal skills. When students have finished the Independent Practice, have them answer the Check Yourself questions in writing. Use their answers to assess their understanding of the steps of using refusal skills and to assess their use of the steps to solve a problem.

Check Yourself Answers

1. Sample answer: Reanna could say, "I like the bracelet, but I don't want to steal it."
2. Sample answer: Reanna could tell Kelsey that shoplifting is dishonest that that a person could get arrested for doing it.
3. Sample answer: Reanna could avoid going shopping with Kelsey in the future.
4. Sample answer: It was difficult to say no to my friend because I didn't want to disappoint him and I didn't want him to stop being my friend.

Act 2: On Your Own

This additional scenario gives students an opportunity to apply what they have learned in both the Guided Practice and the Independent Practice to a new situation.

Suggest to students that they use the Check Yourself questions as a starting point for using refusal skills in the new situation. Encourage students to be creative and to think of ways to improve their use of refusal skills.

Assessment

Review the comic strips that students have created as part of the On Your Own activity. The comic strips should show that the students applied one or more refusal skills in a realistic and effective manner. Display the comic strips around the room. If time permits, ask student volunteers to act out the dialogues of one or more of the comic strips. Discuss the comic strip's dialogue and the use of refusal skills.

CHAPTER 3
Building Self-Esteem
Chapter Planning Guide

PACING	CLASSROOM RESOURCES	ACTIVITIES AND DEMONSTRATIONS
BLOCK 1 • 45 min pp. 48–53 **Chapter Opener**	**CRF** Health Inventory * ■ GENERAL **CRF** Parent Letter * ■	**SE** Health IQ, p. 49 **CRF** At-Home Activity * ■
Lesson 1 Self-Esteem and Your Life	**CRF** Lesson Plan * **TT** Bellringer * **TT** What Influences Your Self-Esteem *	**TE** Activities The Effect of Advertising on Self-Esteem, p. 47F **TE** Group Activity Positive Postures, p. 51 GENERAL **TE** Demonstration Self-Esteem Balloon, p. 51 ◆ GENERAL **SE** Hands-on Activity, p. 52 ◆ **CRF** Datasheets for In-Text Activities * GENERAL **TE** Activity Self-Esteem on TV, p. 52 GENERAL **CRF** Life Skills Activity * ■ GENERAL **CRF** Enrichment Activity * ADVANCED
BLOCK 2 • 45 min pp. 54–59 **Lesson 2** Your Self-Concept	**CRF** Lesson Plan * **TT** Bellringer *	**TE** Activity Poster Project, p. 54 GENERAL **CRF** Enrichment Activity * ADVANCED
Lesson 3 Keys to Healthy Self-Esteem	**CRF** Lesson Plan * **TT** Bellringer * **TT** Examples of Positive Self-Talk *	**TE** Activities Assessing Your Self-Esteem, p. 47F **TE** Activity Role-playing, p. 56 ADVANCED **SE** Language Arts Activity, p. 57 **TE** Group Activity Practicing Positive Self-Talk, p. 58 GENERAL **SE** Life Skills in Action Coping, pp. 62–63 **CRF** Life Skills Activity * ■ GENERAL **CRF** Enrichment Activity * ADVANCED

BLOCKS 3 & 4 • 90 min **Chapter Review and Assessment Resources**

- **SE** Chapter Review, pp. 60–61
- **CRF** Concept Review * ■ GENERAL
- **CRF** Health Behavior Contract * ■ GENERAL
- **CRF** Chapter Test * ■ GENERAL
- **CRF** Performance-Based Assessment * GENERAL
- **OSP** Test Generator
- **CRF** Test Item Listing *

Online Resources

Visit **go.hrw.com** for a variety of free resources related to this textbook. Enter the keyword **HD4SE7**.

Students can access interactive problem solving help and active visual concept development with the *Decisions for Health* Online Edition available at **www.hrw.com**.

CNN Student News
cnnstudentnews.com
Find the latest health news, lesson plans, and activities related to important scientific events.

Compression guide:
To shorten your instruction because of time limitations, omit Lesson 2.

KEY

- **TE** Teacher Edition
- **SE** Student Edition
- **OSP** One-Stop Planner
- **CRF** Chapter Resource File
- **TT** Teaching Transparency
- ***** Also on One-Stop Planner
- ■ Also Available in Spanish
- ◆ Requires Advance Prep

SKILLS DEVELOPMENT RESOURCES	LESSON REVIEW AND ASSESSMENT	STANDARDS CORRELATION
		National Health Education Standards
TE Life Skill Builder Assessing Your Health, p. 52 BASIC **CRF** Cross-Disciplinary * GENERAL **CRF** Decision-Making * GENERAL **CRF** Directed Reading * BASIC	**SE** Lesson Review, p. 53 **TE** Reteaching, Quiz, p. 53 **TE** Alternative Assessment, p. 53 GENERAL **CRF** Concept Mapping * GENERAL **CRF** Lesson Quiz * ■ GENERAL	1.2, 1.4, 4.2
TE Reading Skill Builder Reading Hint, p. 55 BASIC **TE** Inclusion Strategies, p. 55 GENERAL **CRF** Cross-Disciplinary * GENERAL **CRF** Refusal Skills * GENERAL **CRF** Directed Reading * BASIC	**SE** Lesson Review, p. 55 **TE** Reteaching, Quiz, p. 55 **CRF** Concept Mapping * GENERAL **CRF** Lesson Quiz * ■ GENERAL	1.2
TE Reading Skill Builder Paired Summarizing, p. 57 GENERAL **TE** Life Skill Builder Practicing Wellness, p. 57 GENERAL **TE** Inclusion Strategies, p. 57 ADVANCED **SE** Life Skills Activity Using Refusal Skills, p. 58 **TE** Life Skill Builder Setting Goals, p. 58 GENERAL **CRF** Decision-Making * GENERAL **CRF** Refusal Skills * GENERAL **CRF** Directed Reading * BASIC	**SE** Lesson Review, p. 59 **TE** Reteaching, Quiz, p. 59 **TE** Alternative Assessment, p. 59 GENERAL **CRF** Lesson Quiz * ■ GENERAL	1.2, 3.4, 6.4

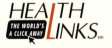

www.scilinks.org/health

Maintained by the
National Science Teachers Association

Topic: Building Healthy Self-Esteem
HealthLinks code: HD4020

Technology Resources

One-Stop Planner
All of your printable resources and the Test Generator are on this convenient CD-ROM.

 Guided Reading Audio CDs

VIDEO SELECT

For information about videos related to this chapter, go to **go.hrw.com** and type in the keyword **HD4SE7V**.

Chapter 3 • Chapter Planning Guide   **47B**

Chapter 3: Building Self-Esteem
Chapter Resources

Teacher Resources

TEACHING TRANSPARENCIES
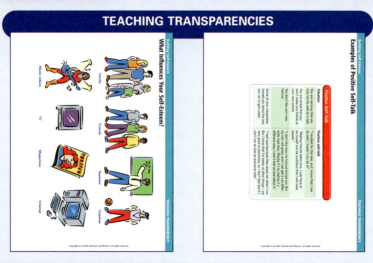

BELLRINGER TRANSPARENCIES
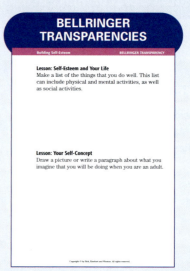

LESSON PLANS
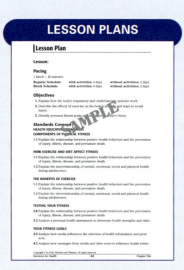

PARENT LETTER
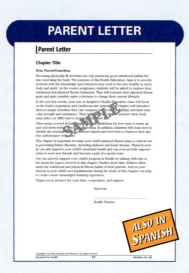

TEST ITEM LISTING
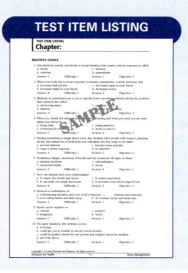

Meeting Individual Needs

DIRECTED READING
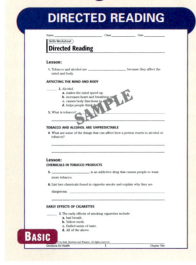

CONCEPT MAPPING
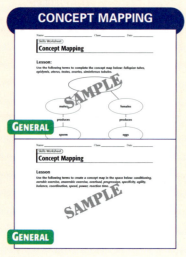

CONCEPT REVIEW
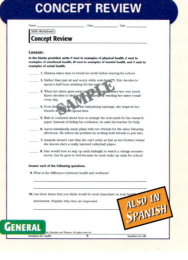

ENRICHMENT ACTIVITIES
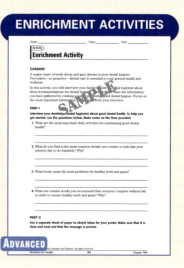

Resources

These worksheet pages can be found in the Chapter Resource File and the One-Stop Planner. The transparencies can be found in the Teaching Transparencies binder and on the One-Stop Planner.

Activities

LIFE SKILLS ACTIVITIES
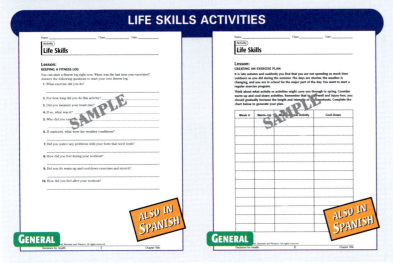

AT-HOME ACTIVITY
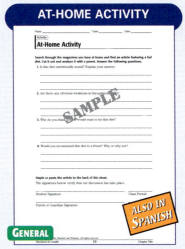

DATASHEETS FOR IN-TEXT ACTIVITIES
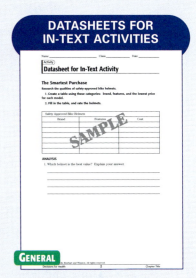

Applications

DECISION-MAKING
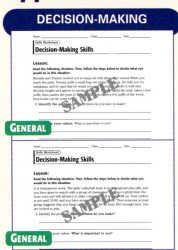

REFUSAL SKILLS
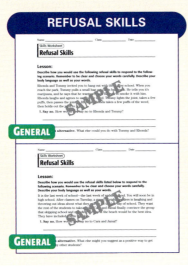

CROSS-DISCIPLINARY
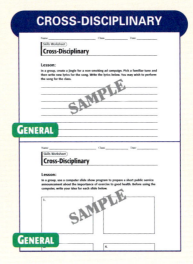

HEALTH BEHAVIOR CONTRACT
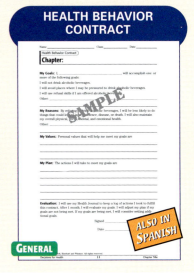

Assessments

HEALTH INVENTORY
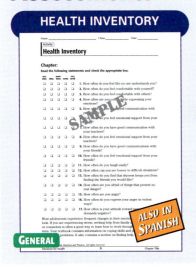

LESSON QUIZZES
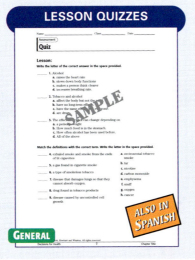

CHAPTER TEST
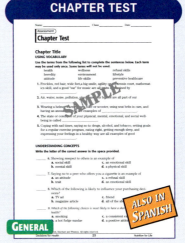

PERFORMANCE-BASED ASSESSMENT
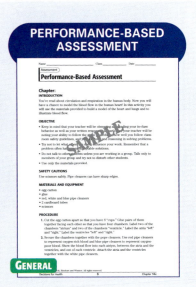

Chapter 3 • Chapter Resources and Worksheets 47D

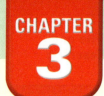

Background Information

The following information focuses on factors that influence self-esteem. This material will help prepare you for teaching the concepts in this chapter.

Influences on Self-Esteem

- The development of self-esteem begins in early childhood. The ways in which parents react to their children make a difference in the development of their children's self-esteem. Young children who are close to their parents are more likely to have high self-esteem. These children tend to be close to their parents because their parents are loving and involved in their lives. These parents also teach and expect appropriate behavior and thus encourage their children to become competent individuals.

- A sense of competence increases with self-esteem. By the age of four, children begin to judge themselves according to their cognitive, physical, and social competence. Children who know that they are good at something usually have higher self-esteem than others. Children may feel good about themselves if they are good at puzzles or counting (cognitive skills), if they are good at tying their shoelaces or swinging (physical skills), or if they have many friends (social skills).

- Both heredity and environment play roles in individual differences in skills. Some people are more physically coordinated than others and therefore are naturally good at sports. Other people may take lessons and train to improve their athletic abilities. Part of becoming competent is setting realistic goals. Warmth and encouragement from parents and teachers can help children reach high levels of competence and self-esteem.

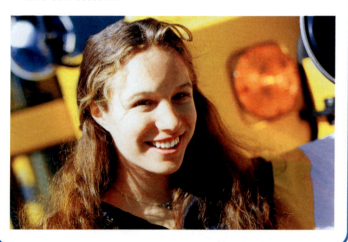

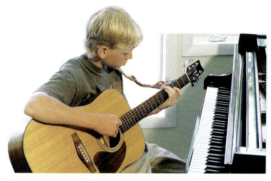

Gender and Self-Esteem

- Between the ages of 5 and 7, children begin to value themselves on the basis of their physical appearance and performance in school. Once in grade school, girls tend to display greater competence, and thus self-esteem, in the areas of reading and general academic skills. Boys tend to display competence and self-esteem in math and physical skills. Psychologists believe this occurs because the people around them have suggested that girls and boys are *supposed* to be good at these skills.

- Girls often predict that they will do better at tasks that are considered feminine. Likewise, boys usually predict that they will do better at tasks that are considered masculine. When people feel they will do well at a particular task, they often do.

Age and Self-Esteem

- Children gain competence as they grow older. Through experience they acquire more skills and become better at these skills. Even so, their self-esteem tends to decline during the elementary school years. Self-esteem seems to reach a low point at about age 12 or 13 and increases again during adolescence.

- It appears that young children assume that others see them as they see themselves. Thus, if they like themselves, they assume that other people like them too. As children develop, however, they begin to realize that some people might not see them the way they see themselves. They also begin to compare themselves to their peers. If they see themselves as less competent in some areas, their self-esteem may decrease.

For background information about teaching strategies and issues, refer to the *Professional Reference for Teachers*.

ACTIVITIES

CHAPTER 3

Consider using the activities on this page as students explore the lessons of this chapter. Look for other activities throughout the Student Edition chapter.

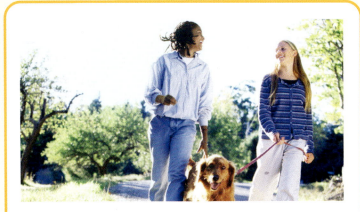

Assessing Your Self-Esteem

Procedure Have each student rate the following statements from 1 to 10, with 10 being "I completely agree" and 1 being "I completely disagree."

1. My family praises me when I try new things.
2. I am always honest with other people.
3. I confront my problems directly.
4. I like to help other people.
5. It is difficult to make me angry.
6. I make eye contact with people when I speak with them.
7. I am not a risk taker.
8. I hardly ever get sick.
9. I tell people how I feel when they make me angry.
10. I always speak my mind about something that I have strong feelings about.

Analysis

- Once students have rated each of the statements, have them add all of their ratings together to come up with their overall score.
- Students with a score of 90–100 points have very high self-esteem.
- Students with a score of 50–90 have average but healthy self-esteem. These students may benefit from activities that improve how they feel about themselves.
- Students with a score below 50 have low self-esteem. These students should consider different ways they could improve their self-esteem.

The Effect of Advertising on Self-Esteem

Hands on

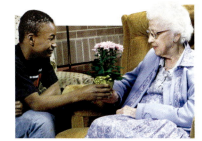

Procedure Instruct students to bring to class advertisements that are aimed at teenagers including magazine ads, videotapes of TV commercials, or recordings from the radio. Have the class discuss how the advertisements might influence a teenager's self-esteem.

Analysis Ask students the following questions:

- What techniques are the advertisers using to sell their products? (Answers may vary. Sample answer: Advertisers use teens who look happy and who are pretty or handsome to imply that their product will make you feel more accepted among your peers.)

- What assumptions does the advertisement make about teenagers? (Answers may vary. Sample answer: In response to a fast-food restaurant advertisement, students may claim that advertisers assume teens have busy lives and need food that is quick and convenient.)

- Could this advertisement affect the way a teenager feels about himself or herself? (Answers may vary. Sample answer: An advertisement for a particular brand of clothing may make a teen feel bad about himself or herself if he or she cannot afford to buy that brand. The teen may feel unaccepted by his or her peers because the teen does not wear that brand.)

- Why might this advertisement appeal more to teenagers than to other age groups? (Answers may vary. Sample answer: The advertisement has a teen spokesperson and the look and feel of the advertisement is trendy and appealing to teens.)

- Does the advertisement target teenagers with low self-esteem? Does the advertisement target teenagers with high self-esteem? (Answers may vary. Advertisements that claim their product will improve a teen's life are usually targeting teens with low self-esteem.)

CHAPTER 3

Overview
Tell students that this chapter will help them understand the concept of self-esteem, learn the characteristics of people who have high and low self-esteem, understand the many influences on self-esteem, and learn strategies for building their self-esteem.

Assessing Prior Knowledge
Students should be familiar with the following topic:
- goal-setting

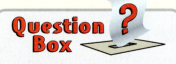

Students may feel more comfortable asking questions if you set up a Question Box to collect their questions. Have students write and anonymously submit their questions about self-esteem. Address these questions during class, or use these questions to introduce lessons that cover related topics.

Current Health
Check out *Current Health* articles and activities related to this chapter by visiting the HRW Web site at **go.hrw.com.** Just type in the keyword **HD4CH18T.**

Chapter Resource File
- Directed Reading BASIC
- Health Inventory GENERAL
- Parent Letter

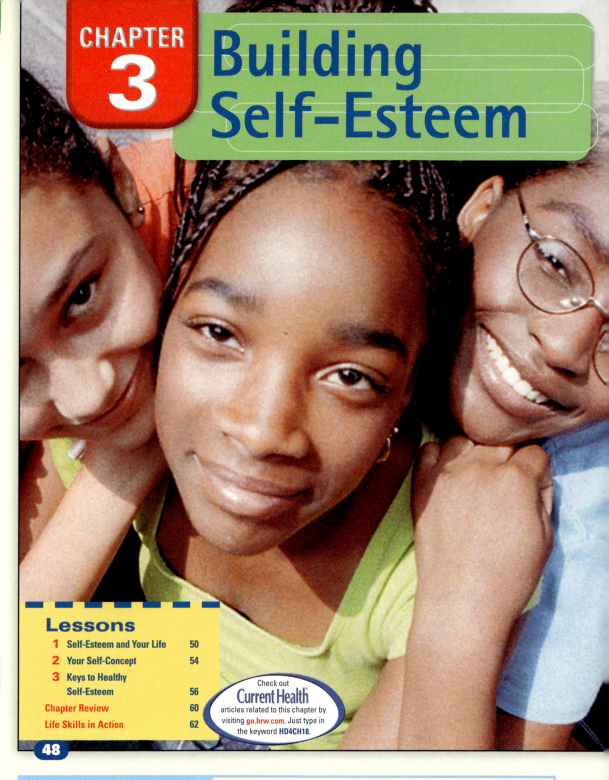

CHAPTER 3 Building Self-Esteem

Lessons
1. Self-Esteem and Your Life — 50
2. Your Self-Concept — 54
3. Keys to Healthy Self-Esteem — 56

Chapter Review — 60
Life Skills in Action — 62

Check out *Current Health* articles related to this chapter by visiting **go.hrw.com.** Just type in the keyword **HD4CH18.**

Standards Correlations

National Health Education Standards

1.2 Describe the interrelationship of mental, emotional, social, and physical health during adolescence. (Lessons 1–3)

1.4 Describe how family and peers influence the health of adolescents. (Lesson 1)

3.4 Demonstrate strategies to improve or maintain personal and family health. (Lesson 3)

4.2 Analyze how messages from media and other sources influence health behaviors. (Lesson 1)

6.4 Apply strategies and skills needed to attain personal health goals. (Lesson 3)

> **" I was upset when I found out that I didn't have any classes with my friends this year.**
> But a few weeks after school started, I began to meet some of my new classmates. I wasn't afraid to make new friends, and now I'm not so sad about going to school. **"**

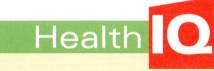

PRE-READING

Answer the following multiple-choice questions to find out what you already know about self-esteem. When you've finished this chapter, you'll have the opportunity to change your answers based on what you've learned.

1. Self-esteem is
   a. a measure of how well you get along with others.
   b. a measure of how much you value and respect yourself.
   c. the way you see yourself.
   d. a measure of how popular you are.

2. Which of the following is a characteristic of a person who has low self-esteem?
   a. accepts himself or herself
   b. has integrity
   c. has little confidence in himself or herself
   d. is not affected deeply by negative comments

3. What is self-concept?
   a. the way you see or imagine yourself as a person
   b. the way you choose to deal with a person who teases you
   c. how you handle your relationships
   d. how much you value yourself as a person

4. Being assertive means that you
   a. take responsibility for your actions.
   b. act on your thoughts and values without hurting others.
   c. are trustworthy.
   d. refuse to take part in activities that you know are wrong.

5. Which of the following might help you build healthy self-esteem?
   a. volunteering your time
   b. setting a goal
   c. accepting yourself
   d. all of the above

ANSWERS: 1. b; 2. c; 3. a; 4. b; 5. d

Using the Health IQ

Misconception Alert

Answers to the Health IQ questions may help you identify students' misconceptions.

Question 1: Students may think self-esteem is a measurement of a person's popularity or a measurement of how well a person gets along with peers rather than a measure of self-worth and self-respect. It may be helpful to point out to students that a person's self-esteem is based on how a person feels about himself or herself.

Question 5: Students may not realize that participating in volunteer work can boost their self-esteem. Some students may not understand that self-acceptance is a part of building self-esteem. It may help to point out to students that there are several ways to boost their self-esteem.

Answers
1. b
2. c
3. a
4. b
5. d

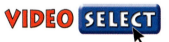

For information about videos related to this chapter, go to **go.hrw.com** and type in the keyword **HD4SE7V**.

Lesson 1

Focus

Overview
Before beginning this lesson, review with your students the objectives listed under the What You'll Do head in the Student Edition. In this lesson, students learn how self-esteem affects their life. Students will learn the characteristics of high self-esteem and low self-esteem, as well as the different influences on self-esteem.

Bellringer
Have students make a list of the things they do well. Remind the students that their list does not have to include just physical or mental activities, it could also include social activities.
LS Intrapersonal

Answer to Start Off Write
Accept all reasonable answers. Sample answer: Self-esteem is a measure of how much you value and respect yourself. I have high self-esteem.

Motivate

Discussion — GENERAL
Self-Esteem Ask volunteers to define the term *self-esteem* in their own words. Have students discuss the volunteers' definitions. Then, have students brainstorm for words they associate with high self-esteem and words they associate with low self-esteem. (Sample answers: confident, likable, valuable, content, capable, lovable, self-accepting, and secure; unwanted, dissatisfied, weak, useless, inferior, withdrawn, and frustrated) Finally, ask students to use their lists to write a personalized definition of *self-esteem*. **LS** Verbal

Lesson 1 — Self-Esteem and Your Life

What You'll Do
- **Describe** how self-esteem affects your life.
- **Identify** the characteristics of a person who has high self-esteem and a person who has low self-esteem.
- **Describe** five influences on your self-esteem.
- **Describe** how self-esteem and body image are related.

Terms to Learn
- self-esteem
- body image

Start Off Write
What is self-esteem? How would you describe your self-esteem?

It is Jessie's first day at her new school. She is nervous because she doesn't know anyone. She doesn't know her way around. Before she leaves the house, she looks in the mirror and says to herself, "I can do this!"

Have you ever been nervous when faced with a new situation? Even though Jessie is nervous about going to a new school, she is confident about herself. Jessie has high self-esteem.

What Is Self-Esteem?
You may not realize that your self-esteem has a big impact on your life. **Self-esteem** is a measure of how much you value, respect, and feel confident about yourself. Your level of self-esteem determines how you face new challenges. Your level of self-esteem affects your relationships with others. It also affects how you make decisions. Finally, your self-esteem affects your success in anything you choose to do. If you have high self-esteem, you will be more likely to succeed at the new things you try. There will be times when you don't succeed. Having high self-esteem will help you deal with a disappointment better than if you have low self-esteem.

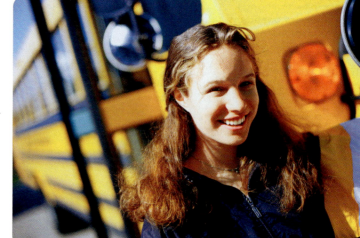

Figure 1 Jessie has high self-esteem. This helps her feel confident about her first day at school.

Background
Girls and Self-Esteem Many television programs and movies show boys having more problems with self-esteem than girls. Inform your students that this is not the case in real-life. Studies of American youths consistently show that adolescent girls tend to have lower self-esteem and more negative assessments of their physical characteristics and intellectual abilities than boys. Psychologists believe that this is the reason why incidences of depression, eating disorders, and suicide-attempts are substantially higher among girls.

Chapter Resource File
- Directed Reading BASIC
- Lesson Plan
- Datasheets for In-Text Activities GENERAL
- Lesson Quiz GENERAL

Transparencies
TT Bellringer
TT What Influences Your Self-Esteem?

50 Chapter 3 • Building Self-Esteem

High Self-Esteem

Having high self-esteem can help a person have a positive outlook on life. High self-esteem can help a person achieve success. People who have high self-esteem share similar traits. They feel good about themselves. They like themselves. They have a high level of confidence. People who have high self-esteem do not feel inferior to others. They are not usually deeply affected by negative comments from other people.

Low Self-Esteem

Low self-esteem may keep a person from enjoying life. People who have low self-esteem do not feel good about themselves. They do not like themselves. Many people have parts of their personality that they do not like. However, people who have low self-esteem often think they have no positive traits. They have a low level of confidence. They may have trouble in their relationships with other people. People who have low self-esteem are often affected by negative comments from other people.

Your self-esteem is likely to change as you change. At times, you may have low self-esteem. Other times you may have high self-esteem. Most people have an overall self-esteem that falls somewhere between high self-esteem and low self-esteem. Aiming to like and accept yourself for who you are can actually help you develop a higher level of self-esteem.

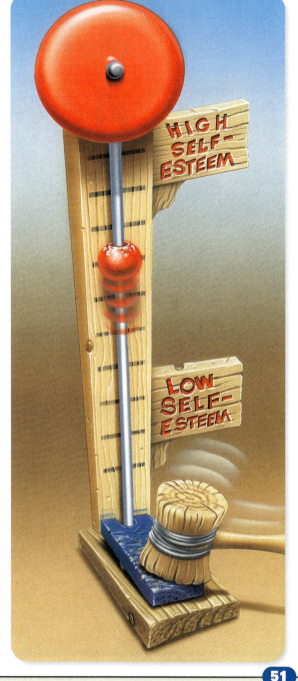

Figure 2 Most people's self-esteem falls between high self-esteem and low self-esteem.

ART CONNECTION — GENERAL

Tell students the following: The Mona Lisa is one of Leonardo da Vinci's most famous paintings. People are fascinated with the Mona Lisa because of her enigmatic expression. Many art critics describe the Mona Lisa as having high confidence and therefore high self-esteem. Other art critics contend that the Mona Lisa seems shy because her gaze is directed slightly to the side. Show a picture of the Mona Lisa to the class, and have them decide whether they think the Mona Lisa portrays high or low self-esteem. **LS Visual**

Teach

Group Activity — GENERAL

Positive Postures Ask students to bring in photos, magazine pictures, or newspaper clippings of people in various postures, gestures, poses, and styles of movement that communicate high self-esteem or low self-esteem. Have students look at each other's images and describe the people who seem to have high self-esteem. *(Sample answers: straight but relaxed posture, energetic walk, firm handshake, sitting forward with hands open and maintaining eye contact)* Then, have students describe the people who seem to have low self-esteem. *(Sample answers: slouching, scuffing floor with each step, averting eyes, stiff, sitting back with arms and legs crossed)*
LS Verbal/Kinesthetic — English Language Learners

Demonstration — GENERAL

Self-Esteem Balloon Bring a large balloon to class and fill the balloon with water. Hold the balloon over a bowl or sink large enough to collect the water. Explain to students that water in the balloon represents a person's self-esteem. Have a volunteer call out something that a person could say or do to him or herself that would lower or "deflate" that person's self-esteem. After the example is called out, use a pin to poke a small hole in the balloon to allow some of the water out. Have another volunteer call out another example. Poke another hole in the balloon. Continue to repeat these steps until there is no water left in the balloon. Have students describe how what happened to the balloon could mirror what happens to a person who develops low self-esteem.
LS Visual

Lesson 1 • Self-Esteem and Your Life 51

Teach, continued

Activity — GENERAL

Self-Esteem on TV Ask students to watch a television program and write about one of the characters. Ask students whether this character exhibited a high or low self-esteem. Have the students explain how they were able to tell if their chosen character had high or low self-esteem. Then, ask the students to give some examples of the way this character's self-esteem was displayed by his or her personal choices and behaviors. Also, have the students describe some of the factors that seemed to influence the person's self-esteem, such as his or her family life, his or her performance at school, or his or her interactions with their friends.
LS Interpersonal

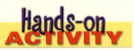

Answers

1. Answers may vary. Sample answer: My classmates pointed out some qualities that I did not realize I had.
2. Answers may vary. Sample answer: I will post this list of positive qualities in my bedroom so I can look at it whenever I need a self-esteem boost.

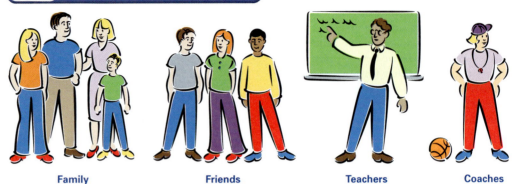

Figure 3 What Influences Your Self-Esteem?

Family   Friends   Teachers   Coaches

Who Can Affect Your Self-Esteem?

Your level of self-esteem is influenced by the people around you. These people include your family, your friends, and people at school. Every person in your life can have a positive or negative effect on your self-esteem.

People who encourage you and give you support will help you feel good about yourself. They will help you develop confidence. People who do not support you may lead you to develop low self-esteem. These people may tease you, or make negative comments about you.

The most important person who influences your self-esteem is you. You can choose to value and like yourself. You can choose to focus on the positive influences on your self-esteem. Similarly, you can choose to deal with negative influences in a positive way.

Hands-on ACTIVITY

SELF-ESTEEM BOOSTER

1. Work in groups of four or five. Each person needs two sheets of paper. On the first sheet of paper, list three positive qualites about yourself. On the second sheet, write your name.
2. Keep the page on which you listed your three qualities. Then, give the sheet with your name on it to a person from your group. On the sheet that another person gives you, list two positive qualities about that person under his or her name.
3. Continue to exchange papers until everyone in the group has had a chance to write under each person's name. Then read your new list.

Analysis
1. How did the list of positive qualities that your classmates wrote compare with the qualities that you listed about yourself?
2. How will you use this list of qualities to boost your self-esteem?

Background

Student-Teacher Interaction Teacher expectations play a vital role in young students' success. One study of grade-school students and teachers involved giving the students an intelligence test. After the test was given, the teachers were told which students ranked in the top 20 percent of the class. In reality, however, the tests were not scored and the names of students in the top 20 percent of the class were chosen at random. Most of the students placed in this "false" top 20 percent had been considered only average students before. Nonetheless, the teachers' attitudes toward these students changed: the teachers became more respectful and confident of the students' success. In the follow-up of this study, the students in the "false" 20 percent tested significantly higher than their classmates on the intelligence test. Their superior performance was attributed mainly to the change in the teachers' attitude.

52 Chapter 3 • Building Self-Esteem

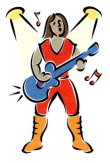 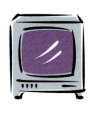 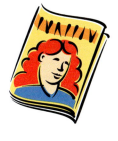 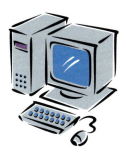

Music videos　　　TV　　　Magazines　　　Internet

The Media and Your Self-Esteem

Did you know that the media can influence your self-esteem? The media includes TV, magazines, movies, and music videos. The media tends to show only people who are very successful or glamorous. The media also tends to show only people who are unusually thin or muscular. Some people may compare themselves to the people they see in the media. This comparison can cause a person to develop an unhealthy body image. **Body image** is the way you see and imagine your body. Your body image can affect your self-esteem. If you are uncomfortable with your body, you probably won't feel good about yourself. Therefore, if you have an unhealthy body image, you may develop low self-esteem. But having a healthy body image can boost your self-esteem. If you feel good about your body, you will probably feel good about yourself.

Health Journal
Write a paragraph describing which forms of media you think influence teens the most.

Lesson Review

Using Vocabulary
1. In your own words, describe the term *self-esteem*.

Understanding Concepts
2. Describe how self-esteem affects your life.
3. Describe the characteristics of a person who has high self-esteem.
4. Identify five influences on your self-esteem.

Critical Thinking
5. **Analyzing Ideas** Explain how having an unhealthy body image can affect your self-esteem. How would having a healthy body image affect your self-esteem?

Answers to Lesson Review
1. Answers may vary. Sample answer: Self-esteem is having pride in myself and having a sense of self-worth.
2. Answers may vary. Sample answer: Self-esteem can affect your level of confidence, your ability to succeed at the things you try to do, and can even affect how well you do in school.
3. People with high self-esteem have a positive outlook on life, feel good about themselves, are confident, and are not affected deeply by the negative comments of others.
4. friends, family, teachers and coaches, and the media, and me
5. People who are not happy or comfortable with their body may not be able to think positive thoughts about themselves. Also, they may be uncomfortable around other people. People with poor body image probably also have low self-esteem. People with positive body image are usually more comfortable with their body and therefore more confident about themselves and more comfortable around other people. People with healthy body image probably also have high self-esteem.

Answer to Health Journal
Answers may vary. This Health Journal may be a good way to close the lesson.

Close

Reteaching — BASIC
Self-Esteem Strengths Have students make a list of activities they perform well. Then, have them write down how these activities affect their self-esteem.
LS Intrapersonal

Quiz — GENERAL
1. Describe what you have learned about your own self-esteem. (Answers may vary. Answers should reflect the students' individual evaluations of self-esteem.)
2. Do you think poverty could cause a person to have low self-esteem? Why? (Answers may vary. Sample answer: Yes, the inability to buy expensive clothes and other material items that the media or peers deem necessary could lower a person's self-esteem.)

Alternative Assessment — GENERAL
Writing **Letter for the Future** Have students imagine that they are adults with their own children. Tell students to write a letter about self-esteem to their children. Have students tell the children how they felt about themselves when they were adolescents and how those feelings changed as they grew older. They should also discuss the things they experienced that made them feel bad about themselves and the things that made them feel good about themselves. The students should end the letter with some advice that will help the child develop high self-esteem. **LS** Verbal

Lesson 2 Focus

Overview
Before beginning this lesson, review with your students the objectives listed under the What You'll Do head in the Student Edition. In this lesson, students will learn the differences between self-esteem and self-concept. Students will also learn about three areas of self-concept.

Bellringer
Have students draw a picture of or write a paragraph about what they imagine they will be doing when they are adults. (Students may draw pictures of or write about themselves doing a certain job or excelling at a certain activity.) **LS Intrapersonal**

Answer to Start Off Write
Accept all reasonable answers. Sample answer: Self-concept is how you see yourself as a person. I see myself as a good athlete.

Motivate

Activity —————— GENERAL
Poster Project Have students imagine that they have to introduce themselves to a stranger. Have students make a list of points explaining who they are. Then, have them use that list to create a poster that represents their overall personalities. When students have completed their posters, volunteers may present them to the class and explain any symbolism or imagery used to represent different aspects of themselves. Encourage students learning English to label their poster in English and in their native language. **English Language Learners**
LS Visual

Lesson 2

What You'll Do
- **Describe** how self-concept and self-esteem are different.
- **Identify** three areas of self-concept.

Terms to Learn
- self-concept

Start Off Write
What is your self-concept?

Your Self-Concept

> Steven tried out for the track team last week. Today he found out that he did not make the team. Steven felt disappointed, but he knows he's good at music. He decided to try out for the band too.

Steven did not let the fact that he didn't make the track team affect his self-esteem. In fact, Steven sees himself more as a musician than a track star. This helped him overcome his disappointment.

Self-Concept and Self-Esteem

Self-concept is a building block of self-esteem. **Self-concept** is the way you see and imagine yourself as a person. Self-concept is different from self-esteem. Self-esteem is the way you value and respect yourself. To find out more about your self-concept, ask yourself the following question: How would you describe yourself to a stranger? Perhaps you see yourself as an athlete. And you see yourself as a good student. Some people may describe themselves as a nice person who makes friends easily.

Imagine that you see yourself as an artist because you like to draw. This image of yourself is your self-concept. However, sometimes you may not feel confident around the people at school. This feeling is your self-esteem. Your self-concept can affect your self-esteem. Because you see yourself as an artist, you may choose to think to yourself, I like to draw, and I am good at it. This makes me feel more confident about myself.

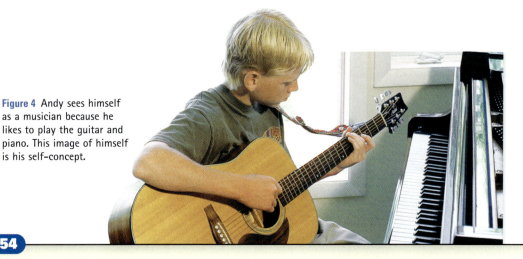

Figure 4 Andy sees himself as a musician because he likes to play the guitar and piano. This image of himself is his self-concept.

MISCONCEPTION ALERT

Some students may think that nobody likes to be around people who say good things about themselves. Tell them that people react positively to individuals who recognize their own good qualities and show self-confidence without being egotistical.

Chapter Resource File
- Directed Reading **BASIC**
- Lesson Plan
- Lesson Quiz **GENERAL**

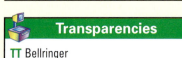

Transparencies
TT Bellringer

---

54 Chapter 3 • Building Self-Esteem

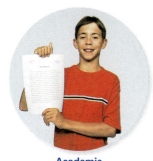
Academic

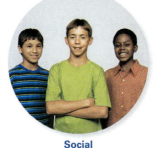
Social

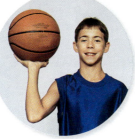
Physical

How Self-Concept Develops

Your self-concept can develop from many areas. Three very important areas are your academic self-concept, your physical self-concept, and your social self-concept.

Your academic self-concept is the way you see yourself as a student. You may see yourself as a good student. Or you may see yourself as an average student.

Your physical self-concept is the way you see your physical abilities. Some people see themselves as good athletes. Other people don't see themselves as athletes, but they are comfortable with their abilities.

Your social self-concept is the way you see yourself in your relationships. Some people see themselves as being very friendly, and they may have a lot of friends. Other people may see themselves as shy. They may have only a few close friends.

These three areas of self-concept contribute to your overall self-concept. As you get to know yourself better, your self-concept will change. In turn, your level of self-esteem may change, too. The way you see yourself in these three areas can help you find your positive traits. Finding your positive traits can boost your self-esteem.

Figure 5 How you see yourself academically, physically, and socially affects your overall self-concept.

Lesson Review

Using Vocabulary
1. What is self-concept?

Understanding Concepts
2. How is self-concept different from self-esteem?
3. What are three areas of self-concept?

Critical Thinking
4. **Making Inferences** Claudia sees herself as a good student who has a lot of friends. However, she does not feel that she is good at sports. Claudia does not let this feeling bother her. Instead she focuses on her strengths. What is Claudia's self-concept? What level of self-esteem does she have?

Lesson 3 Focus

Overview
Before beginning this lesson, review with your students the objectives listed under the What You'll Do head in the Student Edition. This lesson introduces students to the basic keys to developing healthy self-esteem and how to build and maintain healthy self-esteem.

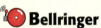 Bellringer
Have students write a paragraph about one of their personal characteristics that they consider a strength. (Answers may vary.)
LS Intrapersonal

Answer to Start Off Write
Accept all reasonable answers. Sample answers: say positive things to myself, do activities that I enjoy, or remind myself that nobody is perfect

Motivate

Activity ———— ADVANCED
Role-Playing Have groups of students role-play different situations that could affect a person's self-esteem. Students should choose situations that might have a positive effect and situations that might have a negative effect on a person's self-esteem. Students should perform the situation in front of the class showing an unhealthy way to react to the situation. The class should suggest healthier ways to deal with the situation in order to maintain high self-esteem.
LS Kinesthetic Co-op Learning

Lesson 3 — Keys to Healthy Self-Esteem

What You'll Do
- **Describe** three keys to healthy self-esteem.
- **Identify** eight strategies for building healthy self-esteem.

Start Off Write
What can you do to boost your self-esteem?

Nicole got mad and yelled at her best friend. Nicole felt very sorry later and apologized to her friend. She asked her best friend for help in thinking of ways to behave when she gets mad in the future.

Everybody makes mistakes. It is easy to apologize, but it takes a healthy attitude to do something about the behavior so that it does not happen again. Doing the right thing helps build healthy self-esteem.

Three Keys to Healthy Self-Esteem
Your actions and behaviors affect the way you feel about yourself. You can have healthy self-esteem by building good character. The first step to developing good character and self-esteem is to have integrity (in TEG ruh tee). Your integrity is your honesty to yourself and others. Integrity is also your ability to take responsibility for your actions. If you are honest and you take responsibility for your actions, you will have a positive image of yourself. Also, the people in your life will be able to trust you.

Second, you must respect yourself to have a healthy self-esteem. Respecting yourself means knowing what is right for you and what is wrong for you. You are respecting yourself if you refuse to join in an activity that you know is wrong, even if it is the popular thing to do.

Third, being assertive can help you build a healthy self-esteem. Being assertive means acting on your thoughts and values in a firm but positive way. You are being assertive when you communicate your feelings clearly and with respect. For example, your friend may ask you to ride bikes one afternoon. But you need to study for a quiz. You can be assertive by telling your friend that you can't ride bikes because you have to study.

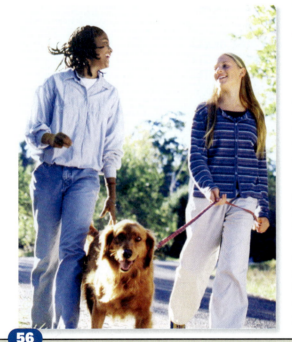

Figure 6 When you have healthy self-esteem, other people see you in a positive way and trust you.

Cultural Awareness
Acculturation is the process of adapting to a new or different culture. Many people who immigrate to the United States undergo acculturation. Research suggests that people who are able to integrate their native customs and values successfully with American customs and values tend to have a higher self-esteem than people who maintain only their native customs and values or completely adopt American customs and values.

Chapter Resource File
- Directed Reading **BASIC**
- Lesson Plan
- Lesson Quiz **GENERAL**

Transparencies
TT Bellringer
TT Examples of Positive Self-Talk

56 Chapter 3 • Building Self-Esteem

Eight Ways to Build Self-Esteem

You know what self-esteem is and how it affects your life. So, how do you build healthy self-esteem? Eight ways to build a healthier level of self-esteem are listed below.

Get to know yourself. Getting to know yourself sounds simple. Do you know yourself simply because you are you? One of the best things to do to improve your self-esteem is to understand who you are. This includes knowing what types of things you like and what things you don't like. For example, you may like to read scary stories. But, you may not like science fiction stories. Getting to know yourself also means knowing what your strengths and weaknesses are. What are you good at? What things could you improve on? You may be really good at math. However, sometimes you get really angry at your little brother, and you would like to improve your behavior towards him. Once you know who you are, it will be easier to know what is right for you and what isn't.

Learn to like yourself. Another step to building healthy self-esteem is learning to like yourself. You need to focus on what you like best about yourself. Imagine that a friend told you that you are a good listener. You like yourself for being a good listener. Liking yourself for your positive qualities helps you be assertive and confident. Liking yourself also means accepting all of your qualities, whether they are good or bad. Accepting and liking yourself helps you build high self-esteem.

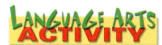

Write a story about a teen who chooses to do one of the items listed in this lesson to build self-esteem. In your story, describe what your character decided to do and how it helped your character improve his or her self-esteem.

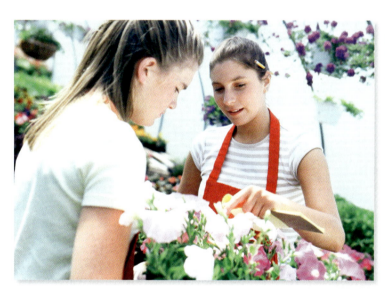

Figure 7 Jen knows that gardening is one of her strengths. This makes her feel good about herself.

Teach, continued

Answer to Life Skills Activity

Answers may vary. Sample answer: I will refuse to let him use my homework to cheat because he should have done his own homework. Showing integrity will increase my self-esteem.

Life SKILL BUILDER — GENERAL

Setting Goals Explain to students that setting small, short-term goals before setting big, long-term goals is the best way to become comfortable with setting goals and building self-esteem. Ask students to think of a small goal they would like to reach within one week. Then, have students make a plan to reach their goal. After one week, have students write a brief paragraph describing how setting and reaching a goal affected their self-esteem. **LS Logical/Verbal**

Group Activity — GENERAL

Practicing Positive Self-Talk

Assign pairs of students to role-play the positive side of a hypothetical personality and the negative side of the same personality. Have each actor pretend to be one side of the personality and respond to various situations with suitable statements. Be sure students have a chance to play both roles. Sample situation: *joining a group at lunch*

Negative: What am I doing? They don't want me with them! I'll probably say something stupid and they won't like me.

Positive: They look friendly, and there's space at their table. This is a great opportunity to find out about their interests. I'll bet we have a lot of things in common. **LS Auditory**

Co-op Learning

LIFE SKILLS ACTIVITY

USING REFUSAL SKILLS

Imagine a classmate approached you before math class. He asked if he could borrow your homework because he didn't do his homework. What will you tell your classmate? How will your actions affect your self-esteem?

MISCONCEPTION ALERT

Students may think that copying the mannerisms of someone in the "in crowd" may cause them to lose their own personality. Explain to students that the teenage years are an important time for both conformity and experimenting with self-expression. Experimenting by copying the actions of someone they admire is normal. However, help students understand that if copying the actions of others leads them to do things that go against their basic values, they must reevaluate their own behavior.

Be good at something. One way to feel good about yourself is to be good at something. Find something you enjoy doing. It could be a hobby, a sport, an activity at school, or anything. In your free time, focus your efforts on the activity you choose. If you really enjoy what you are doing, you can try to become better at your activity. You will develop more confidence and higher self-esteem if you know you are good at something.

Set a goal. Setting goals helps you build self-esteem because reaching goals gives you a sense of accomplishment. When you try hard to reach a goal, you feel good about yourself. Once you reach your goal, you will feel successful. Start by setting small goals. When you feel more confident about setting and reaching goals, you can try to set higher goals. When you set a higher goal, you will have to stretch yourself to reach it. In turn, you will grow as a person. You will also discover your hidden strengths.

Be positive. Did you know that just believing in yourself can help you build self-esteem? Thinking positive thoughts when you are feeling unsure of yourself can help you be more confident in many situations. You can use positive self-talk to be your own cheerleader. Positive self-talk is a way of encouraging yourself by saying or thinking positive statements to yourself. The table below shows you some examples of positive self-talk. The next time you feel nervous in a situation, try using positive self-talk to give yourself a boost of confidence.

TABLE 1 Positive Self-Talk

Situation	Positive self-talk
You are nervous that you may not do well on a test.	"I studied for this test, and I know that I can do well. I know I can do it!"
You are afraid that you won't make any friends at your new school.	"Making friends takes time. I just have to be myself and be confident that I will meet people."
You don't like your new haircut.	"I don't like how my haircut turned out. But my hair will grow, and I can get it cut differently next time. Maybe if I try styling it a different way, I won't feel so bad about it."
Some of your classmates teased you about the way you run in gym class.	"I feel bad because they tease me when I run. But I know that I'm better at other things. I am very good at swimming, so I don't feel bad if I can't run as fast as everyone else."

Career

Cognitive Therapists Health professionals that are trained to help people learn the skill of positive self-talk are called *cognitive therapists*. Cognitive therapists teach clients to talk positively to themselves to change the way they think about things and to affirm their feelings. Cognitive therapists also help clients break problems down into manageable parts and work on one aspect at a time. This helps their clients avoid perceiving the problem as a catastrophe and as something that cannot be overcome.

Chapter 3 • Building Self-Esteem

Find a mentor. A mentor is someone who can give you support and encouragment. Often, a mentor is older than you. A mentor should have qualities that you would like to have. This person can be your role model. A mentor can help you set goals and discover your abilities. In this way, a mentor can help you build self-esteem.

Do something for others. Helping people who are less fortunate than you is a great way to build your self-esteem. It also gives you a chance to share your abilities with other people. Try volunteering at your local charity organization, such as a soup kitchen. Or participate in a food and clothing drive.

Have a sense of humor. People who have a high level of self-esteem are not usually deeply affected by negative comments from others. In fact, people who have high self-esteem are able to laugh at themselves. Having a sense of humor means you are able to laugh at yourself. Having a sense of humor helps you accept some of your weaknesses. For example, suppose you are not a great basketball player. But when you play basketball, you have a sense of humor about yourself. You have a good time no matter what your abilities are. Approaching life with a sense of humor is a great way to build healthy self-esteem.

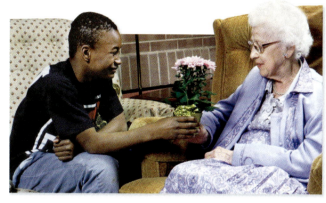

Figure 8 Participating in volunteer activities is a great way to boost your self-esteem.

Lesson Review

Understanding Concepts
1. Describe three keys to self-esteem.
2. How can having a mentor help you build self-esteem?
3. How can volunteer work help you build self-esteem? List three volunteer activities you would like to try.
4. Name an activity that you enjoy. What steps can you take to become better at this activity? How can being better at the activity help your self-esteem?

Critical Thinking
5. **Making Inferences** How does having integrity, respecting yourself, and being assertive help you to have high self-esteem?

internet connect
www.scilinks.org/health
Topic: Building Healthy Self-Esteem
HealthLinks code: HD4020
HEALTH LINKS Maintained by the National Science Teachers Association

---

Close

Reteaching — BASIC
Ask students to write their own review questions and answers for this section. Afterwards, students can exchange review questions and try to answer the questions. They should then exchange their answers and grade each other. **LS Verbal**

Quiz — GENERAL
1. What is positive self-talk? (Positive self-talk is a way of talking to yourself in an encouraging manner by saying positive things.)
2. Why does setting a goal help to build your self-esteem? (Setting and reaching a goal gives you a sense of accomplishment.)
3. What does getting to know yourself mean? (It means getting to know and understanding your strengths and weaknesses and your likes and dislikes.)

Alternative Assessment — GENERAL
Self-Help Book Tell students to imagine that they are writing a self-help book for teenagers with low self-esteem. Students should write an outline of the book that includes a paragraph briefly summarizing the contents of each chapter. **LS Verbal**

Answers to Lesson Review
1. Sample answer: Three keys to self-esteem are having integrity, respecting yourself, and being assertive. Having integrity means being honest with myself and others. Respecting myself means doing the right thing. Being assertive means acting on my thoughts and values.
2. A mentor will give you support, encouragement, and advice. Your mentor's actions can help you build healthy self-esteem.
3. Helping people in need helps you better yourself. You will also feel a sense of accomplishment. (Students may suggest that they would like to plant trees, clean up roadways, or spend time with the elderly.)
4. Answers may vary. Sample answer: I enjoy painting. I can take a painting class to learn how to paint better. Being better at painting can help me build my confidence and therefore build self-esteem.
5. Sample answer: Having these qualities helps build your self-esteem by allowing you to trust yourself and giving you a good framework to make decisions with confidence.

Lesson 3 • Keys to Healthy Self-Esteem

CHAPTER 3 REVIEW

Assignment Guide

Lessons	Review Questions
1	2–3, 6, 8, 18–20, 22
2	4–5, 10, 17, 21
3	7, 9, 11–16, 24–26
1 and 2	1
1–3	23

ANSWERS

Using Vocabulary

1. Self-esteem is how you feel about yourself as a person, while self-concept is the way you see and imagine yourself as a person.
2. Self-esteem is how much you value and like yourself as a person, while your body image is they way you see and imagine your body. Your body image can affect your self-esteem.
3. self-esteem
4. body image
5. self-concept

Understanding Concepts

6. negative outlook on life, has very little confidence, not comfortable with himself or herself, unwilling to try new things, has trouble in his or her relationships with other people
7. Being assertive means acting on your thoughts and values without hurting other people's feelings.
8. Sample answer: friends, family, the media
9. Sample answers:
   a. Accepting your strengths and weaknesses allows you to focus on your strengths instead of your weaknesses.
   b. Setting and reaching a goal can give you a sense of accomplishment. Even if you don't reach your goal, you can feel good about the effort you put into reaching your goal.
   c. Having a positive attitude can help you deal with disappointments and with negative comments from others.
   d. Knowing yourself can help you find your strengths. Therefore, you will be able to focus on your strengths.
   e. Having a sense of humor can help you deal with disappointments or uncomfortable situations in a positive way.
10. the way you see yourself as a student
11. Integrity, assertiveness, and self-respect can help a person build self-esteem by building good character. If a person has a good character, he or she will most likely have healthy self-esteem.
12. Sample answer: If I was having a "bad hair day," I could use positive self-talk to make myself feel better before going to school. For example, I could tell myself that my hair doesn't look as bad as I think it does.

CHAPTER 3 REVIEW

Chapter Summary

- Self-esteem is the way you value, respect, and feel about yourself. ■ Self-esteem affects your relationships with other people and how you face new situations. ■ Influences on your self-esteem include family, friends, teachers, coaches, and the media. ■ Self-concept is how you see yourself as a person. ■ There are three areas of self-concept: academic self-concept, social self-concept, and physical self-concept. ■ Three keys to healthy self-esteem include having integrity, respecting yourself, and being assertive.

Using Vocabulary

For each pair of terms, describe how the meanings of the terms differ.

1. self-esteem/self-concept
2. self-esteem/body image

For each sentence, fill in the blank with the proper word from the word bank provided below.

   self-concept   body image
   self-esteem

3. How you feel about yourself as a person is your ___.
4. Your ___ is the way you see and imagine your body.
5. How you see yourself as a person is called your ___.

Understanding Concepts

6. What are the characteristics of a person who has low self-esteem?
7. What does being assertive mean?
8. Name three influences on your self-esteem.
9. How can the following actions help you build a healthy self-esteem?
   a. accepting yourself
   b. setting a goal
   c. being positive
   d. knowing yourself
   e. having a sense of humor
10. What is academic self-concept?
11. How do integrity, self-respect, and assertiveness help you have healthy self-esteem?
12. Give an example of how you would use positive self-talk to boost your self-esteem.
13. Discovering your strengths and weaknesses can help you build healthy self-esteem. Explain why this may be true.
14. What does having integrity mean?
15. What is a mentor?
16. List eight things you can do to boost your self-esteem.
17. What is physical self-concept?

Critical Thinking

Analyzing Ideas

18. Can the media affect a person's self-esteem? Explain your answer.
19. Why is it healthier to have high self-esteem rather than low self-esteem?
20. Explain how a classmate who teases you may affect your self-esteem.
21. How does your overall self-concept develop?
22. Why do you think you are the most important influence on your self-esteem?

Making Good Decisions

23. Use what you have learned in this chapter to set a personal goal. Write your goal, and make an action plan by using the Health Behavior Contract for building healthy self-esteem. You can find the Health Behavior Contract at **go.hrw.com**. Just type in the keyword **HD4HBC05**.

Interpreting Graphics

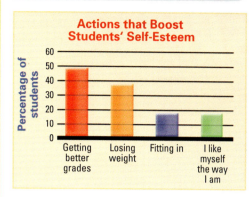

Actions that Boost Students' Self-Esteem

Use the figure above to answer questions 24–26.

24. Several teenagers were interviewed for a survey. The graph above shows the results of the survey. According to the graph, what percentage of teens like themselves as they are?
25. Which of the actions above would make the most teens feel better about themselves?
26. If 200,000 teens were interviewed for this survey, how many students feel that losing weight will help them feel better about themselves?

Reading Checkup

Take a minute to review your answers to the Health IQ questions at the beginning of this chapter. How has reading this chapter improved your Health IQ?

---

13. If you know your strengths, you can focus on them and feel confident in the things you do well. If you know your weaknesses, you can try to overcome them.
14. Having integrity means being honest with yourself and with others.
15. A mentor is someone who is usually older than you, who shares similar interests to you, and can provide you with encouragement and support.
16. get to know yourself, accept yourself, set a goal, develop a hobby, be positive, find a mentor, have a sense of humor, volunteer your time
17. Your physical self-concept is how you see yourself physically and how you see your physical abilities.

Critical Thinking
Analyzing Ideas

18. Answers may vary. Sample answer: The media tend to show people who are unusually thin or muscular and who are unusually successful. Some people may not be satisfied with themselves when they compare themselves to people on TV. Therefore, they begin to develop low self-esteem.
19. Answers may vary. Sample answer: People who have high self-esteem are more likely to overcome disappointments, try new things, take better care for themselves, and do better in school than people who have low self-esteem. So, it is better for a person's health to have high self-esteem.
20. Answers may vary. Sample answer: Negative comments from a classmate can cause you to feel bad about yourself. You may even feel embarrassed. If you let yourself feel bad, you may develop a low self-esteem.
21. Answers may vary. Sample answer: Your overall self-concept develops from many areas. Three important areas of self-concept include academic, social, and physical self-concept.
22. Answers may vary. Sample answer: I think that I am the most important influence on my self-esteem because I can choose to focus on my strengths, I can choose to stay positive when I am feeling down, and I can choose to deal with negative comments in a positive way.

Making Good Decisions

23. Accept all reasonable responses. **Note:** A Health Behavior Contract for each chapter can be found in the Chapter Resource File and at the HRW Web site, go.hrw.com.

Interpreting Graphics

24. 18 percent
25. getting better grades
26. 76,000 students (0.38 × 200,000 students = 76,000 students)

Chapter Resource File
- Concept Review GENERAL
- Concept Mapping GENERAL
- Performance-Based Assessment GENERAL
- Chapter Test GENERAL

Model

Introduce this activity by reminding students that using this Life Skill will help them take personal responsibility for their behavior. Then, review the scenario with the class.

Prepare students for this activity by modeling each of the steps of the skill. Make sure students understand each step before you move on to the next one.

Guided Practice: Practice with a Friend

Guided Practice is the stage in which you and the students analyze their approach to solving the problem given in the scenario and analyze their coping skills. Have students read Act 1. Discuss with the class the situation described and the way students are to act it out. Organize the class into groups of three. In each group, one person plays the role of Brent, another person plays Brent's science teacher, and the third person is the observer.

Proper pacing during the Guided Practice is important. The suggestions listed below will help you control the pace.

1. Stop after completing each step of coping.
2. Discuss with each group the observer's comments.
3. Ask the other members of each group to listen to the observer's suggestions and to suggest ways to improve their coping skills.
4. Instruct students to repeat the steps that need improvement and to include their modifications.

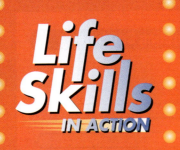

Coping

At times, everyone faces setbacks, disappointments, or other troubles. To deal with these problems, you have to learn how to cope. Coping is dealing with problems and emotions in an effective way. Complete the following activity to develop your coping skills.

The Big Test

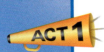

Setting the Scene

Brent has never been a great student in science, but he always works hard enough to get a passing grade. This year, however, Brent is enjoying his science class and is determined to earn a B or better in it. He had his first big test in the class on Friday, and he studied very hard for it. Unfortunately, when Brent gets his test back, he learns that he failed it and is crushed. Brent decides to discuss his grade with his science teacher after school.

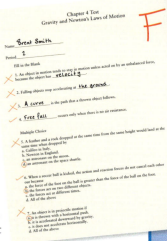

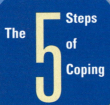

The 5 Steps of Coping

1. Identify the problem.
2. Identify your emotions.
3. Use positive self-talk.
4. Find ways to resolve the problem.
5. Talk to others to receive support.

Guided Practice

Practice with a Friend

Form a group of three. Have one person play the role of Brent and another person play the role of Brent's science teacher. Have the third person be an observer. Walking through each of the five steps of coping, role-play Brent dealing with his failing test grade. Brent can talk to his teacher to receive support. The observer will take notes, which will include observations about what the person playing Brent did well and suggestions of ways to improve. Stop after each step to evaluate the process.

5. Check to make sure that students understand each step before they move on to the next step.
6. If time permits, repeat the exercise three times, switching roles each time. Each student should have the opportunity to play each role. **Co-op Learning**

62 Chapter 3 • Life Skills in Action

Independent Practice

Check Yourself

After you have completed the guided practice, go through Act 1 again without stopping at each step. Answer the questions below to review what you did.

1. What emotions could Brent have after learning what his grade on the test was?
2. What positive self-talk could Brent use to help him cope with his emotions?
3. What are some ways that Brent can resolve his problem?
4. How do you cope when you don't do as well as you had hoped on a test?

On Your Own

With the help of some study tips from his teacher, Brent is able to do better in science. However, to raise his grade, Brent has to spend a lot of time studying. Brent's friends are unhappy because he doesn't spend much time with them anymore. Some of his friends have started calling him a nerd and a teacher's pet. Brent doesn't like the teasing, but his friends won't leave him alone. Write a skit in which Brent uses the five steps of coping to deal with the teasing and name-calling.

Independent Practice: Check Yourself

Instruct students to repeat Act 1 without stopping at each step. Remind students to apply what they learned in the Guided Practice to the Independent Practice. Students do not have to use every step to cope successfully, nor do they have to follow steps 2–5 in order.

Encourage students to use the Check Yourself questions as a starting point for reviewing and analyzing their Independent Practice. Remind students that as they change roles, the answers to these questions may change for each actor. Encourage students to create additional questions for checking their coping skills. When students have finished the Independent Practice, have them answer the Check Yourself questions in writing. Use their answers to assess their understanding of the steps of coping and to assess their use of the steps to solve a problem.

Check Yourself Answers

1. Sample answer: Brent may have felt anger, sadness, frustration, or disappointment.
2. Sample answer: Brent could tell himself that he is a good student and that he is capable of doing well in his classes.
3. Sample answer: Brent could ask his teacher or a tutor for help. Brent could also learn better study habits.
4. Sample answer: I tell myself that it was only one test and that I will do better on the next one. Then, I talk to my teacher about what I need to work on before the next test.

Act 2: On Your Own

This additional scenario gives students an opportunity to apply what they have learned in both the Guided Practice and the Independent Practice to a new situation.

Suggest to students that they use the Check Yourself questions as a starting point for coping in the new situation. Encourage students to be creative and to think of ways to improve their coping skills.

Assessment

Review the skits that students have written as part of the On Your Own activity. The skits should include a realistic conversation and should show that the students applied their coping skills in a realistic and effective manner. If time permits, ask student volunteers to act out one or more of the skits. Discuss the conversation and the use of coping skills.

CHAPTER 4: Physical Fitness
Chapter Planning Guide

PACING	CLASSROOM RESOURCES	ACTIVITIES AND DEMONSTRATIONS
BLOCK 1 • 45 min pp. 64–67 **Chapter Opener**	CRF Health Inventory * GENERAL CRF Parent Letter *	SE Health IQ, p. 65 CRF At-Home Activity *
Lesson 1 The Parts of Fitness	CRF Lesson Plan * TT Bellringer *	TE Activities Which Endurance Is It?, p. 63F TE Activity Poster Project, p. 66 GENERAL CRF Enrichment Activity * ADVANCED
BLOCK 2 • 45 min pp. 68–73 **Lesson 2** Your Fitness Program	CRF Lesson Plan * TT Bellringer * TT Healthy Fitness Zones for Ages 12 to 14 *	TE Activity, pp. 68, 70 BASIC TE Group Activity Role-Play, p. 69 GENERAL TE Demonstration, p. 70 GENERAL SE Life Skills in Action Assessing Your Health, pp. 90–91 CRF Life Skills Activity * GENERAL CRF Enrichment Activity * ADVANCED
Lesson 3 Energy for Exercise	CRF Lesson Plan * TT Bellringer *	TE Group Activity Sunday Funnies, p. 73 BASIC CRF Enrichment Activity * ADVANCED
BLOCK 3 • 45 min pp. 74–79 **Lesson 4** Sports and Competition	CRF Lesson Plan * TT Bellringer *	TE Activities Working Together, p. 63F TE Activity How-To Guide, p. 75 GENERAL CRF Enrichment Activity * ADVANCED
Lesson 5 Weight Training	CRF Lesson Plan * TT Bellringer * TT Some Weight-Training Exercises *	TE Group Activity Selling Weight Training, p. 76 GENERAL SE Science Activity, p. 77 TE Activity Anabolic Steroids, p. 77 ADVANCED TE Demonstration, pp. 77, 78 BASIC CRF Life Skills Activity * GENERAL CRF Enrichment Activity * ADVANCED
BLOCK 4 • 45 min pp. 80–83 **Lesson 6** Injury	CRF Lesson Plan * TT Bellringer * TT The Overtraining Curve *	CRF Enrichment Activity * ADVANCED
Lesson 7 Common Injuries	CRF Lesson Plan * TT Bellringer *	TE Group Activity Skit, p. 82 GENERAL TE Activity Chronic Injury in Teens, p. 83 ADVANCED CRF Enrichment Activity * ADVANCED
BLOCK 5 • 45 min pp. 84–87 **Lesson 8** Eight Ways to Avoid Injury	CRF Lesson Plan * TT Bellringer *	TE Group Activity Sports Safety, p. 85 GENERAL TE Group Activity Sing It!, p. 86 BASIC TE Activity Physical Activity and Children with Disabilities, p. 86 GENERAL CRF Enrichment Activity * ADVANCED

BLOCKS 6 & 7 • 90 min Chapter Review and Assessment Resources

- SE Chapter Review, pp. 88–89
- CRF Concept Review * GENERAL
- CRF Health Behavior Contract * GENERAL
- CRF Chapter Test * GENERAL
- CRF Performance-Based Assessment * GENERAL
- OSP Test Generator
- CRF Test Item Listing *

Online Resources

Visit **go.hrw.com** for a variety of free resources related to this textbook. Enter the keyword **HD4PF7**.

Students can access interactive problem solving help and active visual concept development with the *Decisions for Health* Online Edition available at **www.hrw.com**.

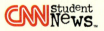

cnnstudentnews.com
Find the latest health news, lesson plans, and activities related to important scientific events.

Compression guide:
To shorten your instruction because of time limitations, omit Lessons 3–5.

KEY

- **TE** Teacher Edition
- **SE** Student Edition
- **OSP** One-Stop Planner
- **CRF** Chapter Resource File
- **TT** Teaching Transparency
- ***** Also on One-Stop Planner
- ■ Also Available in Spanish
- ♦ Requires Advance Prep

SKILLS DEVELOPMENT RESOURCES	LESSON REVIEW AND ASSESSMENT	STANDARDS CORRELATION
		National Health Education Standards
TE Inclusion Strategies, p. 67 `BASIC` **CRF** Directed Reading * `BASIC`	**SE** Lesson Review, p. 67 **TE** Reteaching, Quiz, p. 67 **CRF** Lesson Quiz * ■ `GENERAL`	
TE Life Skill Builder Practicing Wellness, p. 68 **SE** Life Skills Activity Practicing Wellness, p. 70 **CRF** Decision-Making * `GENERAL` **CRF** Directed Reading * `BASIC`	**SE** Lesson Review, p. 71 **TE** Reteaching, Quiz, p. 71 **CRF** Concept Mapping * `GENERAL` **CRF** Lesson Quiz * ■ `GENERAL`	1.1, 3.2, 3.4, 4.3, 6.4
CRF Cross-Disciplinary * `GENERAL` **CRF** Directed Reading * `BASIC`	**SE** Lesson Review, p. 73 **TE** Reteaching, Quiz, p. 73 **CRF** Concept Mapping * `GENERAL` **CRF** Lesson Quiz * ■ `GENERAL`	
CRF Refusal Skills * `GENERAL` **CRF** Directed Reading * `BASIC`	**SE** Lesson Review, p. 75 **TE** Reteaching, Quiz, p. 75 **TE** Alternative Assessment, p. 75 `BASIC` **CRF** Lesson Quiz * ■ `GENERAL`	
TE Life Skill Builder Being a Wise Consumer, p. 77 `ADVANCED` **CRF** Directed Reading * `BASIC`	**SE** Lesson Review, p. 79 **TE** Reteaching, Quiz, p. 79 **TE** Alternative Assessment, p. 79 `GENERAL` **CRF** Lesson Quiz * ■ `GENERAL`	
TE Life Skill Builder Coping, p. 80 `GENERAL` **CRF** Cross-Disciplinary * `GENERAL` **CRF** Directed Reading * `BASIC`	**SE** Lesson Review, p. 81 **TE** Reteaching, Quiz, p. 81 **CRF** Lesson Quiz * ■ `GENERAL`	1.1
TE Inclusion Strategies, p. 83 `BASIC` **CRF** Directed Reading * `BASIC`	**SE** Lesson Review, p. 83 **TE** Reteaching, Quiz, p. 83 **CRF** Lesson Quiz * ■ `GENERAL`	
SE Study Tip, p. 85 **TE** Reading Skill Builder Paired Summarizing, p. 85 `BASIC` **TE** Life Skill Builder Assessing Your Health, p. 85 `GENERAL` **SE** Life Skills Activity Evaluating Media Messages, p. 86 **CRF** Decision-Making * **CRF** Refusal Skills * `GENERAL` **CRF** Directed Reading * `BASIC`	**SE** Lesson Review, p. 87 **TE** Reteaching, Quiz, p. 87 **TE** Alternative Assessment, p. 87 `GENERAL` **CRF** Lesson Quiz * ■ `GENERAL`	1.1, 3.4, 3.5

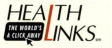

www.scilinks.org/health
Maintained by the **National Science Teachers Association**

Topic: Physical Fitness
HealthLinks code: HD4076

Topic: Aerobic and Anaerobic Exercise
HealthLinks code: HD4004

Topic: Health Benefits of Sports
HealthLinks code: HD4050

Topic: Sports Injury
HealthLinks code: HD4093

Technology Resources

One-Stop Planner
All of your printable resources and the Test Generator are on this convenient CD-ROM.

Guided Reading Audio CDs

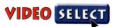

For information about videos related to this chapter, go to **go.hrw.com** and type in the keyword **HD4PF7V**.

Chapter 4 • Chapter Planning Guide   63B

CHAPTER 4

Physical Fitness
Chapter Resources

Teacher Resources

TEACHING TRANSPARENCIES

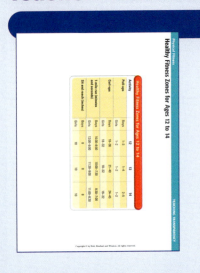
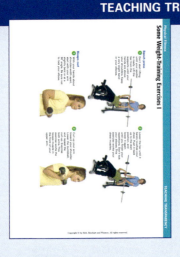
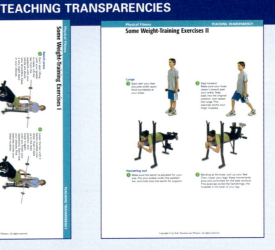
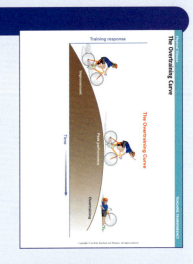

LESSON PLANS
PARENT LETTER
TEST ITEM LISTING
BELLRINGER TRANSPARENCIES

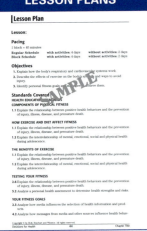
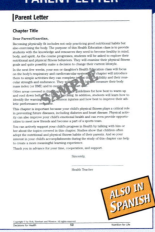
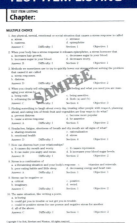

Meeting Individual Needs

DIRECTED READING
CONCEPT MAPPING
CONCEPT REVIEW
ENRICHMENT ACTIVITIES

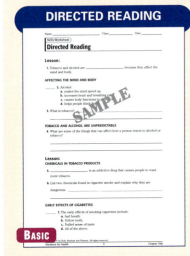
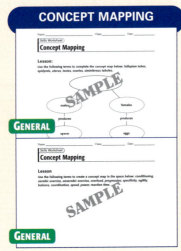
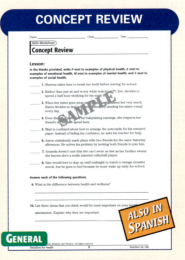
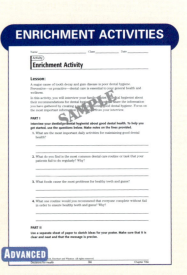

63C Chapter 4 • Physical Fitness

Resources

These worksheet pages can be found in the Chapter Resource File and the One-Stop Planner. The transparencies can be found in the Teaching Transparencies binder and on the One-Stop Planner.

Activities

LIFE SKILLS ACTIVITIES
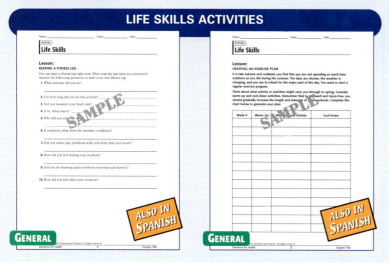

AT-HOME ACTIVITY
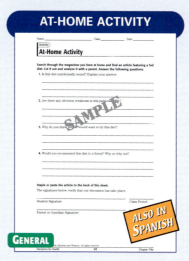

DATASHEETS FOR IN-TEXT ACTIVITIES
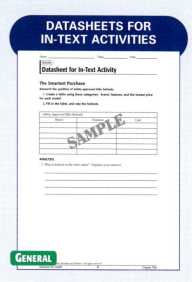

Applications

DECISION-MAKING
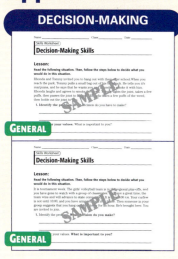

REFUSAL SKILLS
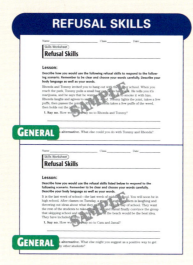

CROSS-DISCIPLINARY
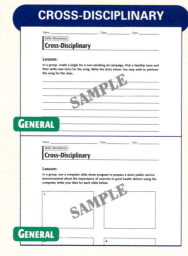

HEALTH BEHAVIOR CONTRACT
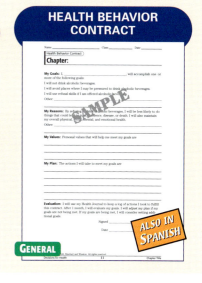

Assessments

HEALTH INVENTORY
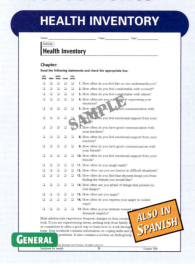

LESSON QUIZZES
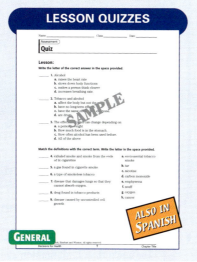

CHAPTER TEST
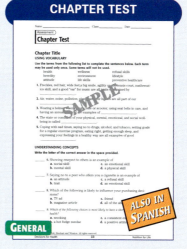

PERFORMANCE-BASED ASSESSMENT
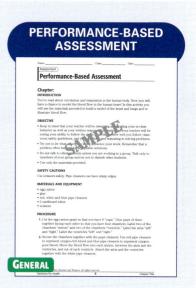

Chapter 4 • Chapter Resources and Worksheets   63D

Background Information

CHAPTER 4

The following information focuses on exercise, weight training, and aerobic and anaerobic energy systems. This material will help prepare you for teaching the concepts in this chapter.

Why Exercise?

- Exercise improves physical fitness. Muscles become stronger. The heart and lungs become more efficient. Exercise can prevent weight gain that may lead to obesity.

- Exercise can help reduce the chances of some non-infectious diseases. Exercise can help prevent some forms of cancer. Because exercise helps prevent obesity, which is linked to heart disease and diabetes, exercise can help prevent these diseases. Exercise also helps prevent osteoporosis by improving bone density.

- Exercise can improve mental and emotional health. A Harvard study revealed that a 10-week strength-training program reduced symptoms of depression more effectively than traditional counseling.

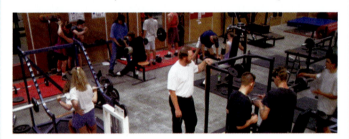

Weight Training

- A regular weight-training program increases resting metabolism, which means you will burn more Calories throughout the day. For each pound of muscle gained, your body uses an extra 35 to 50 Calories a day.

- Isotonic exercises involve free weights, machines, and exercises such as pull-ups, push-ups, and sit-ups. Muscles contract against a constant amount of resistance.

- During isometric exercises, a person contracts muscles against a fixed object. For example, pushing against a wall is an isometric exercise.

- Isokinetic exercises involve special equipment that maintains the speed of an exercise by changing resistance. Isokinetic exercises employ the principle that muscles have variable strength depending on the angle of a joint.

Aerobic and Anaerobic Exercise

- The energy from the food we eat is stored in adenosine triphosphate (ATP), an energy-storage molecule. The amount of ATP in muscles is so small that it must be restored constantly during exercise. The aerobic and anaerobic systems replace this ATP.

- The anaerobic system utilizes two processes for restoring ATP. The first process uses the ATP that is already present in muscles and another molecule called *creatine phosphate*. This process provides energy for about 10 seconds. The second process is called *glycolysis*. ATP is produced from the carbohydrate glycogen, leaving lactic acid as a by-product. Lactic acid fatigues muscles and causes a burning sensation that goes away once activity is stopped. Glycolysis powers activity for 1 to 3 minutes. The anaerobic system doesn't require oxygen to generate ATP.

- When exercising, the body initially uses the anaerobic system. After about 3 minutes, it uses the aerobic system. The aerobic system produces ATP at a slower rate than the anaerobic system, but it can produce much more energy overall than the anaerobic system. In the aerobic system, ATP is made from carbohydrates and fatty acids. This system requires oxygen.

- The anaerobic system is reengaged when the intensity of exercise prevents the body from getting enough oxygen to keep the aerobic system going. For example, when a distance runner is sprinting for the finish, the anaerobic system likely has been engaged.

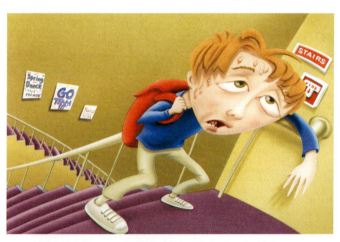

For background information about teaching strategies and issues, refer to the Professional Reference for Teachers.

ACTIVITIES

CHAPTER 4

Consider using the activities on this page as students explore the lessons of this chapter. Look for other activities throughout the Student Edition chapter.

Which Endurance Is It?

Procedure In this activity, students will measure heart rate after four different physical activities. Students should measure their resting heart rates before starting the activity. Make sure students have warmed up before doing any physical activity.

Ask each student to run a lap around the track or the building. Each student should measure his or her heart rate right after finishing the lap. Students should record the results. Have students measure their heart rates again after doing 20 curl-ups, jumping rope for 2 minutes, and doing 10 biceps curls with a 5-pound barbell. Ask students to find the difference between their resting heart rate and their heart rate after the exercises. Have them graph their results.

Safety Caution: Students with health problems should be excused from the activity.

Analysis Ask the following questions:

- Using your graph, which exercise increased your heart rate the most? (Some students will answer that running increased their heart rate the most, but other students may see a bigger increase after jumping rope.)

- Based on your heart rates, which activities will improve your heart and lung endurance? (running and jumping rope) Which improve your muscular endurance? (curl-ups and biceps curls)

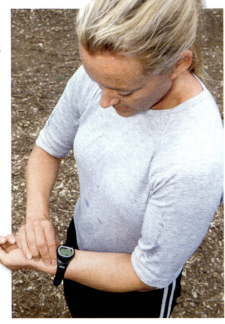

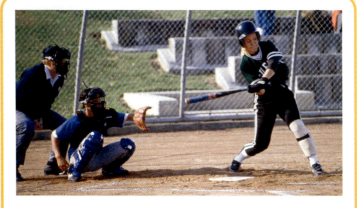

Working Together

Procedure Use this activity to begin a discussion about teamwork.

Set up an obstacle course on a grass field or in the gym. Ask students to work in pairs and hold the opposite ends of a short rope. Ask each pair to run the course and record the amount of time it takes to finish. Students should not let go of the rope. If they do, they should start over.

After pairs are finished, have students work in groups of four. Students should form a chain by holding on to the opposite ends of short pieces of rope. Students should work through the obstacle course without letting go of the ropes. Record the amount of time it takes each group to finish. Do the same for groups of eight students.

Safety Caution: Students with health problems should be excused from the activity.

Analysis Ask the following questions:

- Which time was it easiest for you to run through the obstacle course? (Sample answer: It was easiest when we worked in pairs.)

- Which time was it hardest to run through the obstacle course? Explain. (Sample answer: It was hardest when we went in groups of eight. With more people, it can be harder to work together.)

- What do you think you could have done to make it easier to go through the course with eight people? (Sample answer: We could have communicated more. Also, we could have selected a leader to give directions.)

Chapter 4 • Activities

CHAPTER 4

Overview
Tell students that this chapter will help them learn the parts of fitness. The chapter will discuss starting a fitness program, the two kinds of exercise, and playing sports. This chapter also discusses weight training and illustrates some weight-training exercises. Finally, the chapter describes exercise-related injuries and how to avoid them.

Assessing Prior Knowledge
Students should be familiar with the following topics:
- refusal skills
- setting goals

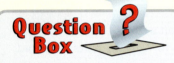

Students may feel more comfortable asking questions if you set up a Question Box to collect their questions. Have students write and anonymously submit their questions about exercise-related injuries, the health benefits of physical fitness, and ways to stay safe when exercising. Address these questions during class, or use these questions to introduce lessons that cover related topics.

Current Health
Check out *Current Health* articles and activities related to this chapter by visiting the HRW Web site at **go.hrw.com**. Just type in the keyword **HD4CH19T**.

Chapter Resource File
- Directed Reading **BASIC**
- Health Inventory **GENERAL**
- Parent Letter

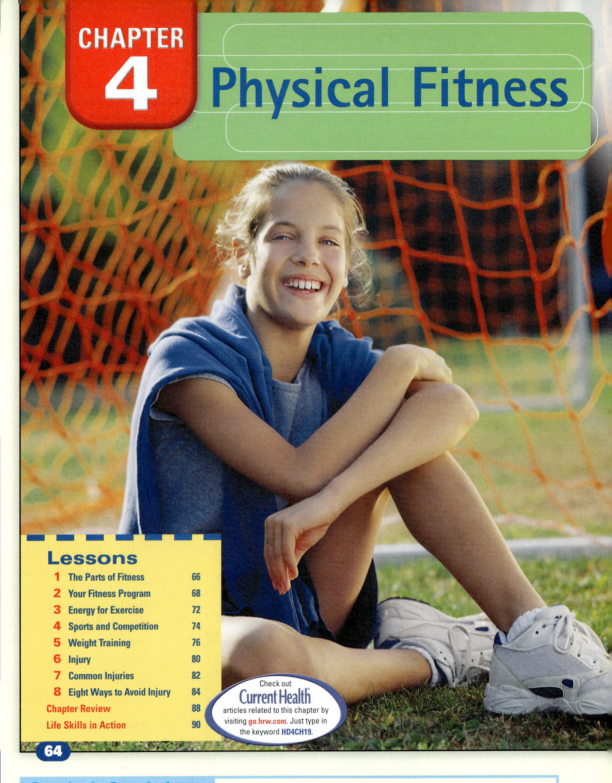

CHAPTER 4 Physical Fitness

Lessons
1	The Parts of Fitness	66
2	Your Fitness Program	68
3	Energy for Exercise	72
4	Sports and Competition	74
5	Weight Training	76
6	Injury	80
7	Common Injuries	82
8	Eight Ways to Avoid Injury	84
	Chapter Review	88
	Life Skills in Action	90

Check out **Current Health** articles related to this chapter by visiting **go.hrw.com**. Just type in the keyword **HD4CH19**.

Standards Correlations

National Health Education Standards

1.1 (partial) Describe the relationship between positive health behaviors and the prevention of injury, illness, disease, and premature death. (Lessons 2, 6, and 8)

3.2 Analyze a personal health assessment to determine strengths and weaknesses. (Lesson 2)

3.4 (partial) Demonstrate strategies to improve or maintain personal and family health. (Lessons 2 and 8)

3.5 (partial) Develop injury prevention and management strategies for personal and family health. (Lesson 8)

4.3 (partial) Analyze the influence of technology on personal and family health. (Lesson 2)

6.4 Apply strategies and skills needed to attain personal health goals. (Lesson 2)

> " I thought I was **pretty fit** until my gym teacher had me do some **fitness tests.** I found out that I **wasn't as fit** as I thought!
>
> My teacher helped me make a fitness plan. It can be hard to stick to sometimes. But I can already tell that I'm getting healthier! "

Health IQ

PRE-READING

Answer the following multiple-choice questions to find out what you already know about physical fitness. When you've finished this chapter, you'll have an opportunity to change your answers based on what you've learned.

1. Which of the following best describes physical fitness?
   a. the ability to do everyday tasks without feeling tired
   b. any physical activity that improves your ability to complete tasks
   c. the way that your body adapts to the stress of exercise
   d. none of the above

2. Which of the following is a component of physical fitness?
   a. strength
   b. body composition
   c. flexibility
   d. all of the above

3. When you get regular exercise, your resting heart rate
   a. increases.
   b. stays the same.
   c. decreases.
   d. None of the above

4. ___ helps you stay safe when you lift weights.
   a. Using machines
   b. Being a spotter
   c. Using proper form
   d. Lifting alone

5. A ___ helps you if you can't finish a lift.
   a. bodybuilder
   b. spotter
   c. weight lifter
   d. good sport

6. Which of the following is NOT a warning sign of injury?
   a. achiness that goes away when you warm up
   b. tenderness in a single area
   c. muscle weakness
   d. numbness or tingling

7. All of the following are weight-training exercises EXCEPT
   a. bench press.
   b. hamstring curl.
   c. sit and reach.
   d. lunge.

ANSWERS: 1. a; 2. d; 3. c; 4. c; 5. b; 6. a; 7. c

Using the Health IQ

Misconception Alert
Answers to the Health IQ questions may help you identify students' misconceptions.

Question 2: While students probably recognize that strength and flexibility are parts of fitness, they may not recognize that body composition is a part of fitness. Body composition compares fat weight to lean weight in the body. A fit person usually has a smaller ratio of fat weight to lean weight.

Question 4: Some students may believe that machines help them stay safe when they lift weights. However, using machines with poor form can lead to injury. So, the best way to avoid an injury is to use proper form, whether using machines or free weights.

Question 6: Many students may think they are hurt after they exercise for the first time or if they exercise harder than usual. The achiness caused by new or harder exercise is not an injury, but a normal result of exercise. It should go away the next time a person exercises. It also occurs less often as a person gets more fit.

Answers
1. a
2. d
3. c
4. c
5. b
6. a
7. c

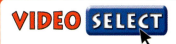

For information about videos related to this chapter, go to **go.hrw.com** and type in the keyword **HD4PF7V**.

Chapter 4 • Physical Fitness

Lesson 1

Focus

Overview
Before beginning this lesson, review with your students the objectives listed under the What You'll Do head in the Student Edition. In this lesson, students will learn about the four parts of physical fitness.

🔔 Bellringer
Ask students to list the physical activities they like to do. **LS Verbal**

Answer to Start Off Write
Accept all reasonable answers. Sample answer: If I'm fit, I don't get tired or feel out of breath when I'm doing physical activities.

Motivate

Activity — GENERAL
Poster Project Ask students to work in groups of four. Groups should make a table with a column for each part of fitness. Ask students to look through magazines for pictures of activities that use each part of fitness. Many activities use multiple parts. For example, students may put dancing under strength and flexibility or running under strength and endurance. Ask groups to present their tables to the class. **English Language Learners** **LS Visual**

Lesson 1 — The Parts of Fitness

Sasha thought dance class would be easy. The class is actually a lot of work. But Sasha knows that she is stronger and more flexible since she started taking the class.

What You'll Do
- Describe four parts of physical fitness.

Terms to Learn
- physical fitness
- strength
- endurance
- flexibility

Start Off Write
How do you know when you are physically fit?

Dance is one of many activities that can improve physical fitness. **Physical fitness** is the ability to do everyday activities without becoming short of breath, sore, or tired. Four parts of fitness are strength, endurance (en DOOR uhns), flexibility (FLEKS uh BIL uh tee), and body composition (KAHM puh ZISH uhn).

Strength
The amount of force that muscles apply when they are used is called **strength.** Strength can be measured by the amount of weight you can lift. You use strength when you lift boxes or push a lawn mower. Strong muscles support bones and joints. Strength also helps prevent injury. Strength can help your body deal with accidents, such as falls.

Endurance
The ability to do activities for more than a few minutes is called **endurance.** There are two types of endurance. Muscular endurance is the ability of your muscles to keep working over time. The ability of your heart and lungs to work efficiently during physical activity is the other type of endurance. Heart and lung endurance keeps you from becoming short of breath.

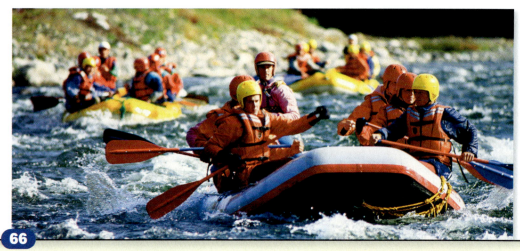

Figure 1 Paddling a boat uses both strength and endurance.

BIOLOGY CONNECTION — ADVANCED
Heart and Lung Endurance Heart and lung endurance is also known as *cardiorespiratory endurance*. Ask interested students to research the effects of exercise on cardiorespiratory endurance. Students should create a pamphlet describing the physiological effects of exercise on the heart and lungs. **LS Verbal/Visual**

Chapter Resource File
- Directed Reading BASIC
- Lesson Plan
- Lesson Quiz GENERAL

Transparencies

TT Bellringer

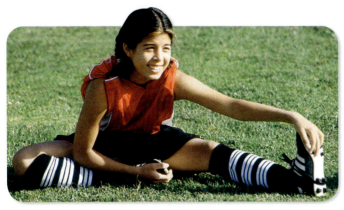

Figure 2 Stretching prevents injury by improving flexibility.

Flexibility

The ability to bend and twist joints easily is called **flexibility**. You use flexibility when you bend down, twist your body, or reach for something. If you are flexible, you are less likely to get hurt during physical activities. To improve your flexibility, you can stretch regularly. *Stretching* is any activity that loosens muscles and joints.

Body Composition

Fat plays an important role in how your body works. However, too much fat may lead to disease. It can also make improving your physical fitness harder. *Body composition* compares the weight of your fat to the weight of your muscles, bones, and organs. Physical activity can improve body composition. It helps your body burn fat.

Myth & Fact

Myth: If you are thin, you are fit.

Fact: Body composition is only one part of physical fitness. If you are thin but do not have good strength, endurance, or flexibility, you are not fit.

Lesson Review

Using Vocabulary

1. Use each of the following terms in a separate sentence: *physical fitness, strength, endurance,* and *flexibility*.

Understanding Concepts

2. What are two types of endurance?
3. What does body composition compare?
4. What part of fitness are you using when you stretch? when you carry your books?

Critical Thinking

5. **Applying Concepts** Josh plays basketball with his friends almost every day. He can run for most of the game. But he can't touch his toes. What part of fitness does Josh need to improve?

internet connect
www.scilinks.org/health
Topic: Physical Fitness
HealthLinks code: HD4076
HEALTH LINKS. Maintained by the National Science Teachers Association

Lesson 2

Focus

Overview
Before beginning this lesson, review with your students the objectives listed under the What You'll Do head in the Student Edition. This lesson explains the importance of exercise, lists fitness standards, and lists influences on fitness goals. The lesson also discusses frequency, intensity, and time (FIT) and heart-rate monitoring.

Bellringer
Ask students to list the adverse effects of not getting enough exercise. **LS** Verbal

Answer to Start Off Write
Accept all reasonable answers. Sample answer: Exercise improves or maintains fitness. It also makes it easier to do everyday activities and can help prevent some diseases.

Motivate

Activity — GENERAL
Selling Exercise Ask students to create television commercials to convince people to become fit. Encourage students to use songs, jokes, or catchy slogans to get their audience to exercise. Have students perform their commercials for the class. **LS** Kinesthetic *English Language Learners*

Lesson 2

Your Fitness Program

What You'll Do
- **Explain** why you should exercise.
- **List** healthy fitness standards for your age group.
- **List** five things that affect your fitness goals.
- **Describe** how increasing frequency, intensity, and time of exercise affects fitness.
- **Estimate** your target heart rate zone.

Terms to Learn
- exercise
- resting heart rate (RHR)
- recovery time

Start Off Write
Why is it important for you to exercise regularly?

Henry has a friend who gets tired walking up a flight of stairs. When they get to the top, Henry has to wait while his friend catches his breath. His friend isn't overweight, but Henry knows that he doesn't go outside much.

Walking up a flight of stairs may not seem like hard work. But for people with poor physical fitness, it can be difficult. In this lesson, you'll learn how you can stay fit.

Why Should You Exercise?
It's pretty easy to spend a lot of time watching TV or using a computer. However, if you spend too much time doing these activities, your fitness could suffer. Regular exercise is important. **Exercise** is any physical activity that maintains or improves fitness. Exercise isn't just jumping jacks and push-ups. The sports you play for fun are also exercise.

Lack of exercise can make doing everyday tasks hard. You might become short of breath easily. Poor fitness can also make dealing with stress more difficult. People who don't get regular exercise increase their chances of diseases such as heart disease, diabetes, and obesity. So, people who don't exercise enough may not live as long.

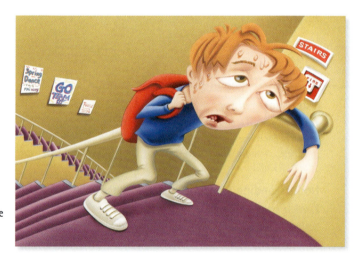

Figure 3 Regular exercise can help prevent shortness of breath.

Life SKILL BUILDER

Practicing Wellness Students who want to improve their physical fitness may find it inspiring to hear these health benefits of exercise:

- Exercise can improve self-esteem, prevent or alleviate the effects of depression, and relieve stress.
- Exercise can improve bone density. So, it can help prevent osteoporosis.
- Exercise reduces the risk of some forms of cancer, such as colon cancer.
- Exercise can improve the quality of life for people with diabetes, arthritis, and asthma.

Chapter Resource File
- Directed Reading BASIC
- Lesson Plan
- Lesson Quiz GENERAL

Transparencies
- TT Bellringer
- TT Healthy Fitness Zones for Ages 12 to 14

---

68 Chapter 4 • Physical Fitness

Testing Your Fitness

When you take a test, you find out how well you know what you were taught. A test can tell you what your strengths and weaknesses are. Then, you can work on your weaknesses to get better. There are also ways to test your physical fitness. Knowing your fitness weaknesses can help you plan to improve your fitness.

There are simple tests for each part of fitness. For example, pull-ups and curl-ups test strength and muscular endurance. The 1-mile run tests heart and lung endurance. The sit-and-reach test measures flexibility.

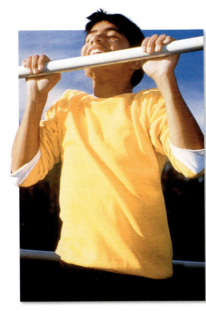

Figure 4 Pull-ups test your strength and muscular endurance.

The table below lists healthy fitness zones for your age group. You should try to meet these fitness standards. If you can meet the lower standard for each zone, then you are doing pretty well. If you meet the higher standard, then your fitness is great! People who are interested in playing sports usually need to reach the higher end of each fitness zone. If you are having trouble meeting any of the fitness standards, talk to your teacher or to your parents. They can help you come up with a plan to improve your fitness.

TABLE 1 Healthy Fitness Zones for Ages 12 to 14

Activity		12	13	14
Pull-ups	Boys	1–3	1–4	2–5
	Girls	1–2	1–2	1–2
Curl-ups	Boys	18–36	21–40	24–45
	Girls	18–32	18–32	18–32
1-mile run (minutes and seconds)	Boys	10:30–8:00	10:00–7:30	9:30–7:00
	Girls	12:00–9:00	11:30–9:00	11:00–8:30
Sit and reach (inches)	Boys	8	8	8
	Girls	10	10	10

SOCIAL STUDIES CONNECTION — ADVANCED

Physical Fitness in the United States
Ask interested students to research the history of fitness testing in the United States. Students could also examine the President's Council on Physical Fitness and Sports, how physical education in the United States compares to physical education in other countries, or how physical education has changed in the United States over time. Have students present their findings to the class. **LS Verbal**

Teach, continued

Activity — BASIC
Poster Project Ask students to create posters that illustrate some of the reasons people do not exercise. Posters should include suggestions about overcoming these obstacles. Have students present their posters to the class. **LS Visual**

Demonstration — GENERAL
Rating of Perceived Exertion (RPE) Scale Tell students that there is a method for evaluating the intensity of exercise. The RPE scale lets you evaluate how hard you are exercising at any given point in your workout. The scale runs from 0 to 10. At level 0, people aren't doing anything. At level 4, people can occasionally talk to their partner, enjoy the scenery, and exercise for a long period of time. At level 7, it is difficult to talk and to exercise for a long time. At level 10, people are near their maximum exercise intensity. Ask students to jog in place or do jumping jacks for two minutes. Ask them to try to rate their exertion level according to the RPE scale.

Safety Caution: Students with health problems should be excused from the activity. **LS Kinesthetic**

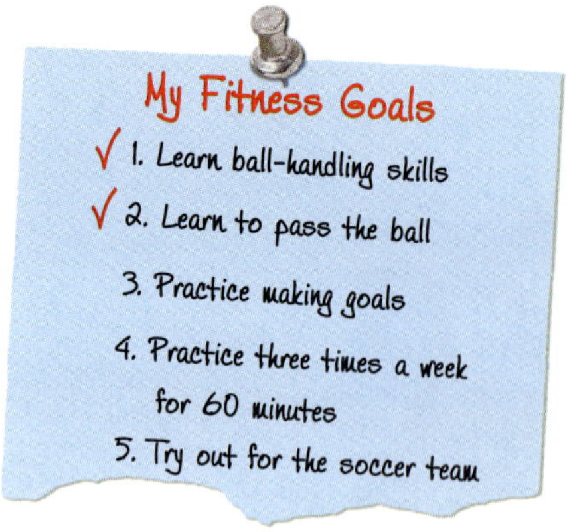

My Fitness Goals
✓ 1. Learn ball-handling skills
✓ 2. Learn to pass the ball
3. Practice making goals
4. Practice three times a week for 60 minutes
5. Try out for the soccer team

Figure 5 Setting short-term goals can make reaching a long-term goal easier.

Your Fitness Goals

Even if you meet healthy fitness standards, it is a good idea to set fitness goals. Setting short-term goals can help you meet a long-term goal.

The activities that you enjoy, your abilities, and the amount of work you want to do can influence your fitness goals. Your goals will also be influenced by how important fitness is to you and the people around you. Finally, there's always a chance you might get hurt during exercise. As you set goals, you need to balance risks against benefits.

A good place to start is to see a doctor. The doctor can make sure it is safe for you to exercise. Also, the doctor may be able to help you with your fitness goals.

FIT

Exercise improves your fitness. However, unless you exercise more over time, your fitness will stop improving. You can influence how quickly your fitness improves by changing three things:

- **Frequency** refers to how often you exercise. If you exercise more often, your fitness can improve faster.
- **Intensity** refers to how hard you exercise. Exercising harder can make you stronger. It can also improve endurance.
- **Time** is how long you exercise. If you spend more time exercising, your fitness can improve.

One way to remember frequency, intensity, and time is to remember that the first letters of the words spell *FIT*. To avoid injury, don't increase more than one part of FIT at a time. Also, don't increase any one part of FIT too much. Your teacher or parents can help you change parts of FIT safely.

LIFE SKILLS ACTIVITY

PRACTICING WELLNESS

Some people keep a fitness log when they exercise. They write down what activity they did, how long they did it, and how they felt during their activity. Try keeping a fitness log for 2 weeks. What are your goals? Do you think you are exercising often enough, hard enough, and long enough to improve your fitness? What parts of FIT do you think you need to change to meet your fitness goals?

LIFE SKILLS ACTIVITY
Answers
Accept all reasonable answers.

Extension: Ask students, "Was it helpful to keep a fitness log?" Ask students to explain their answers.

Career
Personal Trainer Personal trainers work one-on-one with people to develop a personalized fitness program. A personal trainer meets with clients regularly, evaluates fitness, teaches them how to exercise properly, and advises them about nutrition. Personal trainers need an undergraduate degree and certification from a fitness organization, such as the American College of Sports Medicine.

Monitoring Your Heart Rate

One way to see how hard you are exercising is to check your heart rate. Heart rate is the number of times your heart beats per minute. The easiest places to check your heart rate are on your neck and wrist. Use your index and middle fingers to find your heartbeat. Count heartbeats for 10 seconds. Multiply by 6 to find your heart rate.

If you exercise hard enough to improve fitness, you will be in your target heart rate zone. The *target heart rate zone* is 60 percent to 85 percent of your maximum heart rate. *Maximum heart rate (MHR)* is the largest number of times your heart can beat per minute while you exercise. You can use the following equations to estimate your target heart rate zone:

$$MHR = 220 - age$$
$$60\% \text{ of } MHR = MHR \times 0.6$$
$$85\% \text{ of } MHR = MHR \times 0.85$$

For example, a 13-year-old's target heart rate zone is about 124 to 176 beats per minute.

The number of times your heart beats per minute when you are not exercising is called your **resting heart rate (RHR).** RHR decreases as you become more fit. RHR decreases because your heart is stronger. **Recovery time** is the amount of time your heart takes to return to its RHR after exercising. As your fitness improves, your recovery time gets shorter.

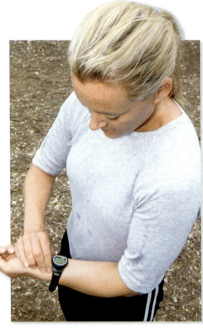

Figure 6 Monitoring your heart rate can help you meet your fitness goals.

Lesson Review

Using Vocabulary
1. What is exercise?

Understanding Concepts
2. List healthy fitness standards for a 12-year-old girl.
3. Name five things that affect your fitness goals.
4. Calculate your target heart rate zone.

Critical Thinking
5. **Making Predictions** If Tanya joins the track team, what may happen to her resting heart rate? to her recovery time?
6. **Applying Concepts** Alejandro isn't doing as well at basketball as he wants. If Alejandro wants to run faster and longer during basketball games, how can he use FIT to do so?

REAL-LIFE CONNECTION — ADVANCED

Karvonen Formula There are several equations that are used to estimate target heart rates. One of those is the Karvonen formula. Ask interested students to research the Karvonen formula and other heart-rate formulas. Students should compare the accuracy of the different formulas. Have students present their findings to the class. Students should show sample calculations during their presentations. **LS** Verbal/Logical

Close

Reteaching — BASIC
Outline Have students outline the lesson. Students should use the headings on each page and create a bulleted list summarizing the material under each heading. **LS** Verbal

Quiz — GENERAL

1. What are the effects of a lack of exercise? (Sample answer: It can make doing everyday tasks harder. You may become short of breath more easily, and you may not be able to deal with stress as well. Also, you can increase your chances of diseases, such as heart disease, diabetes, and obesity.)

2. List exercises that test strength, the two types of endurance, and flexibility. (pull-ups and curl-ups for strength and muscular endurance, 1-mile-run for heart and lung endurance, and sit-and-reach test for flexibility)

3. What can help you meet long-term fitness goals? (Setting short-term fitness goals can help people meet long-term goals.)

Answers to Lesson Review

1. Exercise is any physical activity that maintains or improves physical fitness.
2. 1–2 pull-ups, 18–32 curl-ups, 9:00 to 12:00 minutes for the 1-mile run, and 10 inches for the sit-and-reach test
3. The activities you enjoy, your abilities, the amount of work you want to do, how important fitness is to you and people around you, and the chances of getting hurt all influence fitness goals.
4. Answers may vary. Sample answer for a 13-year-old: 124 to 176 beats per minute (MHR = 220 − 13 = 207; 60% of MHR = 207 × 0.6 = 124; 85% of MHR = 207 × 0.85 = 176)
5. Sample answer: As Tanya gets more fit, her resting heart rate will decrease. Her recovery time will also get shorter.
6. Sample answer: Since Alejandro wants to run longer during basketball games, he can increase how often he runs during practice. He can also try running harder or longer. But he shouldn't do all three at once.

Lesson 3

Focus

Overview
Before beginning this lesson, review with your students the objectives listed under the What You'll Do head in the Student Edition. This lesson compares aerobic and anaerobic exercise and describes when the body uses aerobic and anaerobic energy.

🔔 Bellringer
Ask students to explain the meanings of the terms *aerobic exercise* and *anaerobic exercise*. **LS** Verbal

Answer to Start Off Write
Accept all reasonable answers. Sample answers: A sprinter doesn't have enough energy to sprint an entire marathon. He or she will have to slow down.

Motivate

Discussion — GENERAL
Aerobic Vs. Anaerobic Ask students, "Why is it important to include both anaerobic and aerobic exercise in a fitness program?" (Students should recognize that aerobic exercise improves endurance and anaerobic exercise improves strength. People need both to be fit.) "What are some activities that use both aerobic and anaerobic energy systems?" (Sample answers: soccer, basketball, tennis, and cycling) **LS** Verbal

---

Lesson 3 — Energy for Exercise

What You'll Do
- **Compare** aerobic and anaerobic exercise.
- **Describe** when the body uses aerobic and anaerobic energy.

Terms to Learn
- aerobic
- anaerobic

Start Off Write
Why can't a sprinter keep up his or her pace for an entire marathon?

A world-champion sprinter can run 100 meters in less than 10 seconds. But can a sprinter run a marathon in an hour?

A sprinter can't run a marathon in an hour. The sprinter would run out of energy before he or she could finish. Sprinters and marathon runners use different energy systems when they run.

With and Without Oxygen

Your body gets energy from the food you eat. The sugars in foods, such as fruit and bread, are changed into a sugar called *glucose* (GLOO kohs). Your body uses oxygen to get energy from glucose. When your body uses oxygen to get energy, the process is *aerobic* (er OH bik). **Aerobic exercise** is exercise that uses oxygen to get energy. Endurance exercises, such as long-distance running and swimming, are aerobic exercises.

Glycogen (GLIE kuh juhn) is another sugar made from the food you eat. Your body releases energy from glycogen without using oxygen. A process that doesn't use oxygen is *anaerobic* (AN uhr OH bik). Exercise that is fueled without using oxygen is **anaerobic exercise.** Activities that use strength in short bursts, such as sprinting, are anaerobic exercises. A small amount of glycogen is stored in your muscles. When glycogen runs out, you won't be able to keep going at the same pace. So, a sprinter can't run a marathon in an hour. The sprinter runs out of glycogen and has to slow down.

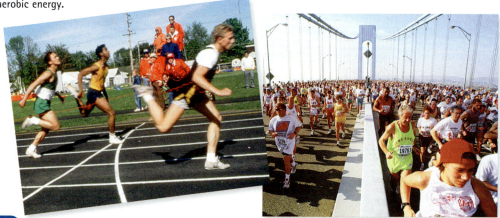

Figure 7 Sprinters use anaerobic energy, while marathon runners use aerobic energy.

BIOLOGY CONNECTION — ADVANCED
Life Without Oxygen *Aerobic* and *anaerobic* don't just describe exercise. These terms are common in biology when discussing how organisms survive. Some organisms are able to live without using oxygen. Ask interested students to research anaerobic organisms. Have students make a pamphlet describing some of these organisms. **LS** Verbal/Visual

Chapter Resource File
- Directed Reading BASIC
- Lesson Plan
- Lesson Quiz GENERAL

Transparencies
TT Bellringer

72 Chapter 4 • Physical Fitness

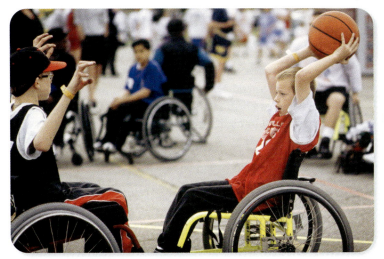

Figure 8 Many sports, such as basketball, require steady aerobic exercise with bursts of anaerobic exercise.

Working Together

How your body uses aerobic and anaerobic energy depends on what you do. For many activities, your body uses both types of energy. For example, tennis players use short bursts of strength when they serve or return a ball. So, they use anaerobic energy. But they also need to be able to play long games. Their bodies use aerobic energy to keep playing.

Fitness improves best if you do both aerobic and anaerobic exercise. Even if you want to do an aerobic exercise, such as distance running, anaerobic exercise can help you improve. Anaerobic exercises, such as sprinting and weight lifting, can improve your strength. Many people who do anaerobic exercise also do aerobic exercise. For example, a sprinter sometimes runs longer distances. This aerobic exercise helps a sprinter practice longer and more efficiently.

Health Journal
Make a list of 10 physical activities. Identify which activities rely on aerobic energy and which rely on anaerobic energy. If an activity uses both types of energy, identify when it uses each.

Lesson Review

Using Vocabulary
1. Compare aerobic and anaerobic exercise.

Understanding Concepts
2. Why can't a sprinter run a marathon in an hour?

Critical Thinking
3. **Identifying Relationships** Theo's track coach wants Theo to run a couple of miles during practice. Theo doesn't know why. He is usually a sprinter. Why would Theo's coach want him to run long distances?

internet connect
www.scilinks.org/health
Topic: Aerobic and Anaerobic Exercise
HealthLinks code: HD4004
HEALTH LINKS. Maintained by the National Science Teachers Association

---

Teach

Group Activity — BASIC
Sunday Funnies Have students work in groups of four. Ask students to draw cartoons illustrating when different sports, such as basketball or soccer, use aerobic energy and anaerobic energy. Have students compile their cartoons into a newspaper. Students can also include activities such as connect-the-dots or crossword puzzles. Have students present their funny pages to the class.
LS Visual
Co-op Learning · English Language Learners

Close

Reteaching — BASIC
Matching Give students pictures of physical activities. On the board, make two columns. Write *aerobic* over one and *anaerobic* over the other. Ask students to place their pictures in the appropriate column.
LS Visual · English Language Learners

Quiz — GENERAL
1. How does your body get energy during aerobic exercise? (Sample answer: Sugars in foods, such as fruit and bread, are changed into glucose. The body uses oxygen to get energy from glucose.)
2. Explain how the body gets energy for anaerobic exercise. (Sample answer: Glycogen is another sugar made from the food you eat. A small amount of glycogen is stored in muscles. The body doesn't use oxygen to release energy from glycogen.)
3. Give two examples of aerobic exercise and two examples of anaerobic exercise. (Sample answer: Running and swimming are aerobic exercises. Sprinting and weight-lifting are anaerobic exercises.)

Answers to Lesson Review
1. Your body uses oxygen to get energy for aerobic exercise. Your body does not use oxygen to get energy for anaerobic exercise. Generally, aerobic exercise lasts a long time while anaerobic exercise lasts a short time.
2. Sprinting is anaerobic exercise, which is fueled by glycogen. A small amount of glycogen is stored in muscles. When glycogen is used up, a sprinter has to slow down. Therefore, he or she can't run a marathon in an hour.
3. Sample answer: Running long distances improves Theo's endurance. If his endurance improves, Theo can practice sprinting longer during practice. Since he can practice sprinting longer, Theo will probably become faster.

Lesson 3 • Energy for Exercise

Lesson 4 Focus

Overview
Before beginning this lesson, review with your students the objectives listed under the What You'll Do head in the Student Edition. This lesson describes five characteristics of a good sport and two ways to start playing sports.

Bellringer
Ask students to write about a time they witnessed bad sportsmanship. Ask students to describe what happened and how the behavior affected other people. 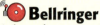 Verbal

Answer to Start Off Write
Accept all reasonable answers. Sample answer: A good sport is someone who treats all players, officials, and fans fairly during competition.

Motivate

Discussion — GENERAL
Poor Sportsmanship Encourage students to discuss poor sportsmanship. Ask students, "Do you think that poor sportsmanship is more common today than it was in the past?" (Answers may vary, but students may say that poor sportsmanship seems more common today.) "Why does poor sportsmanship happen?" (Students may cite pressures from parents, coaches, and peers to win. Students may also discuss the incidence of poor sportsmanship in professional sports as an influence.) "How can poor sportsmanship be avoided?" (Students may suggest stronger rules against poor sportsmanship.) Logical

---

Lesson 4 — Sports and Competition

What You'll Do
- **Describe** five characteristics of someone who is a good sport.
- **List** two places to start playing sports.

Terms to Learn
- competition
- sportsmanship

Start Off Write
What is a good sport?

Rob likes to race on his bicycle. He hasn't won a race, but he still has fun. Rob has even started riding his bike more often. He knows that if he improves his fitness, he might do better at a race.

A bicycle race is a competition. A **competition** is a contest between two or more people or teams. For people like Rob, competition can help them improve fitness. But Rob knows that winning isn't everything. Competition should also be fun!

Competition and Sportsmanship

Have you ever seen a player yell at a game official during a game? Or, have you seen a fight take place at a game? These people weren't practicing sportsmanship. **Sportsmanship** is the ability to treat all players, officials, and fans fairly during competition. Someone who practices sportsmanship is called a *good sport*. A good sports always plays his or her best. A good sport follows the rules of the game. He or she also considers the safety of the other players. A good sport congratulates players for a good job, even if they are on a different team. Finally, a good sport is polite if he or she loses and modest if he or she wins. Sportsmanship makes competition more fun for players, fans, and officials.

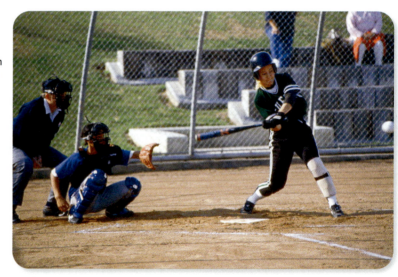

Figure 9 Competition can push you to get fitter and better at your sport.

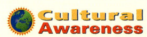 **Cultural Awareness** — GENERAL

National Sportsmanship Day
National Sportsmanship Day was started to raise awareness about sportsmanship. It is held every year on the first Tuesday in March. Schools, colleges, and youth sports leagues in more than 100 countries take part in the event. Ask interested students to research National Sportsmanship Day and find out how schools can get involved. Ask them to write a letter to the school principal suggesting that the school participate. Verbal

Chapter Resource File
- Directed Reading **BASIC**
- Lesson Plan
- Lesson Quiz **GENERAL**

Transparencies
 Bellringer

74   Chapter 4 • Physical Fitness

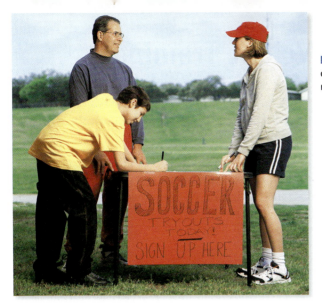

Figure 10 Community organizations sponsor many youth sports.

Getting Started in Sports

You may try several sports in the next few years. You'll probably pick sports that are interesting and fun. Try several sports before deciding which you like most. You may find a new sport that you really like.

Schools and community organizations often have sports teams and clubs. These teams give you a chance to get in shape or to compete against other people. Teams also provide a lot of the equipment you'll need to play your sport. Players are usually organized by age and skill level. Some sports teams may ask you to visit a doctor. A doctor can tell you if it's safe for you to play. Check with your school or local parks and recreation department to find out how you can start playing sports.

Myth: Winning isn't everything. It's the only thing.

Fact: This myth comes from misquoting Vince Lombardi, a famous football coach. What Coach Lombardi actually said was that winning isn't everything but that wanting to win is. He believed that we should always do our best.

Lesson Review

Using Vocabulary
1. What is competition?

Understanding Concepts
2. What are five characteristics of a good sport?
3. List two places to start playing sports.

Critical Thinking
4. **Using Refusal Skills** Katya has a friend who plays roughly and knocks people down during soccer games. Katya's friend wants Katya to do the same thing. How should Katya handle the situation?

internet connect
www.scilinks.org/health
Topic: Health Benefits of Sports
HealthLinks code: HD4050
HEALTH LINKS. Maintained by the National Science Teachers Association

---

Teach

Activity — GENERAL

How-To Guide Have students work in pairs. Ask one student to interview a school coach or a coach at a local recreational center about getting started in sports. Ask the other student to write a how-to guide based on the first student's interview. Have the students present their guides to the class. **LS** Interpersonal Co-op Learning

Close

Reteaching — BASIC

Sportsmanship Draw a line down the middle of the board. Ask students to write the characteristics of a good sport on the left side. Then, ask students to write examples of poor sportsmanship on the right side. **LS** Verbal

Quiz — GENERAL

1. What are the benefits of joining a sports team? (Sample answer: Teams give you a chance to get in shape and to compete against other people. Teams also provide equipment that you'll need to play your sport.)
2. What is sportsmanship? (the ability to treat all players, officials, and fans fairly during competition)
3. List two examples of poor sportsmanship. (Sample answer: a player yelling at a game official and fighting during a game)

Alternative Assessment — BASIC

To Whom It May Concern Ask students to imagine that they are the coach of a soccer team. Have them write a persuasive letter to the team describing the characteristics of a good sport. Students should emphasize that sportsmanship makes competition more fun. **LS** Verbal

---

Answers to Lesson Review

1. Competition is a contest between two or more people or teams.
2. A good sport always plays his or her best. He or she also follows the rules of the game, considers the safety of other players, and congratulates all players for good plays, even if they are on the other team. A good sport is polite when he or she loses and modest when he or she wins.
3. at school or with a community organization
4. Sample answer: Katya can tell her friend that she's not going to play roughly because it is poor sportsmanship and makes the game less fun.

Lesson 4 • Sports and Competition

Lesson 5

Focus

Overview
Before beginning this lesson, review with your students the objectives listed under the What You'll Do head in the Student Edition. This lesson describes two types of weight training, compares free weights and machines, describes how to stay safe while lifting weights, and illustrates four weight-training exercises.

Bellringer
Ask students to list and describe some weight-training exercises and equipment. (Sample answers: lunge, bench press, and free weights.)
LS Verbal

Answer to Start Off Write
Accept all reasonable answers. Sample answer: Not everyone develops big muscles. For some people it is easy, while for others, it is difficult. In fact, it is usually easier for boys to develop big muscles than it is for girls.

Motivate

Group Activity ——— GENERAL
Selling Weight Training Have students work in groups of four. Ask students to design an advertisement for weight training. They should describe the two types of weight training in their advertisements. Students could write a magazine ad or television commercial. **English Language Learners**
LS Visual

Lesson 5

What You'll Do
- **Describe** two types of weight training.
- **Compare** free weights and machines.
- **List** seven safety tips for lifting weights.
- **Describe** four weight-training exercises.

Terms to Learn
- weight training

Start Off Write
Does everyone who lifts weights develop big muscles? Why or why not?

Weight Training

Todd wants to lift weights to get in shape. But he doesn't want huge muscles. His coach said that lifting weights doesn't always build big muscles.

Sometimes, people lift weights to get bigger muscles. But Todd's coach is right. Weight training can improve strength without making muscles bigger. **Weight training** is the use of weight to make muscles stronger or bigger. Weight training improves strength and muscular endurance.

Types of Weight Training

There are two basic kinds of weight training: strength development and bodybuilding. How you lift weights depends on your fitness goals. Some people, like Todd, want to strengthen their muscles without making them bigger. Other people spend a lot of time making their bodies stronger and their muscles bigger. These people are bodybuilders. A bodybuilder usually lifts more weight, does fewer repetitions, and does a different number of sets than someone who doesn't want big muscles. *Repetitions* are the number of times you do an exercise. A *set* is a group of repetitions.

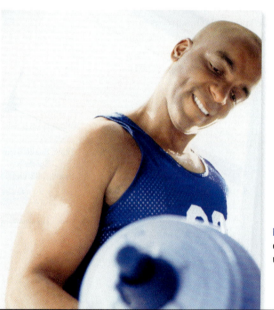

For some people, it doesn't matter how much they lift weights. They will have a hard time getting big muscles. For other people, developing big muscles is very easy. In fact, increasing muscle size is usually easier for boys than it is for girls. To get bigger muscles, female bodybuilders follow very specific weight-training programs.

Figure 11 Biceps curls are one way to strengthen the upper arm.

MISCONCEPTION ALERT
Some girls may think that if they start lifting weights, they will develop big muscles. However, women do not develop muscles as easily as men do. Muscle development is facilitated by the male hormone *testosterone*. Because women have smaller concentrations of testosterone, they usually don't develop muscles as easily as men do.

Chapter Resource File
- Directed Reading **BASIC**
- Lesson Plan
- Lesson Quiz **GENERAL**

Transparencies
TT Bellringer
TT Some Weight-Training Exercises

Chapter 4 • Physical Fitness

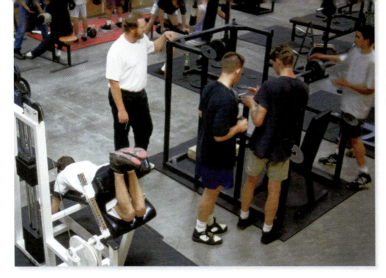

Figure 12 A variety of machines and free weights are used in weight training.

Equipment

There are two types of weight-training equipment: free weights and machines. Free weights include dumbbells, barbells, and curl bars. To use free weights, you add weight to an empty bar and secure the weight with a collar. You can usually do a greater variety of exercises with free weights than with machines. Machines use a system of pulleys to let you control the weight as you lift it. Machines are designed for a specific muscle group. The number of exercises you can do with a machine is often limited. But a machine ensures that a specific muscle group is exercised correctly.

Safety

Safety is very important. To lift weights safely, you should follow several simple rules:

- Use a spotter. A spotter is someone who can take weight away if you can't finish a lift.
- Lift weights in pairs or in small groups. Take turns to rest.
- Make sure that free weights are secured to the bar.
- Make sure you understand how a machine works. Adjust machines to your size.
- Lift only as much weight as you can lift with the correct form.
- Exercise both sides of a joint to prevent injury. For example, if you exercise your chest, you should exercise your shoulders.
- Always use correct form. If necessary, use a weight belt to support your back. But a weight belt is never a substitute for good form.

SCIENCE ACTIVITY

Weight training can be divided into three types of exercises: *isotonic* (IE soh TAHN ik), *isometric* (IE soh MET rik), and *isokinetic* (IE soh ki NET ik). Research the three types of weight-training exercises. Create a poster defining each type and describing how each type affects muscles.

Attention Grabber

Many students may think that weight training just improves outward appearance. The following facts may surprise them:

- Weight training can increase metabolic rates. So, the body burns more Calories during the day.
- Weight training can increase bone density, preventing diseases, such as osteoporosis.
- Weight training prevents injury by strengthening joints and areas that may not be used normally during other exercise.
- Weight training prevents loss of muscle due to the aging process.

Answer to Science Activity

Extension: Ask students to demonstrate examples of each type of weight-training exercise.

Teach

Activity — ADVANCED

Anabolic Steroids Ask interested students to research the use of anabolic steroids among teenagers. Ask students to identify the prevalence of steroid use and the side-effects of steroids. Have students present their findings to the class. **LS Verbal**

Debate — GENERAL

Teens and Bodybuilding Ask interested students to research and debate whether bodybuilding is safe for teenagers. **LS Logical**

Demonstration — BASIC

Weight Room Ask a school coach, personal trainer, or bodybuilder to come to class. Ask the speaker to describe the basics of weight training, the equipment he or she uses, and general safety tips. Ask the speaker to relate some of the injuries that can occur if weight training is not done properly. **LS Visual**

Life SKILL BUILDER — ADVANCED

Being a Wise Consumer Many serious bodybuilders use nutritional supplements and other substances to enhance the results of their weight training. Some of these substances are illegal, such as anabolic steroids. Many, such as protein powders and creatine, are legal and claim to be effective ways to increase muscle size and performance. Ask interested students to research the effectiveness of nutritional supplements for bodybuilders. Students should examine and compare the benefits and risks of these substances. **LS Verbal**

Lesson 5 • Weight Training

Teach, continued

Demonstration — BASIC

Weight Training If possible, take your class to a weight room. Demonstrate the exercises shown in the figure on these pages or ask a school coach or bodybuilder to do so. Students should understand how to do each exercise and how to stay safe while lifting weights. Have the students try out some of the exercises. If time permits, demonstrate other weight-training exercises in addition to those in the figure. Afterwards, ask students, "Why is good form so important?" (Sample answer: It prevents injury. Also, muscles may not get stronger if form is incorrect.)

Safety Caution: Students with health problems should be excused from the activity.
LS Kinesthetic/Visual

English Language Learners

Debate — GENERAL

Weight Belts Ask interested students to research and debate the effectiveness of weight belts while weight training. **LS Logical**

Discussion — BASIC

Getting Started Ask students, "Why do weight training programs start with exercises such as push-ups, pull-ups, and curl-ups?" (Sample answer: Push-ups, pull-ups, and curl-ups strengthen muscles in preparation for free weights and machines.) "What is the weight in these exercises?" (These exercises rely on the weight of the body to make muscles stronger.) **LS Verbal**

Figure 13 Some Weight-Training Exercises

Bench press

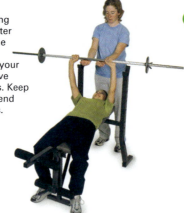

1. Don't start lifting until your spotter is ready. Lift the bar from the supports until your hands are above your shoulders. Keep a very slight bend in your elbows.

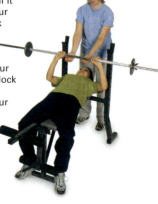

2. Lower the bar until it barely touches your chest. Push it back up to the start position, and lower it again until you finish your repetitions. Don't lock your elbows. This exercise works your chest muscles.

Biceps curl

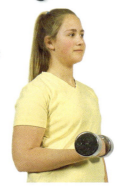

1. With your hands about shoulder-width apart, start with your arm slightly bent or at a 90° angle. Be sure not to lock your elbow.

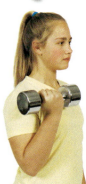

2. Curl up your arm toward your shoulder. Lower the dumbbell, and repeat the curl-up. Exercise both arms. This exercise works the biceps muscle in the front of your upper arm.

Getting Started

It is important to lift weights correctly. If your form is wrong, you can hurt yourself. You may also make it less likely for your muscles to get stronger. To ensure that you're lifting correctly, ask someone who knows. Ask a physical education teacher, coach, or fitness trainer. Any of these people can show you how to do the exercises correctly. They can also help you set goals for your training. And they can tell you which exercises will help you reach those goals. They may also suggest that you talk to your doctor first. Visiting your doctor before starting an exercise program is a good idea.

Weight training often starts with exercises that use body weight to make muscles stronger. These exercises include push-ups, pull-ups, and curl-ups. These exercises get your body ready to use free weights and machines.

BIOLOGY CONNECTION — ADVANCED

How Do They Grow? Ask interested students to research how muscles develop. Students should examine the physiological reaction of skeletal muscles to weight training. Students may also want to examine the effects of anabolic steroids on muscles. Have students write a magazine article about their findings. **LS Verbal**

Lunge

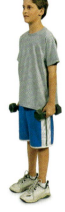

1. Start with your feet shoulder-width apart. Hold dumbbells at your sides.

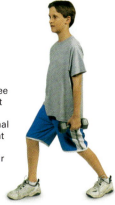

2. Step forward. Make sure your knee doesn't extend past your ankle. Step back into the original position, and repeat the lunge. This exercise works your thigh muscles.

Hamstring curl

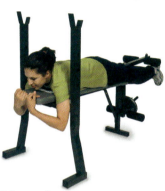

1. Make sure the bench is adjusted for your size. Put your ankles under the padded bar, and hold onto the bench for support.

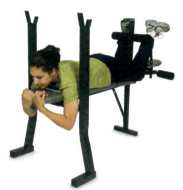

2. Bending at the knee, pull up your feet. Then, lower your legs. Keep movements slow and controlled for the best workout. This exercise works the hamstrings, the muscles in the back of your leg.

Lesson Review

Using Vocabulary
1. What is weight training?

Understanding Concepts
2. How do free weights and machines differ?
3. What are seven safety tips for lifting weights?
4. Describe four weight-training exercises.

Critical Thinking
5. **Making Inferences** Georgia wants to start lifting weights. She wants to get stronger so that she can do better on the swim team. She really wants to focus on her arms and shoulders but worries about getting big muscles. Should she worry? Explain your answer.

Close

Reteaching — BASIC
Comparisons Ask students to discuss the following comparisons: weight training for strength development versus bodybuilding and free weights versus machines. **LS Verbal**

Quiz — GENERAL
1. What are sets and repetitions? (Repetitions are the number of times you do an exercise. A set is a group of repetitions.)
2. Describe two types of weight training. (People who want stronger muscles without building bigger muscles will do strength development. People who want bigger muscles are bodybuilding.)
3. Why would someone use machines over free weights? (Machines ensure that a specific muscle group is exercised correctly.)
4. Why would someone use free weights rather than machines? (You can usually do a greater variety of exercises with free weights than you can with machines.)

Alternative Assessment — GENERAL
Poster Project Have students make a poster listing safety tips for weight training. Students should make their posters colorful and exciting. Consider hanging the posters in a school or community weight room. **LS Visual**

Answers to Lesson Review
1. Weight training is the use of weight to make muscles stronger or bigger.
2. Sample answer: Free weights include dumbbells, barbells, and curl bars. Machines use a system of pulleys to control the weight as you lift it.
3. Use a spotter. Lift in pairs or in small groups. Make sure free weights are secure. Understand how a machine works. Lift only as much weight as you can with correct form. Exercise both sides of a joint. Always use correct form.
4. For the bench press, lower the bar to your chest and raise it again. For the biceps curl, start with the arm slightly bent and curl the dumbbell toward your shoulder. For the lunge, start with feet shoulder-width apart and hold dumbbells at your sides. Step forward without extending the knee past the ankle. For the hamstring curl, start with ankles under the padded bar and bend legs at the knee, raising the bar.
5. Sample answer: Georgia shouldn't worry. First, girls usually don't develop large muscles as easily as boys do. Also, if she lifts a small amount of weight for more repetitions, she's less likely to develop big muscles than someone who lifts a larger amount of weight.

Focus

Overview
Before beginning this lesson, review with your students the objectives listed under the What You'll Do head in the Student Edition. This lesson discusses the warning signs of injury and overtraining.

Bellringer
Have students describe a time when they were hurt. Ask students to describe what caused the injury and what they had to do for the injury to heal properly. Remember that some students may be uncomfortable sharing personal information. **LS** *Verbal*

Answer to Start Off Write
Accept all reasonable answers. Sample answer: An injury is usually painful. Also, the injured area may swell or be hard to move.

Motivate

Discussion — GENERAL
Does It Really Hurt? Discuss the difference between muscle soreness and injury. Ask students, "Have you ever experienced muscle soreness?" (Answers may vary.) "When?" (Students should relate that it happens a day or two after hard exercise. Some students may notice that it happens when they change activities or if they haven't exercised much.) "Have you ever been injured because of exercise?" (Answers may vary.) "If so, how did you know?" (Students should recognize that they had one or more of the warning signs of injury.) **LS** *Verbal*

Lesson 6 Injury

What You'll Do
- **Describe** six warning signs of injury.
- **List** five signs of overtraining.

Terms to Learn
- overtraining

Start Off Write
How can you tell if you have a sports injury?

Health Journal
Write about a time when you were injured or thought you were injured. Describe what you did to treat the injury.

Kelly twisted her ankle during practice. She didn't want to tell her coach. But the ankle became swollen and bruised. She didn't want to stop playing, but the ankle was too painful.

There is a chance of injury whenever you exercise. Your chances of injury increase if you exercise often. You should watch for warning signs of injury. Swelling, bruising, and pain were signs that Kelly was hurt. So, she should stop playing.

Warning Signs of Injury

You should not experience pain when you exercise. Pain is an indication of injury. Six common warning signs of injury are

- sharp pain
- tenderness in a single area
- swelling
- a reduced range of motion around a joint
- muscle weakness
- numbness or tingling

Don't mistake muscle soreness for an injury. *Muscle soreness* is achiness that happens a day or two after hard exercise. It is normal. Muscle soreness usually goes away the next time you exercise. However, pay attention to muscle soreness that turns into sharp pain. If you experience any of the warning signs of injury, tell your parents or teacher. You may need to see a doctor.

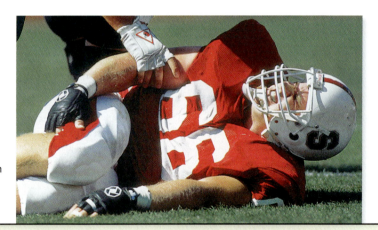

Figure 14 Pain is one sign of injury.

Life SKILL BUILDER — GENERAL
Coping For many people, exercise-related injury keeps them from participating in physical activity for a long period of time. Some of these people may experience depression because they can't exercise. Ask volunteers to relate how they dealt with exercise-related injury. Remember that some students may be uncomfortable sharing personal information. **LS** *Intrapersonal*

Chapter Resource File
- Directed Reading **BASIC**
- Lesson Plan
- Lesson Quiz **GENERAL**

Transparencies
- TT Bellringer
- TT The Overtraining Curve

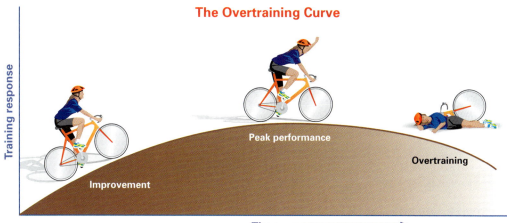

Figure 15 Once you have trained to your peak performance, more training may lead to overtraining.

Overtraining

Most people need to exercise only three to four times a week. However, some people exercise too much. **Overtraining** is a condition that happens when you exercise too much. To recover from overtraining, people need to take a break from exercise. The following are signs of overtraining:

- You feel tired all the time.
- You aren't doing as well during games and practice.
- You are less interested in the activity. You start making excuses to avoid practice.
- Your resting heart rate increases.
- You may get hurt more often. Your body hasn't had a chance to heal from past injuries.

Lesson Review

Using Vocabulary

1. What is overtraining?

Understanding Concepts

2. What are six warning signs of injury, and how do they compare with muscle soreness?

3. Why does someone who has overtrained experience more injuries?

Critical Thinking

4. **Making Good Decisions** Connie has been playing soccer 6 days a week. She has had some injuries in the past, but doesn't have any right now. However, she feels tired a lot. She is also not playing as well as she usually does. What do you think she should do?

Lesson 7

Focus

Overview
Before beginning this lesson, review with your students the objectives listed under the What You'll Do head in the Student Edition. This lesson discusses acute and chronic injuries.

Bellringer
Ask students to discuss a time when they saw someone get hurt. Ask them to describe the first aid for the injury. **LS Verbal**

Answer to Start Off Write
Accept all reasonable answers. Sample answer: Chronic injuries are caused by too much exercise, poor form, exercising on uneven surfaces, and using the wrong equipment.

Motivate

Group Activity —— GENERAL

Skit Have students work in groups of two to four. Ask students to write a skit involving an athlete and a coach. The athlete should be injured. The coach should use RICE to care for the athlete. Have students perform their skits for the class.
LS Kinesthetic Co-op Learning

Lesson 7 — Common Injuries

What You'll Do
- **Describe** acute and chronic sports injuries.
- **List** three examples of acute injuries.
- **List** two examples of chronic injuries.

Terms to Learn
- acute injury
- chronic injury

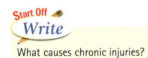
What causes chronic injuries?

Li hurt a muscle in his thigh during a volleyball game. The injury was really painful, and he had trouble using his leg. He told his mom. She made him stop playing until the muscle healed.

Li suffered from an acute (uh KYOOT) injury. An **acute injury** is an injury that happens suddenly.

Acute Injuries

Strains, sprains, and fractures (FRAK churz) are three types of acute injuries. A *strain* happens when a muscle or tendon is overstretched or torn. A tendon is tissue that attaches a muscle to a bone. Strains are painful. The injured area may feel weak. *Sprains* happen when a joint is twisted suddenly. The ligaments (LIG uh muhnts) that connect the bones in the joint are stretched or torn. Sprains are painful and usually cause swelling. A *fracture* is a cracked or broken bone. A fracture is painful. The injured area can feel weak, can swell, and can bruise.

You should report an acute injury to your parents or teacher right away. You may need to see a doctor. First aid includes rest, ice, compression, and elevation. These steps reduce swelling and pain. You rest the injured limb. Then, you put ice on it. You compress the injury by wrapping it in bandages. Finally, you elevate the injury on a chair or stool. To remember rest, ice, compression, and elevation, remember that the first letters of the words spell *RICE*.

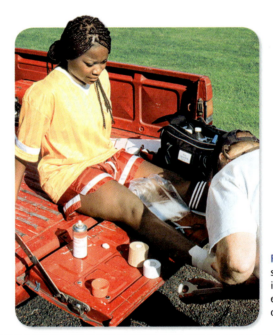

Figure 16 RICE reduces swelling and pain. This girl is using compression and elevation to ease the pain of her injury.

Career

Physician A physician diagnoses and treats disease and injury to maintain the health of individuals. Exercise-oriented physicians may focus on primary care for athletes, orthopedics, or cardiology. Orthopedic medicine deals with bones, joints, and muscles. Cardiology focuses on the heart. A physician needs a 4-year undergraduate degree, 3 to 5 years of medical school, and at least 2 years of fellowship in the medical field he or she wants to focus on.

Chapter Resource File
- Directed Reading **BASIC**
- Lesson Plan
- Lesson Quiz **GENERAL**

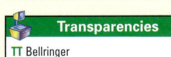
Transparencies
TT Bellringer

Chronic Injuries

Not all injuries happen suddenly. A **chronic injury** is an injury that develops over a long period of time. Two examples of chronic injuries are stress fractures and tendinitis. A stress fracture is a tiny fracture. Tendinitis is an irritation of a tendon. Increasing physical activity too quickly or exercising too much can cause chronic injuries. They can also happen when you use the wrong equipment or exercise on uneven surfaces.

Your doctor should treat chronic injuries. He or she may ask you to do special exercises. Otherwise, the best treatment for chronic injuries is usually rest. Some chronic injuries can take a few months to heal fully.

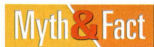

Myth: More exercise is better.

Fact: Too much exercise can lead to chronic injuries. To avoid injury, set reasonable goals and listen to your body when you exercise.

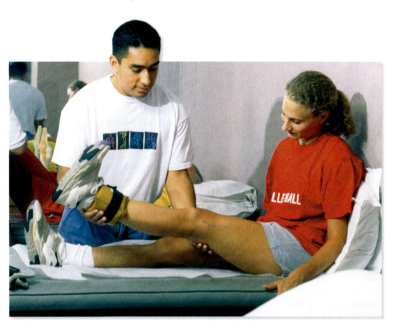

Figure 17 To recover from a chronic injury, you may need to do special exercises.

Lesson Review

Using Vocabulary
1. Compare acute and chronic injuries.

Understanding Concepts
2. What type of injury is a sprain? What type of injury is tendinitis?

Critical Thinking
3. **Making Inferences** Larissa has been running for three months. Recently, she noticed that her knee hurts. If she has new shoes and has been running on even surfaces, what could have caused her injury?

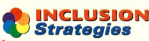

www.scilinks.org/health
Topic: Sports Injury
HealthLinks code: HD4093

HEALTH LINKS. Maintained by the National Science Teachers Association

Lesson 8 Focus

Overview
Before beginning this lesson, review with your students the objectives listed under the What You'll Do head in the Student Edition. This lesson describes eight ways to avoid injury while exercising.

🔔 Bellringer
Ask students to list several strategies they use to avoid injury when they exercise. (Answers may vary.)
LS Verbal

Answer to Start Off Write
Accept all reasonable answers. Sample answer: Stretching relaxes muscles. Stretching can also improve flexibility. Relaxed muscles and flexible joints are less likely to get injured.

Motivate

Discussion — GENERAL
Exercise-Related Injuries Tell students that millions of people are hurt each year while participating in physical activities. Ask students, "Have you ever been hurt during physical activity?" (Answers may vary.) "Could you have avoided your injury?" (Answers may vary.) "How?" (Answers may vary.)
LS Verbal

Lesson 8 — Eight Ways to Avoid Injury

What You'll Do
- **List** eight ways to avoid injury while exercising.

Terms to Learn
- active rest

Start Off Write
How does stretching reduce the chances of injury during warm-up?

Have you ever seen someone get hurt during a football game or basketball game? If you do physical activities, there is always a chance that you will get hurt.

In this lesson, you will learn eight ways to lower your chances of getting hurt during physical activities.

Warm Up and Cool Down
A *warm-up* is any activity that gets you ready for exercise. Exercising without warming up can lead to acute injuries, such as strains. A warm-up loosens your muscles and increases your heart rate. A warm-up also prepares you mentally for the activity. Walking, jogging, or jumping rope are common warm-ups. You should warm up until you break a light sweat.

A *cool-down* helps the body return to normal after exercise. During a cool-down, the heart returns to its resting rate. A cool-down also keeps muscles from getting tight and sore. Like warm-ups, cool-downs are activities such as jogging or walking.

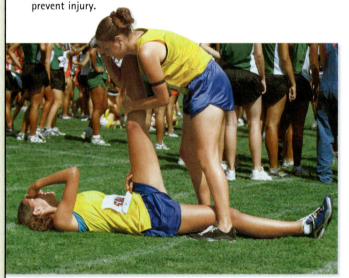

Figure 18 Stretching helps prevent injury.

Stretch
Stretching helps prevent injury and can improve flexibility. Stretching prevents injury by relaxing muscles and improving how far your joints can move. You should stretch only after a warm-up or cool-down. Stretching muscles that haven't been warmed up can lead to strains. Many people stretch as part of their cool-downs. Stretch slowly, and do not bounce. Once you feel a mild stretch in a muscle, hold your position. Stretches should be held for about 10 to 30 seconds. Don't hold a stretch if it hurts.

MISCONCEPTION ALERT
Many students may think that they should "work through the pain" if they get hurt. However, continued exercise may not only make the injury worse but may also cause it to become a permanent condition. Remind students that if they want to continue playing their favorite sports, they should take injuries seriously and give them time to heal.

Chapter Resource File
- Directed Reading **BASIC**
- Lesson Plan
- Lesson Quiz **GENERAL**

Transparencies
TT Bellringer

84 Chapter 4 • Physical Fitness

Don't Go Too Fast

To improve your physical fitness, you need to change the frequency, intensity, and time of your workouts. However, increasing these three things too much or too soon can lead to injury. It's also a bad idea to increase all three at once.

If you exercise too frequently, your body doesn't have time to recover between workouts. So you may develop a chronic injury. Increasing intensity too much can make you work too hard or do an exercise wrong. Long workouts cause injury when the body gets too tired to deal with the impact of exercise. You can also lose focus and have an accident. These situations increase your risk of injury.

Improve Your Form

Sometimes, the way you do a physical activity can lead to injury. Poor form can cause injury over time. For example, many runners get stress fractures or tendinitis because they have poor form. Poor form puts more stress on muscles, bones, and joints. Improving your form can keep you from getting hurt.

Weight lifters and dancers use mirrors to watch their form. For other activities, a coach or trainer can make suggestions for improvement. A training partner can watch what you do and tell you how you're doing. It takes a lot of practice to learn how to use the correct form. But improving your form can keep you from getting hurt. It may also help you do better in a sport or activity.

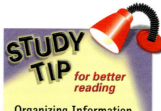

STUDY TIP *for better reading*

Organizing Information
A *mnemonic device* (nee MAHN ik di VIES) is a word or phrase that can help you remember long lists. Sometimes, you can make a word using the first letter of each word or phrase in a list. If you can't make a word, try inventing a silly phrase that uses the first letter of each word in the list. Create a mnemonic device to remember the eight ways to avoid injury!

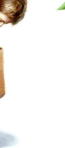
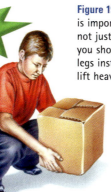

Figure 19 Using the right form is important in any activity, not just exercise. For example, you should always use your legs instead of your back to lift heavy objects.

Teach

READING SKILL BUILDER — BASIC

Paired Summarizing Ask students to read silently in pairs. Have students take turns summarizing the material they read. **LS** Verbal

Group Activity — GENERAL
Sports Safety Have students work in groups of four. Ask groups to make a safety guidebook for a sport. The guidebook should describe some common injuries of the sport and what causes them. Tell students that they should include information on preventing these injuries. Have groups present their guidebooks to the class.
LS Visual Co-op Learning

REAL-LIFE CONNECTION — ADVANCED
How Fast Is Too Fast? Ask interested students to research and describe a 6-week exercise program for someone who doesn't get regular exercise. The program should use FIT to improve the person's fitness for a 10-kilometer race.
LS Verbal

Life SKILL BUILDER — GENERAL
Writing **Assessing Your Health** Ask interested students to speak with a physical education teacher, coach, or parents about their form during physical activities. Have students discuss how their form is incorrect and ways to improve it. Ask students to write a contract with themselves to improve their form. **LS** Interpersonal

---

Attention Grabber

Many students may not realize how many exercise-related injuries young people sustain each year. The following 1997–1998 statistics from the Centers for Disease Control and Prevention about emergency room visits for people aged 5 to 24 may surprise them:
- Baseball and softball: 245,000 visits
- Basketball: 447,000 visits
- Cycling: 421,000 visits
- Football: 271,000 visits
- Gymnastics and cheerleading: 146,000 visits
- Soccer: 95,000 visits

Lesson 8 • Eight Ways to Avoid Injury   85

Teach, continued

Debate — ADVANCED
Elite Training and Teens More and more adolescents are involved in elite training for sports. They often train as much as an adult professional does. Ask interested students to research and debate whether adolescents should be involved in elite training programs.
LS Logical

Group Activity — BASIC
Sing It! Ask students to work in small groups to write a jingle about wearing the right clothing while exercising. Tell students that their songs should inform people about how the right clothing can decrease the chance of injury. Have groups perform their songs for the class. **LS Auditory**

Activity — GENERAL
Physical Activity and Children with Disabilities Ask interested students to research safety concerns specific to disabled children participating in physical activity. Encourage students to look into local organizations that fund and plan sports programs for disabled children. Have students present their research to the class.
LS Verbal

LIFE SKILLS ACTIVITY
Answer
Accept all reasonable answers.

Extension: Ask students whether advertisers should be more responsible with how they portray physical activity. Students should explain their answers.

Take a Break
Rest and recovery are important parts of a fitness program. Getting enough rest gives the body time to repair itself. You should plan rest along with exercise in your fitness program.

You don't have to stop all physical activity to rest. **Active rest** is a way to recover from exercise by reducing the amount of activity you do. Active rest lets your body repair itself. A good fitness program will alternate between hard exercise and active rest. If you plan well, you can avoid overtraining and chronic injuries.

Wear the Right Clothes
Almost every physical activity has special clothing. Most physical activities require clothing that lets you move easily. The right clothing will make you more comfortable as you play. It may also protect you from getting hurt.

Don't forget about the weather when you choose what to wear. Special fabrics keep you warm for cold-weather activities. Other fabrics keep you cool in warm weather. For many warm-weather activities, all you need is shorts and a T-shirt. But, if it's cold, you should dress in layers. Use a hat, sunglasses, and sunscreen to protect yourself from sunburn, even on cloudy days. This tip is very important if you're at the beach or hiking in the mountains.

Shoes are one of the most important pieces of clothing you will use for some activities. Wearing shoes that don't fit correctly or aren't designed for your sport can lead to injury. Most sports shoe stores will have the right shoe for what you do.

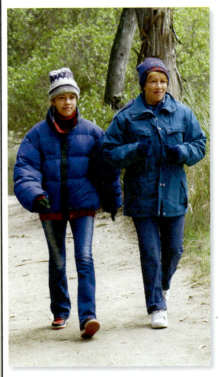

Figure 20 Be sure to wear warm clothes and layers on a cold day!

LIFE SKILLS ACTIVITY
EVALUATING MEDIA MESSAGES

1. Search through popular magazines and Internet sites for an advertisement that uses physical activity to attract customers.

2. How is the physical activity related to this product? If the physical activity is not related, why is the advertiser using it?

3. What age group do you think the advertiser is trying to attract? Why?

4. Is the physical activity being done safely in the ad? If not, what is missing? Why might advertisers leave out safety equipment?

5. Would you buy this product? Why or why not?

REAL-LIFE CONNECTION — GENERAL
Helping Others Responsible and caring students can volunteer for programs, such as Special Olympics, that help disabled children stay physically active. These organizations often need people to help disabled children train or compete for a specific event safely. Have interested teens find out if local organizations for disabled people need volunteers.
LS Interpersonal

86 Chapter 4 • Physical Fitness

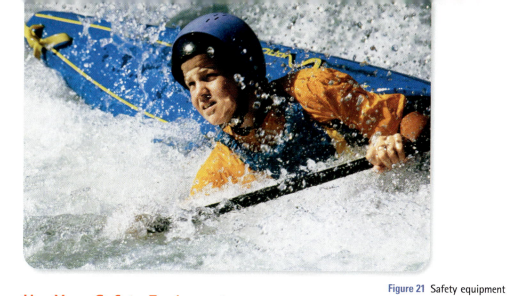

Figure 21 Safety equipment helps protect you from injury during activities.

Use Your Safety Equipment

Many sports have safety equipment. Safety equipment helps protect you from injury. You should always use your safety equipment. For sports such as football and hockey, falls and collisions are common. So, it's dangerous not to use safety equipment. For other activities, accidents happen when you don't expect them. Safety equipment increases enjoyment of physical activities by lowering your chances of injury.

Don't Exercise Alone

Exercising with friends is a good way to protect yourself in case of an accident. If you get hurt and no one is around to help you, an injury can become life threatening. Friends can also make physical activity more exciting. Friends motivate you to continue exercising.

Lesson Review

Using Vocabulary

1. What is active rest?

Understanding Concepts

2. What could happen if you changed the frequency, intensity, and time of your workouts too much? Explain your answer.

3. If someone has poor form, what might happen?

Critical Thinking

4. **Making Good Decisions** Imagine that it's a cold, sunny day. What do you need to wear to protect yourself if you play soccer with your friends?

Close

Reteaching — BASIC

Outlining Have students create an outline of the lesson. Ask them to use the headings as a guideline to summarize the material regarding injury prevention. **LS** Verbal

Quiz — GENERAL

1. How does a warm-up affect the body? (It loosens muscles and increases heart rate.)
2. What does a cool-down do? (It helps the body return to normal after exercise. The heart returns to its resting rate. A cool-down keeps muscles from getting tight and sore.)
3. Why are shoes so important to exercise? (Wearing shoes that don't fit correctly or aren't designed for an activity can lead to injury.)
4. How does exercising with friends help keep you safe? (Friends can help you if you get hurt. They also motivate you to keep exercising.)

Alternative Assessment — GENERAL

Newspaper Reporter Have students interview school coaches, personal trainers, or other fitness professionals about safety during exercise. Students should address the ways these people make sure exercise is safe. Ask students to write a newspaper article about their interview. **LS** Verbal

---

Answers to Lesson Review

1. Active rest is a way to recover from exercise by reducing the amount of activity you do.
2. Sample answer: Increasing FIT too much can cause injury. If you exercise too frequently, your body can't recover from workouts properly. If you exercise too intensely, you may work too hard or do an exercise incorrectly. Exercising for long periods of time can make you tired. Your body may not be able to handle the exercise or you may lose focus and have an accident.
3. Poor form puts more stress on muscles, bones, and joints, so the person may get hurt.
4. Sample answer: Since it is cold, I should dress in layers to stay warm. I should wear sunscreen to protect myself from sunburn.

4 CHAPTER REVIEW

Assignment Guide

Lesson	Review Questions
1	5–6, 9
2	7, 10, 17–19, 21–22, 28–31
3	1
4	2, 11
5	12–14
6	4, 15, 24–26
7	3, 16, 27
8	8, 20, 23

ANSWERS

Using Vocabulary

1. Aerobic exercise is exercise that uses oxygen and lasts a long time. Anaerobic exercise doesn't require oxygen and lasts a short time.
2. A competition is a contest between two or more people or teams. Sportsmanship is the ability to treat all players, officials, and fans fairly during a competition.
3. Acute injuries happen suddenly. Chronic injuries develop over a long period of time.
4. Overtraining
5. Flexibility
6. Endurance
7. Recovery time
8. Active rest

Understanding Concepts

9. Strength is the amount of force muscles apply when they are used. Endurance is the ability to do activities for more than a few minutes. Flexibility is the ability to bend and twist joints easily. Body composition compares the weight of fat in the body to the weight of muscles, bones, and organs.

---

4 CHAPTER REVIEW

Chapter Summary

■ Physical fitness is the ability to do everyday activities without becoming short of breath, sore, or very tired. ■ Four parts of physical fitness are strength, endurance, flexibility, and body composition. ■ Exercise is any physical activity that maintains or improves physical fitness. ■ Frequency, intensity, and time of exercise can be adjusted to help improve fitness. ■ Aerobic exercise uses oxygen to get energy. ■ Anaerobic exercise doesn't use oxygen to get energy. ■ Competition is a contest between two or more people or teams. ■ Weight training is the use of weight to make muscles stronger or bigger. ■ Overtraining happens when someone exercises too much. ■ The two types of injury are acute injuries and chronic injuries.

Using Vocabulary

For each pair of terms, describe how the meanings of the terms differ.

1. aerobic exercise/anaerobic exercise
2. competition/sportsmanship
3. acute injury/chronic injury

For each sentence, fill in the blank with the proper word from the word bank provided below.

body composition   overtraining
active rest   endurance
recovery time   flexibility

4. ___ is a condition that happens when you exercise too much.
5. ___ is the ability to move joints easily.
6. ___ is the ability to do an activity for more than a few minutes.
7. ___ is the amount of time your heart takes to return to its resting heart rate after you exercise.
8. ___ is a fitness technique in which you rest by reducing the intensity of your physical activity.

Understanding Concepts

9. Describe four parts of physical fitness.
10. What five things influence your fitness goals?
11. How do you recognize a good sport?
12. How does weight training for strength development differ from bodybuilding?
13. List seven safety tips for weight training.
14. Describe two weight-training exercises for your upper body.
15. List five warning signs of overtraining.
16. List three examples of acute injuries and two examples of chronic injuries.
17. How does increasing frequency, intensity, and time of exercise affect fitness?
18. How do you avoid injury when changing the parts of FIT?
19. What is the target heart rate zone for a 13-year-old?
20. List eight ways to avoid injury while exercising.
21. How are resting heart rate and recovery time related?

---

10. the activities you enjoy, your abilities, the amount of work you want to do, how important physical fitness is to you and the people around you, and the risk of injury
11. A good sport always plays his or her best, follows the rules, considers the health and safety of other players, congratulates all players for good plays, and is polite when he or she loses and modest when he or she wins.
12. Weight training for strength development makes muscles stronger. Bodybuilding makes muscles stronger and bigger.
13. Use a spotter. Lift weights in pairs or small groups. Make sure free weights are secured properly. Understand how a machine works. Lift only as much weight as you can with correct form. Exercise both sides of a joint. Always use correct form.
14. For the bench press, lift the bar from the supports and lower it to your chest. Then, raise the bar again. For the biceps curl, start with your arm slightly bent or at a 90° angle. Curl your arm toward your shoulder.
15. feeling tired all the time, not doing as well at games and practice, feeling less interested in the activity, an increase in your resting heart rate, and getting hurt more often

Critical Thinking

Applying Concepts

22. Julio is 14 years old. He can do 6 pull-ups and 40 curl-ups. He can run a mile in a little over 7 minutes. He can also reach past 8 inches on the sit-and-reach test. Based on his results, do you think Julio can try out for the soccer team? Explain your answer.

23. Maria has decided to hike in the mountains by herself. Maria claims that she will be safe because no other people are on the trail. Why is hiking by herself a bad idea?

24. One way to avoid overtraining is to make sure that you get plenty of rest between workouts. What can you do to make sure that you get the rest you need?

Making Good Decisions

25. Your friend has been making excuses for not wanting to play basketball lately. When he does show up to practice, he doesn't play as hard as he used to, and he gets hurt easily. What should your friend do?

26. You played tennis with some friends for the first time last night. This morning, your muscles ached and felt sore. Should you play tennis again tonight? Explain your answer.

27. At the ice-skating rink, your friend shows you a jump that she just learned. But she falls as she lands. She seems to have sprained her ankle. What type of injury does she have? What can you do to help?

Interpreting Graphics

Fitness Test Results for Three 13-Year-Old Boys

Exercise	Boy A	Boy B	Boy C
Pull-ups	3	1	4
Curl-ups	35	20	42
1-mile run (minutes and seconds)	8:46	10:24	7:59
Sit and reach (inches)	6	8	9

Use the table above to answer questions 28–31.

28. Which boy has the best fitness? the worst fitness?

29. Which boy needs to improve his flexibility? his heart and lung endurance?

30. How can the boy who needs to improve his flexibility do so? How can the boy who needs to improve his heart and lung endurance do so?

31. Which boy would be most likely to try out for the soccer team? Explain your answer.

Reading Checkup

Take a minute to review your answers to the Health IQ questions at the beginning of this chapter. How has reading this chapter improved your Health IQ?

---

16. Sprains, strains, and fractures are acute injuries. Stress fractures and tendinitis are chronic injuries.
17. Increasing FIT can improve fitness.
18. Don't increase more than one part of FIT at a time. Also, don't increase any one part of FIT too much.
19. 124 to 176 beats per minute
20. warm up and cool down, stretch, don't go too fast, improve your form, take a break, wear the right clothes, use your safety equipment, and don't exercise alone
21. Recovery time is the amount of time it takes the heart to resume its resting heart rate after exercise.

Critical Thinking

Applying Concepts

22. Sample answer: Yes. Julio meets the higher standards in the healthy fitness zones, so he should be able to play soccer.
23. Sample answer: Maria shouldn't hike by herself because there is no one around to help her if she gets hurt.
24. Sample answer: I can schedule rest days between hard workouts. Using a calendar can help me do this.

Making Good Decisions

25. Sample answer: My friend may have overtrained because he isn't interested in playing basketball and he's getting hurt more often. So, he should take a break from playing until he can recover.
26. Sample answer: Muscle soreness is achiness that happens a day or two after hard exercise. It is normal, so it should be OK for me to exercise again tonight. In fact, the muscle soreness should go away the next time I exercise.
27. Sample answer: She has an acute injury. I should tell a parent or teacher right away. For first aid, I can use RICE.

Interpreting Graphics

28. Boy C; Boy B
29. Boy A; Boy B
30. Sample answer: The boy who needs to improve his flexibility can do so by stretching regularly. The boy who needs better heart and lung endurance can improve his endurance by running, swimming, or cycling.
31. Sample answer: Boy C would be most likely to try out for the soccer team because he is the most fit.

Chapter Resource File

- Concept Review GENERAL
- Concept Mapping GENERAL
- Performance-Based Assessment GENERAL
- Chapter Test GENERAL

Model

Introduce this activity by reminding students that using this Life Skill will help them take personal responsibility for their behavior. Then, review the scenario with the class.

Prepare students for this activity by modeling each of the steps of the skill. Make sure students understand each step before you move on to the next one.

Guided Practice: Practice with a Friend

Guided Practice is the stage in which you and the students analyze their approach to solving the problem given in the scenario and analyze their ability to assess their health. Have students read Act 1. Discuss with the class the situation described and the way students are to act it out. Organize the class into groups of three. In each group, one person plays the role of Sonya, another person plays the swim team coach, and the third person is the observer.

Proper pacing during the Guided Practice is important. The suggestions listed below will help you control the pace.

1. Stop after completing each step of assessing your health.
2. Discuss with each group the observer's comments.
3. Ask the other members of each group to listen to the observer's suggestions and to suggest ways to improve the way they assess their health.
4. Instruct students to repeat the steps that need improvement and to include their modifications.

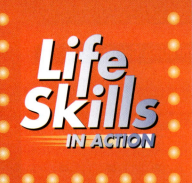

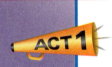

The 4 Steps of Assessing Your Health

1. Choose the part of your health you want to assess.
2. List your strengths and weaknesses.
3. Describe how your behaviors may contribute to your weaknesses.
4. Develop a plan to address your weaknesses.

Assessing Your Health

Assessing your health means evaluating each of the four parts of your health and examining your behaviors. By assessing your health regularly, you will know what your strengths and weaknesses are and will be able to take steps to improve your health. Complete the following activity to improve your ability to assess your health.

Swim Team Tryouts

Setting the Scene

Sonya has gone swimming frequently since she was a little girl. She has always thought of herself as a strong swimmer. So this year, Sonya decides to try out for the school's swim team. Because making the team is so important to her, Sonya wants to make sure she is in good physical condition before the tryouts. She decides to talk to the swim team coach about preparing for the tryouts.

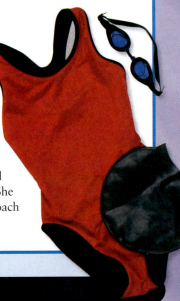

Guided Practice

Practice with a Friend

Form a group of three. Have one person play the role of Sonya and another person play the role of the swim team coach. Have the third person be an observer. Walking through each of the four steps of assessing your health, role-play Sonya assessing her health. The swim team coach can help Sonya by offering advice. The observer will take notes, which will include observations about what the person playing Sonya did well and suggestions of ways to improve. Stop after each step to evaluate the process.

5. Check to make sure that students understand each step before they move on to the next step.
6. If time permits, repeat the exercise three times, switching roles each time. Each student should have the opportunity to play each role. Co-op Learning

Independent Practice

Check Yourself

After you have completed the guided practice, go through Act 1 again without stopping at each step. Answer the questions below to review what you did.

1. What are some of Sonya's possible strengths and weaknesses?
2. What behaviors may contribute to Sonya's weaknesses?
3. What can Sonya do to overcome her weaknesses?
4. What are some weaknesses in your physical health? How can you address your weaknesses?

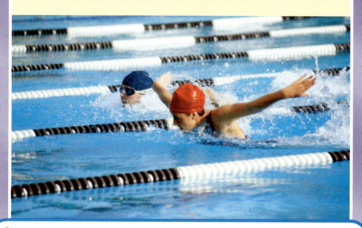

On Your Own

Sonya's efforts to prepare for the swim team tryouts paid off when she made the team. She was very excited during her first swim meet. However, at the end of her race, Sonya was surprised to learn that she lost and that her finishing time was not very good. Since then, Sonya has been very depressed about her race results. She thinks about her failure all the time and has trouble concentrating on her schoolwork. Make an outline showing how Sonya could use the four steps of assessing your health to assess her health.

Independent Practice: Check Yourself

Instruct students to repeat Act 1 without stopping at each step. Remind students to apply what they learned in the Guided Practice to the Independent Practice.

Encourage students to use the Check Yourself questions as a starting point for reviewing and analyzing their Independent Practice. Remind students that as they change roles, the answers to these questions may change for each actor. Encourage students to create additional questions for checking their ability to assess their health. When students have finished the Independent Practice, have them answer the Check Yourself questions in writing. Use their answers to assess their understanding of the steps of assessing their health and to assess their use of the steps to solve a problem.

Check Yourself Answers

1. Sample answer: Sonya's strengths are that she has been swimming for a long time and that she has confidence in her abilities. One of Sonya's weaknesses is that she might not be in the physical condition needed to make the swim team.
2. Sample answer: Sonya may not be in the physical condition needed to make the swim team because she may not have practiced swimming fast and may not have timed herself as she swam.
3. Sample answer: Sonya can train according to the swim team coach's advice. She can find out what times she needs to make the swim team and set goals to make those times.
4. Sample answer: I can't do very many push-ups. I can address this weakness by lifting weights to build upper-body strength and by doing push-ups three times a week.

Act 2: On Your Own

This additional scenario gives students an opportunity to apply what they have learned in both the Guided Practice and the Independent Practice to a new situation.

Suggest to students that they use the Check Yourself questions as a starting point for assessing their health in the new situation. Encourage students to be creative and to think of ways to improve their ability to assess their health.

Assessment

Review the outlines that students have written as part of the On Your Own activity. The outlines should show that the students followed the steps of assessing their health in a realistic and effective manner. If time permits, ask student volunteers to write one or more of their outlines on the blackboard. Discuss the outlines and the way the students used the steps of assessing their health.

Chapter 5 — Nutrition and Your Health
Chapter Planning Guide

PACING	CLASSROOM RESOURCES	ACTIVITIES AND DEMONSTRATIONS
BLOCK 1 • 45 min pp. 92–97 **Chapter Opener**	CRF Health Inventory * GENERAL CRF Parent Letter *	SE Health IQ, p. 93 CRF At-Home Activity *
Lesson 1 Nutrition and Diet	CRF Lesson Plan * TT Bellringer *	TE Demonstration Treats, p. 94 ♦ GENERAL SE Social Studies Activity, p. 96 TE Activity Influences on Food Choices, p. 96 GENERAL CRF Enrichment Activity * ADVANCED
BLOCK 2 • 45 min pp. 98–101 **Lesson 2** The Six Essential Nutrients	CRF Lesson Plan * TT Bellringer *	TE Activities Mystery Tasting Party, p. 91F TE Group Activity Types of Nutrients, p. 99 GENERAL SE Hands-on Activity, p. 100 CRF Datasheets for In-Text Activities * GENERAL TE Group Activity Vitamin Supplements, p. 100 ♦ ADVANCED TE Activity Mineral Deficiencies, p. 100 GENERAL CRF Life Skills Activity * GENERAL CRF Enrichment Activity * ADVANCED
BLOCK 3 • 45 min pp. 102–105 **Lesson 3** Balancing Your Diet	CRF Lesson Plan * TT Bellringer * TT The Food Guide Pyramid * TT The Nutrition Facts Label *	TE Activities Nutrition Survey, p. 91F TE Group Activity Poster Project, p. 102 GENERAL TE Activity Fast Foods, p. 105 ♦ GENERAL SE Life Skills in Action Making Good Decisions, pp. 112–113 CRF Life Skills Activity * GENERAL CRF Enrichment Activity * ADVANCED
BLOCK 4 • 45 min pp. 106–109 **Lesson 4** Building Healthful Eating Habits	CRF Lesson Plan * TT Bellringer *	TE Group Activity Snacking Skit, p. 106 GENERAL TE Activity Show Your Snack, p. 107 GENERAL TE Activity Diet Critique, p. 108 GENERAL TE Group Activity Health Food Directory, p. 108 GENERAL CRF Enrichment Activity * ADVANCED

BLOCKS 5 & 6 • 90 min — Chapter Review and Assessment Resources

- SE Chapter Review, pp. 110–111
- CRF Concept Review * GENERAL
- CRF Health Behavior Contract * GENERAL
- CRF Chapter Test * GENERAL
- CRF Performance-Based Assessment * GENERAL
- OSP Test Generator
- CRF Test Item Listing *

Online Resources

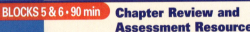

Visit **go.hrw.com** for a variety of free resources related to this textbook. Enter the keyword **HD4NU7**.

Holt Online Learning
Students can access interactive problem solving help and active visual concept development with the *Decisions for Health* Online Edition available at **www.hrw.com**.

CNN Student News
cnnstudentnews.com
Find the latest health news, lesson plans, and activities related to important scientific events.

Compression guide:
To shorten your instruction because of time limitations, omit Lesson 4.

KEY

TE Teacher Edition	**CRF** Chapter Resource File	***** Also on One-Stop Planner
SE Student Edition	**TT** Teaching Transparency	■ Also Available in Spanish
OSP One-Stop Planner		◆ Requires Advance Prep

SKILLS DEVELOPMENT RESOURCES	LESSON REVIEW AND ASSESSMENT	STANDARDS CORRELATION
		National Health Education Standards
SE Study Tip Reviewing Information, p. 95 **TE** Reading Skill Builder Reading Organizer, p. 95 GENERAL **TE** Reading Skill Builder Discussion, p. 96 BASIC **CRF** Decision-Making * GENERAL **CRF** Cross-Disciplinary * GENERAL **CRF** Directed Reading * BASIC	**SE** Lesson Review, p. 97 **TE** Reteaching, Quiz, p. 97 **TE** Alternative Assessment, p. 97 GENERAL **CRF** Lesson Quiz * ■ GENERAL	1.1, 1.4, 4.1
TE Reading Skill Builder Reading Hint, p. 99 BASIC **CRF** Cross-Disciplinary * GENERAL **CRF** Directed Reading * BASIC	**SE** Lesson Review, p. 101 **TE** Reteaching ◆, Quiz, p. 101 **TE** Alternative Assessment, p. 101 GENERAL **CRF** Concept Mapping * GENERAL **CRF** Lesson Quiz * ■ GENERAL	1.1
TE Life Skill Builder Assessing Your Health, p. 103 GENERAL **TE** Inclusion Strategies, p. 103 ADVANCED **TE** Life Skill Builder Practicing Wellness, p. 104 ADVANCED **CRF** Decision-Making * GENERAL **CRF** Refusal Skills * GENERAL **CRF** Directed Reading * BASIC	**SE** Lesson Review, p. 105 **TE** Reteaching, Quiz, p. 105 **CRF** Lesson Quiz * ■ GENERAL	3.4
SE Life Skills Activity Practicing Wellness, p. 107 **TE** Life Skill Builder Evaluating Media Messages, p. 107 ADVANCED **TE** Life Skill Builder Practicing Wellness, p. 107 **TE** Inclusion Strategies, p. 107 ADVANCED **SE** Life Skills Activity Making Good Decisions, p. 108 **CRF** Refusal Skills * GENERAL **CRF** Directed Reading * BASIC	**SE** Lesson Review, p. 109 **TE** Reteaching, Quiz, p. 109 **TE** Alternative Assessment, p. 109 GENERAL **CRF** Concept Mapping * GENERAL **CRF** Lesson Quiz * ■ GENERAL	3.4

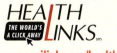

www.scilinks.org/health

Maintained by the **National Science Teachers Association**

Topic: Nutrition
HealthLinks code: HD4072
Topic: Nutrients
HealthLinks code: HD4071
Topic: Food Pyramids
HealthLinks code: HD4043

Technology Resources

 One-Stop Planner
All of your printable resources and the Test Generator are on this convenient CD-ROM.

 Guided Reading Audio CDs

VIDEO SELECT
For information about videos related to this chapter, go to go.hrw.com and type in the keyword **HD4NU7V**.

Chapter 5 • Chapter Planning Guide **91B**

CHAPTER 5
Nutrition and Your Health
Chapter Resources

Teacher Resources

TEACHING TRANSPARENCIES

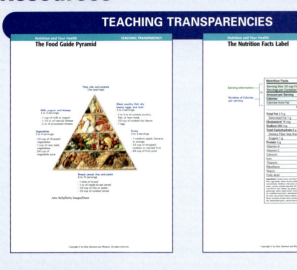

BELLRINGER TRANSPARENCIES

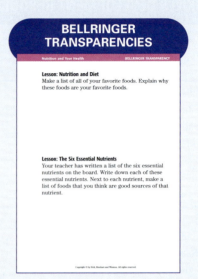

LESSON PLANS

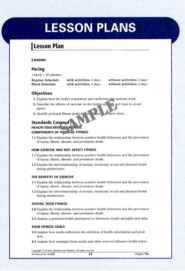

PARENT LETTER

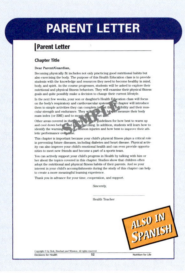

TEST ITEM LISTING

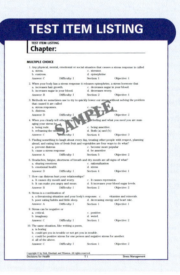

Meeting Individual Needs

DIRECTED READING

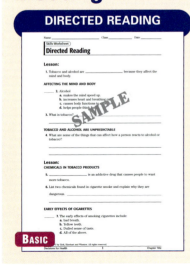

BASIC

CONCEPT MAPPING

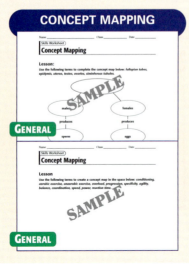

GENERAL

CONCEPT REVIEW

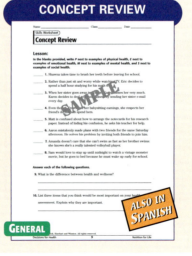

GENERAL

ENRICHMENT ACTIVITIES

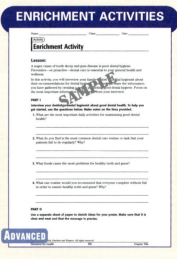

ADVANCED

Resources

These worksheet pages can be found in the Chapter Resource File and the One-Stop Planner. The transparencies can be found in the Teaching Transparencies binder and on the One-Stop Planner.

Activities

LIFE SKILLS ACTIVITIES
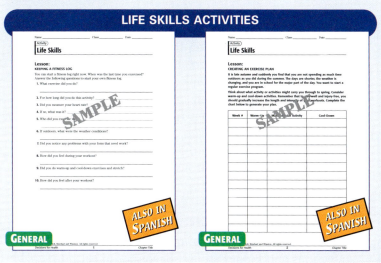

AT-HOME ACTIVITY
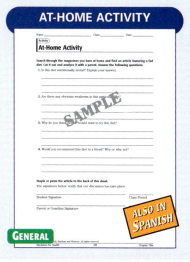

DATASHEETS FOR IN-TEXT ACTIVITIES
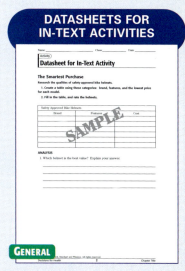

Applications

DECISION-MAKING
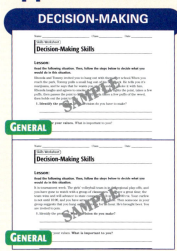

REFUSAL SKILLS
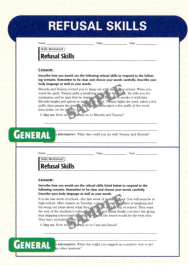

CROSS-DISCIPLINARY
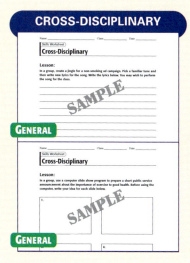

HEALTH BEHAVIOR CONTRACT
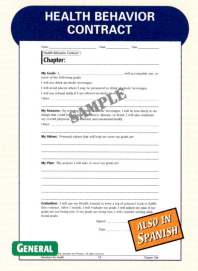

Assessments

HEALTH INVENTORY
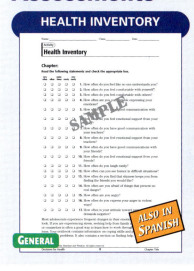

LESSON QUIZZES
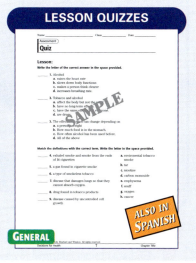

CHAPTER TEST
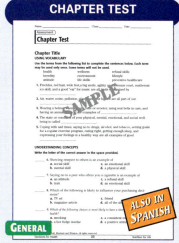

PERFORMANCE-BASED ASSESSMENT
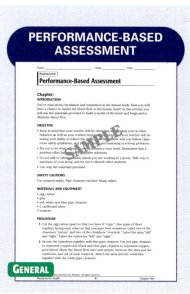

Chapter 5 • Chapter Resources and Worksheets

Chapter 5: Background Information

The following information focuses on the digestive and urinary systems. This material will help prepare you for teaching the concepts in this chapter.

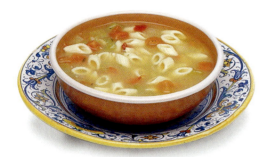

The Digestive System

- The digestive system is a group of organs that work together to digest food so that it can be used by the body. Digestion occurs in the digestive tract, which is a series of tubelike organs that are joined end to end. The digestive tract includes the mouth, throat, esophagus, stomach, small intestine, large intestine, rectum, and anus.

- Food is broken down by mechanical digestion and chemical digestion. Mechanical digestion is the breaking, crushing, and mashing of food by the teeth, tongue, and stomach. Chemical digestion occurs when enzymes in the saliva, stomach, and other organs break down the food.

- The liver and the gallbladder are also involved in digestion. The liver produces bile which is used in fat digestion. The bile is stored temporarily in the gallbladder until it is secreted into the small intestine. The liver also stores excess nutrients. The liver will release the nutrients when the body needs them.

The Urinary System

- The urinary system removes waste products from the bloodstream and is composed of the kidneys, ureters, bladder, and urethra.

- The kidneys are a pair of bean-shaped organs that constantly clean the blood. Kidneys filter about 2,000 L of blood each day. Inside each kidney are more than 1 million microscopic filters called nephrons that remove a variety of harmful substances from the body. Among the most important of these substances is urea, which contains nitrogen and is formed when cells use protein for energy.

- The urinary system ensures that the amount of water taken in and the amount of water leaving the body are equal. For example, if your body loses too much water from sweating, a hormone signals the kidneys to take back water from the nephrons and return it to the bloodstream. If you drink too much water, a hormone signals the kidneys to allow more water to stay in the nephrons and leave the body as urine.

Urinary and Digestive Ailments

- Common urinary system ailments include bacterial infections and kidney stones. Bacteria can get into the bladder and ureters through the urethra and cause painful infections. Sometimes salts and wastes collect inside the kidneys and form kidney stones. Kidney stones usually pass naturally from the body, but sometimes a medical procedure is necessary.

- Common digestive system ailments include heartburn, constipation, diarrhea, and gastric ulcers. The burning pain associated with heartburn is a result of backflow of stomach acid to the esophagus. Common causes of heartburn include eating too much, eating right before going to bed, or eating very acidic foods. When the body does not get enough fiber, water, or exercise, the contents of the large intestine can become too dry. This causes constipation. Diarrhea is often caused by microbial infections of the digestive tract and can result in dehydration. Gastric ulcers are open sores in the stomach. They can be caused by bacteria and exacerbated by a high-fat diet, smoking, caffeine, and alcohol.

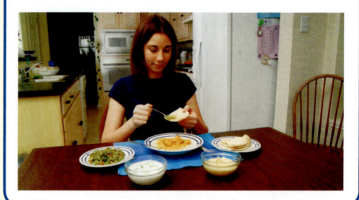

For background information about teaching strategies and issues, refer to the *Professional Reference for Teachers*.

ACTIVITIES

CHAPTER 5

Consider using the activities on this page as students explore the lessons of this chapter. Look for other activities throughout the Student Edition chapter.

Nutrition Survey

Procedure Have students conduct a survey of their friends' nutrition habits. Have each student copy down the following questions and have five of their friends answer them:

1. Do you eat five or more servings of fruits and vegetables every day?
2. Do you eat breakfast every day?
3. Do you drink 8 to 10 glasses of water every day?
4. Do you eat a lot of high-fat foods?
5. Do you eat a lot of high-sugar foods?

Tell students to encourage their friends to answer the questions as honestly as possible. Have the students record how many yes answers and how many no answers they get. The class should then combine their data and record the survey information in a table. Calculate the percentage of people who answered yes to questions 1–3 and no to questions 4 and 5.

Analysis Ask students the following questions:

- What percentage of students answered yes to questions 1–3? What percentage of students answered no to questions 4 and 5? **(Answers may vary.)**
- What do you think these percentages indicate? **(Sample answer: These percentages show the number of students who have healthy eating habits.)**
- How healthy are the surveyed students' eating habits? **(Answers may vary.)**
- Do you think the surveyed students have similar eating habits to other students nationwide? **(Sample answer: Yes, most American adolescents have similar eating habits.)**

When you finish discussing the questions, have students make a list of improvements that the surveyed students could consider making to their eating habits.

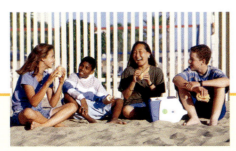

Mystery Tasting Party

Hands on

Procedure Instruct each student to bring in a mystery fruit. Students should research what sort of nutrients their fruit contains, where it is grown, and what sort of recipes it is used in. They should bring the fruit to class in a paper sack so that the other students are not able to see the fruit. Ask volunteers to take turns being blindfolded. Give the blindfolded students a piece of the fruit to taste and have them guess what fruit it is. The student who brought the fruit can use his or her research to give the blindfolded students hints about the fruit.

Analysis After all the fruits have been guessed, ask the students to do the following:

- Draw a table that will list all the fruits brought to class and the nutrients each fruit contains.
- With the help of the student who brought each fruit, have the class list the main nutrients present in each fruit.

Discussion Questions

The following discussion questions may be helpful when teaching the chapter:

- Why do you think eating right is important?
- How is the food you eat related to your weight?
- Why do you think there are so many advertisements for quick weight-loss diets?
- How do you healthfully manage your weight?
- Why is it important to understand what nutrients are and what they do for your body?

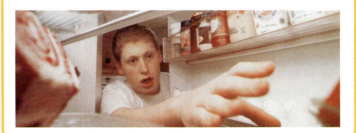

Chapter 5 • Activities

CHAPTER 5

Overview
Tell students that this chapter will help them understand what nutrients are, which foods contain each type of nutrient, and how to plan and maintain a well-balanced diet. Students will learn that eating a well-balanced diet requires making good decisions about food. This chapter will teach students the basics of nutrition so they will be able to make healthy choices in the future.

Assessing Prior Knowledge
Students should be familiar with the following topic:
- decision making

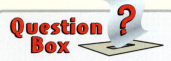

Students may feel more comfortable asking questions if you set up a Question Box to collect their questions. Have students write and anonymously submit their questions about nutrition, dieting, and eating habits. Address these questions during class, or use these questions to introduce lessons that cover related topics.

Current Health
Check out *Current Health* articles and activities related to this chapter by visiting the HRW Web site at **go.hrw.com**. Just type in the keyword **HD4CH20T**.

Chapter Resource File
- Directed Reading BASIC
- Health Inventory GENERAL
- Parent Letter

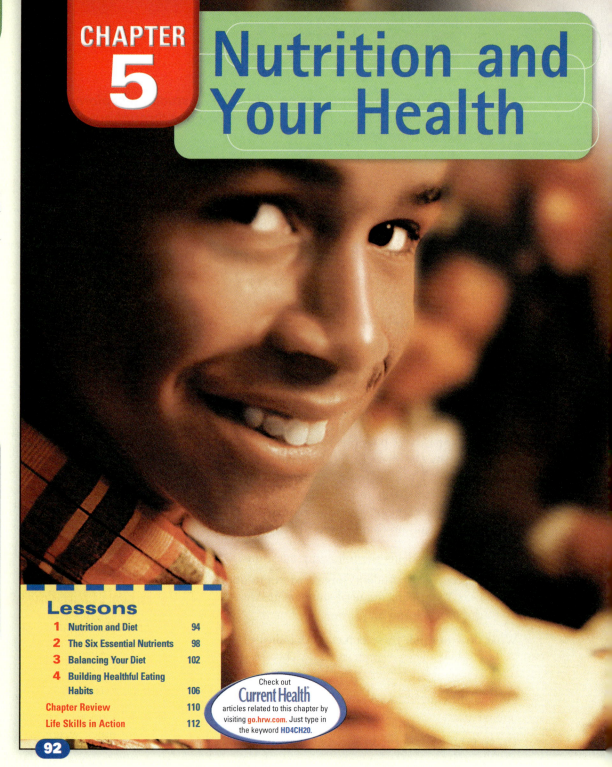

CHAPTER 5 Nutrition and Your Health

Lessons
1	Nutrition and Diet	94
2	The Six Essential Nutrients	98
3	Balancing Your Diet	102
4	Building Healthful Eating Habits	106
Chapter Review		110
Life Skills in Action		112

Check out *Current Health* articles related to this chapter by visiting **go.hrw.com**. Just type in the keyword **HD4CH20**.

92

Standards Correlations

National Health Education Standards

1.1 Explain the relationship between positive health behaviors and the prevention of injury, illness, disease, and premature death. (Lessons 1–2)

1.4 Describe how family and peers influence the health of adolescents. (Lesson 1)

3.4 (partial) Demonstrate strategies to improve or maintain personal and family health. (Lesson 3–4)

4.1 (partial) Describe the influence of cultural beliefs on health behaviors and the use of health services. (Lesson 1)

> "I am usually **hungry** by the end of school. I have **soccer practice** after school, so I just grab something from the **vending machine**. The snack that I buy doesn't usually last very long, and I'm starving by the end of practice. What can I do to make sure that I'm not hungry all the time?"

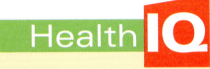

PRE-READING

Answer the multiple-choice questions to find out what you already know about nutrition. When you've finished this chapter, you'll have the opportunity to change your answers based on what you've learned.

1. Your body needs energy to
   a. grow.
   b. repair tissues.
   c. fight germs.
   d. All of the above

2. The process in which your body breaks down food into a form your body can use is called
   a. hunger.
   b. digestion.
   c. metabolism.
   d. indigestion.

3. The process in which your body changes nutrients into usable energy is called
   a. hunger.
   b. digestion.
   c. metabolism.
   d. sleeping.

4. Tofu and ____ are good sources of protein.
   a. fruit
   b. vegetables
   c. peanut butter
   d. water

5. There are ____ different groups in the Food Guide Pyramid.
   a. five
   b. six
   c. seven
   d. four

6. The Nutrition Facts label states
   a. the number of Calories in each serving of food.
   b. the number of servings in a container of food.
   c. the amount of nutrients in each serving of food.
   d. All of the above

ANSWERS: 1. d; 2. b; 3. c; 4. c; 5. b; 6. d

Using the Health IQ

Misconception Alert
Answers to the Health IQ questions may help you identify students' misconceptions.

Question 1: Students may think that the body needs energy only to grow. Make sure students understand that the body needs energy to perform all bodily functions.

Question 4: Students may not realize that dry beans and nuts, in addition to meat, poultry, and fish, are good sources of protein. Tofu is made from dried soybeans and peanut butter is made from peanuts. Soybeans and tofu are considered good sources of low-fat protein. Although peanuts and peanut butter contain higher amounts of fat than soybeans and tofu, they are still considered to be good sources of protein.

Question 5: Students may not realize that fruits and vegetables are two separate food groups on the Food Guide Pyramid. In addition, students may not realize that fats, oils, and sweets form their own group. In fact, students may not consider fats and oils to be foods, since these products are used mostly in the production of foods and not usually eaten alone.

Answers
1. d
2. b
3. c
4. c
5. b
6. d

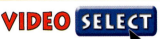

For information about videos related to this chapter, go to **go.hrw.com** and type in the keyword **HD4NU7V**.

Lesson 1 Focus

Overview
Before beginning this lesson, review with your students the objectives listed under the What You'll Do head in the Student Edition. In this lesson, students will learn how their nutrition affects their overall health, about the digestive process, and about the influences on their food choices.

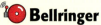 Bellringer
Ask students to make a list of all their favorite foods, including an explanation of why those foods are their favorites. **LS** Intrapersonal

Answer to Start Off Write
Accept all reasonable answers. Sample answer: Practicing good nutrition means eating the right amount of healthy foods every day.

Motivate

Demonstration —— GENERAL
Treats Bring a package of cookies or candies to class and offer the treats to students. As the students are eating, ask them the following:

- Why do people eat? (Answers may include hunger or the need for energy.)
- Why did you choose to eat the treat I offered you? (Sample answers: I like how it tastes; I was hungry.)
- What are some reasons that people eat other than hunger? (Samples answers: cravings, boredom, nervousness, excitement)

LS Kinesthetic

Lesson 1

What You'll Do
- **Explain** how nutrition affects your overall health.
- **Explain** how your body uses food.
- **Identify** six factors that affect your food choices.
- **Explain** how your feelings may affect your food choices.

Terms to Learn
- digestion
- nutrient
- diet

Start Off Write
What does it mean to practice good nutrition?

Nutrition and Diet

Josh's grandfather recently survived a heart attack. Now, all of Josh's family members are talking about eating better and improving their diets. Josh wonders how much food can really affect someone's health.

Like Josh, many people may be confused about how food can affect a person's overall health. After all, you need to eat to stay alive, right? The truth is that food contains substances that your body needs to stay healthy. *Nutrition* is the study of how your bodies use the substances in food to maintain our health.

Nutrition and Your Health
Practicing good nutrition means eating foods that are good for you and eating them in the right amounts. Your nutrition affects many of the things you do every day. The substances in food give you the energy you need for learning, studying, staying active, and hanging out with your friends. Your body uses the same substances to grow, repair tissues, and fight germs that cause sickness.

Think about Josh's grandfather. The foods he ate may have played a part in causing his heart attack. Practicing good nutrition will help Josh's grandfather stay healthy from now on.

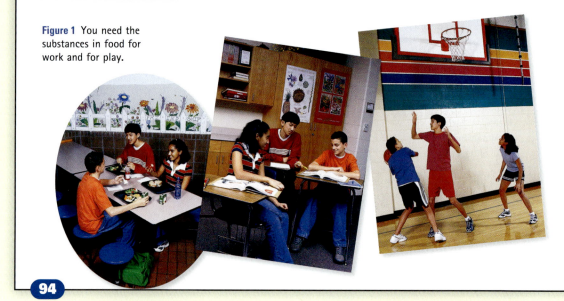

Figure 1 You need the substances in food for work and for play.

Background
Malnutrition An improper or unhealthy diet may lead to malnutrition, which is poor nourishment caused by a lack of nutrients. Malnutrition can lead to a number of vitamin and mineral deficiencies. These deficiencies include iron, vitamin A, and iodine deficiencies. A lack of iron may lead to severe anemia, and a lack of vitamin A may lead to a loss of eyesight. Perhaps the worst of all, a lack of iodine may result in brain damage.

Chapter Resource File
- Directed Reading **BASIC**
- Lesson Plan
- Lesson Quiz **GENERAL**

Transparencies
TT Bellringer

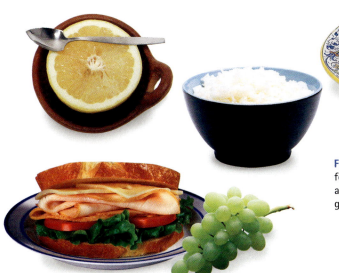

Figure 2 Although these foods are very different, they all contain nutrients that give your body energy.

How Your Body Uses Food

Your body uses food for energy. However, your body can't use food directly for energy. The food must be broken down into a form that your body can use. **Digestion** is the process in which food is broken down into a form your body can use.

Digestion begins when you chew your food. After the food you eat is chewed and swallowed, it passes into the stomach. In the stomach, the food is broken down by a strong acid and other substances. This step turns your food into a thick liquid. The liquid passes into the small intestine, where it is broken down further into nutrients (NOO tree uhnts). **Nutrients** are the substances found in food that your body needs to function properly. The nutrients are absorbed and sent to the liver to be processed into energy for the body. Your body turns the nutrients into usable energy through a process called *metabolism*.

Your body can make some nutrients. But most nutrients come from the foods you eat. For example, your body needs nutrients to fight germs that cause sickness. One way you can get these nutrients is by drinking orange juice. Because not every food has every nutrient, eating a variety of foods is important. This way, you will get all the nutrients you need.

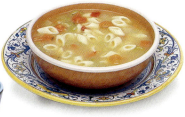

STUDY TIP for better reading

Reviewing Information Make up a story to help you remember how your body breaks down and uses food.

Career

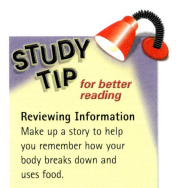

Chefs Many chefs specialize in preparing certain types of cuisine, but all chefs must be familiar with the chemistry and composition of a large variety of foods. At many restaurants, the chefs plan the entrees on the menu. To do this, chefs use their knowledge of food to design an enticing and fulfilling meal.

Teach, continued

Sensitivity ALERT

A discussion of eating behaviors may be embarrassing or uncomfortable for students who are overweight or underweight (or who have overweight or underweight family members). Be sensitive in how you address these topics. Maintain a classroom and school culture that fosters respect, sensitivity, and empathy for self and others.

Activity —— GENERAL
Influences on Food Choices
Have students make a list of the foods they ate yesterday. Next to each food, have students write down any factors that may have had an impact on their choice to eat that food. For example, if a student ate a sugar cookie for a snack, he or she may write "my personal taste" next to that entry. Or, if another student ate chicken curry for dinner, he or she may write "family tradition."
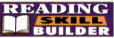 Intrapersonal

READING SKILL BUILDER —— BASIC
Discussion Have students read this page, and then organize students into small groups. Have each group discuss the influences that affect their food choices. Ask students to discuss which influences have more of an impact than others on their individual and their family's food choices.

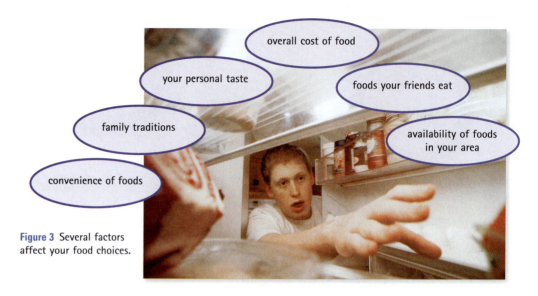

Figure 3 Several factors affect your food choices.

Social Studies ACTIVITY
Interview an elderly friend or relative about what types of food he or she ate while growing up. After your interview, create a poster that compares the foods that your friend or relative ate with the foods that you eat today. Which foods are the same? Which foods are different?

Your Diet and Food Choices

Most people think of a diet as a way of eating to lose weight. Actually, a **diet** is a pattern of eating. Your pattern of eating includes what you eat, how much you eat, and how often you eat. Because your diet includes what kinds of foods you eat, it is affected by your food choices. Many factors influence both your diet and your food choices.

Your personal taste has a lot to do with what you decide to eat. You may eat some foods because they are convenient. For example, you may choose to eat a fast-food burger one night. It is convenient because you can eat it in the car on the way to soccer practice. Often, the cost of food determines the kinds of foods your family buys. Your family traditions or your cultural background may affect the types of foods you decide to eat. You may eat certain foods because your friends like them and because you have come to like these foods, too. Finally, you may eat certain foods because they are available in your local area. The following list shows you six factors that affect your food choices:

- your personal taste
- family traditions
- convenience of foods
- overall cost of food
- foods your friends eat
- availability of foods in your area

Attention Grabber
Children and Food Some students may think that their culture has nothing to do with the types of foods they find disgusting. However, all societies have differences in which foods they see as untouchable. Some studies have shown that toddlers have no inhibitions about eating grasshoppers, imitation dog feces, and other items that their parents would find disgusting. However, by the time the toddler turns three and has been exposed to his or her parents' culture, his or her willingness to try new foods diminishes.

Answer to Social Studies Activity
Answers may vary.

Extension: After students have completed this activity, ask students to discuss the results of their interviews. Ask students if they found any similarities between their subjects' answers. Ask students if they found any differences.

96 Chapter 5 • Nutrition and Your Health

Food and Feelings

Most people know when their bodies need nutrients because they get hungry. Feeling hungry is the way your body tells you that it needs more food for energy. Sometimes, people eat even though they are not hungry.

Often, people's feelings can affect how and what they choose to eat. Some people may eat when they are sad or upset. Others may eat when they are happy or want to celebrate. Some people may skip meals if they are nervous. Others may like to eat when they are nervous. Many people like to eat when they are with friends in a social setting. Have you ever gone to a party and eaten snacks even though you had already eaten dinner?

If a person's feelings affect his or her food choices once in a while, it is not a bad thing. However, some people's feelings may affect their food choices all the time. This behavior can be unhealthy because a person may want to eat every time he or she has a particular emotion. Also, the person may choose to eat foods that are unhealthy. By understanding what feelings affect your food choices, you can avoid eating unhealthy foods. You can also avoid eating when you know you are not hungry.

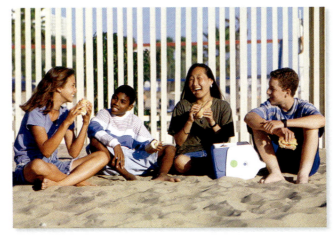

Figure 4 How do your feelings affect what you eat?

Health Journal
Write down everything you eat and drink for one day. Next to each entry, describe how you are feeling when you eat. The next day, take a look at your list. Do you eat only when you are hungry?

Lesson Review

Using Vocabulary
1. Use each of the following terms in a separate sentence: *nutrient*, *diet*, and *digestion*.

Understanding Concepts
2. List six factors that influence your food choices.
3. Explain how your nutrition affects your overall health.
4. How does your body use the food you eat?

Critical Thinking
5. **Making Good Decisions** Your best friend eats large servings of ice cream when she is upset. Lately, she has been eating a big bowl of ice cream every day. You know this behavior may be unhealthy for her. Should you say something to her? If so, what would you tell her?

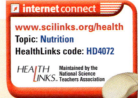

internet connect
www.scilinks.org/health
Topic: Nutrition
HealthLinks code: HD4072
HEALTH LINKS. Maintained by the National Science Teachers Association

Lesson 2

Focus

Overview
Before beginning this lesson, review with your students the objectives listed under the What You'll Do head in the Student Edition. In this lesson, students will learn about the six essential nutrients, how the body uses each nutrient, and which foods are good sources of each nutrient.

Bellringer
On the board, write the names of each of the six essential nutrients. Then, ask students to make a list of foods that they think are good sources of each nutrient. After students complete their lists, collect the lists. Use students' lists to address any misconceptions. **LS Visual** **English Language Learners**

Answer to Start Off Write
Accept all reasonable answers. Sample answer: Vitamins are organic compounds that control many body functions, while minerals are elements that are essential to several body functions.

Motivate

Discussion — GENERAL
Tell students to describe a well-balanced breakfast. (Answers may vary but should describe a breakfast that has a variety of nutrients.) Then, ask volunteers to recall what they ate for breakfast. Have students discuss how balanced their breakfasts were. (Answers may vary.) Then, ask students to explain why breakfast is so important. (Sample answer: It is important to eat a healthful breakfast so that your body has enough energy until lunchtime.) **LS Interpersonal**

Lesson 2 — The Six Essential Nutrients

What You'll Do
- **List** the six essential nutrients.
- **Explain** what each essential nutrient does for your body.
- **Identify** foods that are good sources of the essential nutrients.

Terms to Learn
- carbohydrate
- fat
- protein
- vitamin
- mineral

Start Off Write
What is the difference between vitamins and minerals?

The nutrients in food help your body function properly. But what are these nutrients, and where do you get them? Read on to find out!

The Nutrients You Need

Your body can make some of the nutrients it needs. However, most of the nutrients your body needs come from the food you eat. The nutrients that you get from food are called the *essential nutrients*. The six classes of essential nutrients are carbohydrates (KAHR boh HIE drayts), fats, proteins (PROH TEENZ), vitamins (VIET uh minz), minerals (MIN uhr uhlz), and water. Each of these nutrients plays a special role in your body. Your body uses carbohydrates, fats, and proteins as direct sources of energy. Vitamins and minerals control many body functions. They also help your body use the energy from the other nutrients. Your body uses water to control your body temperature. Water is also used to transport other nutrients throughout your body. The essential nutrients are necessary for your body to function properly. So, eating a variety of foods that contain these nutrients is very important.

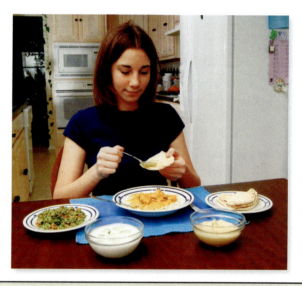

Figure 5 Every food contains different nutrients. It's important to eat a variety of foods so that you get all the nutrients that you need.

SOCIAL STUDIES CONNECTION
The Western World Inform students that some Americans and Western Europeans suffer nutritional problems stemming from improper diets. For example, people in developed countries, on average, consume about 20 times more salt than their bodies need. Such excess salt has been correlated to high blood pressure.

Chapter Resource File
- Directed Reading **BASIC**
- Lesson Plan
- Datasheets for In-Text Activities **GENERAL**
- Lesson Quiz **GENERAL**

 Transparencies

TT Bellringer

Carbohydrates

Carbohydrates provide energy for your body. A **carbohydrate** is a chemical composed of one or more simple sugars. Carbohydrates can be sugars or starches. Sugars are found in foods such as fruit, honey, table sugar, candy, and desserts. Starches are found in foods such as rice, pasta, and bread. Starches are carbohydrates that are made up of many simple sugars. If you put a piece of spaghetti in your mouth and keep it there for a while, substances in your saliva will break down the starches into sugars. The pasta will taste sweet. All sugars are eventually broken down to give you energy.

Fats

Believe it or not, it's important to have a small amount of fat in your diet. **Fats** are nutrients that store energy and store some vitamins. Fats also help your body produce hormones. Fats can be found in solid or liquid form. Solid fats are found in foods such as butter and margarine. Liquid fats are found in cooking oils and salad dressings. Fats are also found in meats such as steak, pork, or chicken. Fats make some foods taste and smell good. Fried foods and desserts taste good in part because they contain a large amount of fat. Fats contain more Calories than any other nutrient does. If you eat too many foods that are high in fat, you may eat more Calories than you need. In these cases, the unused Calories will be stored as fat in your body. Your body needs only a small amount of fat to function properly. When there is too much fat in your body, it can block the flow of blood to your heart. This blockage may lead to a heart attack when you are older.

Proteins

You can think of proteins as building blocks for your body. **Proteins** are nutrients that supply the body with energy for building, maintaining, and repairing tissues and cells. Proteins help the body break down and use nutrients for energy. Proteins also help protect the body from germs that cause sickness. Meat, poultry, and fish are good sources of proteins. Milk and cheese are also good sources of protiens. You can also get proteins from beans, nuts, tofu, eggs, whole grains, and vegetables.

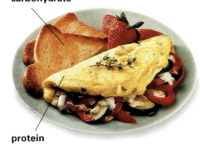

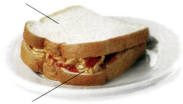

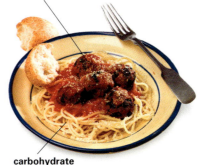

Figure 6 Most foods contain more than one nutrient, but they are often a good source of only one nutrient.

Teach

READING SKILL BUILDER — BASIC

Reading Hint To help students organize the information they will learn from reading this lesson, have them prepare a table with the headings *Carbohydrates, Proteins, Fats, Vitamins,* and *Minerals*. Down the left side, have them write *Functions in the human body, Food sources,* and *Additional comments*. Have students complete the table as they read this section. **LS Verbal/ Logical**

Group Activity — GENERAL

Types of Nutrients Organize the class into small groups. Assign each group one of the following nutrients: carbohydrates, fats, and proteins. Ask each group to design a poster that illustrates important points about the specific nutrient. Have students give a brief presentation to the class and then display all posters around the classroom. **LS Visual**

MISCONCEPTION ALERT

Many students may think that breads contain only carbohydrates, meats contain only proteins, and butter contains only fat. Explain to students that most foods contain two or more essential nutrients. For example, 2 tablespoons of peanut butter contain 16 g of fat, 6 g of carbohydrates, and 7 g of protein.

Attention Grabber

Stomach Growling Students may be interested to know why their stomachs growl when they are hungry. A lack of nutrients in the bloodstream causes a message to be sent to the brain. This message stimulates the stomach and the intestines. The stimulation of the stomach and the intestine causes the sound that is also known as "stomach growling."

Lesson 2 • The Six Essential Nutrients

Teach, continued

Hands-on ACTIVITY

Answers
1. Answers may vary.
2. Answers may vary. Students should find that the foods containing higher amounts of fat left behind the most oil. To avoid misconceptions, tell students to be careful not to mistake water stains from fruits or vegetables with oil.

Group Activity — ADVANCED

Vitamin Supplements Bring a bottle of vitamin supplements to class, and pass it around the classroom. As students pass around the bottle, have them identify vitamins that are not listed in the text. List these additional vitamins on the chalkboard. Have interested groups of students research the vitamins to determine their function, sources, and deficiency information. The groups can share the new information with the class by giving a brief oral report. **LS** Verbal

Activity — GENERAL

Writing **Mineral Deficiencies** Have students research and write a report about the physical effects of mineral deficiencies for at least three minerals. Give students the following examples to help get them started: A deficiency of calcium in later life can lead to osteoporosis. A lack of iodine can cause goiter. An iron deficiency can result in anemia. Phosphorus is needed for bone growth. And both potassium and sodium play key roles in nerve-impulse conduction. **LS** Verbal

Hands-on ACTIVITY

BROWN BAG TEST

1. Cut a brown paper bag into small squares.
2. Gather a variety of foods, such as cookies, fruit, chips, chocolate, and popcorn. Place a piece of each type of food on a different square.
3. Leave the food on the squares overnight.

Analysis
1. Remove each piece of food from its square. How much oil did each food leave behind?
2. Which foods had the most oil? Which foods had the least?

Vitamins and Minerals

Although you need only small amounts of vitamins and minerals, they are very important to your health. **Vitamins** are organic compounds that control many body functions. **Minerals** are elements that are essential for good health. Vitamins and minerals are found in fresh fruits, vegetables, nuts, and dairy products. The figure below shows you foods that are good sources of some vitamins and minerals.

Without vitamins and minerals, your body would not function properly. For example, a lack of vitamin C can cause scurvy, a gum disease. Without vitamin A, you may develop night blindness. You also need minerals for healthy growth. Calcium, phosphorus (FAHS fuh ruhs), iron, sodium, potassium, and zinc are just a few of the minerals that your body needs. You need calcium and phosphorus to build strong bones. Sodium and potassium help regulate blood pressure. Iron is necessary for your blood to deliver oxygen to your cells. To avoid health problems, you should eat plenty of fresh fruits and vegetables every day.

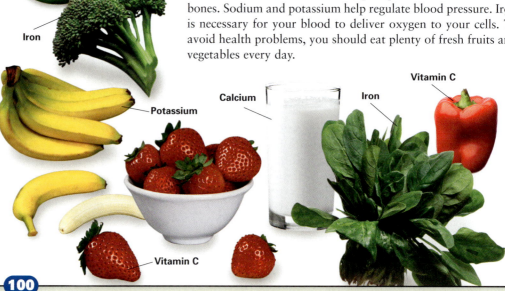

Figure 7 Fruits and vegetables are great sources of vitamins and minerals.

Background

How Vitamins Work Vitamins are important because they enable enzymes to function. Enzymes perform their functions by binding with other body chemicals and either combining the chemicals or breaking the chemicals down. In order for this to happen, vitamins bind to these enzymes. After the vitamins bind to the enzymes, they activate the enzymes by changing the enzymes' shape so that the enzymes bind properly to the chemicals. Without vitamins, many enzymes could not do their jobs.

SOCIAL STUDIES CONNECTION

Scurvy A lack of vitamin C in the diet is the main cause of the deficiency disorder called *scurvy*. Some symptoms of scurvy include bleeding gums, tooth loss, swelling of the face, and sunken eyes. Scurvy was a serious problem in the past, especially for sailors, who did not have access to fresh fruit. Once Dr. James Lind discovered that scurvy could be treated with vitamin C, the British navy began to distribute large amounts of lime juice to British sailors. British sailors were soon referred to as "limeys."

Chapter 5 • Nutrition and Your Health

Water

Water is a very important nutrient. Your body does not get energy from water, but water is needed for most of your body functions. A person can live for several weeks without food. However, without water, the person will die within a few days. The reason is that your body uses water to transport food and nutrients. Water is used to fill the cells and the spaces between the cells in your body. Your body uses water to fill spaces in your joints, and water in your spine is used to absorb shock. Your body uses water to keep your mouth and eyes moist. Your body also uses water to wash away the waste products that your body produces.

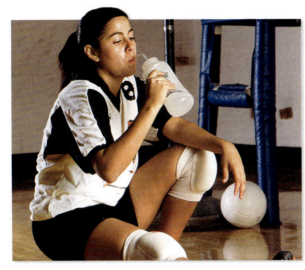

Figure 8 Drinking water is important, especially while you are being physically active.

Water regulates your body temperature. When your body gets too hot, you sweat. As the water evaporates, you feel cooler and your body temperature returns to normal. This keeps you from overheating. If you don't drink enough water each day, you may *dehydrate*, or dry out. If you become dehydrated, your body will not function properly. As a result, you may faint. In extreme cases, you may die. You must drink plenty of water so that you don't dry out.

Drinking water is the best way to replace lost water. But you can get water from other food and drinks. Good sources of water are fruit juices, fruits, vegetables, soups, stews, and milk. A good rule of thumb is to drink 8 to 10 glasses of water every day. If you play sports, you should drink even more.

Lesson Review

Using Vocabulary

1. What are carbohydrates?
2. What are vitamins?

Understanding Concepts

3. List the six essential nutrients. What does each nutrient do for your body?
4. List three foods that are good sources of protein.

Critical Thinking

5. **Analyzing Processes** Your friend asks you to go ride bikes. It is a very hot day. What will happen if you don't drink enough water?

internet connect
www.scilinks.org/health
Topic: Nutrients
HealthLinks code: HD4071
HEALTH LINKS. Maintained by the National Science Teachers Association

---

Answers to the Lesson Review

1. Carbohydrates are chemical compounds that are composed of one or more simple sugars.
2. Vitamins are organic compounds that control many body functions.
3. Carbohydrates provide energy for the body. Fats store energy and some vitamins. Fats also help the body produce hormones. Proteins help the body build, repair, and maintain tissues. Vitamins help control several body functions. Minerals are needed to perform body functions, such as building strong bones. Water is used to transport nutrients throughout the body and is needed to regulate body temperature.
4. Accept all reasonable responses. Sample answers: chicken, steak, and nuts
5. Accept all reasonable responses. Sample answer: If I do not drink enough water, I may become dehydrated and I may feel sick.

ENVIRONMENTAL SCIENCE CONNECTION — ADVANCED

Water and Our World After students have read this page, ask them to think about the importance of clean drinking water. Have interested students do research on areas of the world that do not have clean, accessible drinking water. Ask students to find the answers to the following questions in their research:

- What types of diseases can people get from drinking unclean water? (Sample answer: dysentery and cholera)
- What areas of the world are suffering most from a lack of clean water? (developing nations such as India and China)
- What are some other problems that may be associated with a lack of clean water? (Answers may vary. Sample answer: Contaminated water may harm crops or animals. If crops and animals are harmed, humans may not have enough food to eat.)

Close

Reteaching — BASIC

Nutrients Bring pictures of different foods to class. Hold the pictures up and have students call out the nutrients that are found in each food. **LS** Visual — English Language Learners

Quiz — GENERAL

1. Name the essential nutrient that helps build muscle. (protein)
2. Name the essential nutrient that can be easily converted into sugars. (carbohydrate)
3. What essential nutrient is sodium? (mineral)

Alternative Assessment — GENERAL

Dinner Menu Have students create a dinner menu that contains as many essential nutrients as possible. Students should write out their menu and list all the nutrients found in each type of food they choose to serve. **LS** Logical

Lesson 2 • The Six Essential Nutrients

Lesson 3

Focus

Overview
Before beginning this lesson, review with your students the objectives listed under the What You'll Do head in the Student Edition. In this lesson, students will learn about the Dietary Guidelines for Americans, how to use the Food Guide Pyramid, and how to read a Nutrition Facts label on food packaging.

Bellringer
Ask students to imagine that they found themselves on a deserted desert island and could choose only three different foods to have with them. Tell students to write down what three foods they would choose and why. (Sample answer: I would choose nuts, oranges, and bread so that I would be able to get fat and protein from the nuts, vitamins and simple carbohydrates from the orange, and complex carbohydrates from the bread.) **LS Logical**

Answer to Start Off Write
Accept all reasonable answers. Sample answer: In order to get the nutrients you need to stay healthy, you must eat a balanced diet.

Motivate

Group Activity — GENERAL
Poster Project Organize the class into three groups. Assign each group one of the three dietary guidelines described in the table on this page. The group should work together to make a poster illustrating their assigned dietary guideline. Display the completed posters in the classroom. **LS Visual** **Co-op Learning**

Lesson 3 — Balancing Your Diet

You know that your body needs the nutrients in food to stay healthy. However, you may not know which foods to eat or how much of them to eat to get all the nutrients you need.

What You'll Do
- **Describe** the Dietary Guidelines for Americans.
- **Describe** how to use the Food Guide Pyramid.
- **Explain** how to read a Nutrition Facts label.
- **Explain** the difference between a serving and a portion.

Terms to Learn
- Dietary Guidelines for Americans
- Food Guide Pyramid
- Nutrition Facts label

Start Off Write
Why is eating a balanced diet important?

Fortunately, there are many tools you can use to help you make healthy food choices. These tools include the Dietary Guidelines for Americans, the Food Guide Pyramid, and the Nutrition Facts label.

The Dietary Guidelines for Americans
A healthy lifestyle involves many steps. These steps include eating a healthful diet and staying physically active every day. The <mark>Dietary Guidelines for Americans</mark> are a set of suggestions to help you develop a healthy lifestyle. These guidelines were developed by the U.S. Department of Agriculture and the U.S. Department of Health and Human Services. Following the dietary guidelines will help you develop healthy eating habits. Having healthy eating habits can help you get enough nutrients every day.

You can think of the dietary guidelines as the ABCs for good health. The ABCs are **a**im for fitness, **b**uild a healthy base, and **c**hoose sensibly. The table below provides more information about these guidelines.

TABLE 1 The Dietary Guidelines for Americans

Aim for fitness	Aim to stay at a healthy weight by being physically active every day.
Build a healthy base	Choose healthy foods by using the Food Guide Pyramid. Eat plenty of fresh fruits and vegetables.
	Keep foods safe to eat by cooking your food fully. Store foods properly by keeping cold foods cold and refrigerating hot foods soon after you are finished with them.
Choose sensibly	Choose foods that are low in salt, sugar, and fat.

Background
Adolescents and Nutrition When children reach adolescence, their dietary guidelines change. Energy needs vary depending on growth rate, body composition, and activity level. For example, an adolescent's increased growth rate increases the adolescent's caloric needs. In general, boys have a larger proportion of lean body mass to fat and require more Calories than girls do.

Chapter Resource File
- Directed Reading **BASIC**
- Lesson Plan
- Lesson Quiz **GENERAL**

Transparencies
- TT Bellringer
- TT The Food Guide Pyramid
- TT The Nutrition Facts Label

102   Chapter 5 • Nutrition and Your Health

The Food Guide Pyramid

To build a healthy diet, you must be able to choose foods that give you the proper nutrients. The Food Guide Pyramid is a tool that shows you which foods to eat and how much of each type of food you should eat every day. The pyramid is made up of food groups. A food group is made up of foods that contain similar nutrients. Each food group has its own block, and each block is a different size. A bigger block means you should eat more food from that food group. The number of servings for each group tells you how much food from each food group you should eat daily.

The bread group has the largest block. So, you need more foods from the bread group in your daily diet than you need from any other group. The exact amount you should eat depends on your age and weight. But the Food Guide Pyramid suggests you should eat 6 to 11 servings of bread each day.

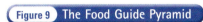

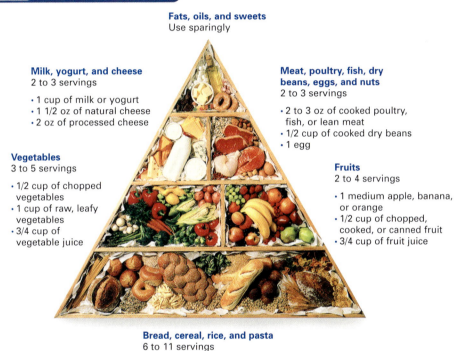

Figure 9 The Food Guide Pyramid

Fats, oils, and sweets
Use sparingly

Milk, yogurt, and cheese
2 to 3 servings
- 1 cup of milk or yogurt
- 1 1/2 oz of natural cheese
- 2 oz of processed cheese

Meat, poultry, fish, dry beans, eggs, and nuts
2 to 3 servings
- 2 to 3 oz of cooked poultry, fish, or lean meat
- 1/2 cup of cooked dry beans
- 1 egg

Vegetables
3 to 5 servings
- 1/2 cup of chopped vegetables
- 1 cup of raw, leafy vegetables
- 3/4 cup of vegetable juice

Fruits
2 to 4 servings
- 1 medium apple, banana, or orange
- 1/2 cup of chopped, cooked, or canned fruit
- 3/4 cup of fruit juice

Bread, cereal, rice, and pasta
6 to 11 servings
- 1 slice of bread
- 1 oz of ready-to-eat cereal
- 1/2 cup of rice or pasta
- 1/2 cup of cooked cereal

Background

The Food Guide Pyramid The serving sizes recommended by the Food Guide Pyramid are listed as ranges. The number of servings for each food group a person should eat daily varies with the age and sex of the person. For example, teen girls should eat about nine servings of the bread group, four servings of vegetables, three servings of fruit, two or three servings of the milk group, and two servings of the meat group. Teen boys should eat about eleven servings of the bread group, five servings of vegetables, four servings of fruit, two or three servings from the milk group, and three servings of the meat group.

Teach

Using the Figure — BASIC

Have students identify each of the foods shown in the Food Guide Pyramid as a carbohydrate, protein, or fat. Be sure they recognize that the base of the pyramid consists of foods that are complex carbohydrates, while those towards the top are simple carbohydrates and fats.
LS Visual

Life SKILL BUILDER — GENERAL

Assessing Your Health Have students keep track of all the food they eat in a day. Have them determine how many servings from each of the food groups they consume. Then, have them determine the percentage of recommended servings these numbers represent. For example, two glasses of milk and a grilled cheese sandwich represents 100 percent of the recommended dairy servings. One medium apple is 25 percent of the recommended fruit servings. Encourage students to identify how they could change their diet to make it more healthful.
LS Logical

INCLUSION Strategies — ADVANCED

- **Gifted and Talented**

Ask students to compare portion sizes of foods served in local restaurants to the serving sizes listed on the Food Guide Pyramid. Have students create a table with two columns. The first column should list the foods they wish to compare. The second column should list the number of servings that each food provides. For example, a 1/2 pound burger with lettuce, onions, tomatoes, and a large side of fries provides 3 servings of meat, 2 servings of bread, 1 serving of vegetables, and so forth.

Lesson 3 • Balancing Your Diet

Teach, continued

Life SKILL BUILDER — ADVANCED

Practicing Wellness Have students bring empty packaging of different snack foods and drinks to class. Have students list five of their favorite snack foods and then record the following information from the nutrition labels: the serving size, number of Calories per serving, number of fat grams per serving, and the amount of carbohydrates and proteins per serving. Then, have students construct a comparison table to illustrate their findings. Afterwards, have students write a paragraph detailing how many snack Calories they typically consume in a day and if they are going to reconsider their snack choices. **LS Logical**

Debate — GENERAL

Vegetarians Tell the class that many people around the world choose to be vegetarians. Vegetarians do not eat meat products. Some of the students may themselves be vegetarians. If so, give students who are vegetarians the opportunity to voice the reasons why they have chosen this lifestyle. Then, have the students research the benefits and disadvantages of both eating meat products and not eating meat products. When the students have completed their research, organize the class into two groups. Have the groups debate whether a vegetarian lifestyle is healthier than an omnivore lifestyle. **LS Verbal/Intrapersonal**

Brain Food

Many teens in the United States do not get enough calcium or iron in their daily diet. They also do not get enough of vitamins A and C. Drinking milk and eating leafy green vegetables and fresh fruit will help you get these nutrients.

The Nutrition Facts Label

A useful tool for finding out what nutrients are in a food is the Nutrition Facts label. The **Nutrition Facts label** is a label found on the outside packages of food and states the number of servings in the container, the number of Calories in each serving, and the amount of nutrients in each serving. The Daily Values section states what amount of your daily nutrient need is in one serving of the food. For example, the chicken soup below has 15 percent of your daily need of vitamin A. You can tell whether a food is high or low in a nutrient by looking at its daily value. A daily value of 5 percent or less means that the food is low in that nutrient. A daily value of 20 percent or more means that the food is high in that nutrient. The label also gives you a list of the ingredients for that food.

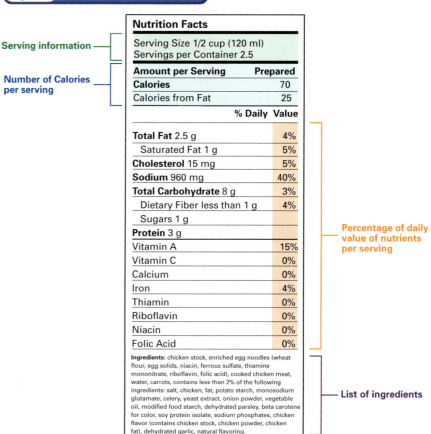

Figure 10 The Nutrition Facts Label

Cultural Awareness

High-Fat Diet In Japan, the incidence of breast cancer is very low. After moving to the United States, however, Japanese women develop the disease nearly as often as American women do. Scientists attribute this to cultural dietary differences. They think that the high-fat diet of many Americans plays a pivotal role in the development of breast cancer.

What Is a Serving Size?

A *serving size* is the amount of food that is considered a healthy amount for an average person. The Food Guide Pyramid and the Nutrition Facts label tell you how much food makes up one serving. For example, 1 cup of milk is one serving of the milk group on the Food Guide Pyramid. One medium apple or 1 cup of orange juice is equal to one serving of the fruit group. A typical serving size of canned soup is 1 cup. A serving size stays the same, but the number of servings that you eat depends on you.

What Is a Portion?

A *portion* of food is the amount of food you want to eat. Often, a portion is not the same as a serving. For example, imagine you are going to eat a can of soup. The Nutrition Facts label states that the can of soup contains two servings. If you eat the whole can of soup, you would be eating two servings. Our portion sizes depend on how much we want to eat. It is important to note that most restaurants provide portions that are larger than one serving. For instance, in some restaurants, one hamburger (or one portion) could equal three servings in the meat group. Be sure to use the Food Guide Pyramid and the Nutrition Facts label to know how many servings of foods from each food group you need. Then, you can choose your portions wisely.

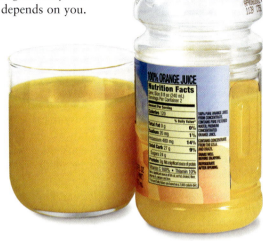

Figure 11 The glass you see here contains a serving of juice. How does that amount compare with the amount in the bottle?

Lesson Review

Using Vocabulary

1. What are the Dietary Guidelines for Americans?
2. What is the Food Guide Pyramid?

Understanding Concepts

3. Use the Food Guide Pyramid to create a menu for 1 day. Be creative by choosing foods that are not shown on the pyramid.

Critical Thinking

4. **Analyzing Ideas** Describe how you would use the Nutrition Facts label to eat foods that are low in fat.
5. **Making Inferences** Suppose you are keeping track of how many Calories you eat. Why is it important to pay attention to the serving size of each food you eat?

internet connect
www.scilinks.org/health
Topic: Food Pyramids
HealthLinks code: HD4043
HEALTH LINKS — Maintained by the National Science Teachers Association

Answers to Lesson Review

1. a set of dietary suggestions to help you develop a healthy lifestyle
2. a tool that shows you which types of foods to eat and how much of these different types of food to eat
3. Answers may vary. Answers should include serving sizes and a variety of food from each group.
4. Sample answer: I could use the Nutrition Facts label to find foods with a low percent daily value of fat.
5. Sample answer: The more you eat of a food, the more Calories you are eating. If one serving of the food has 100 Calories, then 2 servings would have 200 Calories. So, it is important to keep track of the servings you eat in order to count your Calorie intake accurately.

Activity — GENERAL

Fast Foods Obtain a list from a fast-food establishment that describes the nutritional content of its various food products. Have students describe a typical meal at this restaurant. Then, have them compare the nutritional content of this meal with the serving sizes provided on the Food Guide Pyramid. Remind students to look at the difference between a regular meal and a super-sized meal.
LS Logical

Close

Reteaching — BASIC

Pyramid Poem Have students write a poem or a song that will help them remember how many daily servings they need of each food group and what types of food belong in each food group.
LS Auditory

Quiz — GENERAL

1. Name three different food groups. (Sample answer: Fruit; Bread, cereal, rice, and pasta; and Meat, poultry, fish, dry beans, eggs, and nuts)
2. What is a serving size? (The amount of food that is considered a healthy amount for an average person.)
3. How many servings of vegetables does the Food Guide Pyramid recommend that you eat every day? (3–5 servings)

Lesson 4 Focus

Overview
Before beginning this lesson, review with your students the objectives listed under the What You'll Do head in the Student Edition. In this lesson, students will learn why eating breakfast is important, how to choose healthy foods, and how to maintain a healthy diet.

 Bellringer
Write the following snack choices on the board and have students choose which snack is the healthiest:

1. a. candy bar
   b. apple
2. a. a piece of toast with cream cheese
   b. potato chips
3. a. slice of pizza
   b. cup of yogurt
4. a. bowl of pasta
   b. bowl of ice cream

(1. b, 2. a, 3. b, 4. a)

Answer to Start Off Write
Accept all reasonable answers. Sample answer: Eating breakfast will help you concentrate better in school because you will be less likely to feel hungry and irritable, which can be distracting.

Motivate

Group Activity — GENERAL
Snacking Skit Organize the class into groups. Have each group choose a healthy snack food. Then, the group should write a 30-second commercial that makes the food sound as appealing as possible. **LS Kinesthetic**

Lesson 4: Building Healthful Eating Habits

What You'll Do
- **Explain** why eating a healthy breakfast is important.
- **Describe** three strategies for making healthy snack choices.
- **List** seven ways to eat healthily at a fast-food restaurant.
- **List** six ways to eat healthily at home.

Write How does eating breakfast affect your ability to concentrate in class?

Every morning, Jimmy's dad makes Jimmy eat breakfast. But Jimmy isn't always hungry in the morning. Why do you think his dad wants him to eat breakfast?

Breakfast is a very important meal because it gives you the energy you need to start the day.

Eating a Healthy Breakfast
Many teens skip breakfast in the morning. Often, they are too busy to eat, or they do not feel hungry. However, skipping breakfast may affect a person in many ways. First, most people who don't eat breakfast become hungry, irritated, or light-headed by the middle of the morning. They may have trouble concentrating, especially in class. Eating a healthy breakfast usually prevents you from feeling this way. In the morning, your body has been without food all night and needs nutrients from food. The nutrients you get from breakfast will be used for energy at different times. So, if you eat breakfast, you will continue to have energy over a length of time. If you can't eat breakfast in the morning, be sure to bring a healthy, mid-morning snack to school. The figure below shows some ideas for a healthy breakfast.

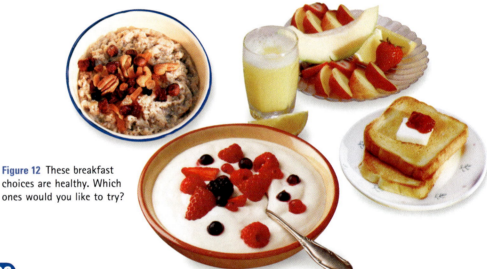
Figure 12 These breakfast choices are healthy. Which ones would you like to try?

 BIOLOGY CONNECTION

Blood Sugar Usually, a person's blood sugar level is lowest in the morning before he or she eats breakfast. After breakfast is eaten, the food is digested and absorbed into the blood. When the blood sugar level is raised to the normal daytime level, the pancreas releases insulin into the bloodstream. Insulin signals the liver to store any extra blood sugar until it is needed later.

Chapter Resource File
- Directed Reading **BASIC**
- Lesson Plan
- Lesson Quiz **GENERAL**

Transparencies
TT Bellringer

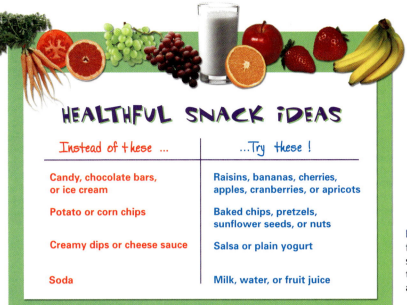

Figure 13 Many snack foods are high in fat, sugar, or salt. Try these snack ideas for a healthy treat.

Snacking Well

Snacks are the foods you eat between meals. Believe it or not, eating snacks is not a bad thing! In fact, eating a snack is a good idea because doing so keeps you from being too hungry at mealtimes. If you are too hungry, you may eat more food than you need. However, the type of snack you choose is important. Unfortunately, many snack foods, such as cookies and chips, are high in fat, sugar, and salt. Also, eating too many snacks may cause you to be full at mealtimes. If you feel full, you may not feel like eating lunch or dinner.

Choosing snacks that are good for you is easy. First, choose to eat sugary or salty snacks only once in a while. These snacks include candy bars, chocolate, hard candies, and chips. Second, choose foods that are low in fat. For example, choose to eat fresh fruit, crackers, yogurt, or vegetables. Bring a snack with you if you know you will be away from home. Bringing a snack from home will keep you from buying a snack from the vending machine. Third, choose healthful snack foods that you will enjoy. You will be more likely to eat healthfully if you are eating something you like! Take a look at the figure above for some healthy snack ideas.

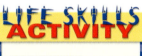

PRACTICING WELLNESS

Try making this great trail mix for a healthy snack!

The ingredients include 1 cup unsalted, shelled nuts, 1 cup sunflower seeds, 1 cup raisins, 1/2 cup dried apricots. Mix all the ingredients together in a large bowl. Store the trail mix in an airtight container, and enjoy!

Practicing Wellness Give students these quick snack hints to encourage them to develop healthy snacking habits:

- Include two to three small snacks during the day to keep your energy level up.
- A glass of fruit or vegetable juice is a great healthy, quick snack.
- Eat snacks full of grains. They have a lot of complex carbohydrates that will keep you energized for longer. Graham crackers, rice cakes, and pretzels are all examples of this type of snack.

INCLUSION Strategies — ADVANCED

- **Behavior Control Issues**

Organize the class into small groups. Make sure each group has only one student with behavior control issues. Ask each group to offer healthy snack suggestions to include in a 16-slot school snack machine (no refrigeration or freezing). Using a spreadsheet program, create a sixteen-row chart. Make one column for each group. Ask students with behavior control issues to add their groups' ideas to the chart. Print out copies and offer your "healthy-vending-machine ideas" to the school administration.

Teach

Activity — GENERAL

Show Your Snack Tell students to bring one of their favorite healthy snacks to class. Each student should do a "show-and-tell" style presentation with their snack, describing the nutritional contents of the snack and why they like it. **LS** Verbal/Visual

Life SKILL BUILDER — ADVANCED

Writing **Evaluating Media Messages** Have students imagine that they are making a concerted effort to improve their eating habits. Then, ask students to watch an hour of TV. They should take notes on what they see. Have students consider the following questions:

- What food products were advertised or discussed?
- In what light was the food displayed in the commercials and shows?
- Was the majority of the food shown healthy or high in fat and/or sugar?

After students finish watching the hour of TV, they should write a report discussing their observations. They should also hypothesize on the psychological effects of watching TV on a person who is trying to maintain a healthy diet. Students can include graphs, tables, and charts in their reports to illustrate the food-related content of the sample hour of TV. **LS** Interpersonal

Teach, continued

Activity — GENERAL
Diet Critique Have students check out a popular diet book from the library. Have them evaluate the diet in terms of its ability to meet the nutrient and energy needs of the body, and encourage them to identify any necessary changes, if any, to make the diet healthful. Have them prepare short reports, and allow them to share their findings with the class. **LS Verbal**

Group Activity — GENERAL
Health Food Directory Tell each student to bring in a list of two or more local restaurants, cafeterias, or cafes that serve healthy foods. They should include in their list some of the healthy entrees served at each restaurant. Use the lists to help students create a local health food directory. When the directory is completed, give each student a copy that they can keep with them when dining out on the town. **Co-op Learning**

Discussion — ADVANCED
Super-Sized? Ask students to think about the benefits and consequences of buying the larger, value-sized meals, or combination meals at fast-food restaurants. (A benefit of ordering a larger portion or a combination meal may be the savings in cost. A consequence may be that a person will consume more Calories, more fat, and more salt than if they had ordered the normal portion.) Then, ask students how they think larger portions and combination meals have affected our society. To prompt more discussion, ask students if they can think of any health trends that are related to the popularity of fast-food restaurants.

LIFE SKILLS ACTIVITY
MAKING GOOD DECISIONS

You and your friends decide to eat dinner at Charlie's Take-Out in the mall. The menu at this restaurant is shown at right. Next to each item, you will find how many grams of carbohydrates (C), protein (P), and fat (F) are found in each food. Based on what you have learned, choose a healthy meal from the menu.

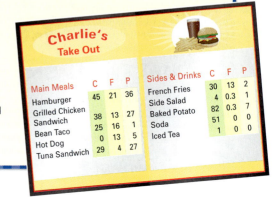

Charlie's Take Out

Main Meals	C	F	P
Hamburger	45	21	36
Grilled Chicken Sandwich	38	13	27
Bean Taco	25	16	1
Hot Dog	0	13	5
Tuna Sandwich	29	4	27

Sides & Drinks	C	F	P
French Fries	30	13	2
Side Salad	4	0.3	1
Baked Potato	82	0.3	7
Soda	51	0	0
Iced Tea	1	0	0

Eating Out

Eating out is a normal part of most people's lives. Many teens choose to eat at fast-food restaurants. It is OK to eat fast-food meals once in a while. But if you eat fast-food meals more than once a week, you may be eating more fat and salt than you need.

If you must eat at fast-food restaurants, choose healthful meals. Many restaurants offer salads or grilled meals. Grilling is a method of cooking that is usually low in fat. If low-fat choices are not available, you can choose not to eat the entire portion.

There are several ways to make your fast-food meal healthier. For example, when you use dressing, ask for one that is low in fat. You can use mustard or ketchup instead of mayonnaise. You should try to avoid using mayonnaise because it is high in fat. Also, you can avoid the extra foods that come with your meal, such as bacon or extra cheese on a hamburger. Try eating salsa instead of cheese sauce. Finally, you can order water with your meal instead of ordering a soda.

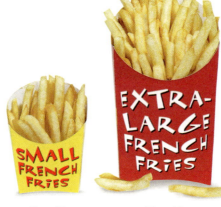

Figure 14 Many fast-food restaurants offer extra-large portions of their meals. These portions are usually very high in fat.

SMALL FRENCH FRIES — 10 g of fat
EXTRA-LARGE FRENCH FRIES — 29 g of fat

LIFE SKILLS ACTIVITY
Answer
Answers may vary. Sample answer: My healthy meal includes a tuna sandwich, a baked potato, and an iced tea.

SOCIAL STUDIES CONNECTION
Ancient Fast Food Fast-food restaurants are not a modern invention. Archaeologists excavating Pompeii found small fast-food and take-out restaurants along many of the city-center streets. The food at these restaurants had been preserved as stone, so the archaeologists were able to identify the soup de jour, so to speak. At one restaurant, the menu included bread with fish paste, vegetable stew, and goose drumsticks.

Eating at Home

Eating healthy meals at home can be fun and easy. Encourage whoever prepares meals at home to make healthy choices by using the Food Guide Pyramid and the Dietary Guidelines for Americans. If you prepare a meal for yourself, you can follow these suggestions, too. Choose whole-wheat bread for a sandwich. Use a tomato sauce on pasta rather than a creamy sauce. Be sure to have plenty of vegetables with your meals. You can easily prepare a salad with lettuce, tomatoes, carrots, and other fresh vegetables that you like. If you like eggs, choose to eat an omelet or scrambled eggs instead of fried eggs. You can also try jam on breads and bagels instead of butter. Finally, try drinking water, milk, or juice instead of soda.

Health Journal
For 1 day, write down everything that you eat. Then, on a second day, plan what you are going to eat on that day. Follow your plan. Compare what you ate when you didn't plan and what you ate when you did plan. Which day did you eat more healthful foods?

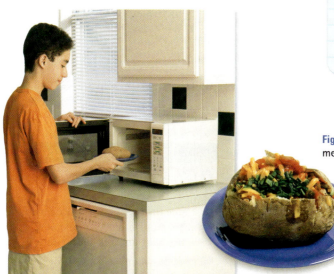

Figure 15 Eating a healthy meal at home can be easy!

Lesson Review

Understanding Concepts
1. Explain why eating a healthful breakfast is important.
2. List three ways to make healthy snack choices.
3. Describe eight ways to make healthy choices at a fast-food restaurant.
4. List six strategies for eating healthily at home.

Critical Thinking
5. Imagine that you have to stay after school for soccer practice. What can you do to make sure that you have a healthy snack before practice?

Answer to Health Journal
Accept all reasonable answers. This Health Journal may be a good way to close the lesson.

Close

Reteaching — BASIC
Healthy Café Tell the class to imagine that they are going to open their own café. Explain to students that they want their café to serve only healthy food. Ask them what they think the café should offer for breakfast, lunch, snacks, and dinner. Write the students' suggestions on the board.

Quiz — GENERAL
Tell students to answer the following questions with "True" or "False."
1. French fries are a healthy snack. false
2. It is important to eat breakfast every morning. true
3. When you go out to eat, you should consider the serving sizes you eat. true
4. Snacking can be a healthy behavior. true

Alternative Assessment — GENERAL
Healthy Eating Brochure Have each student create a brochure about healthy eating habits. The brochure should be similar to one that might be found in a doctor's office. When students are finished with their brochures, have them look at each other's finished products. **LS** Visual

---

Answers to Lesson Review
1. It gives you energy for the rest of the day.
2. Choose snacks that are low in fat, eat sugary or salty snacks only once in a while, and bring a snack with you if you will be away from home.
3. Order a salad, choose a grilled meal, eat only part of the portion, use low-fat dressing, use ketchup instead of mayonnaise, avoid ordering extra foods, use salsa instead of cheese sauce, and order water instead of soda.
4. Eat tomato sauce with pasta instead of creamy sauce, choose whole-wheat bread for sandwiches, use jam instead of butter, eat plenty of vegetables, eat scrambled eggs instead of fried eggs, and drink water or milk instead of soda.
5. Sample answer: bring a healthy snack with me from home

5 CHAPTER REVIEW

Assignment Guide

Lesson	Review Questions
1	3, 7–8
2	2, 4–5, 9–11, 15
3	1, 6, 12, 16–17, 19, 21–27
4	13–14
1–4	18, 20

ANSWERS

Using Vocabulary

1. The Food Guide Pyramid shows me what types of foods I need to eat each day and how much of them to eat, while a Nutrition Facts label explains what nutrients are in a serving of food so that I can follow the Food Guide Pyramid more closely.
2. A carbohydrate is a chemical composed of sugars which is used for energy, and a protein is a nutrient used to build and repair tissues.
3. diet
4. proteins
5. fats
6. Food Guide Pyramid
7. digestion

Understanding Concepts

8. Sample answer: When feeling sad, stressed, excited, or any kind of emotion, we tend to crave certain foods.
9. Sample answer: water—fruit juice, carbohydrates—bread, protein—eggs, fat—butter, minerals—salt, vitamins—oranges
10. Water helps regulate body temperature, transport nutrients, and keep you from drying out.
11. carbohydrates, proteins, and fat
12. A serving is the recommended amount of a food that an average person eats and a portion is the amount of that food you actually eat.
13. Snacks can keep your energy levels up during the day.
14. Sample answer: cereal and fruit juice
15. 8 to 10 glasses

5 CHAPTER REVIEW

Chapter Summary

■ Nutrition is the study of how your body uses the food you eat to maintain your health. ■ Your diet is a pattern of eating that includes what you eat, how often you eat, and how much you eat. ■ The six essential nutrients are carbohydrates, fats, proteins, minerals, vitamins, and water. ■ The Dietary Guidelines for Americans, the Food Guide Pyramid, and the Nutrition Facts label are tools you can use to make healthy food choices. ■ Eating a healthy breakfast prevents you from feeling hungry, irritated, or lightheaded during the first half of the school day. ■ Eating a healthy snack between meals prevents you from eating too much at mealtimes. ■ Choosing foods low in fat and salt when you eat out will help you maintain a healthy diet. ■ Including plenty of fruits and vegetables in your meals at home will help you maintain a healthy diet.

Using Vocabulary

For each pair of terms, describe how the meanings of the terms differ.

1. Food Guide Pyramid/Nutrition Facts label
2. carbohydrate/protein

For each sentence, fill in the blank with the proper word from the word bank provided below.

nutrients digestion
diet carbohydrate
fats proteins
vitamin mineral
Dietary Guidelines for Americans Nutrition Facts label
 Food Guide Pyramid

3. A ___ is a pattern of eating.
4. Nutrients that supply the body with energy for building and repairing tissues are ___.
5. Nutrients that store energy and some vitamins are ___.
6. A tool that shows you which foods to eat and how much of each type of food you should eat every day is the ___.
7. The process in which food is broken down into a form your body can use is called ___.

Understanding Concepts

8. Explain how your feelings may affect your food choices.
9. Name the six essential nutrients. For each nutrient, give one example of a food in which that nutrient can be found.
10. Explain what water does for your body.
11. Which nutrients provide your body with energy?
12. What is the difference between a serving and a portion?
13. Why can eating a snack between meals be good for you?
14. What are some healthy breakfast choices?
15. How many glasses of water should you drink every day?

Chapter Resource File

- Concept Review GENERAL
- Concept Mapping GENERAL
- Performance-Based Assessment GENERAL
- Chapter Test GENERAL

Critical Thinking

Applying Concepts

16. Imagine that you are using the Food Guide Pyramid to plan a meal to eat before your volleyball game. From which food groups will you choose most of your foods?

17. Explain how you can use the Nutrition Facts label to choose a food that is high in calcium.

18. Given what you now know about eating healthfully, list two habits that you would like to change. Then, list two ways you could change your eating habits.

19. If 1 cup of milk is considered a serving, and you buy a gallon of milk, how many servings of milk do you have? According to the Food Guide Pyramid, how many days will the gallon of milk last you?

20. The cheeseburger you ate for lunch today contained 14 grams of fat, 35 grams of carbohydrate, and 12 grams of protein. If 1 gram of carbohydrate contains 4 Calories, 1 gram of fat contains 9 Calories, and 1 gram of protein contains 4 Calories, how many Calories did the cheeseburger contain?

Making Good Decisions

21. You are trying to decide what to eat for a snack. After looking around the kitchen, you find a bag of potato chips, a bagel, some strawberries, and a banana. Suppose that you have basketball practice in 1 hour. Which foods will you choose for your snack? Which foods will give you the most energy for basketball practice?

Interpreting Graphics

Nutrition Facts
Serving Size 1 cup (228 g)
Servings per Container 2

Amount per Serving
Calories 250

	% Daily Value
Total Fat 12 g	18%
Cholesterol 30 mg	15%
Sodium 470 mg	20%
Carbohydrates 31 g	10%
Protein 5 g	
Vitamin A	4%
Vitamin C	2%
Calcium	20%
Iron	4%

Use the Nutrition Facts label for Macaroni and Cheese above to answer questions 22–27.

22. How many Calories are in the entire box of macaroni and cheese?

23. Which vitamins and minerals are found in this box of macaroni and cheese?

24. Would a serving of macaroni and cheese from this package of be considered high in sodium or low in sodium?

25. Is this food high in calcium? Explain your answer.

26. How many total grams are in this box of macaroni and cheese?

27. Is this food high in iron? Explain your answer.

Reading Checkup

Take a minute to review your answers to the Health IQ questions at the beginning of this chapter. How has reading this chapter improved your Health IQ?

Critical Thinking

Applying Concepts

16. Sample answer: the bread group
17. Sample answer: choose a food that has a high percent daily value of calcium
18. Answers may vary.
19. I have 16 servings that will last about eight days.
20. (14 g × 9 Cal/g) + (35 g × 4 Cal/g) + (12 g × 4 Cal/g) = 314 Calories

Making Good Decisions

21. Sample answer: I'd choose the bagel and the banana to get the most long-term energy for basketball practice.

Interpreting Graphics

22. 500 Calories
23. vitamin A, vitamin C, calcium, and iron
24. high in sodium
25. Yes, it is high in calcium because it has a 20 percent daily value of calcium.
26. 456g
27. No, this food is not considered high in iron. This food has less than a 5 percent daily value of iron, so this food is considered low in iron.

Chapter 5 • Chapter Review

Model

Introduce this activity by reminding students that using this Life Skill will help them take personal responsibility for their behavior. Then, review the scenario with the class.

Prepare students for this activity by modeling each of the steps of the skill. Make sure students understand each step before you move on to the next one.

Guided Practice: Practice with a Friend

Guided Practice is the stage in which you and the students analyze their approach to solving the problem given in the scenario and analyze their decision-making skills. Have students read Act 1. Discuss with the class the situation described and the way students are to act it out. Organize the class into groups of three. In each group, one person plays the role of Simon, another person plays Tabitha, and the third person is the observer.

Proper pacing during the Guided Practice is important. The suggestions listed below will help you control the pace.

1. Stop after completing each step of making good decisions.
2. Discuss with each group the observer's comments.
3. Ask the other members of each group to listen to the observer's suggestions and to suggest ways to improve their decision-making skills.
4. Instruct students to repeat the steps that need improvement and to include their modifications.

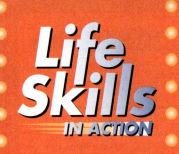

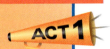

Making Good Decisions

You make decisions every day. But how do you know if you are making good decisions? Making good decisions is making choices that are healthy and responsible. Following the six steps of making good decisions will help you make the best possible choice whenever you make a decision. Complete the following activity to practice the six steps of making good decisions.

What's for Lunch?

Setting the Scene

Simon and his friend Tabitha need to eat a quick lunch before returning to their volunteer jobs at the hospital. The line in the hospital cafeteria is very long, so they decide to go to the fast-food restaurant next door. As they look over the menu, Tabitha says that she wants to eat something healthy. Simon agrees but is unsure of what to pick.

Frank's Take Out

Main Meals		Sides & Drinks	
Hamburger	1.00	French Fries	1.00
Cheeseburger	1.50	Side Salad	1.50
Grilled Chicken Sandwich	1.50	Baked Potato	1.00
		Soda	1.00
Hot Dog	1.00	Iced Tea	1.25
Tuna Sandwich	1.00	Chocolate Brownie	.75
		Frozen Yogurt	.75

The 6 Steps of Making Good Decisions

1. Identify the problem.
2. Consider your values.
3. List the options.
4. Weigh the consequences.
5. Decide, and act.
6. Evaluate your choice.

Guided Practice

Practice with a Friend

Form a group of three. Have one person play the role of Simon and another person play the role of Tabitha. Have the third person be an observer. Walking through each of the six steps of making good decisions, role-play Simon and Tabitha deciding what to eat for lunch. Use the menu shown above when you reach step 3. The observer will take notes, which will include observations about what the people playing Simon and Tabitha did well and suggestions of ways to improve. Stop after each step to evaluate the process.

5. Check to make sure that students understand each step before they move on to the next step.
6. If time permits, repeat the exercise three times, switching roles each time. Each student should have the opportunity to play each role. Co-op Learning

Independent Practice

Check Yourself

After you have completed the guided practice, go through Act 1 again without stopping at each step. Answer the questions below to review what you did.

1. What values should Simon and Tabitha consider before choosing what to eat?
2. What are the healthy food options that Simon and Tabitha can choose from?
3. What are some possible consequences of selecting an unhealthy food option?
4. How can you evaluate the food choices at a restaurant?

On Your Own

After eating lunch, Tabitha tells Simon that she is tired and doesn't want to go back to work at the hospital. She asks Simon to tell their supervisor that she got sick at lunch and had to go home. Simon doesn't want to do it, but Tabitha offers to buy him dessert if he does. Write a short story describing how Simon could use the six steps of making good decisions in this situation.

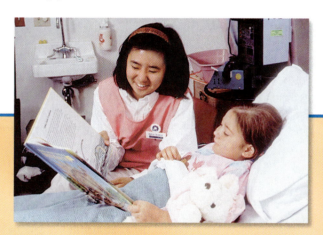

Chapter 6: A Healthy Body, a Healthy Weight
Chapter Planning Guide

PACING	CLASSROOM RESOURCES	ACTIVITIES AND DEMONSTRATIONS
BLOCK 1 • 45 min pp. 114–119 **Chapter Opener**	CRF Health Inventory * GENERAL CRF Parent Letter *	SE Health IQ, p. 115 CRF At-Home Activity *
Lesson 1 What Is Body Image?	CRF Lesson Plan * TT Bellringer *	TE Activity Creative Writing, p. 116 GENERAL TE Group Activity Commercial, p. 117 GENERAL CRF Life Skills Activity * GENERAL CRF Enrichment Activity * ADVANCED
Lesson 2 Building a Healthy Body Image	CRF Lesson Plan * TT Bellringer * TT Staying Positive with "I" Statements *	TE Activities Body Image in the Media, p. 113F CRF Enrichment Activity * ADVANCED
BLOCK 2 • 45 min pp. 120–123 **Lesson 3** Eating Disorders	CRF Lesson Plan * TT Bellringer * TT Some Causes of Eating Disorders *	TE Activity Poster Project, p. 120 GENERAL TE Group Activity Role-Playing Dieting, p. 122 GENERAL CRF Enrichment Activity * ADVANCED
BLOCK 3 • 45 min pp. 124–127 **Lesson 4** Managing Your Weight	CRF Lesson Plan * TT Bellringer *	TE Activities Exercise Survey, p. 113F TE Demonstration Muscle vs. Fat, p. 124 GENERAL TE Demonstration Healthy Balance, p. 125 BASIC TE Activity Weight Management Brochure, p. 125 GENERAL TE Demonstration Why Do We Eat?, p. 126 BASIC TE Group Activity Healthy Diet, p. 126 GENERAL SE Math Activity, p. 127 TE Activity Exercise Education, p. 127 GENERAL SE Life Skills in Action Practicing Wellness, pp. 130–131 CRF Life Skills Activity * GENERAL CRF Enrichment Activity * ADVANCED

BLOCKS 4 & 5 • 90 min Chapter Review and Assessment Resources

- SE Chapter Review, pp. 128–129
- CRF Concept Review * GENERAL
- CRF Health Behavior Contract * GENERAL
- CRF Chapter Test * GENERAL
- CRF Performance-Based Assessment * GENERAL
- OSP Test Generator
- CRF Test Item Listing *

Online Resources

go.hrw.com — Visit go.hrw.com for a variety of free resources related to this textbook. Enter the keyword HD4WMT.

Holt Online Learning — Students can access interactive problem solving help and active visual concept development with the *Decisions for Health* Online Edition available at www.hrw.com.

CNN Student News — cnnstudentnews.com. Find the latest health news, lesson plans, and activities related to important scientific events.

Compression guide:
To shorten your instruction because of time limitations, omit Lesson 4.

KEY

- **TE** Teacher Edition
- **SE** Student Edition
- **OSP** One-Stop Planner
- **CRF** Chapter Resource File
- **TT** Teaching Transparency
- ***** Also on One-Stop Planner
- ■ Also Available in Spanish
- ◆ Requires Advance Prep

SKILLS DEVELOPMENT RESOURCES	LESSON REVIEW AND ASSESSMENT	STANDARDS CORRELATION
		National Health Education Standards
CRF Cross-Disciplinary * GENERAL **CRF** Directed Reading * BASIC	**SE** Lesson Review, p. 117 **TE** Reteaching, Quiz, p. 117 **CRF** Lesson Quiz * ■ GENERAL	
SE Life Skills Activity Evaluating Media Messages, p. 119 **TE** Inclusion Strategies, p. 119 BASIC **CRF** Decision-Making * GENERAL **CRF** Directed Reading * BASIC	**SE** Lesson Review, p. 119 **TE** Reteaching, Quiz, p. 119 **CRF** Lesson Quiz * ■ GENERAL	3.4, 4.2
TE Inclusion Strategies, p. 120 ADVANCED **TE** Life Skill Builder Assessing Your Health, p. 121 GENERAL **SE** Study Tip Organizing Information, p. 122 **TE** Reading Skill Builder Discussion, p. 122 BASIC **SE** Life Skills Activity Making Good Decisions, p. 123 **CRF** Cross-Disciplinary * GENERAL **CRF** Refusal Skills * GENERAL **CRF** Directed Reading * BASIC	**SE** Lesson Review, p. 123 **TE** Reteaching, Quiz, p. 123 **TE** Alternative Assessment, p. 123 GENERAL **CRF** Concept Mapping * GENERAL **CRF** Lesson Quiz * ■ GENERAL	5.3
TE Reading Skill Builder Reading Organizer, p. 125 GENERAL **TE** Life Skill Builder Practicing Wellness, p. 125 GENERAL **CRF** Decision-Making * GENERAL **CRF** Refusal Skills * GENERAL **CRF** Directed Reading * BASIC	**SE** Lesson Review, p. 127 **TE** Reteaching, Quiz, p. 127 **CRF** Concept Mapping * GENERAL **CRF** Lesson Quiz * ■ GENERAL	3.4

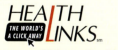

www.scilinks.org/health

Maintained by the **National Science Teachers Association**

Topic: Body Image
HealthLinks code: HD4019
Topic: Eating Disorders
HealthLinks code: HD4034

Technology Resources

 One-Stop Planner
All of your printable resources and the Test Generator are on this convenient CD-ROM.

 Guided Reading Audio CDs

VIDEO SELECT
For information about videos related to this chapter, go to **go.hrw.com** and type in the keyword **HD4WMTV**.

Chapter 6 • Chapter Planning Guide

CHAPTER 6
A Healthy Body, a Healthy Weight
Chapter Resources

Teacher Resources

TEACHING TRANSPARENCIES

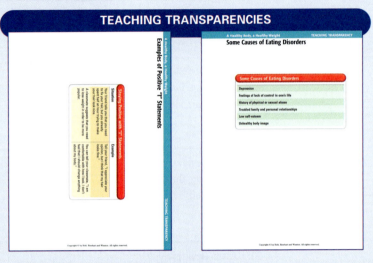

BELLRINGER TRANSPARENCIES

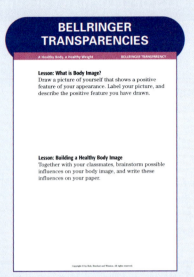

LESSON PLANS

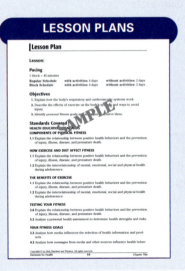

PARENT LETTER

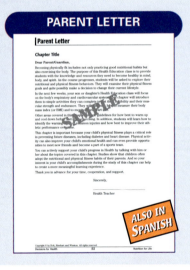

TEST ITEM LISTING

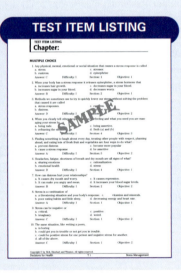

Meeting Individual Needs

DIRECTED READING

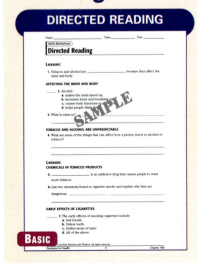

CONCEPT MAPPING

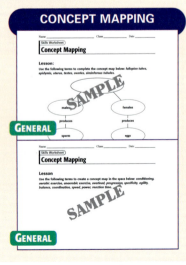

CONCEPT REVIEW

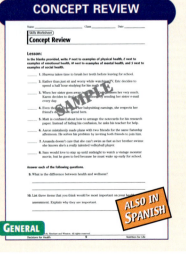

ENRICHMENT ACTIVITIES

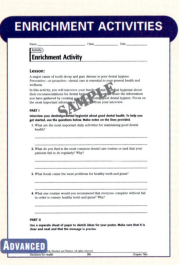

Resources

These worksheet pages can be found in the Chapter Resource File and the One-Stop Planner. The transparencies can be found in the Teaching Transparencies binder and on the One-Stop Planner.

Activities

LIFE SKILLS ACTIVITIES

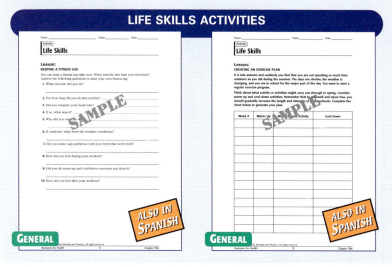

AT-HOME ACTIVITY

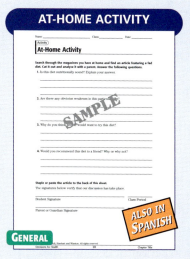

DATASHEETS FOR IN-TEXT ACTIVITIES

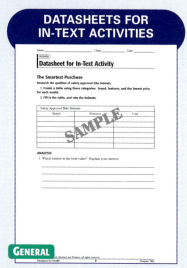

Applications

DECISION-MAKING

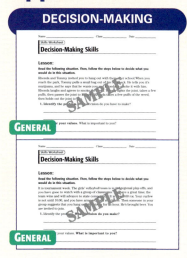

REFUSAL SKILLS

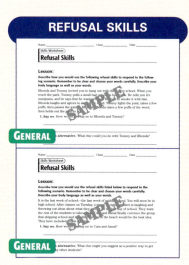

CROSS-DISCIPLINARY

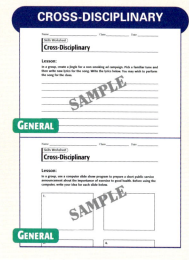

HEALTH BEHAVIOR CONTRACT

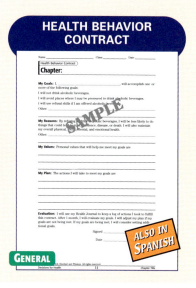

Assessments

HEALTH INVENTORY

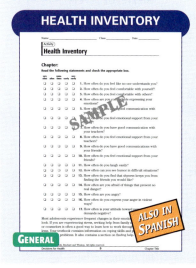

LESSON QUIZZES

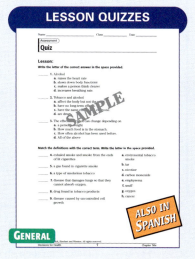

CHAPTER TEST

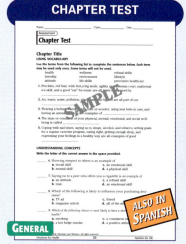

PERFORMANCE-BASED ASSESSMENT

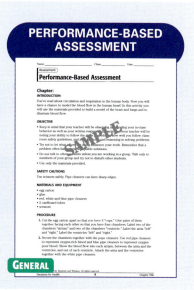

Chapter 6 • Chapter Resources and Worksheets   113D

CHAPTER 6

Background Information

The following information focuses on fats and their effect on the body. This material will help prepare you for teaching the concepts in this chapter.

How Fats are Used

- Fats store a lot of energy. One gram of fat holds 9 Calories of energy, as opposed to the 4 Calories of energy stored in a gram of protein or carbohydrate. Because fat stores so much energy, it is found between muscle cells to provide a ready source of energy.

- Fat does not conduct heat well. A layer of fat just beneath the skin insulates internal organs from extreme heat and cold.

- Fat cushions and protects many organs, including the kidneys, liver, and eyes.

- Fat is necessary for the construction of certain types of tissues, such as the myelin sheaths that insulate nerves.

- Fats are needed in the body to absorb fat-soluble vitamins, such as vitamins A, D, E, and K. Fats also transport these vitamins in the bloodstream to cells that need them.

- Fats keep the skin soft and prevent dryness.

- Fats are used to make body chemicals, including male and female sex hormones.

Types of Fats

- Cholesterol is one well-known type of fat. Cholesterol is found in bile, blood, and the brain.

- About 95 percent of the fats in a typical diet are triglycerides. A triglyceride is a fat molecule made from three fatty acids that are attached to a molecule of glycerol.

- Fats can be saturated or unsaturated. Saturated fats are solids at room temperature. Unsaturated fats are liquid at room temperature. Oils are unsaturated fats. Oils usually come from plant sources.

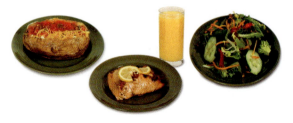

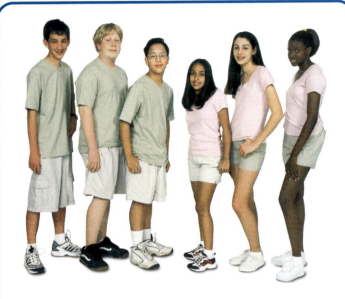

Health Hazards Associated with Fats

- An adult needs only about a tablespoon of fat in his or her daily diet. However, the average American eats around six to eight tablespoons of fat every day. High-fat diets lead to obesity, and obesity can lead to many other health problems, including high blood pressure and diabetes.

- High-fat diets are associated with colon, prostate, lung, and breast cancer.

- A high-fat diet may lead to atherosclerosis. Atherosclerosis is a disease in which plaque builds up on the walls of the arteries. Plaque is composed of fatty substances, cholesterol, and debris in the blood. Atherosclerosis causes heart attacks and strokes. Atherosclerosis is directly related to the amount of cholesterol in the blood. Blood cholesterol levels under 200 mg/dL are healthy. Many Americans have blood cholesterol levels of 200 mg/dL or higher.

- Studies have shown that people who lower their blood cholesterol levels can reverse some of the damage caused by atherosclerosis, such as the build-up of plaque.

- Most blood cholesterol comes from the liver, not the diet. Furthermore, a person's genes go a long way in determining how the person's body handles cholesterol.

For background information about teaching strategies and issues, refer to the *Professional Reference for Teachers*.

ACTIVITIES

CHAPTER 6

Consider using the activities on this page as students explore the lessons of this chapter. Look for other activities throughout the Student Edition chapter.

Body Image in the Media

Procedure Have students bring their favorite magazines to class. Tell students to go through the magazine, including the cover. As they go through the magazine, they will gather information in three charts. In the first chart, students should keep track of the number of male versus female models they see. In addition, students should note whether each model is large, average, or thin. In the second chart, students should track the types of articles in the magazine. The chart should reflect the amount of articles that cover diet, exercise, fashion, and self-esteem, respectively. In the third chart, students should track the amount of the following types of advertisements, respectively: weight loss, weight gain, food, and exercise. Finally, have students write a brief paragraph that explains their magazine's overall message about a normal body image. The class should pool its data together.

Analysis Ask students the following questions:

- What patterns do you see when looking at data collected by all of the students? (Answers may vary. Some patterns may include a high number of thin women and girls.)

- Were men and women represented differently? (Answers will vary.)

- Were the people shown in the magazines average looking? Did they look like people in your school? (Answers may vary. Students are likely to find that the people shown in magazines don't look like the people in their school.)

- How do you think these magazines affect a reader's perception of his or her body image? (Answers may vary.)

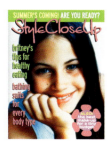 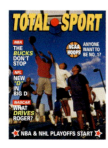 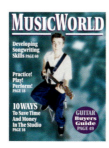

Exercise Survey

Procedure Organize students into pairs. Each pair should research the amount of physical activity necessary for good health for different age groups. Then, ask each pair to design a physical-activity survey. The survey should help students determine the level of activity of the people in their community. Once they've written the survey, each pair should distribute the survey to at least 10 people. The following is a sample survey:

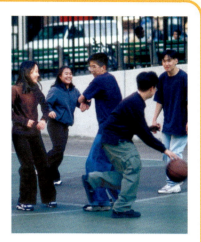

1. How old are you?
2. What is your gender?
3. Do you feel you are physically fit?
4. Do you participate in a regular exercise program? If so, what types of activities do you do? How often do you do these activities?
5. Are you physically active but do not participate in a regular exercise program? If so, how are you physically active and how often are you physically active?
6. If physical activity is not important to you, why not?

Analysis

- Have students compare the results of their surveys with the research they completed on the healthy amount of physical activity for different age groups.

- Then, have students draw graphs, tables, or charts to illustrate their comparisons.

- The class should pool their data and make a diagnosis of their community's level of physical activity.

- If students find that the members of their community do not get enough physical activity, have students write a proposal that suggests different ways to encourage the members of their community to get more exercise.

- If students find that the members of their community get enough physical activity, they should create a brochure that describes the community's resources that encourage physical activity.

Chapter 6 • Activities 113F

CHAPTER 6

Overview
Tell students that this chapter will help them understand what body image is, how to have a healthy body image, and what types of disorders a poor body image can cause. This chapter also discusses effective weight management methods and the importance of a healthy diet and physical activity.

Assessing Prior Knowledge
Students should be familiar with the following topics:
- nutrition
- decision making

Question Box

Students may feel more comfortable asking questions if you set up a Question Box to collect their questions. Have students write and anonymously submit their questions about body image, eating disorders, and weight management. Address these questions during class, or use these questions to introduce lessons that cover related topics.

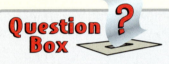

Check out *Current Health* articles and activities related to this chapter by visiting the HRW Web site at **go.hrw.com.** Just type in the keyword **HD4CH21T.**

Chapter Resource File
- Directed Reading BASIC
- Health Inventory GENERAL
- Parent Letter

CHAPTER 6
A Healthy Body, a Healthy Weight

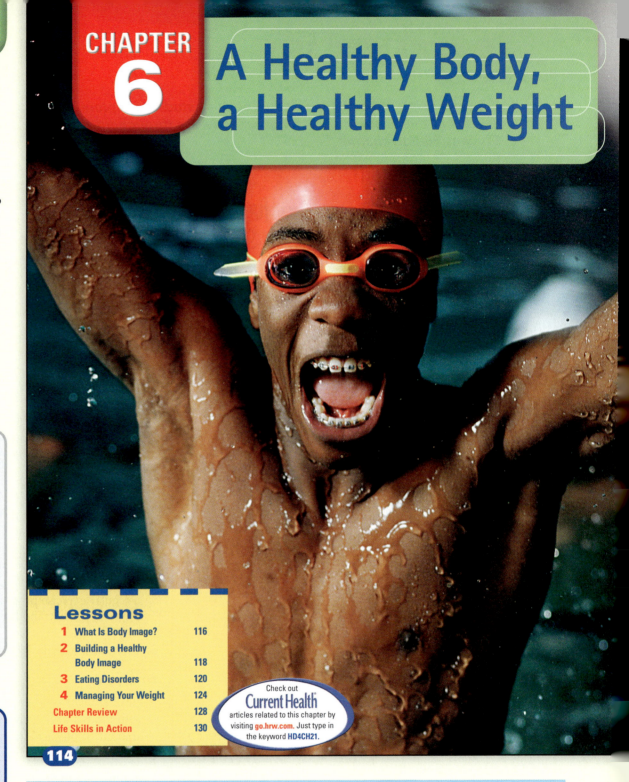

Lessons
1. What Is Body Image? — 116
2. Building a Healthy Body Image — 118
3. Eating Disorders — 120
4. Managing Your Weight — 124

Chapter Review — 128
Life Skills in Action — 130

Check out *Current Health* articles related to this chapter by visiting **go.hrw.com.** Just type in the keyword **HD4CH21.**

Standards Correlations

National Health Education Standards

3.4 Demonstrate strategies to improve or maintain personal and family health. (Lessons 2 and 4)

4.2 Students will analyze the influences of culture, media, technology, and other factors on health. Students will analyze how messages from media and other sources influence health behaviors. (Lesson 2)

5.3 Students will demonstrate the ability to use interpersonal communication skills to enhance health. Students will demonstrate healthy ways to express needs, wants, and feelings. (Lesson 3)

> " I used to think I was **too skinny.** So, I decided to join the **swim team** to build more **muscle.** Now, I feel much better about my body, and I am keeping a healthy weight. "

Health IQ

PRE-READING

Answer the following true/false questions to find out what you already know about body image and eating disorders. When you've finished this chapter, you'll have the opportunity to change your answers based on what you've learned.

1. Eating disorders affect only girls and women.
2. Too much exercise can be bad for you.
3. You can maintain your weight by eating well and staying physically active.
4. Your body image is important only when you are going out with your friends.
5. A person with a healthy body image wants to change his or her body in some way.
6. Following fad diets is not harmful to your health.
7. Your body image affects how you face new challenges.
8. The photographs you see on TV and in magazines can influence your body image.
9. If you eat more food than your body needs to get energy for your daily activities, you will gain weight.
10. Eating disorders are only a phase, and most people don't suffer from them for a long time.
11. Having a healthy body image can boost your confidence.
12. Your body image does not affect your self-esteem.
13. Unhealthy eating behaviors can lead to eating disorders.
14. Obesity may result in health problems such as diabetes or stroke.

ANSWERS: 1. false; 2. true; 3. true; 4. false; 5. false; 6. false; 7. true; 8. true; 9. true; 10. false; 11. true; 12. false; 13. true; 14. true

Using the Health IQ

Misconception Alert
Answers to the Health IQ questions may help you identify students' misconceptions.

Question 1: Eating disorders are usually presented as being a problem for females only. This is not the case. Boys and men are also at risk for developing eating disorders.

Question 4: A person's body image can affect his or her life at any time. A poor body image tends to cause people to think badly of their own appearance constantly. A negative body image may lead to an eating disorder.

Question 10: An eating disorder is a serious medical condition that may need long-term treatment.

Answers
1. false
2. true
3. true
4. false
5. false
6. false
7. true
8. true
9. true
10. false
11. true
12. false
13. true
14. true

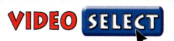

For information about videos related to this chapter, go to **go.hrw.com** and type in the keyword **HD4WMTV**.

Lesson 1

Focus

Overview

Before beginning this lesson, review with your students the objectives listed under the What You'll Do head in the Student Edition. In this lesson, students will learn about body image and how body image affects a person's health. Students will also learn how to distinguish between a healthy and an unhealthy body image.

Bellringer

Ask students to draw a picture which depicts a positive feature of their own appearance. Students should label their pictures, describing the positive attribute they have illustrated. Have students learning English label the picture in English and in their native language.
LS Visual

Answer to Start Off Write

Accept all reasonable answers. Sample answer: If you are uncomfortable with your body, you may not feel like participating in class and calling attention to yourself. Not being active in class may hurt your grades.

Motivate

Activity — GENERAL

Creative Writing Direct students' attention to the photo on this page. Have students write a brief story based on this picture. Ask one or two volunteers to read their stories aloud to the class.
LS Verbal

Lesson 1

What You'll Do

- **Describe** how body image affects your life.
- **Explain** the difference between healthy body image and unhealthy body image.

Terms to Learn

- body image

Start Off Write

How can your body image affect your grades?

What Is Body Image?

Sudeep is shorter and thinner than most of the boys at school. The day of the big race in gym class, some of his classmates laughed at him because he's so small. Sudeep ignored them and focused on running as fast as he could.

Instead of letting the comments about his small size bother him, Sudeep focused on his goal. He is comfortable with his body. Sudeep has a healthy body image.

Your Body Image

Your **body image** is the way you see and imagine your body. Your body image is important because it affects many aspects of your life.

How you feel about your body can affect the way you handle many situations. If you feel comfortable with yourself and your body, you will be more likely to have confidence when you are faced with new challenges. For example, you may have more confidence when trying a new activity, or you may feel more confident in class. If you are uncomfortable with your body, you may want to change how your body looks. The desire to change can lead to unhealthy behaviors.

Your body image is especially important at your age because your body is changing a lot. You will most likely grow taller and develop more muscle mass. Most teens gain weight as they grow and as their body changes. Feeling good about your body will help you deal with these changes in a positive way.

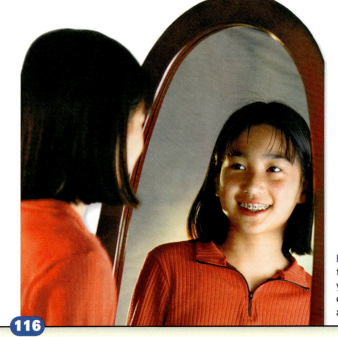

Figure 1 Your body image is the way you see and imagine your body. This teen is comfortable with her body and has a healthy body image.

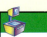

Background

Body Image and Girls Overall, girls are more likely than boys to develop unhealthy body image. Tell students that a national survey of high school students showed that slightly more than thirty-three percent of the girls identified themselves as overweight, while less than 15 percent of the boys did. Almost half the girls in the survey indicated that they were on a diet. Almost one-quarter of the girls on the diet did not think they were overweight.

Chapter Resource File

- Directed Reading BASIC
- Lesson Plan
- Lesson Quiz GENERAL

Transparencies

TT Bellringer

---

116 Chapter 6 • A Healthy Body, a Healthy Weight

What Is a Healthy Body Image?

To have a healthy body image is to accept and feel good about your body. People who have a healthy body image are comfortable with their appearance. They like and accept their bodies. They do not constantly compare themselves to other people in their lives. Nor do they always compare themselves to the people they see on TV or in magazines. People who have a healthy body image do not usually want to change their bodies. And their healthy body image gives them more confidence to handle new challenges.

What Is an Unhealthy Body Image?

To have an unhealthy body image is to feel uncomfortable with your body. People who have an unhealthy body image often compare their body with others. And people who have an unhealthy body image are very unhappy with their appearance. In fact, they may not see themselves accurately.

Many people feel somewhat unhappy with their body. They may feel unhappy with their weight, their hair, their legs—any part of their body. This is normal. However, some people are extremely unhappy about their body. Their body image keeps them from spending time with other people or from trying new things. Their body image may also keep them from being active in class, which can hurt their grades. Often, these people want very much to change their bodies. They may drastically change their eating habits, which can be dangerous.

Health Journal

Each day for the next three days, write down two things that you like about your appearance. Think about the items on your list when you feel down about your appearance.

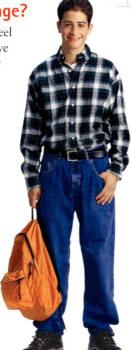

Figure 2 Jon feels good about his appearance, which helps him feel confident at school.

Lesson Review

Using Vocabulary
1. What is body image?

Understanding Concepts
2. Describe the characteristics of a person who has an unhealthy body image.

Critical Thinking
3. **Making Inferences** How can your body image affect how you feel on your first day at a new school?

internet connect
www.scilinks.org/health
Topic: **Body Image**
HealthLinks code: **HD4019**
HEALTH LINKS. Maintained by the National Science Teachers Association

Lesson 2

Focus

Overview
Before beginning this lesson, review with your students the objectives listed under the What You'll Do head in the Student Edition. In this lesson, students will learn about the factors that influence body image and how to maintain a healthy body image.

Bellringer
Have students brainstorm a list of possible influences on their body image. Ask the students to think about who or what can affect their body image. Then, have students call out influences from their list as you write them on the board. (Answers may vary. Sample answers: culture, family, peers, media)
LS Intrapersonal

Answer to Start Off Write
Accept all reasonable answers. Sample answer: Your friends can positively affect your body image by supporting you when you feel uncomfortable about your body. Your friends can negatively affect your body image if they make negative comments about your appearance.

Motivate

Discussion — GENERAL
Show the class pictures of different celebrities and have the class think about how the media might influence a person's body image. Then, discuss what it means to have a healthy body image and ask students to suggest healthy ways to enhance body image.
LS Interpersonal

Lesson 2 — Building a Healthy Body Image

What You'll Do
- **Identify** three influences on your body image.
- **Describe** how I statements can help you build a healthy body image.

Start Off Write
How can your friends affect your body image?

Lexi loves teen magazines. She enjoys reading about celebrities and looking at the latest fashion trends. Sometimes, though, Lexi thinks that she'll never be thin enough to look good in the clothes that the models wear.

Lexi tends to compare herself to the models she sees in magazines. She thinks that if she doesn't look like the models, she doesn't look good.

The Media and Your Body Image

Did you know that the media can influence your body image? The media includes TV, movies, magazines, and music videos. TV shows and magazines usually show unrealistic images of men and women. Many magazines and TV programs show girls and women who are unusually thin. They also show boys and men who are unusually muscular.

Some people think that they should look like the models in magazines or the actors on TV. They may even feel ugly or fat compared with the models and actors. But the people shown on TV and in magazines are not typical. In fact, if you look around your classroom, you will probably find that most of your classmates do not look like models or actors. Most of your classmates are not that thin or that muscular. The unrealistic images of people that magazines and TV tend to show can lead a teen to develop an unhealthy body image.

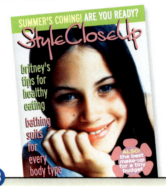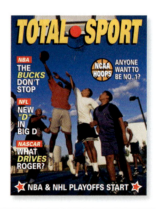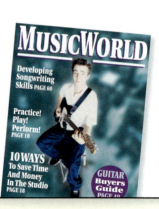

Figure 3 Often, the images in magazines and on TV give us the wrong impression of what is "normal."

 Cultural Awareness
A society's ideal body image for women varies around the world. Western societies tend to promote tall, thin bodies for women. Arab societies idealize more plump, petite women. Central African societies admire women with wide hips and thighs. And in China, women with small, sloped shoulders are considered the most beautiful.

Chapter Resource File
- Directed Reading **BASIC**
- Lesson Plan
- Lesson Quiz **GENERAL**

Transparencies
TT Bellringer
TT Staying Positive with "I" Statements

---

118   Chapter 6 • A HEALTHY BODY, a Healthy Weight

Family, Friends, and Body Image

You will face many physical and emotional changes as a teen. When you go through periods of change, you may be sensitive to the comments of others. Your family, friends, and even your teachers and coaches may make comments about your appearance. Most likely, these people do not want to hurt you. But sometimes these comments can hurt your feelings. If you already feel bad about your body, hearing negative comments may lead you to develop an unhealthy body image. If you feel good about your body, you can deal with these comments in a positive way. Also, remember that your family, friends, teachers, and coaches are usually very supportive when you are feeling uncomfortable about your body.

"I" Statements

So, what do you do when someone teases you about your appearance? One of the best things to do is to share your feelings by using "I" statements. An "I" statement tells someone how you feel by using a statement that begins with the word *I* instead of the word *you*. The table below shows some examples of "I" statements.

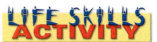

EVALUATING MEDIA MESSAGES

In small groups, cut out pictures of people who have "ideal" bodies from several magazines. Together, paste your clippings to create a collage. Do these people look like most of the people you know? Do you think that the media influences the way you think of yourself? Why or why not?

TABLE 1 Staying Positive with "I" Statements

Situation	Example
Your friend tells you that you need to fix your hair, but you already spent half an hour trying to make your hair look nice.	Tell your friend, "I appreciate your opinion, but I think that my hair looks fine."
A classmate suggests that you need to lose weight in order to be more popular.	You can tell your classmate, "I am comfortable with how I look. I don't feel that I should change anything about my body."

Lesson Review

Understanding Concepts

1. Explain how magazines and TV can influence your body image.
2. Write an "I" statement you would use if your brother told you that your nose was big.

Critical Thinking

3. **Analyzing Ideas** Explain how having a healthy body image can help you handle negative comments in a positive way.

Answers to the Lesson Review

1. Sample answer: Magazines and TV show images of men and women with "perfect" bodies. If I compare myself to these images, I may develop an unhealthy body image.
2. Sample answer: I think my nose is fine. I like the way I look.
3. Sample answer: If I am comfortable with my body, and someone makes a negative comment about my body, I will be less likely to let the comment bother me. Or I will be confident enough to tell the person how I feel about his or her comment.

Teach

LIFE SKILLS ACTIVITY

Answers
Answers may vary.
Extension: Ask students to list both the negative and positive effects that the media has on body image. Ask students how the media could change in order to promote more positive effects on body image.

INCLUSION Strategies — BASIC

• **Visually Impaired**

Students who are partially-sighted can more easily handle reading materials that are enlarged. Sometimes, students can read the text but not the charts and tables, such as the the table on this page. Smaller fonts and dense text can create additional reading difficulties. Try copying the table on this page onto the board, enlarging it so that visually impaired students can read it more easily. **LS** Visual

Close

Reteaching — BASIC

Body-Image Builder Have students role-play different ways to stay positive about their body image. Students should enact situations that would build a healthy body image and situations that could hurt a person's body image. In each situation, the students should find a positive way to behave. **LS** Kinesthetic

Quiz — GENERAL

1. Name three things that could affect your body image. (Sample answer: friends, media, family)
2. Write a skit in which someone teases you about your appearance and you react in a positive manner. (Answers may vary.)

Lesson 2 • Building a Healthy Body Image

Lesson 3

Focus

Overview
Before beginning this lesson, review with your students the objectives listed under the What You'll Do head in the Student Edition. In this lesson, students will learn about unhealthy eating behaviors, fad diets, and eating disorders.

🔔 Bellringer
Ask students to write down details about a diet they have seen advertised. Have students write a brief paragraph discussing the probable effectiveness of this diet. (Answers may vary.) **LS Logical**

Answer to Start Off Write
Accept all reasonable answers. Sample answer: Eating disorders may develop from a poor body image or from unhealthy eating behaviors.

Motivate

Activity ——————— GENERAL
Poster Project Tell students that a 1996 study of college students found that 58 percent of the women and 38 percent of the men were identified as being at risk for developing an eating disorder. In addition, the study discovered that 45 percent of the women believed that they should have less than 12 percent body fat, when in fact the healthy amount of body fat for young women is 20 percent to 30 percent of body weight. Organize the class into groups and ask the groups to use this information to design an eating disorder information poster to be placed in the school's locker rooms and gyms. **LS Visual**

Lesson 3 — Eating Disorders

What You'll Do
- **Identify** two characteristics of a fad diet.
- **Describe** three possible causes of eating disorders.
- **Describe** three types of eating disorders.

Terms to Learn
- fad diet
- eating disorder
- anorexia nervosa
- bulimia nervosa
- binge eating disorder

Start Off Write
How do eating disorders develop?

Johanna went on a fasting diet to lose 10 pounds. She wanted to look thinner for the school dance. Johanna did not think about how unhealthy she was being by not eating.

Johanna did not realize that she was developing an *unhealthy eating behavior*. Fasting to lose weight is one example of an unhealthy eating behavior.

Unhealthy Eating Behavior
Many people feel the need to have a perfect body to be accepted or popular among their peers. Some people may change their eating habits to become thinner or more muscular. For example, people may skip meals, eat only certain foods, or eat large amounts of food at one time. They may also use diet pills or follow unhealthy diets. These types of eating habits are called *unhealthy eating behaviors* and can be very harmful.

The most common unhealthy eating behavior is following a fad diet. **Fad diets** are eating plans that promise quick weight loss with little effort. Most fad diets require you to buy special products, such as pills or shakes. Fad diets often require you to avoid many foods that are good sources of essential nutrients.

Unhealthy eating behaviors can affect a teen's growth, development, and ability to learn. Unhealthy eating behaviors may develop into an eating disorder. Eating disorders are illnesses that severely affect a person's body image and eating habits.

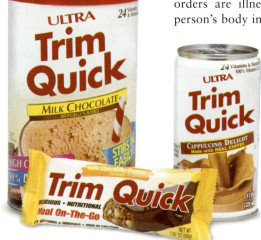
Figure 4 Fad diets usually require you to buy special products, which can be expensive.

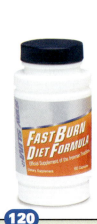
• **Gifted and Talented**
Ask students to go on the Internet and research fad diets such as the Grapefruit Diet, the Protein Diet, and the Banana Diet. Have them make charts explaining each of the diets, and then lead a class discussion about which of the diets are most/least healthy and why. **LS Logical**

Chapter Resource File
- Directed Reading **BASIC**
- Lesson Plan
- Lesson Quiz **GENERAL**

 Transparencies
TT Bellringer
TT Some Causes of Eating Disorders

---

120 Chapter 6 • A Healthy Body, a Healthy Weight

Overexercising

In addition to changing their eating habits, some people increase their physical activity to lose weight. Regular exercise is healthy, but some people exercise too much. When a person exercises harder and for a longer period of time than is healthy, that person is *overexercising*. People may overexercise because they are concerned about their weight or because they feel the need to be better at athletics. These people risk getting injured and usually feel tired all the time. They may also feel depressed. Unfortunately, most people don't realize that too much exercise can be dangerous.

What Is an Eating Disorder?

Both unhealthy eating behaviors and overexercising can be dangerous. They can harm a person's growth and development. Or they can develop into an eating disorder. An **eating disorder** is a disease in which a person has an unhealthy concern with his or her body weight and shape. Eating disorders are very complex. They can be caused by many factors. Three factors are low self-esteem, emotional problems, and poor body image. Other factors are pressure from peers to be thin and a history of physical or emotional abuse.

Eating disorders are dangerous to a person's physical and emotional health. Some physical effects of eating disorders include dangerous digestive problems and heart failure. Some emotional effects are depression and anxiety. Eating disorders can affect anyone—boys, girls, men, and women of all cultures and ethnicities. Examples of eating disorders are anorexia nervosa (AN uh REKS ee uh nuhr VOH suh), bulimia nervosa (boo LEE mee uh nuhr VOH suh), and binge eating disorder. People who develop anorexia nervosa or bulimia nervosa often suffer from poor body image and low self-esteem. People who develop binge eating disorder often suffer from emotional problems and low self-esteem.

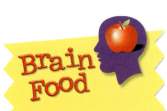

Brain Food

In the United States, 5 million to 10 million girls and women and 1 million boys and men struggle with eating disorders.

TABLE 2 Some Causes of Eating Disorders
Depression
Feelings of lack of control in one's life
History of physical or sexual abuse
Troubled family and personal relationships
Low self-esteem
Unhealthy body image

Teach, continued

Group Activity — GENERAL

Role-Playing Dieting Organize students into pairs. Have one student play the role of someone engaged in a dangerous dieting practice, and have the other play the role of a sympathetic but worried friend. The first student should disagree with the fact that dieting can be dangerous. The second student should express his or her concerns and tell the first student that dieting can lead to a serious eating disorder. As a class, discuss why a person with an eating disorder needs more help than a friend can provide and what teens can do if they have serious concerns about a friend. **LS Kinesthetic**

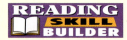 — BASIC

Discussion Have students read the sections on anorexia nervosa and bulimia nervosa. Then, have students discuss what they have read in groups. In addition, ask them to talk about how they would feel if one of their friends had an eating disorder. **LS Interpersonal**

Myth & Fact

Myth: Eating disorders are only phases of heavy dieting.

Fact: Eating disorders are illnesses, not phases. Professional help from a psychiatrist or other doctor is necessary to recover from an eating disorder.

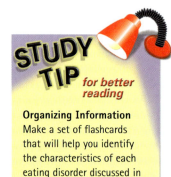

STUDY TIP for better reading

Organizing Information Make a set of flashcards that will help you identify the characteristics of each eating disorder discussed in this lesson.

Anorexia Nervosa

Anorexia nervosa is a disease in which a person has a great fear of gaining weight. **Anorexia nervosa** is an eating disorder that includes self-starvation, an unhealthy body image, and extreme weight loss. People who develop anorexia nervosa also suffer from low self-esteem. They are very scared of becoming fat even though they are very thin. They usually starve themselves or eat only foods that are low in Calories and fat. They may spend more time playing with food than eating it. They may also wear many layers of clothing to hide their weight loss. If left untreated, a person with this disease may develop kidney and heart problems. In severe cases, a person suffering from anorexia nervosa may starve to death.

Bulimia Nervosa

Bulimia nervosa is a disease in which a person has difficulty controlling how much he or she eats. **Bulimia nervosa** is an eating disorder in which a person eats a large amount of food and then tries to rid their body of the food. A person who has this disease usually eats large amounts of food at one time, which is called *bingeing* (BINJ ing). After bingeing, the person may make himself or herself vomit. Or he or she may take laxatives or diuretics to eliminate some of the food. The act of ridding the body of food is called *purging* (PUHRJ ing). This "binge and purge" cycle damages a person's health. The person will suffer from a lack of nutrients. And the acid that comes up from the stomach when a person vomits eats away at the gums and teeth. A person with bulimia may also have swollen jaws and cheeks and stained teeth.

TABLE 3 Some Symptoms of Anorexia Nervosa and Bulimia Nervosa

A person with anorexia nervosa may…	A person with bulimia nervosa may…
eat only low-fat or low-Calorie foods	spend a lot of time thinking about food
play with his or her food but not eat it	steal food or hide food in strange places
wear baggy clothes to hide his or her thinness	take trips to the bathroom immediately after eating
overexercise	make himself or herself throw up after eating
	overexercise

Background

Understanding Bulimia Unlike someone with anorexia nervosa, a person with bulimia nervosa may appear healthy. However, there are some warning signs. These include depression, an inability to sleep well, talking about suicide, a fear of appearing fat, and purchasing large quantities of food. Bulimia nervosa can lead to malnutrition and other health problems.

MISCONCEPTION ALERT

Students may think that a person with anorexia nervosa just doesn't want to listen to those offering help. People who suffer from anorexia nervosa are incapable of recognizing the danger of their condition. Medical intervention is imperative.

Binge Eating Disorder

People who have binge eating disorder often feel as though they cannot stop themselves from eating. **Binge eating disorder** is a disease in which a person has difficulty controlling how much he or she eats but does not purge. In many cases, a person who has this disease suffers from depression as well. People who suffer from this disease usually become very overweight. In many cases, a person may become obese. *Obesity* is a condition in which a person has a large percentage of body fat. Obesity results in many health problems such as increased cholesterol levels, high blood pressure, diabetes, and increased risk for heart disease, stroke, and cancer.

Giving and Getting Help

If you think you or a friend may have an eating disorder, it is very important that you tell a trusted adult about your feelings. This adult may be a parent or teacher. You can also talk to the school nurse, school counselor, or even a doctor. An adult can help you or a friend get professional help as soon as possible. Eating disorders are serious diseases that can damage your health. Even though getting help may be very hard, it is the best decision for your health.

MAKING GOOD DECISIONS

Imagine you think that your friend may have an eating disorder. How would you help your friend?

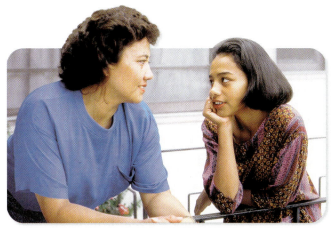

Figure 5 The first step in getting help for an eating disorder is to talk to a parent or other trusted adult.

Lesson Review

Using Vocabulary

1. What are two characteristics of a fad diet?
2. What is an eating disorder?

Understanding Concepts

3. Describe three types of eating disorders.
4. Why are eating disorders dangerous to a person's health?
5. What are three possible causes of eating disorders?

Critical Thinking

6. **Making Good Decisions** You notice that your friend has been exercising a lot lately. He is also very concerned about how his body looks. You think that he is developing unhealthy eating behaviors. Would you talk to your friend? If so, what would you say?

internet connect
Topic: Eating Disorders
HealthLinks code: HD4034
HEALTH LINKS. Maintained by the National Science Teachers Association

Answers to Lesson Review

1. Fad diets may require you to buy expensive products and to avoid foods that are high in essential nutrients.
2. An eating disorder is a disease in which a person has an unhealthy concern with his or her body weight and shape.
3. Anorexia nervosa is an eating disorder in which a person starves himself or herself in order to be thin; bulimia nervosa is an eating disorder in which a person eats a large amount of food and then purges the food from his or her body; and binge eating disorder is an eating disorder in which a person eats a large amount of food at one time but does not purge.
4. Some eating disorders, such as anorexia nervosa and bulimia nervosa, prevent a person from getting the nutrients he or she needs to survive. But, all of these illnesses may result in death.
5. Answers may vary. Sample answer: Three causes of eating disorders may be poor body image, depression, or troubled family relationships.
6. Sample answer: Yes, I would talk to him about his problem and tell him where he could go for help. If he did not stop his behavior, I would go to talk to his parents.

LIFE SKILLS ACTIVITY

Answer
Answers may vary.

Extension: Ask students to write down what they would do if they felt that they had an eating disorder.

Close

Reteaching — BASIC

Role-Play Have students role-play a discussion between a counselor and a student. The student should pretend to have an eating disorder and should describe the symptoms of the eating disorder until the counselor can make a correct diagnosis. Once the counselor has diagnosed the disorder, he or she should give the student advice about what to do to treat the eating disorder. **LS** Logical

Quiz — GENERAL

1. What are the health risks of bulimia nervosa? (tooth and gum decay, swollen jaw and cheeks, not getting enough nutrients to perform regular body functions)
2. What eating disorder leads to obesity? (binge eating disorder)
3. What eating disorder is characterized by self-starvation? (anorexia nervosa)

Alternative Assessment — GENERAL

Public Service Announcement Have students write a radio public service announcement discussing the dangers of eating disorders and telling people how to get help if they think they may have an eating disorder. Students can read their announcement on tape and play the tape to the class. **LS** Auditory

Lesson 3 • Eating Disorders

Lesson 4 Focus

Overview
Before beginning this lesson, review with your students the objectives listed under the What You'll Do head in the Student Edition. In this lesson, students will learn ways to stay within their healthy weight range. Students will learn what affects their weight and how diet and physical activity play a role in weight management.

Bellringer
Have students describe what they think would be the most safe and effective way to lose weight. (Answers may vary.) **LS Verbal**

Answer to Start Off Write
Accept all reasonable answers. Sample answer: You can maintain your weight healthfully by eating the right amount of food and by staying physically active everyday.

Motivate

Demonstration — GENERAL
Muscle vs. Fat Tell students that muscle weighs more than fat. To help students visualize the difference in mass between fat and muscle, bring a cut of beef rimmed with fat to class. Cut out a 1-cm² cube of the beef and a 1-cm² cube of the fat. Weigh each cube. (The fat will weigh less than the beef.) Have students use the weights of the two cubes to calculate the amount of fat needed to equal the weight of the 1-cm² cube of meat. Then, have students use this information to explain why weight is not a perfect indicator of body composition. **LS Visual**

Lesson 4

What You'll Do
- **Describe** how to find your healthy weight range.
- **Describe** five factors that affect your weight.
- **Describe** how to keep a healthy weight.
- **Explain** how your feelings can affect your eating habits.
- **List** five ways to make healthy food choices.

Terms to Learn
- healthy weight range

Start Off Write
How can you maintain your weight healthfully?

Managing Your Weight

Lauren wants to maintain her weight. She is often confused about which foods to eat and which foods to avoid. Lauren wishes that she didn't have to worry about food so much.

Many teens wonder how to maintain, gain, or lose weight. However, most of these teens do not consider how to manage their weight healthfully.

Your Healthy Weight Range
The first step in managing your weight healthfully is to determine your healthy weight range. Your **healthy weight range** is an estimate of how much you should weigh depending on your height and your body frame. Every person has a unique body shape and size. So, determining exactly how much a person should weigh is impossible. There is no ideal weight for a person.

So, how do you determine your healthy weight range? The body mass index, or BMI, is a calculation that can help you find your healthy weight range. You can find a BMI table in the appendix of this book. You can also ask your family doctor to help you determine what weight range is healthy for you.

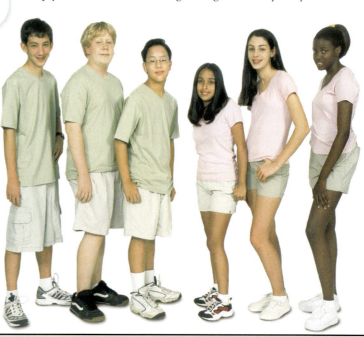

Figure 6 There is no such thing as a normal body shape or size.

BIOLOGY CONNECTION
Explain to students that adult BMI guidelines are unsuitable for teenagers because of the physical changes taking place during puberty. During puberty, an average healthy girl's body fat changes from about 16 percent body fat to about 27 percent body fat. An average healthy boy's body fat changes from about 5 percent body fat to about 11 percent body fat.

Chapter Resource File
- Directed Reading **BASIC**
- Lesson Plan
- Lesson Quiz **GENERAL**

Transparencies
TT Bellringer

What Affects Your Weight?

Many factors affect your weight. You inherit traits for body size and shape from your parents. These traits play a role in your height and weight as you become an adult. Here are some other factors that may affect your weight:

- Teens go through a period of rapid growth, which can cause a natural, healthy weight gain.
- Hormonal changes, especially in girls, can cause changes in a teen's weight.
- The types of food you eat can affect your weight.
- Your level of physical activity can affect your weight.

Keeping a Healthy Weight

Eating a healthy diet and balancing the food you eat with physical activity will help you keep a healthy weight. Your body uses the food you eat for energy. You use some of this energy to keep your body systems working. You use some of it for exercise, such as riding your bike or playing sports.

If you eat more food than your body can use for your daily activities, you will gain weight. If you eat the same amount of food that your body needs daily, you will maintain your weight. Similarly, if your body uses more energy than the energy you get from the food you eat, you will lose weight.

After you find your healthy weight range, you should balance the amount of food you eat with enough physical activity to stay in your healthy weight range.

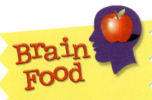

About 54 percent of teens describe their weight as "about right." Twenty-five percent of teens view themselves as overweight. About 58 percent of teens exercise to maintain their weight, while about 40 percent try to control how much food they eat.

Figure 7 Balancing the food you eat with physical activity helps you stay in your healthy weight range.

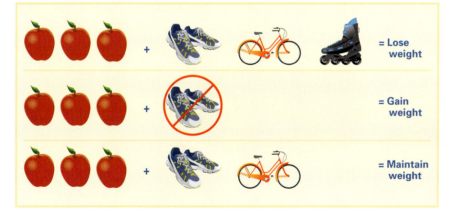

Background

Body Fat Distribution and Health The risks associated with being overweight and obese are related to the location of the excess fat in the body. Some people carry their excess fat around and above the waist. This body shape often is called an *apple* body shape. Others carry it below the waist in the hips and thighs. This is called the *pear* body shape. Studies have shown that people with apple-shaped bodies are more likely to develop heart disease, high blood pressure, stroke, diabetes, and breast cancer than people with pear-shaped bodies.

Teach

READING SKILL BUILDER — GENERAL

Reading Organizer Have students make an outline of the material on this page by using the heads provided in the text. Then, as students read this page, have them fill in their outlines with information from the text. **LS Logical**

Life SKILL BUILDER — GENERAL

Practicing Wellness Have students prepare a sample day's diet and physical activity program. They should suggest foods for breakfast, lunch, dinner, and snacks, and then recommend physical activities. Students should include "lifestyle" activities, such as taking the stairs, as well as more structured exercise routines. Students can post their plans for others to review. **LS Logical**

Demonstration — BASIC

Healthy Balance Tell students' that the information in the figure on this page can be represented by a see-saw. Build a model of a seesaw using cardboard. Label one end of the seesaw "Gain Weight" and the other end of the seesaw "Lose Weight." Explain to students that if the seesaw is balanced, it represents "Maintain Weight." Then, have different students call out different daily activities that might make the seesaw move back and forth. Activities can include several things such as eating meals, taking the stairs, playing in sports, or playing with friends.
LS Kinesthetic

Activity — GENERAL

Weight Managment Brochure Have each student write a brochure about healthy weight management. The brochure should be similar to one that might be found in a doctor's office. When students are finished with their brochures, they should share each other's finished products. **LS Visual**

Lesson 4 • Managing Your Weight

Teach, continued

Answer to Health Journal
This Health Journal can be used to begin a class discussion on food and feelings. Remember that some students may be uncomfortable sharing personal information.

Demonstration — BASIC
Why Do We Eat? Before students read this section, bring some cookies or candies to class and offer them to students. As the students are eating their treats, ask them why people eat. (The most likely answers will be hunger and the need for sustenance.) If students fail to mention desire, rather than a need, as a reason for eating, ask them why they chose to eat the treat you just offered them. Have students consider the reasons people eat foods that are not healthy. (Answers may include taste, the influence of food advertisements, and pleasant sensations caused by the food.) **LS Kinesthetic**

Group Activity — GENERAL
Healthy Diet Have groups of students use the information under the Eating Healthfully head to design a healthy menu for a week. After the groups create a menu, they should write a brief paragraph explaining their choices. **LS Verbal**

Health Journal
Keep an eating journal for 2 days. Each day, write down everything you eat or drink. Next to each entry, write down your reasons for eating. For example, did you eat because you were bored, upset, or excited, or because you were hungry? After the 2 days, look at your entries. Did you eat only when you were hungry? If not, which emotions made you feel like eating? How can you change your emotional eating patterns?

Why Do You Eat?
Do you know why you eat when you eat? You may think that the answer is because you are hungry. Most people eat when they are hungry. However, other reasons may affect your decision to eat. Sometimes, your emotions may make you feel like eating even if you are not hungry. Or they may make you feel like not eating at all. Here are some situations that may affect your decision to eat:

- nervousness
- anger
- sadness
- happiness
- a family gathering or a friend's party
- a holiday, such as Thanksgiving

Sometimes, when your feelings affect the way you eat, your food choices may be unhealthy. If you know how your feelings affect your eating habits, you can make healthful food choices.

Eating Healthfully
Eating a well-balanced diet is a good way to keep a healthy weight. Here are some tips for making good nutritional choices:

- Eat plenty of fresh fruits and vegetables every day.
- Drink water or juice rather than soda with each meal.
- Eat lean meat, chicken, or fish.
- Limit the amount of fried foods that you eat, such as french fries and potato chips.
- Limit the amount of sweets that you eat, such as candies, cookies, and cakes.

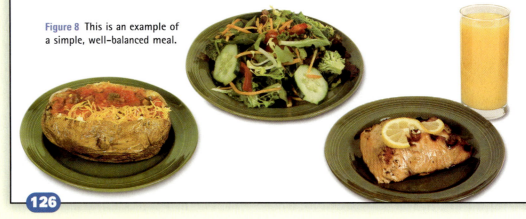

Figure 8 This is an example of a simple, well-balanced meal.

Career
Dietitians Health professionals that help people make good food choices are called *dietitians*. Dietitians take courses in college to train them in nutrition, food chemistry, and diet planning. These health professionals work closely with physicians to create diets specifically designed for their patients. Many people suffering from lifestyle illnesses, such as heart disease, must use dietitians to regain their health.

126 Chapter 6 • A HEALTHY BODY, a HEALTHY WEIGHT

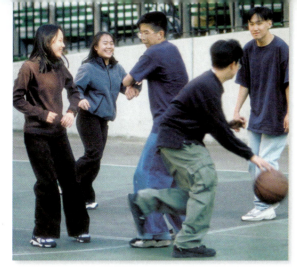

Figure 9 Going outside and having fun with your friends is a great way to stay physically active.

Staying Physically Active

Being physically active is a great way to keep a healthy weight. Being physically active does not mean you have to play sports. You don't even have to follow an exercise routine to be physically active. Activities such as in-line skating and riding bikes are great ways to stay physically active. You can also stay physically active by helping out around the house, gardening, or walking around the neighborhood. It is great if you enjoy playing sports or exercising. However, you don't have to be an athlete to enjoy being physically active. Regular physical activity can help you feel good about your body. These feelings will help you build a healthy body image. Being regularly active will also help you keep a healthy weight.

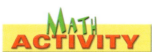

The energy you get from food is measured in units called Calories. Suppose you ate a cheeseburger for lunch. The cheeseburger contained 300 Calories. If running around the track uses 480 Calories an hour, how long would you have to run to use all the energy you got from the cheeseburger?

Lesson Review

Vocabulary

1. How do you find your healthy weight range?

Understanding Concepts

2. Explain how to stay within your healthy weight range.
3. Explain how your feelings may affect your eating habits.
4. Describe five factors that influence your weight.

Critical Thinking

5. **Applying Concepts** Imagine your family doctor told you that you are below your healthy weight range. Make a plan that will help you get to a healthy weight. Suppose your doctor said that you are over your healthy weight range. How would your plan change?

Activity — GENERAL

Exercise Education Have students research different sports or other forms of exercise. Students should then give the class a presentation about the exercise. The presentation should include the level of difficulty of the exercise, the benefits of the exercise, and a demonstration of how to safely perform the exercise. **LS Kinesthetic**

Answer to Math Activity
If running around the track requires 480 Calories per hour, a person running around the track burns 8 Calories per minute (480 Calories ÷ 60 minutes = 8 Calories/minute). So, if a person wanted to burn 300 Calories, he or she would have to run around the track for 37.5 minutes (300 Calories ÷ 8 Calories/minute = 37.5 minutes).

Close

Reteaching — BASIC

Poster Project Organize students into groups. Have each group create a poster that discusses the different ways a person can manage his or her weight. The poster should include suggestions for eating healthfully and staying active. **LS Logical**

Quiz — GENERAL

Tell students to answer the following true/false questions.

1. Dried fruit is a healthy snack. (true)
2. Exercising only once in a while can help you maintain your weight. (false)
3. Only hunger encourages you to eat. (false)
4. The amount of food you eat and your level of physical activity should balance out for you to maintain your current weight. (true)

Answers to Lesson Review

1. You can use the body mass index, or BMI, table to find your healthy weight range.
2. Sample answer: If I eat as much food as I need for the energy I use to exercise and maintain my body functions, I will keep my weight within my healthy weight range.
3. Sample answer: Feeling angry, depressed, nervous, or excited may lead a person to eat. Being in social situations may also lead a person to eat. Our feelings may make us eat even if we aren't hungry.
4. The traits you inherit from your parents, periods of growth, hormonal changes, your level of physical activity, and the types of food you eat can influence your weight.
5. Sample answer: I would ask my doctor about which healthful foods I would need to eat in order to gain weight, and I would make sure that I am eating a balanced diet. Also, I would try to eat more food than I would need for my daily activites. If my doctor told me I was over my healthy weight range, I would try to eat smaller meals and be more physically active.

CHAPTER 6 REVIEW

Assignment Guide

Lesson	Review Questions
1	3, 10, 15
2	11, 16–17
3	1–2, 4–6, 8, 18–20
4	7, 9, 12–14, 21–23

ANSWERS

Using Vocabulary

1. A person who has anorexia nervosa forces himself or herself to eat very little food. A person who has bulimia nervosa eats a lot of food at one time, and then he or she purges afterwards.
2. A fad diet promises fast weight loss with little effort. People follow fad diets because they want to lose weight quickly. An eating disorder is a disease in which a person has an unhealthy concern with his or her weight. An eating disorder is far more dangerous than a fad diet.
3. body image
4. Bulimia nervosa
5. eating disorder
6. fad diet

Understanding Concepts

7. Sample answer: You can maintain your weight by eating a balanced diet and exercising enough to use the energy you received from the food you ate.
8. Sample answer: It is very important to tell a trusted adult about a friend who may have an eating disorder because that person may not recognize his or her own problem and may need professional help.

CHAPTER 6 REVIEW

Chapter Summary

- Your body image is the way you see and imagine your body. Your body image can affect many aspects of your life. ■ If you have a healthy body image, you will be less likely to want to change your body for unhealthy reasons. ■ Your body image is influenced by the media, your family, and friends, and your teachers and coaches. ■ You can maintain your healthy body image by using "I" statements to deal with unkind remarks from other people. ■ Unhealthy eating behaviors, such as dieting, can develop into an eating disorder. ■ Eating disorders are very dangerous and may result in death. ■ Each person has a different healthy weight range. You can keep a healthy weight by eating well and staying active.

Using Vocabulary

For each pair of terms, describe how the meanings of the terms differ.

1. anorexia nervosa/bulimia nervosa
2. fad diet/eating disorder

For each sentence, fill in the blank with the proper word from the word bank provided below.

> healthy weight range
> fad diet
> bulimia nervosa
> binge eating disorder
> eating disorder
> body image

3. The way you see, imagine, and feel about your body is called your ___.
4. ___ is an illness in which a person eats a large amount of food and then purges.
5. An illness in which a person is overly concerned about his or her body weight and shape is a(n) ___.
6. An eating plan that promises quick weight loss is called a(n) ___.

Understanding Concepts

7. Explain how to keep a healthy weight by eating well and staying physically active.
8. Describe the importance of telling an adult if you suspect your friend has an eating disorder.
9. How can your level of physical activity affect your weight?
10. Why is having a healthy body image important?
11. Describe three factors that influence your body image. How do these factors influence you?
12. What is a healthy weight range? Does every person have the same healthy weight range? Explain your answer.
13. What are some feelings that may affect your eating habits?
14. List five ways to make healthy food choices.
15. Explain the difference between healthy body image and unhealthy body image.
16. Explain how using "I" statements can help you build a healthy body image.

---

9. If you eat the same amount of food every day, and you aren't physically active, you will gain weight because you are not being active enough to use the extra Calories from the food you ate. However, if you exercise only enough to use the Calories you got from food, then you will maintain your weight. If you have a high level of physical activity, you will use more Calories than you received from the food you ate, so you will lose weight.

10. A healthy body image helps a person have high self-esteem and confidence. It also keeps a person from developing an eating disorder.

11. Answers may vary. Sample answer: Family, friends, and the media all influence your body image.

12. A healthy weight range is an estimate of how much you should weigh depending on your height and body frame. Since different people have different body frames, different people have different healthy weight ranges.

13. Sample answer: Some feelings that may affect my eating habits include nervousness, anger, or excitement.

14. Sample answer: eat lean meats, eat low-fat foods, eat fruits and vegetables, drink plenty of water, limit sweets

Critical Thinking

Making Inferences

17. Megan compares herself to the teens she sees in magazines. She thinks that she needs to look like the teen models in order to be popular at school. She decides to go on a diet. Does Megan have a healthy body image? What could happen to Megan if she continues to diet?

18. Michael admits to you that he has a problem controlling how much he eats. He tells you that sometimes he just can't stop eating, and afterwards he feels ashamed of himself. Michael asks you to not tell anyone about his problem. What kind of problem does Michael have? What will happen to him if he does not get help from an adult? What can you do to help him?

Using Refusal Skills

19. Tracy tells you that she purges after she eats lunch. She tells you that if you purge every day after lunch for the next week, you will be thinner for the school dance. Tracy tells you that purging is okay because you are going to do it for only a short period of time. What will you say to Tracy?

20. Rebecca brings diet pills to school. You overhear Rebecca telling your best friend that one pill will help your friend burn more Calories than if she exercised for 1 hour. Your friend is tempted to try the pills. How can you help your friend refuse Rebecca's diet pills?

Interpreting Graphics

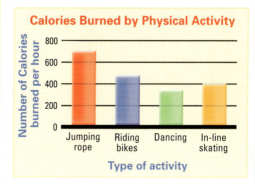

Use the figure above to answer questions 21–23.

21. Imagine that you are trying to maintain your healthy weight. Your food intake for the day was 2,500 Calories. How many hours would you have to jump rope to burn half of these Calories?

22. Your friend Rachel dances for 1 hour every day after school. She does not dance on the weekends. How many Calories does Rachel use for dancing in 1 week?

23. Tom in-line skates for 2 hours each week. He also rides his bike for 3 hours each week. How many Calories does Tom use for these two physical activities each week?

Reading Checkup

Take a minute to review your answers to the Health IQ questions at the beginning of this chapter. How has reading this chapter improved your Health IQ?

15. A person who has a healthy body image feels comfortable with himself or herself, has high self-esteem, and is more likely to feel confident in new situations. A person who has a negative body image has low self-esteem, doesn't like to try new things, is uncomfortable with his or her body, and tends to not do well in school.

16. Using "I" statements can help me build a healthy body image by helping me express my feelings. If someone says something about my appearance, I can use "I" statements to tell that person how I feel about my body.

Critical Thinking

Making Inferences

17. Sample answer: Megan does not have a healthy body image. She is comparing herself to unrealistic images. If she tries to force herself to look like a model, she may develop a serious eating disorder.

18. Sample answer: Michael suffers from binge eating disorder. If he keeps binge eating, he may become obese. I should tell Michael to get help. If he doesn't get help on his own, I should go to a trusted adult and have him or her help Michael.

Using Refusal Skills

19. Sample answer: I would tell her that purging can be damaging to her body even if she does it only a few times. Also, I would tell her that she may not be able to stop purging, even if she does it only a few times.

20. Sample answer: I would tell my friend that the pills may cause serious damage to her body. Also, I would explain to her that there is no proven way to lose weight quickly. The best way to lose weight is through eating a balanced diet and exercising.

Interpreting Graphics

21. 1.78 hours

22. 1,750 Calories (350 Cal/hr × 5 hours = 1,750 Calories)

23. 2,225 Calories per week ([400 Cal/hr × 2] + [475 Cal/hr × 3] = 2,225 Calories)

Chapter Resource File

- Concept Review GENERAL
- Concept Mapping GENERAL
- Performance-Based Assessment GENERAL
- Chapter Test GENERAL

Model

Introduce this activity by reminding students that using this Life Skill will help them take personal responsibility for their behavior. Then, review the scenario with the class.

Prepare students for this activity by modeling each of the steps of the skill. Make sure students understand each step before you move on to the next one.

Guided Practice: Practice with a Friend

Guided Practice is the stage in which you and the students analyze their approach to solving the problem given in the scenario and analyze their ability to practice wellness. Have students read Act 1. Discuss with the class the situation described and the way students are to act it out. Organize the class into groups of three. In each group, one person plays the role of Alan, another person plays the dietitian, and the third person is the observer.

Proper pacing during the Guided Practice is important. The suggestions listed below will help you control the pace.

1. Stop after completing each step of practicing wellness.
2. Discuss with each group the observer's comments.
3. Ask the other members of each group to listen to the observer's suggestions and to suggest ways to improve the way they practice wellness.
4. Instruct students to repeat the steps that need improvement and to include their modifications.

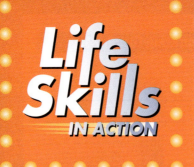

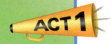

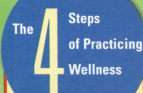

The 4 Steps of Practicing Wellness

1. Choose a health behavior you want to improve or change.
2. Gather information on how you can improve that health behavior.
3. Start using the improved health behavior.
4. Evaluate the effects of the health behavior.

Practicing Wellness

Practicing wellness means practicing good health habits. Positive health behaviors can help prevent injury, illness, disease, and even premature death. Complete the following activity to learn how you can practice wellness.

The Junk Food Junkie

Setting the Scene

Alan loves eating junk food. He uses all of his allowance to buy pizza, chips, and other junk food. One day, a dietitian gives a talk to his health class. During her talk, the dietitian shows the class how much fat is in a serving of french fries and how much sugar is in a can of soda. Alan is surprised to learn how unhealthy junk food is and begins to think about changing his eating habits.

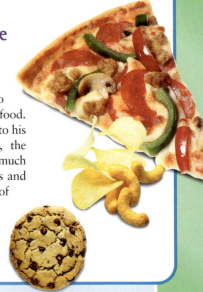

Guided Practice

Practice with a Friend

Form a group of three. Have one person play the role of Alan and another person play the role of the dietitian. Have the third person be an observer. Walking through each of the four steps of practicing wellness, role-play Alan learning to improve his eating habits. Alan can talk to the dietitian to gather information about nutrition. The observer will take notes, which will include observations about what the person playing Alan did well and suggestions of ways to improve. Stop after each step to evaluate the process.

5. Check to make sure that students understand each step before they move on to the next step.
6. If time permits, repeat the exercise three times, switching roles each time. Each student should have the opportunity to play each role. Co-op Learning

Independent Practice

Check Yourself

After you have completed the guided practice, go through Act 1 again without stopping at each step. Answer the questions below to review what you did.

1. In addition to talking with the dietitian, how can Alan find information about good eating habits?
2. What are some specific examples of what Alan could do to improve his health behavior?
3. How could Alan evaluate the effects of changing his eating habits?
4. What are some ways that you can improve your eating habits?

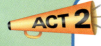

On Your Own

Alan has been eating better for a month, and he is feeling great. Improving his eating habits has caused him to think about his overall health. Alan wonders if he is getting enough exercise. He spends most of his afternoons watching TV or playing video games. Make a poster showing how Alan could use the four steps of practicing wellness to begin an exercise program.

Independent Practice: Check Yourself

Instruct students to repeat Act 1 without stopping at each step. Remind students to apply what they learned in the Guided Practice to the Independent Practice.

Encourage students to use the Check Yourself questions as a starting point for reviewing and analyzing their Independent Practice. Remind students that as they change roles, the answers to these questions may change for each actor. Encourage students to create additional questions for checking their ability to practice wellness. When students have finished the Independent Practice, have them answer the Check Yourself questions in writing. Use their answers to assess their understanding of the steps of practicing wellness and to assess their use of the steps to solve a problem.

Check Yourself Answers

1. Sample answer: Alan can read books on nutrition or search reliable Web sites to find information about good eating habits.
2. Sample answer: To improve his health behavior, Alan could eat foods that are low in fat, eat plenty of fruits and vegetables, and drink fewer sodas.
3. Sample answer: To evaluate his eating habits, Alan could keep a journal of what he eats and how he feels each day. Alan could also compare his food intake with the suggested guidelines shown in the Food Pyramid.
4. Sample answer: I could eat fewer candy bars and eat less fried foods.

Act 2: On Your Own

This additional scenario gives students an opportunity to apply what they have learned in both the Guided Practice and the Independent Practice to a new situation.

Suggest to students that they use the Check Yourself questions as a starting point for practicing wellness in the new situation. Encourage students to be creative and to think of ways to improve their ability to practice wellness.

Assessment

Review the posters that students have created as part of the On Your Own activity. The posters should show that the students followed the steps of practicing wellness in a realistic and effective manner. Display the posters around the room. If time permits, discuss some of the posters with the class.

CHAPTER 7: Mental and Emotional Health
Chapter Planning Guide

PACING	CLASSROOM RESOURCES	ACTIVITIES AND DEMONSTRATIONS
BLOCK 1 • 45 min pp. 132–137 **Chapter Opener**	CRF Health Inventory * ■ GENERAL CRF Parent Letter * ■	SE Health IQ, p. 133 CRF At-Home Activity * ■
Lesson 1 Kinds of Emotions	CRF Lesson Plan * TT Bellringer * TT Emotional Spectrum *	SE Social Studies Activity, p. 135 ◆ TE Activity Drawing Spectrums, p. 135 BASIC TE Group Activity Basic Emotions, p. 137 BASIC CRF Enrichment Activity * ADVANCED
BLOCK 2 • 45 min pp. 138–143 **Lesson 2** Expressing Emotions	CRF Lesson Plan * TT Bellringer *	TE Activities Body Language, p. 131F TE Activity A Picture Is Worth 1000 Words . . . , p. 138 GENERAL SE Life Skills in Action Communicating Effectively, pp. 154–155 CRF Life Skills Activity * ■ GENERAL CRF Enrichment Activity * ADVANCED
Lesson 3 Managing Your Emotions	CRF Lesson Plan * TT Bellringer * TT Positive Self-Talk *	TE Activities Thinking Positively, p. 131F TE Activity Comic Strip, p. 140 GENERAL TE Demonstration Stress Relief, p. 141 BASIC SE Hands-on Activity, p. 142 CRF Datasheets for In-Text Activities * GENERAL CRF Enrichment Activity * ADVANCED
BLOCK 3 • 45 min pp. 144–147 **Lesson 4** Mental Illness	CRF Lesson Plan * TT Bellringer *	TE Demonstration Filtering Stimuli, p. 146 ◆ ADVANCED CRF Enrichment Activity * ADVANCED
BLOCK 4 • 45 min pp. 148–151 **Lesson 5** Getting Help	CRF Lesson Plan * TT Bellringer *	TE Activity Skit, p. 148 GENERAL TE Group Activity Community Mental Health Resources, p. 150 GENERAL CRF Life Skills Activity * ■ GENERAL CRF Enrichment Activity * ADVANCED

BLOCKS 5 & 6 • 90 min
Chapter Review and Assessment Resources

- SE Chapter Review, pp. 152–153
- CRF Concept Review * ■ GENERAL
- CRF Health Behavior Contract * ■ GENERAL
- CRF Chapter Test * ■ GENERAL
- CRF Performance-Based Assessment * GENERAL
- OSP Test Generator
- CRF Test Item Listing *

Online Resources

Visit **go.hrw.com** for a variety of free resources related to this textbook. Enter the keyword **HD4ME7**.

Students can access interactive problem solving help and active visual concept development with the *Decisions for Health* Online Edition available at **www.hrw.com**.

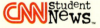

cnnstudentnews.com

Find the latest health news, lesson plans, and activities related to important scientific events.

Compression guide:
To shorten your instruction because of time limitations, omit Lesson 4.

KEY
- **TE** Teacher Edition
- **SE** Student Edition
- **OSP** One-Stop Planner
- **CRF** Chapter Resource File
- **TT** Teaching Transparency
- ✱ Also on One-Stop Planner
- ■ Also Available in Spanish
- ◆ Requires Advance Prep

SKILLS DEVELOPMENT RESOURCES	LESSON REVIEW AND ASSESSMENT	STANDARDS CORRELATION
		National Health Education Standards
TE Life Skill Builder Assessing Your Health, p. 135 TE Inclusion Strategies, p. 135 `GENERAL` TE Life Skill Builder Evaluating Media Messages, p. 136 `ADVANCED` CRF Cross-Disciplinary * `GENERAL` CRF Directed Reading * `BASIC`	SE Lesson Review, p. 137 TE Reteaching, Quiz, p. 137 CRF Lesson Quiz * ■ `GENERAL`	1.2, 5.8
SE Life Skills Activity Communicating Effectively, p. 139 TE Inclusion Strategies, p. 139 `GENERAL` CRF Refusal Skills * `GENERAL` CRF Directed Reading * `BASIC`	SE Lesson Review, p. 139 TE Reteaching, Quiz, p. 139 CRF Lesson Quiz * ■ `GENERAL`	3.4, 5.1, 5.3, 5.5, 7.1, 7.2
SE Life Skills Activity Coping, p. 141 TE Life Skill Builder Assessing Your Health, p. 141 `BASIC` TE Reading Skill Builder Discussion, p. 142 `BASIC` CRF Decision-Making * `GENERAL` CRF Refusal Skills * `GENERAL` CRF Directed Reading * `BASIC`	SE Lesson Review, p. 143 TE Reteaching, Quiz, p. 143 TE Alternative Assessment, p. 143 `ADVANCED` CRF Concept Mapping * `GENERAL` CRF Lesson Quiz * ■ `GENERAL`	1.2, 1.6, 3.4, 3.7, 5.8
TE Life Skill Builder Making Good Decisions, p. 145 `BASIC` TE Life Skill Builder Coping, p. 145 CRF Cross-Disciplinary * `GENERAL` CRF Directed Reading * `BASIC`	SE Lesson Review, p. 147 TE Reteaching, Quiz, p. 147 TE Alternative Assessment, p. 147 `ADVANCED` CRF Lesson Quiz * ■ `GENERAL`	1.1, 1.5, 1.7, 1.8, 2.6, 3.4, 3.5
TE Life Skill Builder Making Good Decisions, p. 149 `GENERAL` SE Study Tip Organizing Information, p. 150 SE Life Skills Activity Making Good Decisions, p. 151 CRF Decision-Making * `GENERAL` CRF Directed Reading * `BASIC`	SE Lesson Review, p. 151 TE Reteaching, Quiz, p. 151 TE Alternative Assessment, p. 151 `GENERAL` CRF Concept Mapping * `GENERAL` CRF Lesson Quiz * ■ `GENERAL`	1.1, 1.4, 1.6, 1.7, 2.2, 2.4, 2.6, 3.4, 3.5, 4.4, 5.2, 7.4

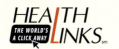

www.scilinks.org/health
Maintained by the **National Science Teachers Association**

Topic: Emotions
HealthLinks code: HD4035
Topic: Schizophrenia
HealthLinks code: HD4085
Topic: Bipolar Disorder
HealthLinks code: HD4014
Topic: Anxiety Disorders
HealthLinks code: HD4010

Technology Resources

 One-Stop Planner
All of your printable resources and the Test Generator are on this convenient CD-ROM.

 Guided Reading Audio CDs

VIDEO SELECT
For information about videos related to this chapter, go to **go.hrw.com** and type in the keyword **HD4ME7V**.

Chapter 7: Mental and Emotional Health
Chapter Resources

Teacher Resources

TEACHING TRANSPARENCIES

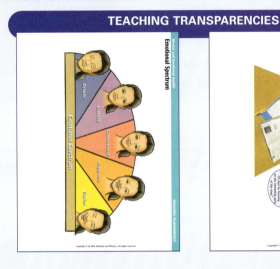
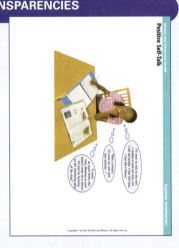

BELLRINGER TRANSPARENCIES

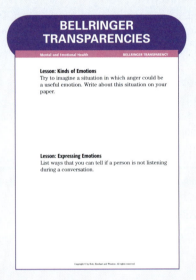

LESSON PLANS

PARENT LETTER
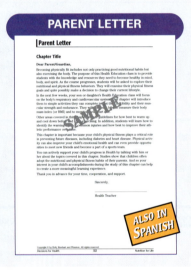
ALSO IN SPANISH

TEST ITEM LISTING
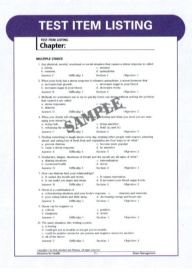

Meeting Individual Needs

DIRECTED READING
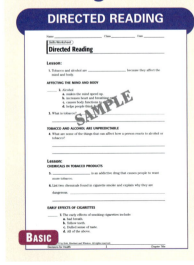
BASIC

CONCEPT MAPPING
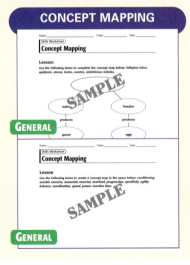
GENERAL

CONCEPT REVIEW
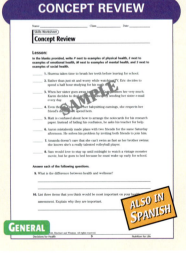
GENERAL — *ALSO IN SPANISH*

ENRICHMENT ACTIVITIES
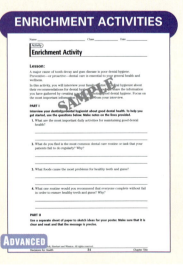
ADVANCED

Resources

These worksheet pages can be found in the Chapter Resource File and the One-Stop Planner. The transparencies can be found in the Teaching Transparencies binder and on the One-Stop Planner.

Activities

LIFE SKILLS ACTIVITIES
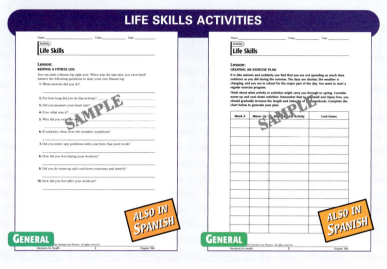

AT-HOME ACTIVITY
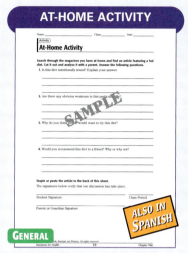

DATASHEETS FOR IN-TEXT ACTIVITIES
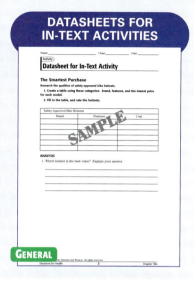

Applications

DECISION-MAKING
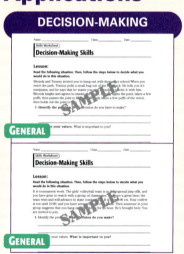

REFUSAL SKILLS
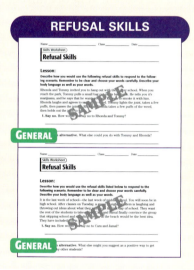

CROSS-DISCIPLINARY
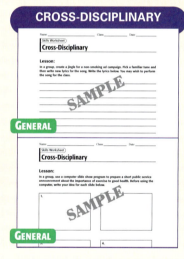

HEALTH BEHAVIOR CONTRACT
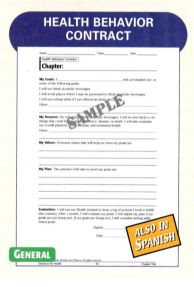

Assessments

HEALTH INVENTORY
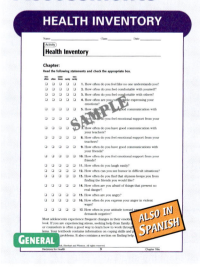

LESSON QUIZZES
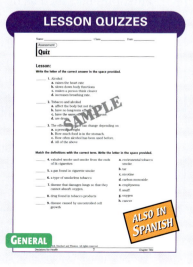

CHAPTER TEST
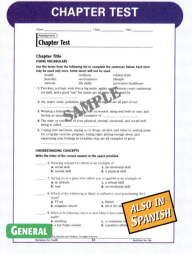

PERFORMANCE-BASED ASSESSMENT
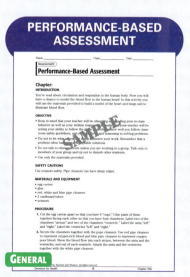

Chapter 7 • Chapter Resources and Worksheets   131D

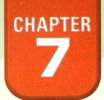

Background Information

The following information focuses on mental illness. This material will help prepare you for teaching the concepts in this chapter.

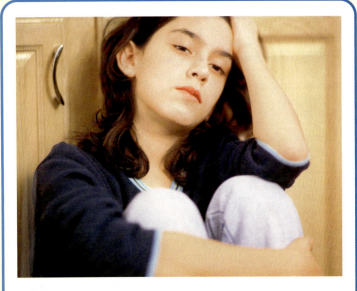

Mood Disorders and Suicide

- About 18.8 million Americans suffer from mood disorders, such as depression and bipolar disorder. Most of these people can be helped through therapy and medication. Unfortunately, many people who suffer from mood disorders do not seek treatment.

- Treatment often includes therapy and medication. Sometimes medications or viral infections cause symptoms that mimic depression. These causes should be ruled out before a person is treated for depression.

- The cause of mood disorders is not clearly understood. Some types, including bipolar disorder, appear to have a genetic link. However, these problems can also occur in people who have no family history of the disease.

- Young people who have substance abuse problems may be suffering from depression. Some people suffering from depression abuse alcohol or other drugs in an attempt to feel differently or forget the problem. It is important to remember that anyone can be depressed—high achievers and class clowns may also suffer from depression.

- Although women experience depression about twice as often as men, men are less likely to admit that they are depressed. The rate of successful suicide in men suffering from depression is three to four times that of depressed women. This is because women who attempt suicide often choose less lethal methods than those methods chosen by men.

- More than 30,000 Americans commit suicide successfully every year. The incidence of suicide among young adults and teenagers nearly tripled in the 30 years between 1965 and 1995. More young adults and teenagers die from suicide than die from the combined effects of AIDS, chronic drug use, birth defects, pneumonia, influenza, stroke, heart disease, and cancer.

- The two most important things someone can do for a depressed person are to 1) help the person get an appropriate diagnosis and treatment, and 2) offer emotional support throughout the treatment cycle.

Schizophrenia

- Schizophrenia affects about 2.2 million Americans. Although schizophrenia can affect people at any age, most cases develop between the late teens and the middle 30s. The cause of schizophrenia is not known. However, as with many mental illnesses, schizophrenia appears to have a genetic link in some cases. In some cases, life experiences trigger the illness in an individual.

- Changes in certain neurotransmitters, such as serotonin and dopamine, play a role in the development of schizophrenia. Often, medications that are used to treat schizophrenia try to control the levels of these neurotransmitters in the brain. In many cases, antipsychotic medications can relieve symptoms of schizophrenia, such as disorganized thinking, delusions, and hallucinations.

- Suicide is the number one cause of death among people who have schizophrenia. About 10 to 13 percent of people who suffer from schizophrenia commit suicide. Educating people about the cause, experience, and treatment of mental illness may help reduce these numbers. It is important that people understand that treatment often relieves the symptoms of mental illnesses, including schizophrenia. Medication and therapy can have a dramatic effect on schizophrenia.

For background information about teaching strategies and issues, refer to the *Professional Reference for Teachers*.

ACTIVITIES

CHAPTER 7

Consider using the activities on this page as students explore the lessons of this chapter. Look for other activities throughout the Student Edition chapter.

Body Language

Procedure Organize students into groups of six. Give each group six slips of paper that have the following emotions written on them: anger, fear, sadness, happiness, love, and surprise. Have each student pick one slip of paper without showing the other students what their slip says. Tell students that body language expresses thoughts and emotions by moving the face and parts of the body, but does not involve speech or words. Ask students to use only body language to communicate the emotion listed on his or her slip of paper. The other students in the group should guess what emotion is being communicated. Have students continue the activity until all members of the group have had a chance to communicate the emotion they picked.

Analysis Ask the following questions to each group:

- Were you tempted to speak when communicating emotions? (Answers will vary.) Why or why not? (Some students may say that speaking would make it easier to communicate.)

- Are some emotions easier to communicate through body language than others? (Answers will vary. Some students will find that certain emotions, such as love, are harder to communicate than others.)

- Do you think body language is a good way to communicate emotions? (Answers will vary. Some students may say that a combination of body language and spoken language is the most effective way to communicate emotions.)

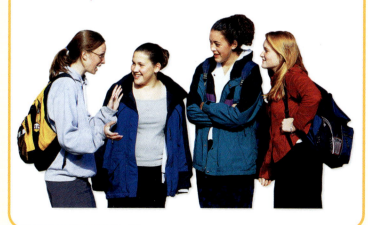

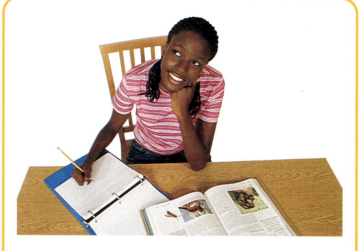

Thinking Positively

Procedure Tell students to take out a piece of paper and fold it lengthwise to make two columns. At the top of one column, have students write "Negative Thought." Ask students to choose one of the following statements and fill in the blank. "I have trouble with my ___ class," "My brother/sister/friend really bugs me when ___," or "I don't think I'll ever be able to ___." The students should write the statement in the "Negative Thought" column. Then have students use positive self-talk to change how a person might think about the negative thought. Next to the negative thought, students should write a positive statement that would help someone think differently about the negative idea. For example, to address a negative thought such as, "I don't think I'll ever be able to make the baseball team," a student could write, "I enjoy playing and watching baseball. I can practice after school to get better." Give more examples if students appear to have trouble with positive thinking.

Analysis Ask students the following questions:

- How could acting on the positive thoughts help a person stop having negative thoughts? (Acting on a positive thought can often solve the problem that caused the negative thinking. Once the problem is removed, the negative thoughts will go away.)

- Do you think you could use positive thinking on your own when problems come up? (Answers may vary. Most would say yes.)

Chapter 7 • Activities 131F

CHAPTER 7

Overview
Tell students that this chapter will help them learn about mental and emotional health. Students will learn how to express emotions constructively and how to seek help for emotional problems. Students will also learn about mental illness and about the work done by mental health professionals.

Assessing Prior Knowledge
Students should be familiar with the following topics:
- refusal skills
- decision making
- physical health
- self-esteem

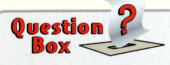

Students may feel more comfortable asking questions if you set up a Question Box to collect their questions. Have students write and anonymously submit their questions about mental and emotional health, mental illness, or finding help for emotional problems. Address these questions during class, or use these questions to introduce lessons that cover related topics.

Current Health
Check out *Current Health* articles and activities related to this chapter by visiting the HRW Web site at **go.hrw.com**. Just type in the keyword **HD4CH22T**.

Chapter Resource File
- Directed Reading BASIC
- Health Inventory GENERAL
- Parent Letter

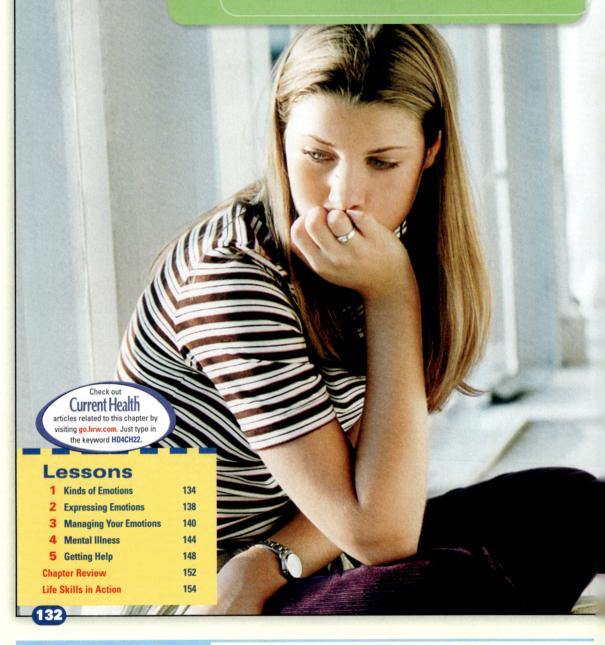

CHAPTER 7
Mental and Emotional Health

Check out **Current Health** articles related to this chapter by visiting **go.hrw.com**. Just type in the keyword **HD4CH22**.

Lessons
1	Kinds of Emotions	134
2	Expressing Emotions	138
3	Managing Your Emotions	140
4	Mental Illness	144
5	Getting Help	148
Chapter Review		152
Life Skills in Action		154

Standards Correlations

National Health Education Standards

1.2 Describe the interrelationships of mental, emotional, social, and physical health during adolescence. (Lessons 1 and 3)

1.4 Describe how family and peers influence the health of adolescents. (Lesson 5)

1.5 Analyze how environment and personal health are interrelated. (Lesson 4)

1.6 Describe ways to reduce risks related to adolescent health problems. (Lessons 3 and 5)

1.7 Explain how appropriate health care can prevent premature death and disability. (Lessons 4–5)

1.8 (partial) Describe how lifestyle, pathogens, family history, and other risk factors are related to the cause or prevention of disease and other health problems. (Lesson 4)

2.2 Demonstrate the ability to utilize resources from home, school, and community that provide valid health information. (Lessons 5)

2.4 (partial) Demonstrate the ability to locate health products and services. (Lesson 5)

2.6 Describe situations requiring professional health services. (Lessons 4–5)

> "I never knew that **depression** could be so **serious** until my dad was **diagnosed** with it. He said that it was different from just feeling **sad.** He goes to therapy and takes medicine, and he is becoming much more like himself again."

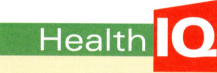

PRE-READING
Answer the following multiple-choice questions to find out what you already know about mental and emotional health. When you've finished this chapter, you'll have the opportunity to change your answers based on what you've learned.

1. Mental illness
   a. is very rare.
   b. happens only to people who have a weak mind.
   c. cannot be treated.
   d. affects thoughts, emotions, and behavior.

2. Which of the following statements is true?
   a. Teens can't manage their emotions.
   b. Hormones have nothing to do with emotions.
   c. Most teens are happy and well adjusted.
   d. It is normal to be depressed when you are a teenager.

3. Which of the following statements is true?
   a. Depression means being sad.
   b. Depression will go away if something good happens.
   c. Depression is a disorder that can lead to suicidal thinking.
   d. People who have depression are lazy.

4. A trigger is
   a. a person, thing, or event that causes an emotional response.
   b. a way of using body language to communicate.
   c. a way of thinking about emotional problems.
   d. a behavior used to cope with emotional stress.

5. Bipolar mood disorder
   a. is an illness that affects moods.
   b. includes a happy period called mania.
   c. is bad only during periods of depression.
   d. is an anxiety disorder.

ANSWERS: 1. d; 2. c; 3. c; 4. a; 5. a

Using the Health IQ

Misconception Alert
Answers to the Health IQ questions may help you identify students' misconceptions.

Question 2: Students may think that all teens are depressed and emotionally out of control, but this is not true. Teens do have to get used to new hormones and responsibilities, but most are well adjusted and take on this challenge successfully. Students should know that depression is not normal and that teens who are depressed should get help.

Question 3: Students may think that a person who is depressed is just sad or in a bad mood. It may be helpful to explain to students that depression is a mental illness that can lead to death when it causes suicidal thinking. Depression will not go away on its own or if something good happens. This illness requires professional treatment.

Answers
1. d
2. c
3. c
4. a
5. a

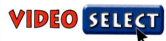

For information about videos related to this chapter, go to **go.hrw.com** and type in the keyword **HD4ME7V**.

3.4 (partial) Demonstrate strategies to improve or maintain personal and family health. (Lessons 2–5)

3.5 (partial) Develop injury prevention and management strategies for personal and family health. (Lessons 4–5)

3.7 Demonstrate strategies to manage stress. (Lesson 3)

4.4 Analyze how information from peers influences health. (Lesson 5)

5.1 Demonstrate effective verbal and non-verbal communication skills to enhance health. (Lesson 2)

5.2 Describe how the behavior of family and peers affects interpersonal communication. (Lesson 5)

5.5 Demonstrate communication skills to build and maintain healthy relationships. (Lesson 2)

5.8 Demonstrate strategies to manage conflict in healthy ways. (Lessons 1 and 3)

7.1 Analyze various communication methods to accurately express health information and ideas. (Lesson 2)

7.2 Express information and opinions about health issues. (Lesson 2)

7.4 Demonstrate the ability to influence and support others in making positive health choices. (Lesson 5)

Lesson 1

Focus

Overview

Before beginning this lesson, review with your students the objectives listed under the What You'll Do head in the Student Edition. In this lesson, students will learn how hormones and life changes affect teen emotions. Students will also learn about emotional spectrums and some specific emotions, such as love and anger. The lesson also describes how emotions can be recognized by the physical feelings that accompany the emotions.

Bellringer

Ask students to imagine and write about a situation in which anger could be a useful emotion. (Answers may vary. Sample answer: Anger at my grade on a test let me know that I should study more for the next test.)

Motivate

Discussion — GENERAL

New Responsibilities Most students are expected to help around their homes by washing dishes or doing other chores. Responsibilities often increase as a person grows more mature. Ask students if any of them have recently taken on any new responsibilities, such as a paper route, babysitting jobs, extra responsibilities around the house, or leadership positions in extracurricular activities. Remind students that these new situations may cause new emotions, problems, and successes in their lives. **LS Verbal**

Lesson 1

What You'll Do
- **Explain** how teens' changing lives and bodies affect their emotions.
- **Describe** how emotions can be pleasant or unpleasant.
- **Explain** how emotions can have physical effects.

Terms to Learn
- mental health
- emotion
- hormone
- emotional health

Start Off Write
How could unpleasant emotions be helpful to a person?

Kinds of Emotions

Hatim is confused about his emotions. Lately, he has been feeling really sensitive about everything. He finds himself arguing with his parents more often. He also gets upset at his friends a lot.

Being confused about new feelings is normal. Dealing with confusing feelings is part of good mental health. **Mental health** is the way people think about and respond to events in their lives.

Teen Emotions

People respond to the world around them with thoughts, actions, and emotions. An **emotion** is a feeling produced in response to a life event. Emotions are caused by chemical changes in the brain that affect how the body feels. Emotional reactions help people understand relationships, danger, success, and loss.

Both personality and experience influence a person's emotional responses. People are born with tendencies to respond to life in a certain way. But as they grow and experience more situations, people learn and change their emotional responses. Much of this learning happens during the teen years. Teens take on many new roles and responsibilities as they grow and mature. Reacting to these changes can produce unfamiliar feelings. Teens can learn and mature from these experiences and the emotions the experiences produce.

Teen emotions are also affected by the changes happening in their bodies. During the early teen years, the body produces new hormones. A **hormone** is a chemical that helps control how the body grows and functions. These chemicals can affect the brain and sometimes cause mood swings. Most teens find healthy ways to deal with the emotional changes they experience.

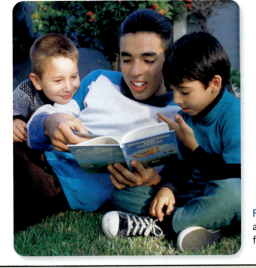

Figure 1 New responsibilities, such as babysitting, can cause teens to feel new emotions.

Answer to Start Off Write

Accept all reasonable answers. Sample answer: Unpleasant emotions, such as sadness, can help us appreciate losses and realize when we need to make changes in our lives.

Chapter Resource File
- Directed Reading **BASIC**
- Lesson Plan
- Lesson Quiz **GENERAL**

Transparencies
TT Bellringer
TT Emotional Spectrum

From Sadness to Happiness

Moods can range from very sad to very happy. Having such a wide range of moods is normal. Feeling a range of emotions is part of good emotional health. Emotional health is the way a person experiences and deals with feelings. Experiencing one emotion all the time—even happiness—would be unhealthy.

Unpleasant emotions, such as sadness, can be valuable. Sadness can help us remember and appreciate a loss. If a pet dies, sadness can help you understand how important the pet was to you. Sadness can also help you realize when you need to make changes in your life. Sadness about not doing well in school can help you decide to study more often or ask for help.

Emotions become unhealthy when they get in the way of relationships and responsibilities. For example, sadness is healthy. But skipping class because you are sad is unhealthy. Dealing with emotions in healthy ways keeps them from becoming unhealthy. Talking with someone when you are sad is a healthy way to deal with sadness.

Recognizing your emotions can help you deal with them in healthy ways. Your emotions can be easier to recognize when you know where they lie on an emotional spectrum. An *emotional spectrum* is a range of emotions organized by how pleasant they are. The figure below shows an emotional spectrum.

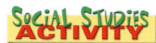

Do you think emotions are the same around the world? Many emotions can be expressed by a person's face and body language. Look through magazines that have pictures of people from different cultures. Can you recognize emotions in people all around the globe?

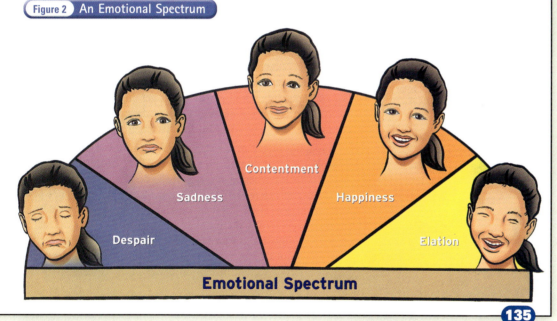

Figure 2 An Emotional Spectrum

Despair • Sadness • Contentment • Happiness • Elation

Emotional Spectrum

Life SKILL BUILDER

Assessing Your Health Sometimes emotional problems have physical causes. Anxiety is often a normal reaction to life events such as upcoming exams, the loss of a loved one, or a serious illness. But anxiety that is not related to stress may have a physical cause, such as an overactive thyroid gland. This is especially possible if feelings of anxiety are accompanied by weight loss and heavy perspiration. In cases where emotional problems do not have obvious causes, you should consult a physician to see if there may be a physical problem affecting your emotions. **LS** Intrapersonal

Answer to Social Studies Activity
Students should be able to recognize many emotions, such as happiness, sadness, anger, and fear, in photos of people all around the globe.

Teach

Activity — BASIC
Drawing Spectrums Have students draw emotional spectrums showing a range of emotions such as from hate to love, from confidence to fear, or from anger to contentment. Students can illustrate their spectrums with faces showing facial expressions. **LS** Visual

REAL-LIFE CONNECTION — GENERAL
Growing Up The new responsibilities taken on by teens can bring out new emotions in their lives. These responsibilities can also help teens feel more mature and maintain high self-esteem. Ask students to create posters full of ideas for how teens can express their maturity. Getting a job, such as doing a paper route or babysitting, is one way teens can express their maturity. Also, volunteering to work with children or with elderly people can help kids improve their self-esteem and encourage healthy emotions as they mature. Ask students to choose a new responsibility that appeals to them and write a paragraph explaining why they chose that responsibility.
LS Intrapersonal

INCLUSION Strategies — GENERAL
• Visually Impaired
Students with visual impairments will not be able to explore different emotions through the Emotional Spectrum graphic. Help them understand the idea of the emotional spectrum by identifying ways (other than facial expressions) that people express the different emotions. For example, you might describe how a person's voice changes with each emotion. Voices often sound more tense when expressing unpleasant emotions. **LS** Auditory

Lesson 1 • Kinds of Emotions

Teach, continued

Discussion — GENERAL

Comprehension Check Tell students to imagine the following scenario: "Your father has just lost his job. He comes home and slams the door, then yells at you to go put your bicycle away. He sits down to read the newspaper, then throws it down when he sees that you cut out an article for a school assignment." Then ask students, "Why might your father be acting this way?" (When people are angry about something, they often direct their anger towards someone or something else. Misdirected anger is causing your father to act this way. He isn't actually angry with you, but that he lost his job.) "What could he do differently to control his anger?" (He could accept that he needs to find another job and figure out a way to work on getting a new job.) **LS Logical**

Debate — GENERAL

Unconscious Prejudice Show students magazine photos of teens doing different activities. Ask the students if they think they'd like the teens in the photos. (Answers will vary.) Ask them why they think that way, and how they can have an impression without meeting that person. (Students may be considering how the teens look, the expressions on their faces, and the activities they are doing.) Point out that students were using prejudice to form their opinions. Then ask students to debate whether prejudice is always a bad thing, or whether it can sometimes be helpful and useful. Ask students to determine when prejudice is bad or unfair. **LS Visual/Logical**

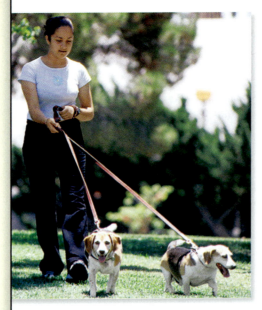

Figure 3 If you like dogs, you might have a good first impression of a person who also likes dogs.

Myth & Fact

Myth: A person can tell if he or she is going to like or dislike another person the first time they meet.

Fact: Many times your impression of a person changes after you get to know the person better.

Love and Hate

The emotions that range from love to hate help us know how we feel about parts of life. Love and like help us understand how much we value objects, events, or relationships. Hate and dislike let us know when we do not value these things.

There are many ways to value something. You might like the taste of chocolate. You might love playing basketball. Or, love can be a reaction to a family member, a friend, or a romantic interest. People can also experience hate in different strengths. You might dislike peas but hate snakes.

Sometimes, feelings of dislike or hate are based on prejudice (PREJ oo dis). *Prejudice* is an unfair judgment made before a person knows anything about someone or something. For example, if a person you don't know reminds you of something that you dislike, you may be tempted to dislike that person. But after you get to know the person, you may find out that you really like him or her. Avoiding prejudice can help you clearly understand your values. You can avoid prejudice by learning more about the differences between people that make them unique.

What's Useful About Anger?

Anger is an emotion of strong disappointment and displeasure that forms when hopes are not met. Anger can be helpful if it is dealt with in healthy ways. But anger can be unhealthy if it is misdirected at people who are not at fault. *Misdirection* is aiming your feelings at a person who did nothing to cause those feelings. For example, a baseball player might get angry if he strikes out. He could react by yelling at a coach or the umpire. These people did not cause him to strike out, so his anger is misdirected.

Managing anger in a healthy way begins with figuring out what hopes or desires were not met. After you figure this out, you can decide whether meeting these desires is possible. If it is possible, you can try to meet them another way. If it is not possible, you can think about a new set of hopes that is within reach. For example, the baseball player could realize that he is angry with himself for not being a better player. He may realize that he cannot expect a home run every time. He may decide to practice harder so that he can do better in the future.

Life SKILL BUILDER — ADVANCED

Evaluating Media Messages Companies that advertise on TV and in magazines use people's emotions to help sell their products. Ask students if they have ever had emotional reactions to advertisements. Point out that some emotions can encourage people to buy a product. Have interested students research the use of emotional statements or images on TV and in magazines. **LS Logical**

Physical Effects of Emotions

During an emotional response, chemical changes in the brain cause changes in the body. For example, when a person is scared, chemicals are released into the blood. These chemicals prepare the body to escape or defend itself. They increase heart and breathing rates, and they prepare the muscles to react quickly. These physical changes can help you recognize that you are afraid.

Many of the physical effects that occur in an emotional response vary from person to person. However, pleasant emotions, such as happiness, usually have comfortable physical effects. These emotions sometimes even improve physical health by lowering blood pressure and heart rate. But sadness and worry can bring headaches or feelings of tiredness. And stressful emotions can increase heart rate, blood pressure, and muscle tension. Anger may even cause hot flashes and shaking. Tension in your body can sometimes be a sign that you should deal with your emotions.

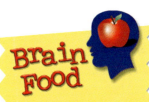

Brain Food

When animals are in stressful or dangerous situations, they show many of the same physical signs of fear as humans do. These signs have led some researchers to wonder if animals have emotions, too.

TABLE 1 Physical Responses to Fear

Increased heart rate, blood pressure, and breathing rate
Hair stands on end
Lightheadedness
Trembling, shaking, and chills or hot flashes
Sweating

Lesson Review

Using Vocabulary
1. What are emotions?
2. How is mental health related to emotional health?

Understanding Concepts
3. What life changes affect teen emotions?
4. How can emotions be pleasant or unpleasant?

Critical Thinking
5. **Analyzing Ideas** What physical signs could tell you that someone is angry?
6. **Making Predictions** Which emotions are more likely to be fair—those based on facts or those based on prejudice? Explain your answer and give an example.

internet connect
www.scilinks.org/health
Topic: Emotions
HealthLinks code: HD4035
HEALTH LINKS. Maintained by the National Science Teachers Association

Answers to Lesson Review
1. Emotions are feelings produced in response to a life event.
2. Mental health is the way people think about and respond to events in their lives. Emotional health is the way a person experiences and deals with feelings. Emotional health is a part of mental health.
3. new roles, responsibilities, and experiences
4. Emotions are pleasant when they make you feel good and unpleasant when they feel bad or uncomfortable.
5. The angry person may look like his or her muscles are tense and shaking.
6. Sample answer: Emotions based on facts are more likely to be fair. Prejudice is based on unfair judgements made before a person knows anything about someone or something. Emotions based on prejudice are likely to change when a person learns more about the situation. For example, feeling dislike for a new school because the building is similar to an old school is an unfair judgement that may change over time.

Group Activity — BASIC

Basic Emotions Write the following list of basic emotions on the board: love, hate, anger, sadness, fear, happiness, surprise, disgust, and shame. Organize students into groups and ask them to brainstorm lists of variations on those basic emotions. For example, variations on happiness include feeling ecstatic, joyful, cheerful, glad, merry, delighted, and elated. If students have trouble, you can provide them with a thesaurus.
LS Verbal

Close

Reteaching — BASIC

Classifying Pass out flashcards that have an emotion written on them. Use happiness, sadness, elation, despair, contentment, hate, love, anger, and fear. Have students group cards into two piles—one for emotions that result in comfortable physical effects, and one for emotions that result in uncomfortable physical effects. Ask them if any emotions could be placed into both piles. (Answers will vary. Some emotions, such as love, can be comfortable or uncomfortable, depending on the situation.)
LS Kinesthetic

Quiz — GENERAL

1. What are hormones? (chemicals that help control how the body grows and functions)
2. How can anger be misdirected? (Misdirected anger involves feeling angry at a person who did nothing to cause the anger.)
3. What are the physical effects of stressful emotions? (increased heart rate, higher blood pressure, muscle tension)

Lesson 1 • Kinds of Emotions

Lesson 2

Focus

Overview
Before beginning this lesson, review with your students the objectives listed under the What You'll Do head in the Student Edition. This lesson describes ways to express emotions. The lesson discusses active listening, body language, and creative expression.

Bellringer
Ask students how they can tell if a person is not listening during a conversation. (Sample answer: The person looks away and says nothing.)

Answer to Start Off Write
Sample answer: Body language expresses emotions through posture, facial expressions, and hand movements.

Motivate

Activity — GENERAL
A Picture Is Worth 1000 Words . . . Without letting the rest of the class know what they are doing, have five students create the following scene using only body language: "A family is posing for a portrait. The family is made up of a mother, father, grandfather, and two teens. The mother and father are angry at each other. One teen ignores the family. The other teen feels close to the grandfather. The grandfather feels protective of the mother." Then tell the class that these students represent a family portrait. Have the class identify the emotions they see. Ask, "How did you identify the emotions?" (body language) **LS** Visual

---

Lesson 2 — Expressing Emotions

What You'll Do
- **Explain** why people express and communicate emotions.
- **List** four effective ways to communicate.
- **Describe** how a person can use creative expression.

Terms to Learn
- verbal communication
- active listening
- body language
- creative expression

Start Off Write
How can body language express emotions?

Amy could tell that Deena was not being honest. Deena insisted she was fine. But her body was slouched, and she was frowning.

Amy knew from Deena's behavior that she was sad. Understanding other people is one part of communication. Being able to express your own emotions is the other part.

Communicating Emotions
Communication allows people to understand each other. When other people understand your emotions, they can share your joy or help you solve problems. People use both verbal and nonverbal communication.

Verbal communication is expressing and understanding thoughts and emotions by talking. Words can be used to express emotions clearly so problems can be resolved. For verbal communication to be effective, someone must hear and understand a speaker. An active listener does this. **Active listening** is not only hearing but also showing that you understand what a person is saying. Asking questions and listening to answers encourages the other person to keep talking. Making eye contact is another signal that you are paying attention.

Body language is a way to express thoughts and emotions with the face, hands, and posture. Body language is nonverbal communication. Eye contact can express your interest in another person. Facial movements, such as smiles and frowns, can express happiness or sadness. And a slouched body posture shows a lack of energy or confidence. By being aware of body language, people can avoid sending others the wrong messages. Someone pacing and clenching his or her fists in anger can be very scary. However, that person may not realize how scary these behaviors look.

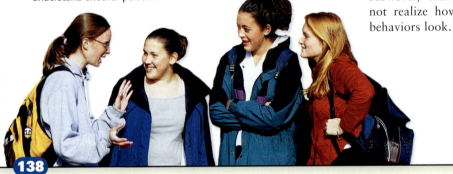

Figure 4 Noticing body language can help you understand another person.

Cultural Awareness
Personal Space Ask students if they have ever felt that someone was standing too close or too far when speaking to them. Individual people have different ideas of what is a comfortable amount of *personal space*, or distance around a person that other people should not enter when talking. Ideas about personal space vary between cultures. **LS** Interpersonal

Chapter Resource File
- Directed Reading BASIC
- Lesson Plan
- Lesson Quiz GENERAL

Transparencies
TT Bellringer

138 Chapter 7 • Mental and Emotional Health

Expression as Release

Why is expressing emotions important? Communication can solve problems and clear up misunderstandings between people. But expressing emotions can feel good even when it does not solve a person's problems. People often feel better after crying or telling someone about feeling sad. Expressing emotions allows people to release physical and emotional tension.

Sometimes, discussing emotions with other people is hard. When communicating with others is difficult, you can express emotions through creative expression. **Creative expression** is using an art to express emotion. This type of expression includes painting, sculpting, acting in a play, dancing, writing a poem, keeping a journal, and playing music. Creative expression is a healthy way to release emotional tensions.

Not all ways of expressing emotions are healthy. Fighting, vandalism, or hurting oneself are unhealthy ways of expressing emotions. Healthy emotional expression never damages oneself, other people, or property.

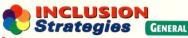

COMMUNICATING EFFECTIVELY

Choose an emotion, and express it through a creative project. The project could be a drawing, a sculpture, or a story.

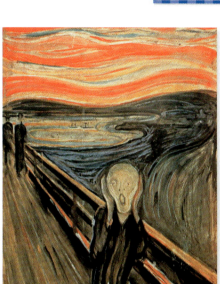

Figure 5 Edvard Munch expressed emotion through his painting, *The Scream*.

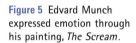

Using Vocabulary
1. What is active listening?

Understanding Concepts
2. What are four effective ways to communicate?
3. Why do people express emotions and communicate?

Critical Thinking
4. **Making Inferences** What emotions do you think Edvard Munch was expressing when he painted *The Scream*? Do you notice any body language in the painting? Consider both facial expression and body posture.

Answers to Lesson Review
1. Active listening means not only hearing, but also showing that you understand what another person is saying.
2. verbal communication, active listening, body language, and creative expression
3. Communicating about emotions helps people understand each other, and helps people to solve problems.
4. Answers may vary. Sample answer: The body language in the picture suggests the artist was expressing the feeling of being scared, overwhelmed, or frustrated.

Lesson 3

Focus

Overview
Before beginning this lesson, review with your students the objectives listed under the What You'll Do head in the Student Edition. In this lesson, students will learn how to overcome negative thinking with positive self-talk. The lesson also explains that defense mechanisms can be either healthy or unhealthy. Students will also learn about triggers and other factors that influence emotions.

Bellringer
Ask students to think of something that makes them angry, and another thing that makes them happy. (Answers will vary.) Tell them these are emotional triggers.

Answer to Start Off Write
Accept all reasonable answers. Sample answer: Emotions can become unhealthy if they are dealt with in unhealthy ways.

Motivate

Activity — GENERAL
Comic Strip Ask students to draw a short comic strip that deals with a situation in which a person has negative thoughts. Tell students to include a positive response to the negative thoughts in the comic strip. For example, the negative thought could be about auditioning for a school play. If the character thinks, "I don't sing well enough to be the lead," a positive response could be, "But I sing well enough to be in the chorus," or "But I paint very well, so I could paint scenery instead." **LS** Visual

---

Lesson 3 — Managing Your Emotions

What You'll Do
- **Explain** how to overcome negative thinking with positive self-talk.
- **Explain** how defense mechanisms can be healthy or unhealthy.
- **Describe** two influences on emotional health.

Terms to Learn
- negative thinking
- positive self-talk
- defense mechanism
- trigger

Write
When is an emotion unhealthy?

Shayla was worried about her friend Ellie. Ellie's parents were getting divorced. Shayla couldn't believe that Ellie wasn't affected, but Ellie didn't act sad.

People deal with stress in many ways. Sometimes, not thinking about unpleasant emotions is easier. But being able to deal honestly with emotions is part of good emotional health.

Dealing with Unpleasant Emotions
It is normal to have unpleasant emotions sometimes. These emotions may help you learn from a situation or motivate you to solve problems. But unpleasant emotions can become unhealthy if they are not dealt with properly.

Sometimes, you can deal with unpleasant emotions by simply thinking about them in a new way. Focusing on only the bad parts of a situation is called **negative thinking**. Trying to think about the good parts of a situation may help you feel differently. **Positive self-talk** is the process of thinking about the good parts of a bad situation. Positive self-talk about a bad situation may include ideas such as these: "This situation won't last forever," "I will have other chances," and "It doesn't always happen like this." Being able to think of a bad situation in a positive way can help you cope until the situation improves. Positive thinking can help you feel better.

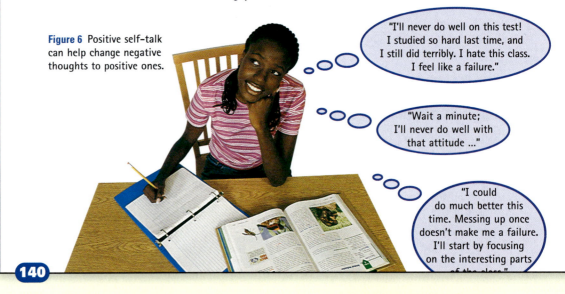
Figure 6 Positive self-talk can help change negative thoughts to positive ones.

"I'll never do well on this test! I studied so hard last time, and I still did terribly. I hate this class. I feel like a failure."

"Wait a minute; I'll never do well with that attitude ..."

"I could do much better this time. Messing up once doesn't make me a failure. I'll start by focusing on the interesting parts of the class."

Chapter Resource File
- Directed Reading **BASIC**
- Lesson Plan
- Lesson Quiz **GENERAL**

Transparencies
TT Bellringer
TT Positive Self-Talk

---

140   Chapter 7 • Mental and Emotional Health

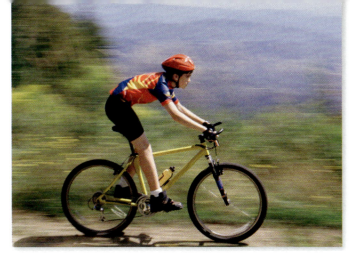

Figure 7 Fun activities, such as riding a bike, can be a good way to cope with stress.

Coping with Stress

Stress is the body's response to new or unpleasant situations. Sometimes, we ignore problems to delay dealing with stress. Other times, we deal with problems immediately. A famous doctor named Sigmund Freud (SIG muhnd FROYD) called our responses to stress defense mechanisms. **Defense mechanisms** are behaviors we use to deal with stress.

Healthy defense mechanisms help you deal with emotions in a useful way. For example, humor can help relieve stress by focusing on the amusing parts of a tough situation. Defense mechanisms are unhealthy if they cause you to ignore your emotions or the issues that cause them. *Devaluation* is a defense mechanism in which someone transfers unpleasant feelings about a situation to specific people. Thinking negatively about others allows that person to ignore the negative situation. If you are aware of defense mechanisms, you can avoid the behaviors that keep you from dealing honestly with emotions.

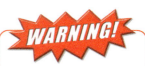

Avoiding Emotions

While it may be easier to ignore unpleasant emotions, avoiding your emotions can prevent you from solving the problems that cause them. In fact, the problems could even get worse.

LIFE SKILLS ACTIVITY

COPING

Imagine that you just moved to a new school, started a new babysitting job, had a fight with your parents, and sprained your wrist. These things have caused you to feel a lot of stress. Write and illustrate a short story showing at least five different ways that you could cope with stress in this situation. Point out which strategies are healthy and which are unhealthy. Explain how the unhealthy strategies could affect you in negative ways.

Background

Defense Mechanisms The following is a list of defense mechanisms:

- Denial: refusing to think about a stressful reality
- Rationalization: inventing a reason to accept something that is not acceptable
- Regression: behaving in an immature or age-inappropriate way
- Projection: attributing one's stressful characteristics to others
- Displacement: shifting stressful feelings from one object to another
- Compensation: using achievement in one area to make up for failure in another area
- Humor: focusing on the amusing aspects of a situation
- Self-observation: reflecting on thoughts, feelings, and behaviors

Teach, continued

Hands-on ACTIVITY

Answers
1. Answers will vary. Most students will have unique ideas in their scripts.
2. Sample answer: Positive self-talk decreases the feeling of anger by focusing on the positive parts of the situation. Sometimes positive self-talk can even help solve the problems that were causing the anger.

READING SKILL BUILDER — BASIC

Discussion Before students read this page, ask them if there are certain people, situations, or events that make them happy or sad. Ask them how they deal with these emotions most of the time. Tell them that this page discusses how to identify people, situations, and events that trigger emotions so that they can deal with their emotions more effectively. **LS Intrapersonal**

Discussion — GENERAL

Healthy Activities Ask student volunteers to describe activities that make them happy. Ask students, "What is it about these activities that makes them enjoyable?" (Answers will vary.) "Are these activities always ones in which you do well?" (Answers will vary.) "Why do some activities make you feel unhappy?" (Answers will vary.) **LS Verbal**

Hands-on ACTIVITY

USING POSITIVE SELF-TALK

1. Think of a situation that triggers anger.
2. Write a positive self-talk script about dealing with anger in that situation.
3. With a partner, act out the script, and show how positive self-talk affects emotions.

Analysis
1. Was your script similar to or different from other students' scripts?
2. How did positive self-talk affect the feelings of anger?

Finding Your Triggers

One way to deal with unpleasant emotions is to avoid situations that cause them. You can do this by figuring out what triggers your different emotions. A **trigger** is a person, situation, or event that influences emotions. If you recognize that certain situations always make you feel badly, you can try to avoid those situations.

Once you know what triggers your emotions, you can also seek out situations that trigger pleasant emotions. For example, if you know that music makes you happy, you could join a music group or listen to music more often. Spending time doing healthy things that you enjoy can improve your emotional health.

Knowing your triggers can also help you to be more aware of your emotions. If you know that a particular situation triggers certain emotions, you can recognize those feelings more easily when they happen. Once you recognize emotions, you can deal with them more effectively. Dealing with emotions quickly can keep them from becoming problems.

Myth & Fact

Myth: A person has no control over his or her emotions. When a person feels angry or sad, that person can't do anything about those feelings.

Fact: You can influence your emotions by changing your thoughts and behaviors.

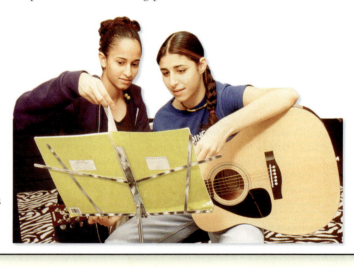

Figure 8 An activity such as playing music may trigger pleasant emotions.

BIOLOGY CONNECTION — ADVANCED

Biofeedback Chronic stress from school, work, or family relationships can result in physical symptoms such as headaches, high blood pressure, and even heart problems. One method used to reduce chronic stress and its physical symptoms is called *biofeedback*. Biofeedback is a way to recognize the body's conscious and unconscious responses to stress. People who study biofeedback consider data collected by sensors attached to the skin. These sensors can monitor body temperature, blood pressure, breathing, skin resistance, heart rate, and muscle tension. As stress increases, changes in these responses can be seen or heard. The goal of biofeedback is to see exactly how the body reacts to stress so that we can understand how to counteract against these effects. Once this is understood, people could learn to relax consciously in response to their level of stress. Biofeedback can help people learn to control anxiety, asthma, migraines, high blood pressure, sleep disorders, and nervousness. Interested students can research biofeedback and try using their findings to reduce the impact of stress in their own lives. **LS Intrapersonal**

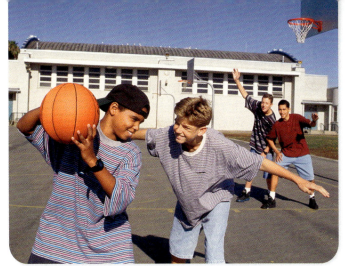

Figure 9 Activites that improve physical health can also improve emotional health.

Influences You Can Control

Everyone has unpleasant emotions from time to time. These emotions can be healthy, but sometimes they are stressful. One way to reduce the impact of stressful emotions is to improve your social and physical health.

Filling your life with people, activities, and healthy habits can improve social and physical health. Building close relationships is valuable. Friends and family members can help you cope with emotional problems. Finding activities that you enjoy can help you express yourself and feel good about yourself. Exercising and eating right can also improve your self-esteem. Improving these aspects of your life will make rough times easier to handle.

Lesson Review

Using Vocabulary
1. What is a defense mechanism?
2. Use the term *trigger* in a sentence.

Understanding Concepts
3. How can defense mechanisms be healthy or unhealthy?
4. Name two habits that can influence emotional health.

Critical Thinking
5. **Making Inferences** Suppose you are disappointed about not doing well on a test. What are three ways to handle the disappointment?
6. **Analyzing Ideas** Your friend just moved away, and you feel terrible. Write a paragraph in which you use positive self-talk to feel better.

REAL-LIFE CONNECTION — GENERAL
Physical and Emotional Health
Tell students that emotional, physical, and social health are all interrelated. Challenge students to exercise the next time they feel sad to see if the physical activity can make them feel better emotionally. **LS** Kinesthetic

Close

Reteaching — BASIC
Reviewing Information Remind students that a trigger is a person, situation, or event that influences emotions. Have students make a list of a person, a situation, and an event that trigger emotions of joy. **LS** Intrapersonal

Quiz — GENERAL
1. What is negative thinking? (focusing on only the bad parts of a situation)
2. What is positive self-talk? (thinking about the good parts of a bad situation)
3. What is stress? (the body's response to new or unpleasant situations)
4. What is a trigger? (a person, situation, or event that influences emotions)

Alternative Assessment — ADVANCED
Poster Project Have students draw a poster showing a person thinking about his or her ability to get a high grade on a math test. Tell students to draw five conversational bubbles and write both positive and negative thoughts about the possibility of getting a high grade on the test. Ask them to identify any bubbles that illustrate defense mechanisms. Then ask students whether the math test is an emotional trigger, and if so, what emotions it triggers. **LS** Visual

Answers to Lesson Review
1. A defense mechanism is a behavior used to deal with stress.
2. Sample answer: Being teased by my brother and having to answer questions in class are two unpleasant emotional triggers for me.
3. Healthy defense mechanisms deal honestly with stressful emotions. Unhealthy defense mechanisms cause people to ignore their emotions and the issues that caused them.
4. Sample answer: Healthy habits such as exercising and eating right can influence emotional health.
5. Sample answer: positive self-talk, healthy defense mechanisms, and improving social and physical health
6. Sample answer: "This doesn't have to mean the end of our friendship. We can still communicate through the Internet and visit each other on school holidays. We can also talk on the telephone. And also, I will make new friends. It's okay to feel sad about this now, but I will feel better soon."

Lesson 3 • Managing Your Emotions

Lesson 4

Focus

Overview
Before beginning this lesson, review with your students the objectives listed under the What You'll Do head in the Student Edition. In this lesson, students will learn about mental illnesses, including depression, bipolar mood disorder, schizophrenia, and anxiety disorders.

 Bellringer
Ask students what they think causes mental illness. (Answers may vary. Nobody understands exactly what causes mental illness, but it is related to changes in brain chemistry caused by life experiences and genetic tendencies.)

Answer to Start Off Write
Accept all reasonable answers. Sample answer: A depressed person acts tired and sad for a long time.

Motivate

Discussion — GENERAL

Living With Mental Illness Ask students what they think life is like for a person with a mental illness. (Answers will vary.) Then tell students that many people with mental illnesses live normal lives because they go through therapy or take medicines that affect their brain chemistry. **LS Verbal**

Lesson 4

What You'll Do
- **List** two factors that can cause mental illness.
- **Explain** how depression is different from sadness.
- **Describe** bipolar mood disorder and schizophrenia.
- **Describe** three anxiety disorders.

Terms to Learn
- mental illness
- depression
- phobia

Start Off Write
How can you tell if someone is depressed?

Mental Illness

> Lana thought something was wrong with her mother. Lana's whole family was going to a party for her brother's graduating class. But Lana's mother refused to go because she was afraid of crowds.

Lana's mother has an intense fear of crowds. Controlling her fear is very difficult because she has a mental illness. Illness can affect mental and emotional health just as it can affect physical health.

What Is Mental Illness?

The brain usually responds to events with normal thoughts and emotions. But sometimes brain chemistry is disrupted, which causes thoughts and emotions to get out of control. This disruption may result in a mental illness. A **mental illness** is a disorder that affects a person's thoughts, emotions, and behaviors.

Nobody knows what causes the changes in brain chemistry that lead to mental illness. Some people may be born with a tendency to have these disorders. Some people develop mental illness when stressful life events cause changes in the brain.

Medicines can help treat mental illness by balancing the brain's chemistry. *Therapy*, or talking about thoughts and changing behaviors, can also help people. With continuing medicine and therapy, many people who have mental illness can live regular lives.

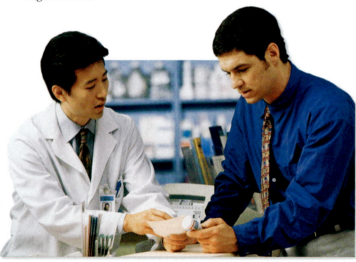

Figure 10 Medicine can be used to help treat mental illness.

Background

Types of Mental Illnesses Mental illnesses can be classified as anxiety, mood, psychotic, eating, and personality disorders along with addictions. Anxiety disorders include phobias, panic disorders, general anxiety disorder, and obsessive compulsive disorder. Mood disorders include depression and bipolar mood disorder. Psychotic disorders include schizophrenia and other psychoses. Eating disorders include anorexia nervosa, bulimia, and sitomania (overeating). Addictions include alcoholism and drug addiction.

Chapter Resource File
- Directed Reading BASIC
- Lesson Plan
- Lesson Quiz GENERAL

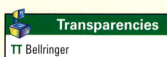
Transparencies
TT Bellringer

144 Chapter 7 • Mental and Emotional Health

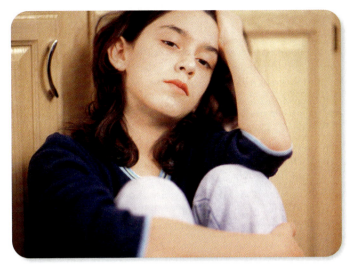

Figure 11 Depression may sometimes lead to suicide. Luckily, there are ways to treat depression.

Depression

A mental illness that affects a person's moods is called a *mood disorder*. **Depression** is a mood disorder in which a person is extremely sad and hopeless for a long time.

Depression differs from healthy sadness. People with depression can become sad or hopeless for no reason. And these feelings last two weeks or longer in a depressed person.

The following behaviors can be signs of depression:

- being unable to enjoy daily activities
- sleeping either more or less than normal
- overeating or not having an appetite
- feeling tired or lacking energy
- moving slowly or being unable to sit still
- having difficulty concentrating or making decisions
- using alcohol or other drugs
- feeling guilty, irritable, or hopeless without cause
- thinking about death or hurting oneself

If you think you or someone you know is depressed, you should find help immediately. The most dangerous part of depression is the possibility of suicide. *Suicide* is the act of killing oneself. Depression can feel so painful and hopeless that a person would rather be dead. However, depression can be treated successfully. With treatment, people who were depressed can feel happy to be alive.

Myth & Fact

Myth: Depressed people are just lazy.

Fact: People that are depressed must cope with unbalanced brain chemistry that keeps their minds and bodies from working properly.

Teach

Life SKILL BUILDER — BASIC

Making Good Decisions Have students apply their decision-making skills to the following scenario: "Your best friend hasn't bathed in a week, rarely eats anything, and seems to have no energy at all. She also is sleeping longer than normal and having difficulty concentrating." Ask students, "What can you do to help this friend?" (Sample answer: Ask the friend what is wrong, tell an adult that the friend may have a problem, and let the friend know that you are there to support him or her.)
LS Interpersonal

BIOLOGY CONNECTION — ADVANCED

Treating Depression
Most people with depression are treated with therapy or a combination of therapy and medication. The most common medications used to treat depression are antidepressants and selective serotonin reuptake inhibitors. Interested students can research what symptoms of depression are relieved by medication. They can also research whether medication for depression has any side effects on the patients who use them. Students can present their research as a paper or in a poster.
LS Verbal/Visual

Life SKILL BUILDER

Coping Tell students that even though sadness is not the same as depression, it is still important to deal with sadness or else that emotion can become unhealthy. Tell students that everyone feels sad sometimes, but that there are ways they can cope with sadness before it becomes overwhelming. For example:

- Focus on what you can do, not on what you can't do. Are you really good at sports, math, listening to others, or unicycle riding? Everyone is good at something.
- Sharing your feelings with others helps you work through those feelings and move on.
- Taking care of your physical health by exercising, eating well, sleeping enough, and getting enough water can do a lot to improve your mood. **LS** Intrapersonal

Lesson 4 • Mental Illness

Teach, continued

Demonstration —ADVANCED

Filtering Stimuli Ask for five volunteers. Tell the first student not to listen while you give the other students their instructions. The second student should read the following sentence repeatedly: "Ten foxes went running by the river and seven foxes fell into the water." The third student should turn a flashlight off and on repeatedly. The fourth student should jump up and down repeatedly while saying "okay" repeatedly. The fifth student should get ready to spray one puff of air spray while tapping his or her foot repeatedly. Then, ask the first student to sit while the other volunteers surround his or her chair and act out their tasks. Allow this to continue for 15 seconds. Then, ask the seated student if he or she can remember what everyone was doing and if he or she can remember the sentence about foxes. (The student will likely be overwhelmed by all the activity and may not be able to remember all the details of the demonstration.) Tell students that normally, humans are only conscious of about 10 percent of the countless stimuli that surround us, such as heat, cold, noise, and odors. If people were aware of more of the stimuli, their brains would become overloaded. Tell students that some people think that schizophrenia involves the inability to filter out sensory perceptions, so that thoughts become confused by overwhelming input to the brain. Interested students can research this idea and present their results to the class. **LS Kinesthetic**

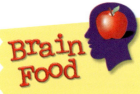

Brain Food

While mental illness can affect many areas of a person's life, other areas remain healthy. John Nash, Jr. received a Nobel Prize in economics for work he performed while suffering from symptoms of schizophrenia.

Bipolar Mood Disorder

Bipolar mood disorder is a mood disorder in which a person has depression sometimes and mania other times. This disorder is commonly known as manic depression. *Mania* is an excited mood that is associated with excessive energy or irritation. During mania, people need very little sleep. Their thoughts may become disorganized. They may talk fast and be difficult to interrupt.

In some cases, people who have bipolar mood disorder break from reality. They may *hallucinate* (huh LOO si NAYT), or hear and see things that do not exist. They may also have *delusions* (di LOO zhuhnz), or false beliefs. For example, they may believe that they know a famous person well. Bipolar mood disorder can often be controlled with medicine and therapy.

Schizophrenia

Schizophrenia (SKIT suh FREE nee uh) is a mental illness that affects thoughts and behaviors more than it affects moods. In fact, people who have schizophrenia may show very little emotion despite the difficulties they face. Schizophrenia causes people to hallucinate and have delusions. It can cause a person's thoughts to become so disorganized that other people cannot understand that person's speech. In some cases, people who have schizophrenia remain "frozen" in one position for a long time.

This disorder can take over a person's life. However, with proper treatment, people who have schizophrenia can often live as regular members of a community.

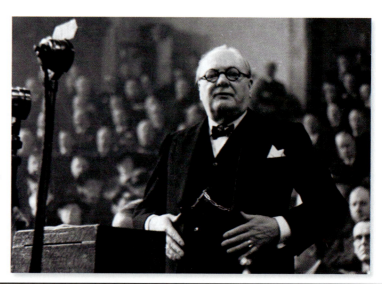

Figure 12 Winston Churchill, who was the prime minister of Great Britain during WWII, had bipolar mood disorder and yet he led an extraordinary life.

Background

Phobias Professionals recognize three types of phobic disorders in humans. These types are:
- agoraphobia: the fear of open spaces
- social phobia: the fear of social situations
- specific phobia: the fear of specific things

There are five types of specific phobia, including fear of 1) an animal; 2) part of the environment; 3) blood; 4) situations (such as being in an elevator); and 5) other specifics (such as clowns or dolls).

Sensitivity ALERT

Discussing mental illness may be difficult for students who have family members who suffer from a mental illness, or for students who suffer from a mental illness themselves. It may be helpful to stress that mental illness can affect any person, and there is nothing shameful about these illnesses. It may also help to point out that therapy and medication can often relieve symptoms of mental illnesses.

146 Chapter 7 • Mental and Emotional Health

Anxiety Disorders

Anxiety (ang ZIE uh tee) *disorders* are mental illnesses that cause extreme nervousness, worry, or panic. There are several types of anxiety disorders. They can be classified by how long the nervous feelings last and by what triggers the feelings.

Feelings of anxiety that happen in brief spurts without a trigger or warning can be signs of *panic disorder*. These brief periods of extreme anxiety are called *panic attacks*. During panic attacks, people get very scared and may think they are having a heart attack. They may shake, feel light-headed, and have a hard time breathing.

If panic attacks are triggered by certain situations, the attacks can be signs of a phobia (FOH bee uh). A 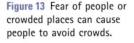 is a strong, abnormal fear of something. Many people have phobias of animals, such as snakes, or situations, such as flying in airplanes. Some people even have phobias of other people.

Some people feel anxiety about thoughts that they have over and over again. These repeating thoughts are called *obsessions*. When people develop repeating behaviors in response to these thoughts, those people have *obsessive-compulsive disorder (OCD)*. For example, a person with OCD might try washing repeatedly to avoid the anxiety of thinking about dirt. OCD and most other anxiety disorders can be treated with medicines and therapy.

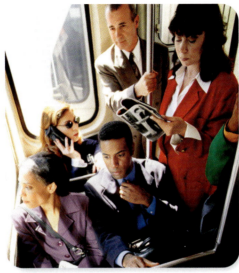

Figure 13 Fear of people or crowded places can cause people to avoid crowds.

Lesson Review

Using Vocabulary
1. What is a phobia?
2. How is depression different from sadness?

Understanding Concepts
3. What are two factors that might cause the brain changes that lead to mental illness?
4. Describe three anxiety disorders.
5. Describe bipolar mood disorder and schizophrenia.

Critical Thinking
6. **Identifying Relationships** What are the similarities and differences between depression and a medical problem that does not affect the brain, such as high blood pressure?

internet connect
www.scilinks.org/health
Topic: Schizophrenia
HealthLinks code: HD4085
Topic: Bipolar Disorder
HealthLinks code: HD4014
Topic: Anxiety Disorders
HealthLinks code: HD4010

HEALTH LINKS. Maintained by the National Science Teachers Association

---

Answers to Lesson Review
1. A phobia is a strong, abnormal fear of something.
2. Depression is a mood disorder in which a person is extremely sad and hopeless for at least two weeks. People with depression can become sad for no obvious reason. Sadness is a healthy emotion that is a response to a life event.
3. Some people may be born with a tendency to have mental illness. Some people develop mental illness when stressful life events trigger changes in their brain chemistry.
4. Anxiety disorders include panic attacks, in which people get very scared and have a hard time breathing; phobias, in which people have a strong, abnormal fear of something; and obsessive-compulsive disorder, in which people have repeating thoughts and behaviors.
5. Bipolar mood disorder is an illness in which a person's moods shift between depression and mania. Schizophrenia is an illness in which a person has delusions, hallucinations, and uncontrolled thinking.
6. Sample answer: Both problems can be caused by environmental and genetic factors. Both can be treated with medications and behavioral changes. Depression includes behavioral changes in a person, while high blood pressure includes physical changes in a person.

Close

Reteaching — BASIC
Vocabulary Have students make an index card for each bold and italic word in this lesson. Have them make index cards with the definitions for these words as well. Then ask students to pair each word with its correct definition. **LS Visual**

Quiz — GENERAL
1. What is a mental illness? (a disorder that affects a person's thoughts, emotions, and behaviors)
2. What is the most dangerous part of depression? (the possibility that the person may commit suicide)
3. What is the difference between hallucinations and delusions? (People who hallucinate see and hear things that do not exist. People with delusions have false beliefs.)

Alternative Assessment — ADVANCED
Comparing Illnesses Have students write a paragraph comparing mental illness to other physical health problems, such as heart attacks or osteoporosis. They should include a comparison of how these health problems are caused, who can suffer from them, and how they are treated. They should conclude with an observation about what they did not realize about mental illness before studying this lesson. **LS Verbal**

Lesson 5

Focus

Overview
Before beginning this lesson, review with your students the objectives listed under the What You'll Do head in the Student Edition. In this lesson, students will learn how to find help for mental and emotional health problems. Students will identify sources of help, including family, friends, and professional help. Students will also learn how to find help for other people who are suffering from emotional problems.

 Bellringer
Ask students to think of three people they could talk to about an emotional problem. (Students may think of friends, family members, adults at school, doctors, or other people they know.)

Answer to Start Off Write
Accept all reasonable answers. Sample answer: I could tell an adult about the depression and tell my friend that I want to support him or her.

Motivate

Activity — GENERAL

 Skit Have groups of students write skits about someone deciding whether or not to seek help for an emotional problem. The person can consider who to talk to and then try speaking with different people until finding someone who makes him or her feel better. The person who has an emotional problem could try speaking with a friend, a family member, and a professional psychologist. **LS Kinesthetic**

Lesson 5

What You'll Do
- **Describe** how to know when you need help for an emotional problem.
- **List** three sources of help for emotional problems.
- **Explain** when to find help for others who have emotional problems.

Terms to Learn
- therapist
- psychiatrist

Start Off Write
What should you do to help a friend who is depressed?

Getting Help

Martin had not slept well for three nights, and he couldn't concentrate at school. He was very sad that his best friend moved across the country. Would he need help getting through this?

Unpleasant emotions that last for a long time can be scary. Asking for help dealing with emotions can only make things better. And sometimes it can keep problems from getting worse.

Knowing When to Get Help

Unpleasant emotions are very uncomfortable. You may sometimes wonder if you need help dealing with these feelings. Asking someone for help is always OK. Finding help is nothing to be ashamed of or embarrassed about.

There are several signs that can help you know when finding help is especially important. You should tell someone if:
- unpleasant emotions last for a long time or happen often
- unpleasant emotions frequently happen for no reason
- your emotions interfere with relationships or responsibilities

It is best to try solving these problems quickly, before they become even more serious.

Emotions and thoughts that cause you to want to hurt yourself or others are serious warning signs. If you have thoughts about hurting yourself or others, you should get help immediately.

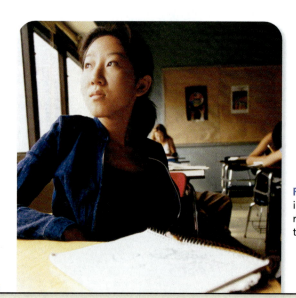

Figure 14 When emotions interfere with duties or relationships, it is time to get help.

Background

Counseling People with mental health problems can seek counseling from a wide variety of organizations, including churches, social service institutions, community mental-health organizations, and private counseling services. Most of these organizations are equipped to offer care for people seeking help with family problems, conflict resolution, and crisis intervention. Counselors who work for such organizations usually have specialized training in psychotherapy. The objectives of psychotherapy are to help each individual find his or her own path to health and emotional balance.

Chapter Resource File
- Directed Reading BASIC
- Lesson Plan
- Lesson Quiz GENERAL

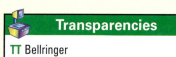 **Transparencies**
TT Bellringer

148 Chapter 7 • Mental and Emotional Health

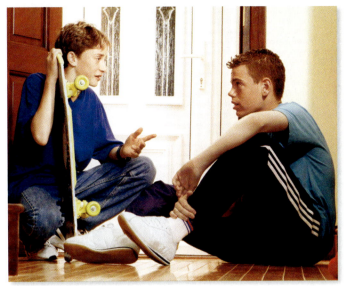

Figure 15 Talking to friends about problems can help you stay emotionally healthy.

Friends and Family

When people have emotional problems, they often turn to people they know for help. Friends, family, and trusted adults can be an important resource for working out emotional problems. These people can help you see your problem from another point of view. They may be able to share stories of similar situations they have experienced. Knowing that others have had similar problems can be comforting.

Sometimes, people are uncomfortable talking to friends or family about personal problems. This can happen when a problem is private or embarrassing. It can also happen when family or friends are part of the problem. In these cases, a friend or family member's involvement could prevent that person from understanding the problem. When family and friends are not a comfortable source of help, people in the community can help. Community resources include teachers, principals, school counselors, doctors, clergy, anonymous hotlines, and peer counseling groups. Because these people are not involved in the situation, their help will be *impartial,* or without prejudice.

Talking about emotional problems can be difficult. It is helpful to prepare a plan of action before you have problems. This preparation includes identifying people that could help you if you had a problem. It can also be helpful to talk with friends and family about emotions when things are going well. This can make you more comfortable discussing emotions with them when problems come up later.

Health Journal
Make a table in your Health Journal. For a week, keep track of all the triggers that make you angry, happy, or sad. Note whether you exercise each day and how much sleep you get each night. Does exercise or sleep affect your emotions? How do you feel after talking to a friend about your emotions?

Answer to Health Journal
Answers will vary. Most students will find that exercise and sleep do affect their emotions. Getting more exercise and getting enough sleep usually helps a person experience more pleasant emotions, or helps people deal with unpleasant emotions more effectively. Most students will feel better after talking to a friend about their emotions.

Teach

Discussion — BASIC
Talking About Problems Ask students what qualities make certain people easy to talk to. (Students may list being a good listener, having ideas about how to solve problems, and sharing their own personal experiences.) Then ask what qualities make certain people difficult to talk to. (Students may list not being an attentive listener, making judgements about personal problems, and changing the subject without considering the problem.) Remind students that being aware of qualities that make a person easy to talk to can help students be good friends and listeners for other people. **LS** Interpersonal

Life SKILL BUILDER — GENERAL
Making Good Decisions Have students apply their decision-making skills to the following scenario: "Your older sister has stopped going out with friends, rarely comes out of her room, and eats very little. Then she gives you some of her most prized possessions. She says she wants to tell you a secret, but you must promise not to tell your parents." Ask students what they would do in this situation. (Students could ask her if anything is wrong and let her know they are there to support her. They could also tell a parent or trusted adult that they were concerned for her.) Ask them what they would do if she said she was going to attempt suicide. (Students could get help from an adult immediately.) Stress that it is important not to keep secrets that can harm a person. If someone tells students a secret about wanting to commit suicide, the students should tell an adult immediately—even if that person will be angry. It could save a life. **LS** Interpersonal

Lesson 5 • Getting Help 149

Teach, continued

Group Activity —— GENERAL

Community Mental Health Resources If your school policy allows, have students explore community mental health resources. One student can interview a school counselor to find out what resources are available at school. Other students can interview local physicians, clergy, or peer counseling groups to identify resources for students with mental health problems. Another student can conduct Internet research on community mental health resources. Several students could prepare posters for a classroom presentation about community resources that are available, and another could lead the presentation. **LS Logical**
Co-op Learning

PHYSICS CONNECTION —— ADVANCED

Light Therapy Therapists have identified a mood disorder related to the lack of sunlight during the winter months. This illness is called Seasonal Affective Disorder (SAD). Light therapy is sometimes used to treat SAD, depression, vitamin D deficiency, and skin disorders. However, light is not always healthy for a person. Ultraviolet (UV) sunlight can cause sunburn and has been linked to the formation of skin cancer. Light therapy should be used only under the supervision of a physician. Interested students can research how light therapy is used, and how effective it is.

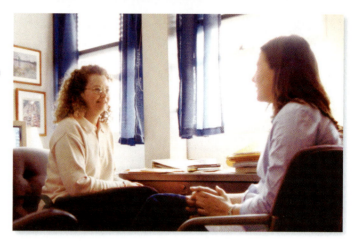

Figure 16 Professionals can give you a fresh point of view on your problems.

Professionals

Sometimes, talking to friends, family, or community members is not enough to solve mental and emotional problems. Trained mental health professionals can help treat serious problems and mental illness.

A **therapist** is a professional who is trained to treat emotional problems by talking about them. Therapists, such as counselors and social workers, try to change the way people think, feel, and act. Through talking, people can learn the cause of their thoughts and feelings or learn new ways to manage their emotions.

Psychiatrists (sie KIE uh trists) are medical doctors that understand how the brain and body affect emotions and behavior. Psychiatrists may use medicine and therapy to treat people who have a mental illness. Often, people who have a mental illness need this treatment to help them recover.

STUDY TIP *for better reading*

Organizing Information Make a table listing sources of help for two categories of emotional problems: temporary emotional problems and mental illness.

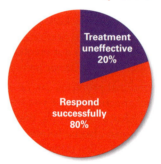

Figure 17 Most people who get professional treatment for depression recover, but many do not get help.

Successful Response to Treatment for Depression

- Treatment uneffective 20%
- Respond successfully 80%

Source: American Psychiatric Association.

Career

Therapists People who help others overcome their emotional and mental health problems an called therapists. They help by working with people to identify and acknowledge problems, discover how the problems formed, and develop opportunities for change. Although therapists build trusting and open relationships with their patients, they remain neutral in other parts of a patient's life. This is because professionals must function independently of a patient's expectations and demands.

150 Chapter 7 • Mental and Emotional Health

Finding Help for Others

People do not always seek help for their emotional problems. This could be because they are embarrassed. Or they could think that they are able to handle the problem on their own. If someone you know suffers from an emotional problem and is not asking for help, you can encourage that person to find help.

When a person has a mental illness, he or she may be unable to get help alone. Letting a serious emotional problem or mental illness go untreated is very dangerous. People with these problems can suffer greatly. They may even end up hurting themselves or others. If you believe that someone might hurt himself or herself or someone else, it is important that you get help for that person. You may save a life.

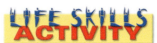

MAKING GOOD DECISIONS

A friend has asked you to keep a secret. The secret is that he or she does not care about anything anymore and is thinking about suicide. What will you do? Weigh the risks of making your friend angry by telling the secret to an adult against the risks of keeping the secret. Write a paragraph explaining how you made your decision.

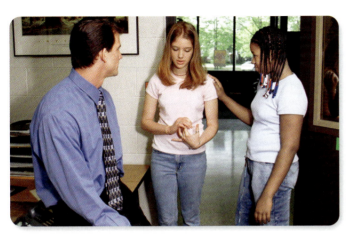

Figure 18 Getting help for a friend with an emotional problem or mental illness can save that friend's life.

Lesson Review

Using Vocabulary
1. What is the difference between a therapist and a psychiatrist?

Understanding Concepts
2. When should you get help for an emotional problem?
3. What are three sources of help for emotional health problems?
4. When should you help a friend who has emotional problems?

Critical Thinking
5. **Applying Concepts** Carlos has had an emotional problem for 1 month. He thought it would go away on its own, but now he feels worse. He talked to his family, but that didn't help either. What should he do now?
6. **Making Predictions** What are possible negative outcomes of not asking for help if a friend is having emotional problems?

Close

Reteaching — BASIC
Planning Ahead Have students make a list of four places that they could go to for help with their emotional problems. Ask them not to list people they know. They should list professional resources and other people from the community. (doctors, counselors at school, therapists, psychologists, etc.) Then ask why it's important to have resources beyond family and friends. (Sometimes friends and family are part of an emotional problem, or sometimes people want help from an impartial listener.)

Quiz — GENERAL
1. When should you solve emotional problems? (quickly, before they get worse)
2. Is talking with friends appropriate treatment for a person with a mental illness? Explain. (Talking with friends is not enough. People who have mental illness need to be treated by psychiatrists. These are doctors who understand how the brain and the body affect emotions and behavior.)
3. Why should you help a person who appears to be suffering from a mental illness as quickly as possible? (These people are in danger of hurting themselves or others.)

Alternative Assessment — GENERAL
Story Writing Have students write a short story in which a teen has emotional problems as a result of his or her parents' divorce, and needs help dealing with those problems. Ask students to be as specific as possible when describing what type of help the teen needs, and where he or she can go for that help.

Answers to Lesson Review
1. A therapist is a professional who is trained to treat emotional problems by talking about them. A psychiatrist is a medical doctor who understands how the brain and body affect emotions and behavior and who can prescribe medicine.
2. when unpleasant emotions last for a long time, happen for no reason, or interfere with relationships or responsibilities
3. Three sources of help include friends and family, professionals, and community resources such as teachers, counselors, doctors, and clergy.
4. Sample answer: I can encourage a friend to find help if the friend has a problem but is not finding help. I can find help for a friend if the friend is in danger of hurting himself or herself or someone else.
5. Now he should look into getting some professional help, from counselors, therapists, or psychiatrists who are trained to help people with their emotional problems.
6. Accept all reasonable answers. Sample answers: The friend might suffer needlessly, have problems with physical health, get bad grades in school, or attempt suicide.

7 CHAPTER REVIEW

Assignment Guide

Lesson	Review Questions
1	1, 3, 9–11, 21
2	2, 4, 12–14, 23
3	5, 7–8, 15, 22, 24
4	6, 16–19
5	20, 25

ANSWERS

Using Vocabulary

1. Mental health is the way people think about and respond to events in their lives. Emotional health is the way a person experiences and deals with feelings.
2. Verbal communication is expressing and understanding thoughts and emotions by talking. Body language is the movements of the face and body that express thoughts and emotions.
3. Hormones
4. Active listening
5. Positive self-talk
6. Depression
7. triggers
8. defense mechanism

Understanding Concepts

9. As teens grow, they begin to produce hormones, chemicals that cause changes in both their bodies and emotions. Taking on new roles and responsibilities provides new opportunities for new and confusing emotions.
10. No; Emotions are only unhealthy when they are dealt with in unhealthy ways.

Chapter Summary

- Emotions are feelings that are produced in response to life events. ■ Hormones and changing responsibilities affect teens' emotions. ■ Having a full range of emotions is healthy. ■ Expressing emotions helps people solve problems, understand others, and release tension. ■ Positive self-talk can overcome negative thinking. ■ Defense mechanisms are ways to cope with stress. ■ Knowing your triggers can help you avoid unpleasant emotions. ■ A mental illness is a disorder that affects emotions, thoughts, and behavior. ■ Family members, friends, community members, and professionals can help people who have emotional problems. ■ Encouraging someone to get help for an emotional problem can save that person's life.

Using Vocabulary

For each pair of terms, describe how the meanings of the terms differ.

1. mental health/emotional health
2. verbal communication/body language

For each sentence, fill in the blank with the proper word from the word bank provided below.

active listening	mental illness
triggers	hormones
defense mechanism	positive self-talk
creative expression	therapist
negative thinking	depression

3. ___ are chemicals that help control how the body grows and functions.
4. ___ is one way to encourage someone to talk and communicate.
5. ___ is a way to think about the good parts of a bad situation.
6. ___ is a mental illness that includes extreme sadness.
7. Knowing your ___ helps you avoid situations that cause unpleasant emotions.
8. Using a(n) ___ is a way to cope with stress.

Understanding Concepts

9. How do changes in teens' bodies and in their lives affect their emotions?
10. Are pleasant emotions healthier than unpleasant emotions? Explain.
11. How can emotions affect a person physically?
12. Why is it helpful to express emotions?
13. What are some effective ways to communicate emotions?
14. When might a person want to use creative expression?
15. How do social and physical health affect mental and emotional health?
16. What are two things that can affect brain chemistry and lead to a mental illness?
17. How is depression different from sadness?
18. What is bipolar mood disorder?
19. What is schizophrenia?
20. How would you know if you needed help for an emotional problem?

---

11. Emotions can cause physical effects such as changing heart and breathing rates, blood pressure, muscle tension, hot flashes, and shaking. Stressful emotions over time can cause major health problems.
12. Expressing emotions allows people to understand one another and help solve problems. Expressing emotions also allows people to release physical and emotional stress.
13. verbal communication, active listening, body language, and creative expression
14. when discussing emotions with others is difficult

15. Good social and physical health make it easier to have good mental and emotional health.
16. Some people may be born with a tendency to have mental illness; others may develop mental illness when life events trigger changes in the brain.
17. Depression is a mood disorder in which a person is extremely sad and hopeless for at least two weeks. Sadness is a healthy emotional response to a life event.
18. Bipolar mood disorder is a mood disorder in which a person experiences both depression and mania.

Critical Thinking

Applying Concepts

21. Julia just turned thirteen. She moved to a new school and had to make new friends. She started babysitting after school, and her parents put her in charge of taking care of the family dog. Lately, Julia has felt emotionally confused and overwhelmed. Why do you think she might feel confused about her emotions?

22. Imagine that you are helping your family get ready for a big reunion. You have been working hard all day, and your sister yelled at you because she thought you weren't helping enough. As you walk home from the grocery store with party supplies, the bag of groceries breaks and milk spills all over the street. How could you use positive self-talk to overcome negative thinking in this situation?

23. Erik really hates it when his friend Robert teases him about his big feet. Robert is just joking and doesn't know that Erik is upset. What might happen if Erik doesn't express his emotions to Robert?

Making Good Decisions

24. Alex went to the park every day after school to play basketball. There were two courts there, and the bigger one was always full of older kids. When Alex tried playing with the older kids, he got really nervous. When he got home after playing with them, he felt sad and exhausted. What could Alex do to avoid this trigger for sadness?

25. Rita's friend Leigh has been sad for several weeks. Rita notices that Leigh doesn't eat much at lunch and that she looks really tired. Rita tries to talk to Leigh about her emotions, but Leigh will not discuss her problem. What can Rita do to help Leigh?

26. Use what you have learned in this chapter to set a personal goal. Write your goal, and make an action plan by using the Health Behavior Contract for mental and emotional health. You can find the Health Behavior Contract at **go.hrw.com**. Just type in the keyword **HD4HBC06**.

Reading Checkup

Take a minute to review your answers to the Health IQ questions at the beginning of this chapter. How has reading this chapter improved your Health IQ?

Chapter Resource File
- Concept Review GENERAL
- Concept Mapping GENERAL
- Performance-Based Assessment GENERAL
- Chapter Test GENERAL

---

19. Schizophrenia is a mental illness that affects thoughts and behaviors more than it affects moods. Schizophrenia causes people to hallucinate and have delusions.

20. when unpleasant emotions last for a long time or happen often, happen for no reason, or interfere with relationships or responsibilities

Critical Thinking

Applying Concepts

21. Julia is experiencing new hormones and new roles and responsibilities. These changes result in unfamiliar and confusing emotions.

22. Accept all reasonable answers. Sample answer: I would tell myself "This situation won't last forever. The family reunion will be fun even if the events leading up to it were bad. My sister is feeling stress and just used a defense mechanism when she yelled at me."

23. Erik needs to express his emotions to his friend, because emotions become unhealthy when they get in the way of relationships. If Erik doesn't let Robert know how he feels about being teased, Robert may continue teasing Erik, and Erik may not want to continue the friendship.

Making Good Decisions

24. Alex should avoid this situation and replace it with one that triggers pleasant emotions. For example, he could find a different place to play basketball.

25. Rita needs to find help immediately because her friend Leigh may be depressed. Rita could suggest that Leigh find help, and if Leigh will not do this, Rita can find it for her by talking to a school counselor or another adult.

26. Accept all reasonable responses. **Note:** A Health Behavior Contract for each chapter can be found in the Chapter Resource File and at the HRW Web site, go.hrw.com.

Model

Introduce this activity by reminding students that using this Life Skill will help them take personal responsibility for their behavior. Then, review the scenario with the class.

Prepare students for this activity by modeling each of the steps of the skill. Make sure students understand each step before you move on to the next one.

Guided Practice: Practice with a Friend

Guided Practice is the stage in which you and the students analyze their approach to solving the problem given in the scenario and analyze their communication skills. Have students read Act 1. Discuss with the class the situation described and the way students are to act it out. Organize the class into groups of three. In each group, one person plays the role of Sean, another person plays Sean's father, and the third person is the observer.

Proper pacing during the Guided Practice is important. The suggestions listed below will help you control the pace.

1. Stop after completing each step of communicating effectively.
2. Discuss with each group the observer's comments.
3. Ask the other members of each group to listen to the observer's suggestions and to suggest ways to improve their communication skills.
4. Instruct students to repeat the steps that need improvement and to include their modifications.

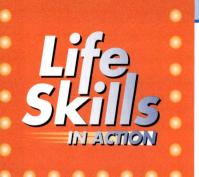

Life Skills IN ACTION

Communicating Effectively

Have you ever been in a bad situation that was made worse because of poor communication? Or maybe you have difficulty understanding others or being understood. You can avoid misunderstandings by expressing your feelings in a healthy way, which is communicating effectively. Complete the following activity to develop effective communication skills.

ACT 1 — Sean's Sadness

Setting the Scene

Sean's parents have been fighting a lot. It seems like they fight every night. Sean hates listening to their fights but doesn't know how to make them stop. All of the anger in the house is upsetting him, and he wonders if he somehow caused his parents' unhappiness. He feels sad all the time, and he is having trouble sleeping and concentrating on his schoolwork. Sean decides to talk to his father about his problems.

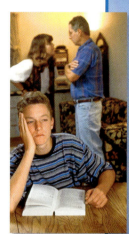

The 4 Steps of Communicating Effectively

1. Express yourself calmly and clearly.
2. Choose your words carefully.
3. Use open body language.
4. Use active listening.

Guided Practice

Practice with a Friend

Form a group of three. Have one person play the role of Sean and another person play the role of Sean's father. Have the third person be an observer. Walking through each of the four steps of communicating effectively, role-play Sean talking with his father about his problems. Sean should tell his father how the fights between him and his mother are affecting his mental and emotional health. The observer will take notes, which will include observations about what the person playing Sean did well and suggestions of ways to improve. Stop after each step to evaluate the process.

5. Check to make sure that students understand each step before they move on to the next step.
6. If time permits, repeat the exercise three times, switching roles each time. Each student should have the opportunity to play each role. Co-op Learning

154 Chapter 7 • Life Skills in Action

Independent Practice

Check Yourself

After you have completed the guided practice, go through Act 1 again without stopping at each step. Answer the questions below to review what you did.

1. Why is it important for Sean to express himself calmly and clearly?
2. What specific body language could Sean use when he is talking with his father?
3. What should Sean's father do to show that he is actively listening to what Sean is saying?
4. Why is it important to use good communication skills when explaining your feelings to someone?

ACT 2 — On Your Own

After several talks with his parents, Sean now understands that their fighting is not his fault. He is starting to feel better mentally and emotionally. One day, Sean's parents tell him that they are getting a divorce and that he will live with his mother. Sean doesn't like the arrangement because he wants to be able to spend time with his father. Make a flowchart showing how Sean could use the four steps of communicating effectively to tell his parents how he feels.

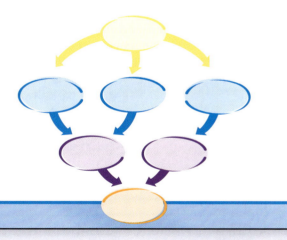

Independent Practice: Check Yourself

Instruct students to repeat Act 1 without stopping at each step. Remind students to apply what they learned in the Guided Practice to the Independent Practice. Students do not have to use the steps in the order listed to communicate effectively.

Encourage students to use the Check Yourself questions as a starting point for reviewing and analyzing their Independent Practice. Remind students that as they change roles, the answers to these questions may change for each actor. Encourage students to create additional questions for checking their communication skills. When students have finished the Independent Practice, have them answer the Check Yourself questions in writing. Use their answers to assess their understanding of the steps of communicating effectively and to assess their use of the steps to solve a problem.

Check Yourself Answers

1. Sample answer: If Sean does not express himself calmly and clearly, his father may not understand what he is saying and he may not get his point across.
2. Sample answer: Sean should maintain eye contact and could keep his hands folded in her lap.
3. Sample answer: Sean's father should look at Sean while he is talking and should ask questions if he doesn't understand what Sean is saying.
4. Sample answer: Using good communication skills while expressing your feelings is important because you want to be sure that the other person understands how you feel. If the other person doesn't understand how you feel, the problem won't be resolved and it could cause more problems.

Act 2: On Your Own

This additional scenario gives students an opportunity to apply what they have learned in both the Guided Practice and the Independent Practice to a new situation.

Suggest to students that they use the Check Yourself questions as a starting point for communicating effectively in the new situation. Encourage students to be creative and to think of ways to improve their communication skills.

Assessment

Review the flowcharts that students have made as part of the On Your Own activity. The flowcharts should show that the students used the communication skills in a realistic and effective manner. If time permits, ask student volunteers to draw one or more of their flowcharts on the blackboard. Discuss the flowcharts and the use of communication skills.

Chapter 7 • Communicating Effectively

CHAPTER 8

Managing Stress
Chapter Planning Guide

PACING	CLASSROOM RESOURCES	ACTIVITIES AND DEMONSTRATIONS
BLOCK 1 • 45 min — pp. 156–161 **Chapter Opener**	**CRF** Health Inventory * ■ GENERAL **CRF** Parent Letter * ■	**SE** Health IQ, p. 157 **CRF** At-Home Activity * ■
Lesson 1 Stress Is Only Natural	**CRF** Lesson Plan * **TT** Bellringer * **TT** Life-Change Stressors *	**TE** Activity Modeling Distress, p. 159 ◆ BASIC **TE** Demonstration Acting Stressed, p. 160 ◆ GENERAL **TE** Activity Singing the Blues, p. 160 ADVANCED **CRF** Enrichment Activity * ADVANCED
BLOCK 2 • 45 min — pp. 162–165 **Lesson 2** The Effects of Stress	**CRF** Lesson Plan * **TT** Bellringer * **TT** The "Fight-or-Flight" Response *	**TE** Activities Modeling a Stress Reaction, p. 155F **TE** Activity Role-Playing, p. 162 GENERAL **SE** Science Activity, p. 163 **CRF** Life Skills Activity * ■ GENERAL **CRF** Enrichment Activity * ADVANCED
Lesson 3 Defense Mechanisms	**CRF** Lesson Plan * **TT** Bellringer *	**TE** Activity Poster Project, p. 164 GENERAL **SE** Hands-on Activity, p. 165 **CRF** Datasheets for In-Text Activities * GENERAL **CRF** Enrichment Activity * ADVANCED
BLOCK 3 • 45 min — pp. 166–169 **Lesson 4** Managing Distress	**CRF** Lesson Plan * **TT** Bellringer *	**TE** Activities Coping with Stress, p. 155F **TE** Demonstration Balloon Stress, p. 166 ◆ GENERAL **SE** Hands-on Activity, p. 167 **CRF** Datasheets for In-Text Activities * GENERAL **TE** Activity Overcoming Procrastination, p. 168 GENERAL **SE** Life Skills in Action Setting Goals, p. 172–173 **CRF** Life Skills Activity * ■ GENERAL **CRF** Enrichment Activity * ADVANCED

BLOCKS 4 & 5 • 90 min — **Chapter Review and Assessment Resources**

- **SE** Chapter Review, pp. 170–171
- **CRF** Concept Review * ■ GENERAL
- **CRF** Health Behavior Contract * ■ GENERAL
- **CRF** Chapter Test * ■ GENERAL
- **CRF** Performance-Based Assessment * GENERAL
- **OSP** Test Generator
- **CRF** Test Item Listing *

Online Resources

Visit **go.hrw.com** for a variety of free resources related to this textbook. Enter the keyword **HD4MS7**.

Students can access interactive problem solving help and active visual concept development with the *Decisions for Health* Online Edition available at **www.hrw.com**.

cnnstudentnews.com

Find the latest health news, lesson plans, and activities related to important scientific events.

Compression guide:
To shorten your instruction because of time limitations, omit Lesson 3.

KEY

TE Teacher Edition	**CRF** Chapter Resource File	* Also on One-Stop Planner
SE Student Edition	**TT** Teaching Transparency	■ Also Available in Spanish
OSP One-Stop Planner		◆ Requires Advance Prep

SKILLS DEVELOPMENT RESOURCES	LESSON REVIEW AND ASSESSMENT	STANDARDS CORRELATION
		National Health Education Standards
TE Life Skill Builder Assessing Your Health, p. 159 `GENERAL` **SE** Life Skills Activity Assessing Your Health, p. 160 **CRF** Cross-Disciplinary * `GENERAL` **CRF** Decision-Making * `GENERAL` **CRF** Refusal Skills * `GENERAL` **CRF** Directed Reading * `BASIC`	**SE** Lesson Review, p. 161 **TE** Reteaching, Quiz, p. 161 **TE** Alternative Assessment, p. 161 `ADVANCED` **CRF** Concept Mapping * `GENERAL` **CRF** Lesson Quiz * ■ `GENERAL`	1.2
TE Inclusion Strategies, p. 163 `BASIC` **CRF** Directed Reading * `BASIC`	**SE** Lesson Review, p. 163 **TE** Reteaching, Quiz, p. 163 **CRF** Lesson Quiz * ■ `GENERAL`	1.2, 3.7, 5.2
TE Inclusion Strategies, p. 165 `ADVANCED` **CRF** Refusal Skills * `GENERAL` **CRF** Cross-Disciplinary * `GENERAL` **CRF** Directed Reading * `BASIC`	**SE** Lesson Review, p. 165 **TE** Reteaching, Quiz, p. 165 **CRF** Lesson Quiz * ■ `GENERAL`	3.7, 5.1, 5.2
TE Reading Skill Builder Anticipation Guide, p. 167 `ADVANCED` **TE** Life Skill Builder Practicing Wellness, p. 167 `GENERAL` **SE** Life Skills Activity Coping, p. 168 **SE** Study Tip Reviewing Information, p. 169 **CRF** Decision-Making * `GENERAL` **CRF** Directed Reading * `BASIC`	**SE** Lesson Review, p. 169 **TE** Reteaching, Quiz, p. 169 **TE** Alternative Assessment, p. 169 `ADVANCED` **CRF** Concept Mapping * `GENERAL` **CRF** Lesson Quiz * ■ `GENERAL`	3.7, 5.1, 5.2

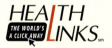

Topic: Fight or Flight
HealthLinks code: HD4040

www.scilinks.org/health

Maintained by the
National Science Teachers Association

Technology Resources

 One-Stop Planner
All of your printable resources and the Test Generator are on this convenient CD-ROM.

 Guided Reading Audio CDs

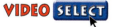
For information about videos related to this chapter, go to **go.hrw.com** and type in the keyword **HD4MS7V**.

Chapter 8 • Chapter Planning Guide

Chapter 8: Managing Stress
Chapter Resources

Teacher Resources

TEACHING TRANSPARENCIES

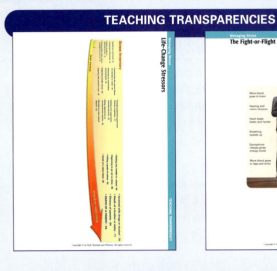
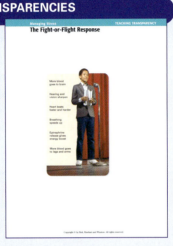

BELLRINGER TRANSPARENCIES

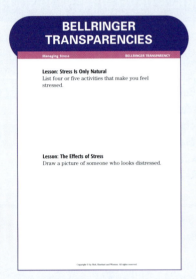

LESSON PLANS

PARENT LETTER

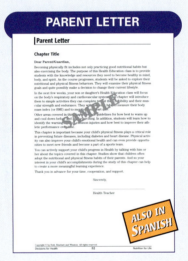

TEST ITEM LISTING

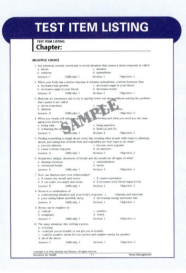

Meeting Individual Needs

DIRECTED READING
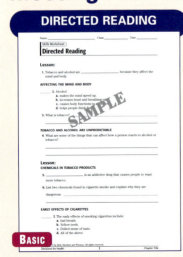
BASIC

CONCEPT MAPPING
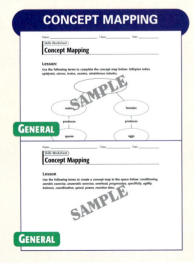
GENERAL

CONCEPT REVIEW
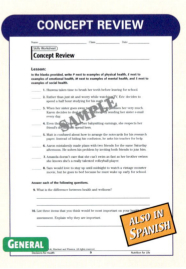
GENERAL

ENRICHMENT ACTIVITIES
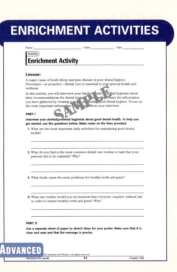
ADVANCED

155C Chapter 8 • Managing Stress

Resources

These worksheet pages can be found in the Chapter Resource File and the One-Stop Planner. The transparencies can be found in the Teaching Transparencies binder and on the One-Stop Planner.

Activities

LIFE SKILLS ACTIVITIES
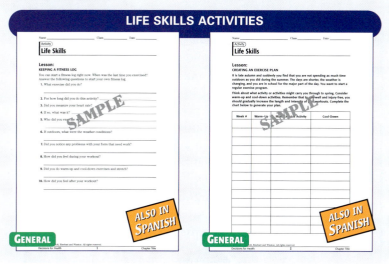

AT-HOME ACTIVITY
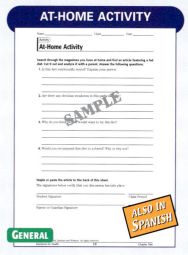

DATASHEETS FOR IN-TEXT ACTIVITIES
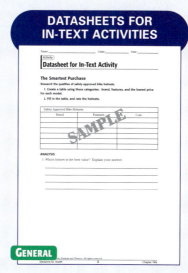

Applications

DECISION-MAKING
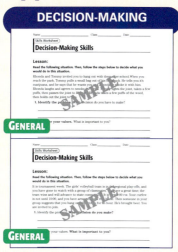

REFUSAL SKILLS
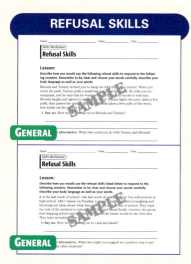

CROSS-DISCIPLINARY
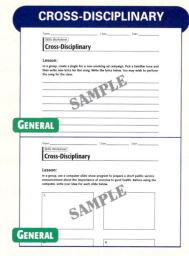

HEALTH BEHAVIOR CONTRACT
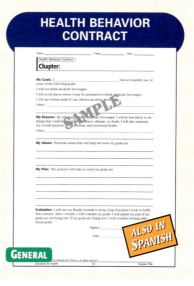

Assessments

HEALTH INVENTORY
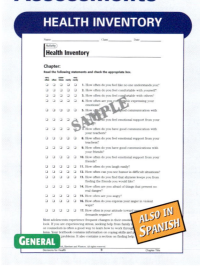

LESSON QUIZZES
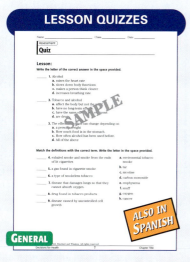

CHAPTER TEST
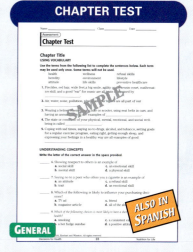

PERFORMANCE-BASED ASSESSMENT
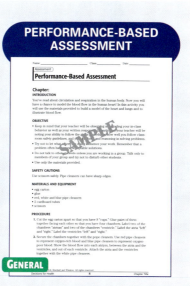

Chapter 8 • Chapter Resources and Worksheets   155D

Chapter 8: Background Information

The following information focuses on four theories that explain why people react differently to stressors. This material will help prepare you for teaching the concepts in this chapter.

Constitutional Theory

- A person's constitution, or genetic and physiological make-up, can influence his or her health a great deal. Many scientists believe genetics also influence a person's ability to cope with stress.
- Identical twins, even when they are raised in different environments, tend to exhibit similar mental stability and nervous habits.
- Among animals, many factors that cause fear and anxiety are instinctive. For example, baby rats will freeze in position if they see a cat even if they have never seen a cat before. And many young animals react with fear when they see a snake for the first time.

Learning-Behavioral Theory

- Not all stress is caused by instinctive reactions or genetic predisposition. For instance, a person could enjoy riding horses, but after being thrown from a horse the same person could feel extreme stress just by being near a horse or seeing a picture of one. This is an example of learned stress.
- One of the most famous learned-stress studies was done by Campbell, Sanderson, & Laverty in 1964. Using medical students as subjects, the researchers administered a drug that caused paralysis at the same time as they showed a light or sounded a tone. The subjects' reaction to the paralysis was absolute terror. After that, whenever the subjects saw the light or heard the tone, they experienced the same overwhelming terror, even though the drug was not administered again.
- A person does not have to have a traumatic experience to develop a learned stress. For example, a person can hear about a plane crash and then develop a total fear of flying.

Cognitive-Humanistic Theory

- Some scientists wonder how a person can gain a fear without having had a traumatic experience first. One theory is that this type of stress is developed from inner conflicts between a person's actual self and his or her ideal self. These conflicts could also manifest as differences between actual reality and perceived reality or differences in held beliefs or values. Basically, this theory states that any thought that challenges a person's ideal state of mind causes stress. In other words, stress is mainly caused not by instinctive reactions or conditioning, but by thought processes.

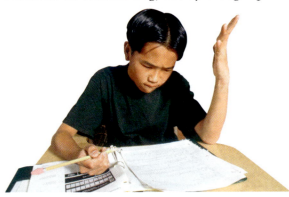

- One of the main arguments behind the cognitive-humanistic theory is that people with more self confidence tend to have lower stress levels. The theory is that self-confident people react to a stressor by thinking, "I can deal with this." A less-confident person would think, "This situation is hopeless," and become dangerously distressed.

Psychoanalytical Theory

- The psychoanalytical theory is based on Freudian psychology. It states that a person's reaction to stressors is directly linked with subconscious memories of childhood.
- Freud believed that the first stressful experience people ever have is their own birth. After birth, the child continues to have more stressful experiences—all of which will affect the child's future reactions to stressors. Freud also believed that defense mechanisms first used by the child to deal with stressors are further enhanced and developed in adulthood.

For background information about teaching strategies and issues, refer to the *Professional Reference for Teachers*.

ACTIVITIES

CHAPTER 8

Consider using the activities on this page as students explore the lessons of this chapter. Look for other activities throughout the Student Edition chapter.

Modeling a Stress Reaction

Hands on

Procedure As students are sitting at their desks, tell them to place their index and middle fingers on the inside of their wrist just below their thumb. Ask them to take their pulse by counting the number of times they feel their wrist veins throb during a 15-second interval. Time the 15 seconds by calling out when to start counting and when to stop. Have students write down their pulse rate. Continue with normal class activities for a while, and then suddenly announce a pop quiz. Have students quickly put their books away and get out paper and a pencil. Immediately after this, ask students to take their pulse again.

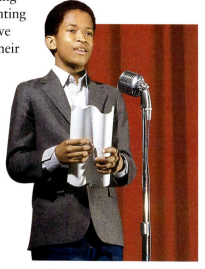

Analysis Ask students the following questions:

- How did your pulse change the second time you took it? (Sample answer: My pulse increased.)
- What do you think caused the change? (Sample answer: The idea of a pop quiz stressed me and my response was that my heart beat faster.)

Explain to students that there is actually no pop quiz and you purposefully created a stressor to help them see some of the effects of stress, such as an increased heart rate. Ask the following questions:

- How does an increased heart rate help a person respond to a stressor? (Sample answer: If a person's heart beats faster, more blood gets to the organs and muscles so the person can react faster to the stressor.)
- What other physical effects did you experience after learning about the pop quiz? (Sample answer: sweaty palms, shortness of breath, clenched teeth.)

Coping with Stress

Procedure Organize the class into four groups. Assign each group one of the following stressors:

- an aggravation (such as failing a test)
- a daily annoyance, such as taking a crowded, noisy bus between school and home
- a life change, such as watching your parents go through a divorce
- a conflict, such as having a fight with your best friend

Have each member of the group brainstorm a list of at least five examples of their assigned situation. Tell students to make sure their examples are relevant to people in their age group. When the group members have finished brainstorming on their own, have them get into their groups and choose one example that they would like to act out. The group should work together to write a short skit that illustrates why the situation is stressful and different ways in which a person could react to the situation. Ask students to show at least one positive and one negative reaction to the situation. When the groups are done writing their skits, have them perform the skits in front of the rest of the class.

Analysis After each skit is performed, ask the audience the following questions:

- Why was the presented situation stressful?
- Which reactions to the situation were positive and which were negative? Why?
- What are some other possible positive reactions to the situation?
- Have any of you ever experienced a similar situation? If so, how did you react? If not, how do you think you would react in this situation?
- If you were facing a similar situation, to whom would you turn for help? Make a list of three people who would help you.

When you finish discussing the skits, have students work in pairs to create a poster illustrating the variety of reactions that the class has discussed.

Chapter 8 • Activities   155F

CHAPTER 8

Overview
Tell students that this chapter will help them to understand what stress is and what steps to take to manage stress. This chapter reassures students that stress is a natural part of life.

Assessing Prior Knowledge
Students should be familiar with the following topics:
- refusal skills
- decision making
- emotional health

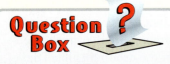

Students may feel more comfortable asking questions if you set up a Question Box to collect their questions. Have students write and anonymously submit their questions about stress and how to manage their stress. Address these questions during class, or use these questions to introduce lessons that cover related topics.

Current Health

Check out *Current Health* articles and activities related to this chapter by visiting the HRW Web site at **go.hrw.com.** Just type in the keyword HD4CH23T.

Chapter Resource File
- Directed Reading BASIC
- Health Inventory GENERAL
- Parent Letter

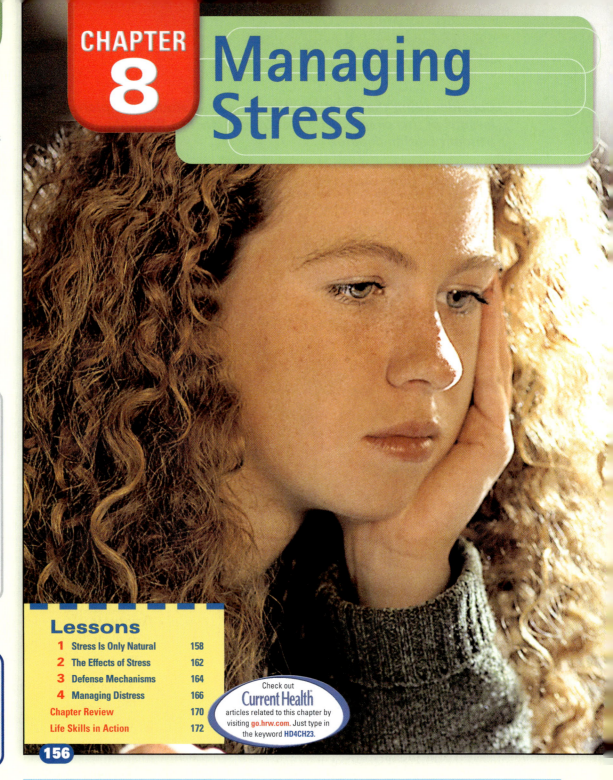

CHAPTER 8 Managing Stress

Lessons
1 Stress Is Only Natural	158
2 The Effects of Stress	162
3 Defense Mechanisms	164
4 Managing Distress	166
Chapter Review	170
Life Skills in Action	172

Check out **Current Health** articles related to this chapter by visiting go.hrw.com. Just type in the keyword HD4CH23.

Standards Correlations

National Health Education Standards

1.2 Describe the interrelationship of mental, emotional, social, and physical health during adolescence. (Lessons 1 and 2)

3.7 Demonstrate strategies to manage stress. (Lessons 3 and 4)

5.1 Demonstrate effective verbal and nonverbal communication skills to enhance health. (Lessons 3 and 4)

5.2 Describe how the behavior of family and peers affects interpersonal communication. (Lessons 2 and 3)

> "When my **grandmother** got **sick**, she came to **live with us**. That was two years ago. I had to give up **my bedroom**, but that was OK. Now, my grandmother needs help all the time. My mom can't do everything, so my sister and I help her. I love my grandmother, and I want to help my mom. But sometimes I just want to get away."

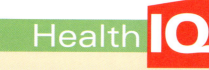

PRE-READING

Answer the following multiple-choice questions to find out what you already know about managing stress. When you've finished this chapter, you'll have the opportunity to change your answers based on what you've learned.

1. Which of the following statements is true?
   a. You can manage much of the stress in your life.
   b. You should avoid all stress.
   c. Good stress does not exist.
   d. Asking other people to help you manage your stress is a bad idea.

2. Ignoring stress
   a. will make the stress go away.
   b. can make the stress worse.
   c. helps a person manage stress.
   d. None of the above

3. Stress can be caused by
   a. schoolwork.
   b. family problems.
   c. running in a race.
   d. All of the above

4. The physical effects of stress include
   a. quick energy boost.
   b. slowed digestion.
   c. an increased heart rate.
   d. All of the above

5. A defense mechanism is
   a. a type of medical procedure that prevents malaria.
   b. a short-term way to handle stress.
   c. used by doctors to stop disease.
   d. a type of play in football.

6. The stress response is
   a. a reaction that occurs only before a big test.
   b. a physical change in your body as a result of puberty.
   c. a natural response to something new or threatening.
   d. always caused by mental problems.

ANSWERS: 1. a; 2. b; 3. d; 4. d; 5. b; 6. c

Using the Health IQ

Misconception Alert
Answers to the Health IQ questions may help you identify students' misconceptions.

Question 1: Living a "stress-free life" is a phrase used in advertising. However, no life can be completely stress free. In fact, some types of stress are beneficial. Students who are athletes probably already know that they use stress to help improve their athletic performance.

Question 6: Stress is often presented in negative terms in the media, so many students may believe that somebody who is experiencing distress has mental problems. However, even the most mentally healthy individuals experience stress. It is a natural reaction to any type of change a person encounters.

Answers
1. a
2. b
3. d
4. d
5. b
6. c

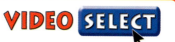

For information about videos related to this chapter, go to **go.hrw.com** and type in the keyword **HD4MS7V**.

Lesson 1

Focus

Overview
Before beginning this lesson, review with your students the objectives listed under the What You'll Do head in the Student Edition. In this lesson, students learn what stress is and the difference between distress and positive stress (also known as *eustress*). Students will also take inventory of their own stressors and determine their stress level.

Bellringer
Have students write a list of five activities that make them feel stressed. (Sample answers: taking a test, giving a speech, having a fight, trying something new, competing in a sport) **LS** Intrapersonal

Answer to Start Off Write
Answers will vary. Sample answer: Stress is when I am under pressure and feel nervous or worried.

Motivate

Discussion — GENERAL
Effects of Stress Ask students what the word *stress* means to them. Have a class discussion about signs of stress. Write the signs on the board as students suggest them, then ask students how they feel when they are not stressed. They may mention feelings of calmness, happiness, or relaxation. Write down these feelings on the other side of the board. Tell students that in this lesson they will learn more about what stress is and what causes it. **LS** Verbal/Intrapersonal

---

Lesson 1

What You'll Do
- **Discuss** stress as a natural part of life.
- **Distinguish** between positive stress and distress.
- **Identify** three sources of stress in your life.

Terms to Learn:
- stress
- stressor
- distress
- positive stress

Start Off Write
What does the word *stress* mean to you?

Stress Is Only Natural

> Kris plays basketball for her school team. Kris is usually very relaxed, but her stomach gets upset right before each game. Sometimes she even throws up.

Waiting for the game to start is stressful for Kris. Her body responds to the tension with an upset stomach. Kris's response is not unusual—everyone experiences stress at one time or another.

Stress Is Part of Life
Stress is the combination of a new or possibly threatening situation and your body's natural response to it. Stress can be physical, mental, emotional, or social. Some situations are stronger stressors than others are. A **stressor** is anything that triggers a stress response. A stressor may be something small, such as not being able to find your favorite shirt. Or a stressor may be something big, such as a serious illness or the death of a parent. You have control over some stressors. For example, you can study more for an upcoming test. But other stressors, such as moving to a new school, cannot be controlled.

How you react to a stressor is important. Different people have different reactions to the same stressor. Something that is not stressful to you may be stressful to one of your friends. Knowing that stressors come in all sizes will help you deal with stress when it comes. And knowing that you can control some stressors but not others may help you react to a stressor in a positive way.

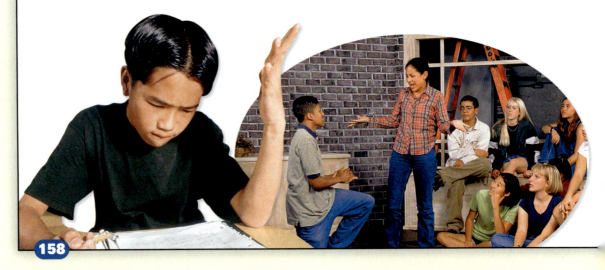

Sensitivity ALERT
Throughout this chapter, different stressful situations are discussed in great detail. Some students may be going through a stressful situation that is mirrored in this book. A discussion about the situation may make the student uncomfortable or distressed. As you teach this chapter, consider inviting the school counselor to speak to the class about distress and ways to manage or relieve stress.

Chapter Resource File
- Directed Reading **BASIC**
- Lesson Plan
- Lesson Quiz **GENERAL**

Transparencies
- TT Bellringer
- TT Life-Change Stressors

158 Chapter 8 • Managing Stress

Distress and Positive Stress

When you hear the word *stress*, you may think of something negative or harmful. **Distress** is any stress that keeps you from reaching your goals or that makes you sick. Distress can leave you feeling tired and depressed or may make you lose sleep. It can keep you from studying properly. Distress may affect your relationships and damage your health. Sometimes, distress is caused by a major stressor, such as fighting with your best friend. But distress is often caused by a collection of minor problems that pile up. If you are rushing to get dressed and are worried because you are late, breaking your shoelace just adds to the stress you already feel.

Some kinds of stress are good for you. **Positive stress** is stress that makes you feel good. It is triggered by something that makes you excited or happy, such as having a special birthday party, winning a speech tournament, or making a basketball team. Positive stress can help you reach your goals. And positive stress usually leaves you feeling relaxed and calm.

A new or changing situation may produce either distress or positive stress. Some changes are more stressful than others. Something that wasn't a stressor in the past can be stressful now if you aren't prepared for it. Or you may find that something that once caused you distress, such as speaking in front of your class, now makes you excited. How you react to a stressor often determines whether you feel distress or positive stress.

Myth & Fact

Myth: All stress is bad.

Fact: Not all stress is bad. Some stress in your life can be healthy. Stress can be either good or bad, depending on how you deal with it.

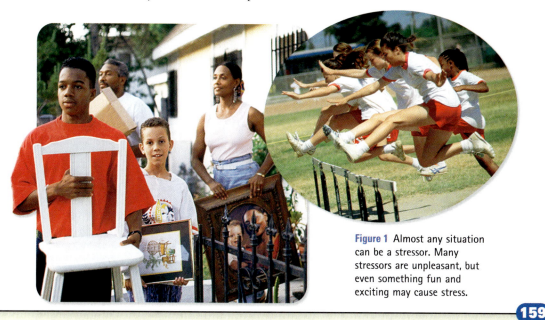

Figure 1 Almost any situation can be a stressor. Many stressors are unpleasant, but even something fun and exciting may cause stress.

SOCIAL STUDIES CONNECTION — GENERAL

Project Mercury For the first manned space program, President Eisenhower's staff at first considered using circus performers or racecar drivers—because of their physical skills and their ability to perform under pressure in dangerous situations—as astronauts. The new space agency, NASA, then decided to use experienced military pilots. After extensive medical evaluations, the candidates were given extremely elaborate and difficult stress tests that examined their physical and mental endurance. The stress endurance tests included forcing candidates to endure rapid acceleration, extreme temperatures, loud noises, high pressures, and long-term isolation. The tests were designed to push the candidates to the point of exhaustion to prepare them for the rigors of space.

Teach, continued

Demonstration — GENERAL

Acting Stressed Find a few scenes in some popular movies that show stressful situations. Caution: The movies should not be R rated and should be age-appropriate for the students. Bring the movies to class one day and show students the scenes. Ask them to describe how the characters are affected by the situation. What signs of stress are the characters showing? Do they think the portrayals of stress were realistic? Why or why not? Finally, ask the students to write down the scenes in order of highest stress levels to lowest stress levels. Then have students compare their lists to see how other students perceived the scenes. Ask students to discuss the criteria they used to rate the scenes.

You can have students continue this activity on their own by asking them to watch one of their favorite movies or television shows and then writing a report discussing the types of stress depicted, how the characters handled the stress, and how the students might handle the same situation differently.
LS Interpersonal

Activity — ADVANCED

Singing the Blues Have interested students explore themes in musical lyrics that deal with distress. Students can create charts to show which stressful situations are dealt with most often. More advanced students can explore the use of instrumental music in movies to portray different feelings of stress. **LS Verbal**

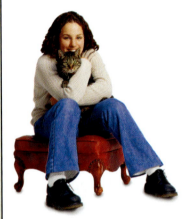

Stress Inventory

- Arguing less with friends - 26
- Arguing less with parents - 29
- Having a brother or sister leave home - 33
- Having another adult, such as a grandparent, move in - 34
- Experiencing the serious illness of a brother or sister - 44
- Achieving an outstanding personal goal - 45
- Beginning middle school - 45
- Arguing with parents more - 46
- Changing physical appearance (braces or glasses) - 47
- Seeing more arguments between parents - 48
- Being rejected for an extracurricular activity - 48
- Moving to a new school district - 52

less stress

Figure 2 Each of the life changes in this stress inventory has been given a point value. When your life changes add up, you may begin to feel the effects of stress.

Figure 3 Accepting responsibility for a new pet may be a stressor to some people. Does this change cause positive stress or distress? Why?

Stress In Your Life

Teens face a variety of stressors. Common stressors are breaking up with a boyfriend or girlfriend, arguing more with your parents, or having trouble with a brother or sister. More-serious stressors include seeing your parents argue more or finding out that your parents are divorcing. If you make a list of stressors in your own life, some will be more serious than others.

The effect that a particular stressor will have on someone may be hard to measure. A change that causes you great distress may seem minor to someone else. For example, moving to a new school may be very stressful to you. Someone else may not mind changing schools at all. But some changes, such as the death of a parent, are very stressful to almost everyone. Some common life changes that cause teenagers stress are listed in Figure 2. These stressors are listed from the least stressful to the most stressful.

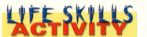

ASSESSING YOUR HEALTH

Use the list of life changes in Figure 2 to total the points for the changes you have gone through in the last year. Analyze your results. Do your stressors come from a particular part of your life, such as family, school, or friends? Are your stressors things over which you have some control, such as schoolwork or relationships? Or are they things that are beyond your control, such as moving to a new city? Can you eliminate any stressors?

160

Background

Stress in Plants and Animals Humans are not alone when it comes to stress. In fact, all organisms can experience stress. Plants experience stress when they are transplanted or undergo a drought. One of the first signs that a plant is stressed is the loss of foliage. Many students may have a dog or cat. Tell them that some common signs of stress in dogs are pacing, nipping, sweaty paws, and loss of appetite. Signs of stress in cats include hiding, excessive shedding, and urinating and defecating outside of the litter box.

LIFE SKILLS ACTIVITY

Answer
Answers will vary.

Extension: Ask students if there are other stressors they would add to the Stress Inventory on this page and the next page.
LS Intrapersonal

- Getting into trouble at school - 54
- Beginning to go out on dates - 55
- Failing a grade at school - 62
- Death of a close friend - 65
- Involved with drugs or alcohol - 70
- Death of a brother or sister - 71
- Divorce of parents - 84
- DEATH OF A PARENT - 94

more stress

Personal Stress Inventory

People suffering from stress sometimes take a personal stress inventory. They list all the life changes they have faced in the last year. Each change, such as those listed in Figure 2, is given a point value. Life changes that are less stressful or are somewhat stressful have lower point values. Stressors that are more stressful or extremely stressful have higher point values.

Doctors know that high levels of stress or stress over a long period of time can increase a person's chances of getting sick. For instance, a score of 300 points or more for a year shows that the person has gone through major life changes. Someone with a score that high has almost certainly experienced stress. He or she must be careful to protect his or her physical and emotional health. Protect your own health. Do a stress inventory occasionally and watch for the warning signs of stress.

Health Journal

Review your list of life changes and the total points for the list. Now think back over the last year. Try to remember if you have had any health problems, such as headaches, colds, or other illnesses. Do you think the health problems may be related to stressful events?

Lesson Review

Using Vocabulary

1. What is stress?
2. Define *stressor*, and identify three stressors in your life.

Understanding Concepts

3. Which is more harmful to your health: positive stress or distress? Explain your answer, and give examples.

Critical Thinking

4. **Identifying Relationships** You and a friend are talking about his personal stress inventory. Most of his stressors are things that he can control or change. Explain how adding stressors beyond his control might affect his health.

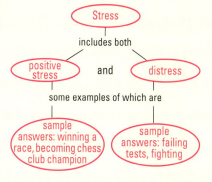

internet connect
www.scilinks.org/health
Topic: Fight or Flight
HealthLinks code: HD4040
HEALTH LINKS. Maintained by the National Science Teachers Association

Close

Reteaching — BASIC

Draw the following concept map on the board—leave the ovals empty—and have volunteers fill it in:

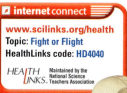

Stress includes both **positive stress** and **distress** some examples of which are sample answers: winning a race, becoming chess club champion / sample answers: failing tests, fighting

Quiz — GENERAL

1. List three stressors over which you would have no control. (Sample answer: beginning middle school, death of a close friend, divorce of parents)
2. List three stressors over which you do have control. (Sample answer: having an outstanding personal achievement, having more arguments with parents, getting in trouble in school)
3. What can you conclude about a person who has a personal stress score of 310 points for the past year? (The person is going through some major life changes and may be showing signs of stress.)

Answer to Health Journal

Answer will vary. This Health Journal may be a good way to close the lesson.

Alternative Assessment — ADVANCED

Picture Book Have students create picture books that illustrate various sources of stress. Each picture should have a caption or description. **LS** Visual   English Language Learners

Answers to Lesson Review

1. Stress is the combination of a new or possibly threatening situation and your body's natural response to it.
2. A stressor is anything that triggers a stress response. Sample answer: My stressors are moving to a new town, fighting with my friends, and winning a soccer game.
3. Distress. Sample answer: Your response to stress can keep you from meeting your goals and may make you sick. Your distress response to situations, such as you might feel after failing a test, can make you worried, angry, and depressed. Your distress response can weaken your immune system and may increase your chances of getting sick.
4. Sample answer: Adding stressors beyond your friend's control may increase his stress inventory, and your friend may become ill.

Lesson 1 • Stress Is Only Natural   161

Lesson 2

Focus

Overview
Before beginning this lesson, review with your students the objectives listed under the What You'll Do head in the Student Edition. In this lesson, students will learn about the physical, mental, emotional, and social effects of stress.

 Bellringer
Have students draw a picture of somebody who looks distressed. When they are done, they can share their pictures with the class. (Pictures might show signs of fatigue, such as dark areas under the eyes or signs of depression, such as a slouched posture.)

Answers to Start Off Write
Answers may vary. Sample answer: My heart beats faster, my muscles get tense, my breathing gets faster, and I want to do something physical.

Motivate

Activity ——————— GENERAL

Role-Playing Ask students to list three serious stressors that people their age may have to face. Divide the class into groups. Have each group select one stressor and brainstorm some ideas about how a teen might handle that stressor. Have students act out their ideas. Have students switch roles to see if there are differences in the way each person handles the stressor.
LS Interpersonal/Kinesthetic

Lesson 2 — The Effects of Stress

Adriana moved to a new city far from her old home and all of her old friends. Now Adriana always seems tired. Her mother thinks Adriana is suffering from stress.

Adriana's mother may be right. Stressors can cause physical and mental reactions, including tiredness. And reactions caused by stressors can be either short-term or long-term.

What You'll Do
- **Describe** the body's response to stress.
- **Distinguish** between physical effects and mental or emotional effects of stress.

Terms to Learn:
- stress response
- fatigue

Start Off Write
Describe how your body responds when something scares you.

Physical Effects of Stress

When you face a stressor, your brain analyzes the situation quickly. For example, imagine that you are walking along and suddenly a strange dog runs up to you and starts barking and growling. Your brain must decide if this stressor is important or not. Is the dog dangerous or just looking you over? If your brain decides the dog is a threat, it orders the release of *epinephrine* (EP uh NEF rin). Epinephrine is a hormone that triggers your body's stress response. The **stress response** is a set of physical changes that prepare your body to act in response to a stressor. The stress response is also called the "fight-or-flight" response because the release of epinephrine gives you a quick burst of energy. This energy boost prepares your body either to fight the stressor physically or to run from it. Figure 4 shows the major physical changes that make up the stress response.

Most of the stress response changes go away when the stressor is gone. But if you do not relieve your stress or eliminate the stressor, you may suffer long-term physical effects.

One common effect of long-term stress is fatigue. **Fatigue** is physical or mental exhaustion. Physical fatigue can cause aches and pains all over your body. It also makes you feel extremely tired. Other long-term effects of stress include stomachaches, headaches, and changes in appetite. Stress can weaken your immune system. It may cause high blood pressure or make asthma worse.

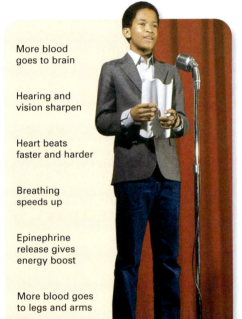

- More blood goes to brain
- Hearing and vision sharpen
- Heart beats faster and harder
- Breathing speeds up
- Epinephrine release gives energy boost
- More blood goes to legs and arms

Figure 4 The stress response produces specific physical reactions.

Career

Army Special Forces Soldiers who qualify for the Army Special Forces must go through rigorous survival training to teach them how to deal with physical and mental stressors. Soldiers are taught that the two most dangerous stressors—not being able to be comfortable and developing a passive attitude—are emotional. If soldiers can harden themselves against discomfort and keep their will to survive, they are well equipped to endure physical stressors such as pain, hunger, thirst, fatigue, and loneliness.

Chapter Resource File
- Directed Reading BASIC
- Lesson Plan
- Lesson Quiz GENERAL

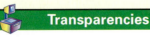 **Transparencies**
TT Bellringer
TT The "Fight-or-Flight" Response

162 Chapter 8 • Managing Stress

Other Effects of Stress

Repeated or long-term stress can also cause mental, emotional, and social effects. Mental effects include confusion and memory problems. Emotional effects include sleeplessness, anxiety, and sadness. One of the most serious long-term effects of stress is psychological (SIE kuh LAHG i kuhl) fatigue. Psychological fatigue is much like physical fatigue. They both make you feel extremely tired or exhausted. Psychological fatigue can be very hard to relieve. It can even lead to depression. More emotional and mental effects of stress are shown in Table 1.

Social effects of stress may be as harmful as other effects. If you are always angry, relationships with your family may be harmed. If you are sad all the time, your friends may not understand why. If you are depressed, you may not want to be around anyone else. Severe stress can be dangerous.

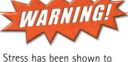

Stress has been shown to lower a person's IQ by 10 to 15 points. You are likely to make more mistakes during a stressful time.

Table 1 Emotional and Mental Effects of Stress

Emotional effects	Mental effects
depression	boredom
anger	confusion
distrust	memory problems
frustration	lack of concentration
guilt	psychological fatigue
sadness and crying	anxiety
sleeplessness, insomnia	poor decision making
irritability, irrational behavior	become accident prone
jealousy	

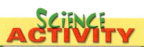

Research the relationship between long-term stress and disease. Make a poster that shows how long-term stress affects the body.

Lesson Review

Using Vocabulary

1. What do you call the set of physical changes that prepare your body to act in response to a stressor?

Understanding Concepts

2. Describe the difference between physical effects of stress and mental or emotional effects of stress.

3. Why is the stress response called the "fight-or-flight" response?

Critical Thinking

4. **Analyzing Ideas** Discuss fatigue and the reasons why it can be so hard to deal with. Include a discussion of how fatigue interacts with other effects of stress.

Answers to the Lesson Review

1. stress response
2. Sample answer: The physical effects of stress, also called the stress response, include changes in your heart rate, digestion, blood flow, and adrenaline level. All these changes prepare you to respond in a physical way to a stressor. If you do not deal with the stressor and the physical effects of stress remain, you may suffer from physical fatigue, headaches, and a weakened immune system. Mental and emotional effects of stress affect your thinking, memory, and feelings. You may become anxious, depressed, sad, or confused.
3. It prepares you to fight the stressor if you must, or for flight from the stressor if you can run away.
4. Sample answer: Fatigue is when your mind or your body is too tired to operate normally. If you respond to a stressor by becoming fatigued, you may be too tired or confused to perform ordinary physical and mental tasks or to deal with other stressors you encounter. Fatigue also weakens your immune system and makes it easier for you to become ill.

Teach

Using the Figure — GENERAL

Use Figure 4 to explain how stress responses prepare the body to flee from or to fight a stressor. For example, epinephrine releases sugar from the liver and helps convert the sugar to energy. **LS** Visual/Verbal

Close

INCLUSION Strategies — BASIC

• Learning Disabled

Give students a chance to learn through a tactile/visual method by having them draw examples of different effects of stress. Have each student choose a different physical, emotional, or mental effect of stress and depict it on a poster. Assign each poster a number and place the posters around the room in numerical order. Ask students to identify the stress effects that are depicted. **LS** Visual/Verbal

Reteaching — BASIC

Work with students to draw a flow chart diagramming the stress response. (stress or adrenaline release, fight-or-flight response, stress goes away OR stress stays, long-term effects) **LS** Visual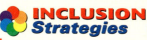

Quiz — GENERAL

1. Imagine that you are sitting in class on Friday afternoon and you are daydreaming about the party you are going to the next afternoon. Suddenly, the teacher calls on you to answer a question. What are three ways that your body might respond? (Your body might show some physical reactions of the stress response, such as increased heart rate, more rapid breathing, and a feeling that you want to run away.)

2. List five mental effects of stress. (Sample answer: boredom, confusion, memory problems, anxiety, and lack of concentration)

Lesson 2 • The Effects of Stress

Lesson 3 Focus

Overview
Before beginning this lesson, review with your students the objectives listed under the What You'll Do head in the Student Edition. In this lesson, students will learn about short-term ways to handle stress and whether these mechanisms are helpful or harmful.

Bellringer
Ask students to list what they think of when they hear the word *defense*. (Sample list: sports, law court, martial arts, suit of armor, and military)

Answer to Start Off Write
Answers will vary. Sample answer: I failed a test in math. I was angry at myself for not studying, but I blamed my teacher for asking things I didn't know.

Motivate

Activity — GENERAL
Poster Project Organize the class into groups. Have each group come up with a stressful situation and discuss different defenses that someone might use in the situation. Have one member of the group make a poster illustrating the situation. Have other members make posters illustrating a defense for the situation and possible consequences of using that defense.
Verbal/Visual — Co-op Learning — English Language Learners

Lesson 3

What You'll Do:
- Describe two defense mechanisms.
- Explain how defense mechanisms can be helpful or harmful.

Terms to Learn:
- defense mechanism

Start Off Write
Describe a time when you were angry at yourself but blamed someone else.

Defense Mechanisms

Doug and Wes were best friends. Now, Wes has a new friend and doesn't spend time with Doug anymore. To cope, Doug acts as if nothing has changed. Wes just ignores Doug.

Losing a friend can be a strong stressor. The loss may affect you emotionally and physically, depending on how you handle it. Some ways of dealing with stress are better than others.

Short-Term Ways to Handle Stress

The best way to end the stress response is to deal with the stressor. If you act to solve the problem, the effects of stress will not pile up. For example, Doug may just need to talk to Wes. The two of them may be able to fix their friendship. In the long term, Doug may have to make new friends. But talking to Wes may relieve Doug's stress right away.

When the release of epinephrine triggers the stress response, the body wants to take action. It wants to do something physical. So, one way to relieve physical effects of stress is to exercise to burn off energy. Exercise helps your body return to normal. That is why exercise also helps relieve mental or emotional effects of stress.

To relieve mental or emotional effects of stress quickly, people sometimes rely on defense mechanisms. A **defense mechanism** is a short-term, automatic way to protect yourself from being hurt emotionally. It is a way of managing distress or coping with distress. Defense mechanisms are ways you have learned to deal quickly with distress. Your defense mechanisms help you maintain your self-esteem. And you may not even realize you are using a defense mechanism.

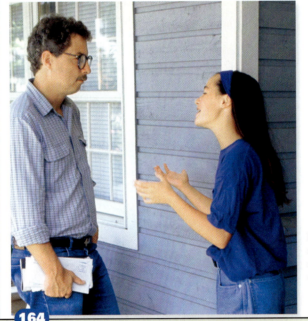

Figure 5 Defense mechanisms, such as rationalization, are short-term ways to handle emotional stress.

Cultural Awareness
Nyakyusa Funerals The Nyakyusa tribe of Sub-Saharan Africa have very ritualized, emotionally intense funerals. When a person dies, the female relatives begin wailing around the clock until the body is buried a few days later. As the wailing ends, the men of the tribe start a dance full of leaps, war cries, and pounding feet. Then the young women join in the dancing. Soon the tribe's mood is transformed from grief to exuberance.

Chapter Resource File
- Directed Reading BASIC
- Lesson Plan
- Datasheets for In-Text Activities GENERAL
- Lesson Quiz GENERAL

Transparencies
TT Bellringer

---

164 Chapter 8 • Managing Stress

TABLE 2 Common Defense Mechanisms

Mechanism	Description
Daydreaming	using your imagination to escape an unpleasant situation
Denial	refusing to accept reality
Projection	putting negative feelings on someone else
Rationalization	making excuses for or justifying behavior to avoid a problem or to gain acceptance
Regression	expressing emotions like anger or disappointment in very childlike ways
Repression	blocking out unpleasant thoughts or memories

Defense Mechanisms—Good or Bad?

Defense mechanisms are unconscious and automatic. Doug and Wes are a good example. Doug uses *denial*, a common defense mechanism, to deal with the changed friendship. Doug, in his mind, denies that anything has changed. He acts as he always has. That way, Doug avoids the hurt feelings and distress from losing a friend. Wes doesn't know that he is hurting Doug's feelings. He doesn't think about Doug at all. Wes blocks out all thoughts about Doug. This is called *repression*.

In the short term, Doug and Wes use defense mechanisms to feel good about themselves. But neither one has faced the real problem—they may end up having no friendship at all. Defense mechanisms can manage your distress. They do not fix the problem. It is important to recognize stress and to know when you are using a defense mechanism. Then you can usually find a way to solve the problem.

Hands-on ACTIVITY

STRESSORS

1. Select one stressor in your life. Identify one or more defense mechanisms you use to cope with the stressor.
2. List the benefits and problems of using the defense mechanisms.
3. Working as a class, do a survey to see how many different defense mechanisms you and your classmates use.

Analysis

1. Make a bar graph that shows all of the defense mechanisms you and your classmates use and the frequency of each one.
2. Discuss why some defense mechanisms are more common than others.

Lesson Review

Using Vocabulary

1. Define *defense mechanism*.
2. Explain the difference between denial and repression.

Understanding Concepts

3. Explain how defense mechanisms can be used in a healthy way.

Critical Thinking

4. **Making Good Decisions** Explain how you can avoid always relying on defense mechanisms to handle distress.
5. **Analyzing Ideas** How can daydreaming be harmful?

Lesson 4

Focus

Overview
Before beginning this lesson, review with your students the objectives listed under the What You'll Do head in the Student Edition. In this lesson, students will learn the signs of stress and how to manage their stress. Students will also learn ways to avoid stress and prevent distress.

Bellringer
Ask students to list three techniques, such as controlling their breathing, that they use to relax before doing something important, such as taking a test or participating in a sports activity. Have them explain how each technique helps them to relax and perform better.

Answer to Start Off Write
Sample answer: By planning ahead, you prepare for stressors and, when they hit, they will not seem as bad.

Motivate

Demonstration — GENERAL
Balloon Stressor Take a party balloon. Ask volunteers to name stressors. As each stressor is named, blow into the balloon. Keep blowing until the balloon pops, then ask students what do they think the balloon symbolized. (a person undergoing distress) The balloon finally blew up because the stress was not released. Ask students how this simulates what may happen to people who do not manage their distress. (People may develop mental or emotional problems if they do not manage or release their distress.) **English Language Learners** Visual

---

Lesson 4

What You'll Do
- **Identify** physical, mental, or emotional signs of distress.
- **Discuss** ways to manage distress.
- **Identify** ways to avoid or prevent distress.

Terms to Learn
- stress management
- relaxation
- redirection
- reframing

Start Off Write
How can planning ahead help you manage stressors?

Managing Distress

Moesha is very shy. In one of her classes, she has to give a speech. Moesha is so worried about the assignment that she cannot sleep and has an upset stomach.

There are many ways to react to stress. Moesha's not being able to sleep is one reaction. But knowing when you are distressed and doing something to relieve the distress is a better reaction.

Signs of Distress
Your stress response usually follows certain steps:
1. A stressor appears, and you interpret it as unpleasant or threatening.
2. You respond physically, mentally, and emotionally to the stressor—this is when you may begin to show signs of distress.
3. If you don't stop distress, the signs of distress may become long-lasting effects.

When you know what causes you distress, you can take steps to solve the problem. Some common warning signs of distress are listed in Table 3. These warning signs can help you learn whether something is a stressor for you. If you have one or more of these signs, you may be distressed. Recognizing your distress will help you deal with it as soon as you can. If you don't deal with it, you may become ill or depressed. Fortunately, there are ways to manage, stop, and even avoid distress. But all good stress management plans start with recognizing the sources of distress in your life.

TABLE 3 Warning Signs of Distress

Physical signs	Emotional and mental signs
headaches	nightmares
teeth grinding	frustration
fatigue	mood swings
heart pounding	depression
	forgetfulness

MISCONCEPTION ALERT
The term *nervous breakdown* is commonly used to refer to somebody who is undergoing serious mental or emotional problems and is not able to function normally. However, *nervous breakdown* is not a medical term. Doctors instead would diagnose somebody with a serious problem as having acute depression, anxiety, or some other definable mental or emotional disorder.

Chapter Resource File
- Directed Reading BASIC
- Lesson Plan
- Datasheets for In-Text Activities GENERAL
- Lesson Quiz GENERAL

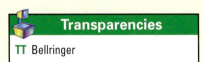
Transparencies
TT Bellringer

166   Chapter 8 • Managing Stress

Managing Your Stress

You can't stop all the stress in your life, but you can manage much of it. **Stress management** is the ability to handle stress in healthy ways. Stress management is part of mental, emotional, and physical health.

Two common ways to manage stress are relaxation and redirection. **Relaxation** is doing something to take your mind off the problem and to focus on something else that is not stressful. Relaxing activities include listening to music, reading a book, and going for a walk. **Redirection** is taking energy from your stress response and directing it into an activity that is not stressful. For example, jogging or riding your bike burn off energy caused by stress.

Another way to manage stress is to reframe the stressor. **Reframing** is looking at the situation from another point of view and changing your emotional response to the situation. Reframing often lets you find something positive about the situation. When you reframe a stressor, you may reduce distress caused by seeing the situation only in a negative way. For example, failing a quiz can be distressful. But if you look at the questions you got wrong, you can study that material and do better on the final test.

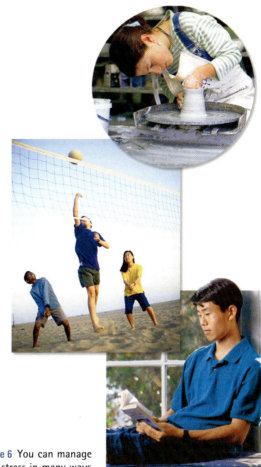

Figure 6 You can manage your stress in many ways.

Hands-on ACTIVITY

STRESS MANAGEMENT

1. Conduct an anonymous class survey in which each student lists three ways that he or she usually manages stress.
2. Compile the class results in a table that shows how often each stress management technique is used.

Analysis
1. Create a bar graph that shows the results of your survey and the information in the table.

2. In a group, select one of the ways of managing stress from the class list. Create a skit that shows a stressful situation and demonstrates the use of the stress management technique that your group selected. Have the class guess which way to manage stress your skit portrays.
3. What other ways to manage stress could you have used in the same situation?

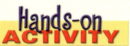

Life SKILL BUILDER — GENERAL

Practicing Wellness Students know that laughter is great medicine. Organize students into groups, and have the groups work together to produce a humorous song, poem, comic strip, skit, video, joke book, or poster about one of the topics in this chapter. Groups can present their completed projects to the class. Afterwards, have the class discuss the physical and emotional effects of laughter.
LS Visual/Verbal/Kinesthetic/Auditory/Interpersonal/Intrapersonal

---

Teach

Debate — ADVANCED

Stress Management or Defense Mechanisms After students have learned about relaxation, redirection, and reframing, ask them to consider how these are related to the defense mechanisms they learned about in the previous section. Have students debate whether stress management techniques might be used in an unhealthy way.
LS Logical/Intrapersonal

READING SKILL BUILDER — ADVANCED

Anticipation Guide Before students read this lesson, ask them to glance over the headings. Then have students answer the following questions:

1. What do you think this lesson will be about? (managing, avoiding, and preventing distress)
2. Think of a stressful situation you recently went through. How could you have avoided the stress? (Answers will vary.)
3. What techniques do you use to manage distress? (Answers will vary.)

LS Intrapersonal

Hands-on ACTIVITY

Answer
Answers will vary.

Extension: Make a class list of other stress management techniques that students suggest. Discuss which ones might be most useful for managing distress. **LS** Logical

Lesson 4 • Managing Distress

Teach, continued

Activity — GENERAL
Overcoming Procrastination
Tell students that one of the major reasons for procrastination is a lack of organization. Have students schedule their time for the upcoming week. Give them suggestions to help with this task. Some tips include: make a to-do list, set priorities, break tasks down into smaller pieces, consider how much time you can reasonably expect each task to take, schedule in rest breaks or down time, and consider rewarding yourself for completing your goals. At the end of the week, have students evaluate their progress. **LS** Logical

REAL-LIFE CONNECTION — BASIC
Sweet Dreams Different people need different amounts of sleep to feel rested. Ask students how much sleep they think they need each night, and how much sleep they actually get. Have students keep a sleep journal for a week. Students should record their activities, including anything they ate or drank, in the hour before they went to bed, what time they went to bed, what time they got up, and the quality of their sleep. At the end of the week, have students analyze their sleeping habits by making charts illustrating sleep duration and sleep quality. Ask them to try and relate their pre-bedtime activities and snacks to their sleep patterns.
LS Logical/Intrapersonal

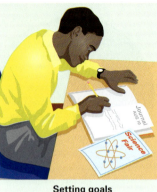
Setting goals

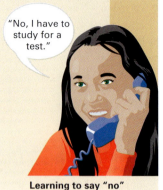
"No, I have to study for a test."
Learning to say "no"

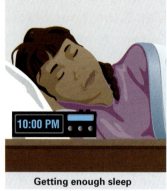
Getting enough sleep

Figure 7 Use these tips to avoid or to prevent distress.

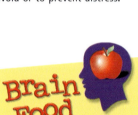
Brain Food
Laughter is a natural way to avoid or relieve stress temporarily. When you are stressed, watching a funny movie or being with people who are laughing and having a good time helps.

Avoiding Distress
A good way to deal with distress is to avoid it. Avoiding distress requires thinking ahead and doing some planning. For example, Moesha knows that she is shy. She can avoid some of her distress by finishing her speech ahead of time and then practicing a few times.

Another way to avoid distress is to build up your confidence. You cannot be an expert at everything, but you can be good at some things. When you develop a skill, such as taking good notes, use it to help you avoid distress whenever you can. Be confident!

Stressors that you face repeatedly—in school, at home, or in another place—are stressors you can plan to avoid. Avoiding stressors takes practice. You have to learn what situations cause you distress. With experience, you can identify potentially stressful situations. Then, you can plan to avoid them. For example, by marking the dates of major tests on a calendar, you can avoid the distress of having to study for the test at the last minute. Other ways to avoid the effects of distress include getting plenty of exercise and sleep, setting goals, and taking some time just for yourself.

LIFE SKILLS ACTIVITY

COPING

Imagine that you have to move to a new city. List 5 to 10 things about moving that may cause you distress. Now list at least one way to manage or to avoid each of the stressors you have listed. For example, imagine that you are moving to a city you have never heard of. What are some ways you could learn more about the city?

REAL-LIFE CONNECTION — GENERAL
Phobias Fear of an object or an activity is sometimes a cause of great distress. These types of fear are called *phobias*. Psychologists have documented and named thousands of different phobias. Some people's phobias keep them from leading a normal life. But, with treatment and medicine, many people can either overcome—or at least learn to manage—their phobias and function normally. Some of the more unusual phobias include ablutophobia (fear of bathing), chromophobia (fear of colors), euphobia (fear of hearing good news), logophobia (fear of words), ouranophobia (fear of heaven), and vestiphobia (fear of clothing).

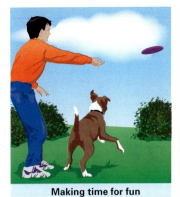
Making time for fun

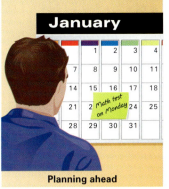
Planning ahead

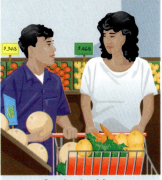
Staying healthy

Preventing Distress

The best way to prevent distress is to be prepared. Think of a situation that causes you distress. What about the situation is so stressful? When you know what the stressor is, make plans to cope with it. For example, you may worry about the first day of school each year. It may be difficult for you to meet new people and start new classes. How can you prevent some of that distress? One way may be to visit the school to learn where your classrooms are. Another way would be to meet a good friend at school and help each other through the first day.

There will always be stress, good and bad, in your life. You cannot live totally stress free. But you can set goals and make choices that keep stress under control. If stress ever becomes more than you can handle by yourself, get help quickly! Stress won't just go away. When stress is bad, find a friend, especially an adult you can trust, to help you. Don't be afraid to ask—everyone needs help sometimes.

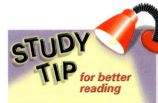

STUDY TIP for better reading

Reviewing Information Use the highlighted vocabulary words and the red headings to create a concept map that summarizes the chapter. Be sure to use connecting words or phrases to link the vocabulary words and important concepts.

Lesson Review

Using Vocabulary
1. Define *stress management*.

Understanding Concepts
2. List six warning signs of distress. Include physical and mental or emotional signs of stress.
3. Explain two ways to manage stress.
4. Explain how planning ahead can help you avoid distress.

Critical Thinking
5. **Making Inferences** Why is learning how to manage distress in our lives a good idea?

Close

Reteaching — BASIC
Have each student create a brochure about stress management similar to one that might be found in a doctor's office. When students are done with their brochures, have them look at each other's finished products. **LS Visual**

Quiz — GENERAL
Tell students to answer the following questions with "True" or "False."
1. All stress can be prevented. (false)
2. You can plan to avoid stress that you face repeatedly. (true)
3. Reframing is directing the energy from a stress response to something else. (false)
4. Relaxation is a form of stress management. (true)
5. Forgetfulness is a sign of stress. (true)

Alternative Assessment — ADVANCED
Board Game Have students create a board game that sends players through stressors and has them choose how best to manage the stress. Players that do not manage the stress well must suffer the effects of stress and lose the game. When the board games are completed, let the students play them. **LS Visual**

Answers to Lesson Review
1. Stress management is the ability to handle stress in healthy ways.
2. Sample answer: headaches, nightmares, teeth grinding, frustration, fatigue, mood swings
3. Sample answer: You can relax and take your mind off of the stress, or you can redirect the energy caused by the stress to something else like running.
4. Sample answer: Planning ahead may help you handle and organize stressful activities better.
5. Sample answer: By learning to manage distress, you can avoid or reduce many of the negative effects of distress on your health. For example, you may avoid the physical and mental fatigue that comes with distress, and you may not make your high blood pressure or your asthma worse.

8 CHAPTER REVIEW

Assignment Guide

Lesson	Review Questions
1	5, 9, 11–12, 18, 21, 24, 26
2	2, 13, 15–16, 19, 25
3	6, 8, 10, 17
4	3–4, 7, 14, 19–20, 23
1, 2, 3, 4	1
3 and 4	22

ANSWERS

Using Vocabulary

1. Sample answer: I felt positive stress when I won the tennis match. I feel fatigue when I worry about things too much. I need to practice relaxation when my muscles are tense from distress. A stressor is something that causes stress.
2. stress response
3. Relaxation
4. redirection
5. stress
6. Repression
7. stress management
8. defense mechanism
9. Positive stress
10. Denial

Understanding Concepts

11. Answers will vary. Accept all reasonable answers.
12. Sample answer: Different people are affected differently by major life changes because they might look at the stressor from a different point of view or be able to better manage their stress.
13. Sample answer: The stress response prepares you to fight with the stressor if necessary, or to run away from the stressor if possible.

---

8 CHAPTER REVIEW

Chapter Summary

■ Stress is a natural part of your life. Stress can come from a wide variety of sources. ■ Stress can be positive or negative. Negative stress is called *distress*. ■ Something that causes stress is called a *stressor*. ■ Stress can cause physical, mental, emotional, and social effects. Some of the effects of stress may be very serious. ■ People often handle stress in the short term by using defense mechanisms. Common defense mechanisms include daydreaming, denial, rationalization, and repression. ■ You can manage most of your distress. Some distress can be avoided, and some distress can even be prevented entirely. ■ An effective way to manage distress is to know what causes your distress and to plan ahead.

Using Vocabulary

❶ Use each of the following terms in a separate sentence: *positive stress, fatigue, relaxation,* and *stressor*.

For each sentence, fill in the blank with the proper word from the word bank provided below.

stress	defense mechanism
distress	stress management
positive stress	relaxation
stress response	redirection
denial	repression

❷ The way your body reacts to a stressor is called the ___.

❸ ___ is taking your mind off your stress and focusing on something that is not stressful.

❹ Taking energy produced by the stress response and using it in a nonstressful activity is called ___.

❺ The combination of an unpleasant situation and your body's natural response to it is called ___.

❻ ___ is blocking out unpleasant thoughts or memories.

❼ When you make plans to handle something stressful, you are doing ___.

❽ A ___ is a way to handle stress in the short term.

❾ ___ is stress that helps you reach a goal and makes you feel good.

❿ ___ is refusing to accept reality.

Understanding Concepts

⓫ Describe three major stressors in your life.

⓬ Explain how major life changes may affect different people differently.

⓭ Why is the stress response called the "fight-or-flight" response?

⓮ Explain why managing and preventing distress are important.

⓯ Explain why relieving stress is important.

⓰ Describe three long-term mental and emotional effects of stress.

⓱ Can defense mechanisms be helpful? harmful? Explain your answers.

⓲ Is all stress bad? Explain your answer.

---

14. Preventing and managing distress are important because a person's response to distress may cause serious physical, mental, emotional, and social effects that can harm his or her health.

15. It is important to relieve stress so that your body does not experience physical or emotional fatigue from the constant presence of stress.

16. Answers will vary. Long-term effects of mental and emotional distress include high blood pressure, depression, memory problems, and insomnia.

17. Defense mechanisms can be both helpful and harmful. They help by giving short-term relief to stress, but they can harm by not forcing a person to face the problem that is causing the stress.

18. Not all stress is bad. Some stress is positive and helps you perform better at certain activities such as sports.

170 Chapter 8 • Managing Stress

Critical Thinking

Identifying Relationships

19. Teresa plays on a softball team. Sometimes she feels that she has extra energy, that she can run faster than usual, and that she can see the ball better when the pitcher pitches it. Explain why Teresa may be experiencing stress.

20. Efrain made a list of stressors in his life. He realized that some of the stressors were beyond his control. Describe ways that Efrain can manage those stressors even though he cannot control them.

21. Jada always seems excited by changes and challenges. Her twin brother, James, gets nervous and can't sleep when he faces the same events. Explain how the way in which Jada and James each view a stressor can affect the way they respond to it.

Making Good Decisions

22. You and your friend have a major test coming up. Both of you are worried about it. Your friend tells you that he is losing sleep and can't concentrate because he is so worried. What can you do to help him?

23. Jimmy is a good student. He and his friend Carlos want to start a band. Jimmy's parents are worried that Jimmy won't have time to do his schoolwork and to play in a band. Jimmy is distressed because his parents may not let him start the band. What can Jimmy do to reassure his parents that his schoolwork won't suffer?

Interpreting Graphics

Brandon's Personal Stress Inventory for the Last 12 Months

Having fewer arguments with his friends	26
Having another adult move into his home	34
Achieving an outstanding personal goal	45
Moving to a new school district	52
Divorce of parents	84

Use the table above to answer questions 24–27.

24. What does this table tell you about Brandon?

25. Based on the information in this table, would you be looking for signs of distress in Brandon? Explain your answer.

26. Which items in the table might help reduce Brandon's distress level?

27. Imagine that another year has gone by. Brandon has made some good friends at his new school, and he has made the basketball team. Brandon still has a good relationship with both his parents. Predict how these factors may affect Brandon's stress level. Explain your prediction.

Reading Checkup

Take a minute to review your answers to the Health IQ questions at the beginning of this chapter. How has reading this chapter improved your Health IQ?

Critical Thinking

Applying Concepts

19. Sample answer: Teresa is experiencing positive stress that allows her body to work at a heightened level.

20. Sample answer: When Efrain experiences those stressors, he can do relaxation exercises, he can redirect the energy produced by the stress, or he can reframe how he views the stressor.

21. Sample answer: Jada responds to certain stressors with positive stress, which is healthier than how her brother James responds. He responds with distress that can cause health problems.

Making Good Decisions

22. Sample answer: Help your friend organize his week so that he has plenty of time to study, but also to exercise and relax. He should also be careful to follow a healthy diet.

23. Sample answer: Jimmy can make a schedule that allows time for both activities, and for any other responsibilities Jimmy has. After he makes the schedule, he can discuss it with his parents to show that he is responsible and to get their approval.

Interpreting Graphics

24. Sample answer: That Brandon's life has had some changes in the last year. For example, his parents got a divorce, and he moved to a different home with one of his parents, who may have a new partner. And for some reason, Brandon has fewer arguments with his old friends.

25. Sample answer: Yes, Brandon's stress score is 241, which is not extraordinarily high, but Brandon's stress level may still lead to some significant health effects.

26. Brandon's distress might have been reduced by his having fewer arguments with his friends and achieving an outstanding personal goal.

27. These changes in Brandon's life a year later will probably reduce his level of stress. Making new friends will help relieve the stress of going to a new school. Being on the basketball team might cause Brandon a small amount of distress if it hurts his grades. But making the basketball team is an important personal achievement that will make Brandon feel better about himself, and in the end will probably be a positive stressor for Brandon. Even though Brandon's parents' divorce causes Brandon distress, he has kept a good relationship with both of his parents, so the distress is not as great as it would be if he were angry or depressed over the divorce.

Chapter Resource File

- Concept Review GENERAL
- Concept Mapping GENERAL
- Performance-Based Assessment GENERAL
- Chapter Test GENERAL

Model

Introduce this activity by reminding students that using this Life Skill will help them take personal responsibility for their behavior. Then, review the scenario with the class.

Prepare students for this activity by modeling each of the steps of the skill. Make sure students understand each step before you move on to the next one.

Guided Practice: Practice with a Friend

Guided Practice is the stage in which you and the students analyze their approach to solving the problem given in the scenario and analyze their ability to set goals. Have students read Act 1. Discuss with the class the situation described and the way students are to act it out. Organize the class into groups of two. In each group, one person plays the role of Zach, and the second person is the observer.

Proper pacing during the Guided Practice is important. The suggestions listed below will help you control the pace.

1. Stop after completing each step of setting goals.
2. Discuss with each group the observer's comments.
3. Ask the other members of each group to listen to the observer's suggestions and to suggest ways to improve their ability to set goals.
4. Instruct students to repeat the steps that need improvement and to include their modifications.

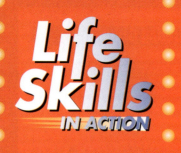

Life Skills IN ACTION

The 5 Steps of Setting Goals

1. Consider your interests and values.
2. Choose goals that include your interests and values.
3. If necessary, break down long-term goals into several short-term goals.
4. Measure your progress.
5. Reward your success.

Setting Goals

A goal is something that you work toward and hope to achieve. Setting goals is important because goals give you a sense of purpose and achieving goals improves your self-esteem. Complete the following activity to learn how to set and achieve goals.

The Procrastinator

Setting the Scene

Zach is a procrastinator—he usually waits until the last minute to do things. He doesn't do his homework until the night before it is due, and he does his chores only after his parents are mad that he hasn't already finished them. It is now 2 weeks until the end of school, and Zach has many projects due in the next week. Zach hasn't started any of them, and he is feeling stressed because he doesn't know if he will be able to finish them all.

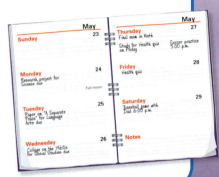

Guided Practice

Practice with a Friend

Form a group of two. Have one person play the role of Zach, and have the second person be an observer. Walking through each of the five steps of setting goals, role-play Zach setting goals to help him finish his projects and manage his stress. The observer will take notes, which will include observations on what the person playing Zach did well and suggestions of ways to improve. Stop after each step to evaluate the process.

5. Check to make sure that students understand each step before they move on to the next step.
6. If time permits, repeat the exercise and have the students switch roles. Each student should have the opportunity to play each role. Co-op Learning

172 Chapter 8 • Life Skills in Action

Independent Practice

Check Yourself

After you have completed the guided practice, go through Act 1 again without stopping at each step. Answer the questions below to review what you did.

1. Suppose one of Zach's projects is a research project for Science. How could Zach divide this project into short-term goals?
2. How could setting short-term goals help Zach reduce his stress?
3. How could Zach measure his progress on his school projects?
4. Think about one of your school projects. What long-term and short-term goals can you set to finish this project?

ACT 2 — On Your Own

Zach managed to finish all of his school projects in time to turn them in. He had to work very hard to finish everything, and he decided never to procrastinate again. At the start of the next school year, Zach's Language Arts teacher gives the class a month-long group project. The other members of Zach's group are worried about the size of the project. Imagine you are Zach, and make a pamphlet for the group members explaining how to use the five steps of setting goals to finish the project without getting stressed.

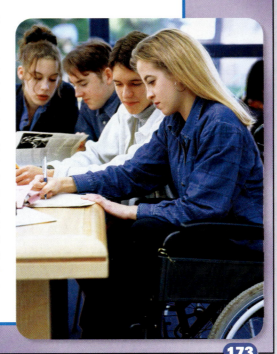

Independent Practice: Check Yourself

Instruct students to repeat Act 1 without stopping at each step. Remind students to apply what they learned in the Guided Practice to the Independent Practice.

Encourage students to use the Check Yourself questions as a starting point for reviewing and analyzing their Independent Practice. Remind students that as they change roles, the answers to these questions may change for each actor. Encourage students to create additional questions for checking their ability to set goals. When students have finished the Independent Practice, have them answer the Check Yourself questions in writing. Use their answers to assess their understanding of steps of setting goals and to assess their use of the steps.

Check Yourself Answers

1. Sample answer: Zach could divide the research project into the following short-term goals: find a subject, research the subject, organize information, and write the paper.
2. Sample answer: Setting short-term goals will reduce Zach's stress because he will see that he is making progress toward finishing his work each time he reaches a short-term goal.
3. Sample answer: Zach could make a checklist of all the short-term goals he needs to accomplish to finish his projects.
4. Sample answer: I have a project to write a play for English. My long-term goal is to write the play and my short-term goals are to develop characters, develop a plot, and write the scenes.

Act 2: On Your Own

This additional scenario gives students an opportunity to apply what they have learned in both the Guided Practice and the Independent Practice to a new situation.

Suggest to students that they use the Check Yourself questions as a starting point for setting goals in the new situation. Encourage students to be creative and to think of ways to improve their ability to set goals.

Assessment

Review the pamphlets that students have made as part of the On Your Own activity. The pamphlets should show that the students followed the steps of setting goals in a realistic and effective manner. If time permits, ask student volunteers to give presentations over one or more of the pamphlets. Discuss the pamphlets and the steps of setting goals.

CHAPTER 9

Encouraging Healthy Relationships
Chapter Planning Guide

PACING	CLASSROOM RESOURCES	ACTIVITIES AND DEMONSTRATIONS
BLOCK 1 • 45 min pp. 174–179 **Chapter Opener**	**CRF** Health Inventory * GENERAL **CRF** Parent Letter *	**SE** Health IQ, p. 175 **CRF** At-Home Activity *
Lesson 1 Building Relationships	**CRF** Lesson Plan * **TT** Bellringer * **TT** Body Language *	**TE** Activities Librarian, p. 173F ♦ **TE** Activity Communicating Effectively, p. 176 GENERAL **SE** Language Arts Activity, p. 178 **TE** Activity Charades, p. 178 ♦ GENERAL **CRF** Enrichment Activity * ADVANCED
BLOCK 2 • 45 min pp. 180–185 **Lesson 2** Family Relationships	**CRF** Lesson Plan * **TT** Bellringer *	**TE** Activities Considering Relationships, p. 173F ♦ **TE** Activity Assigning Roles, p. 180 GENERAL **TE** Group Activity Family Instruction Manual, p. 181 GENERAL **SE** Life Skills in Action Evaluating Media Messages, pp. 194–195 **CRF** Enrichment Activity * ADVANCED
Lesson 3 Healthy Communities	**CRF** Lesson Plan * **TT** Bellringer *	**TE** Activities Pen Pals, p. 173F ♦ **TE** Group Activity Choosing Sides, p. 184 ♦ GENERAL **CRF** Life Skills Activity * GENERAL **CRF** Enrichment Activity * ADVANCED
BLOCK 3 • 45 min pp. 186–191 **Lesson 4** Building Friendships	**CRF** Lesson Plan * **TT** Bellringer *	**TE** Activity Poster Project, p. 187 GENERAL **TE** Group Activity Using Positive Peer Pressure, p. 187 GENERAL **CRF** Life Skills Activity * GENERAL **CRF** Enrichment Activity * ADVANCED
Lesson 5 Practicing Abstinence	**CRF** Lesson Plan * **TT** Bellringer *	**TE** Activity Goals, p. 190 GENERAL **CRF** Enrichment Activity * ADVANCED

BLOCKS 4 & 5 • 90 min — Chapter Review and Assessment Resources

- **SE** Chapter Review, pp. 192–193
- **CRF** Concept Review * GENERAL
- **CRF** Health Behavior Contract * GENERAL
- **CRF** Chapter Test * GENERAL
- **CRF** Performance-Based Assessment * GENERAL
- **OSP** Test Generator
- **CRF** Test Item Listing *

Online Resources

Visit **go.hrw.com** for a variety of free resources related to this textbook. Enter the keyword **HD4RL7**.

Holt Online Learning

Students can access interactive problem solving help and active visual concept development with the *Decisions for Health* Online Edition available at **www.hrw.com**.

cnnstudentnews.com

Find the latest health news, lesson plans, and activities related to important scientific events.

173A Chapter 9 • Encouraging Healthy Relationships

Compression guide:
To shorten your instruction because of time limitations, omit Lesson 3.

KEY

TE Teacher Edition	**CRF** Chapter Resource File	∗ Also on One-Stop Planner
SE Student Edition	**TT** Teaching Transparency	■ Also Available in Spanish
OSP One-Stop Planner		◆ Requires Advance Prep

SKILLS DEVELOPMENT RESOURCES	LESSON REVIEW AND ASSESSMENT	STANDARDS CORRELATION
		National Health Education Standards
TE Life Skill Builder Setting Goals, p. 177 GENERAL **TE** Life Skill Builder Communicating Effectively, p. 178 ADVANCED **TE** Inclusion Strategies, p. 178 BASIC **CRF** Cross-Disciplinary * GENERAL **CRF** Decision-Making * GENERAL **CRF** Directed Reading * BASIC	**SE** Lesson Review, p. 179 **TE** Reteaching, Quiz, p. 179 **CRF** Lesson Quiz * ■ GENERAL	1.4, 1.6, 3.1, 3.4, 3.6, 4.4, 5.1, 5.2, 5.3, 5.4, 5.5, 6.3, 7.4, 7.5
TE Life Skill Builder Practicing Wellness, p. 181 BASIC **TE** Life Skill Builder Communicating Effectively, p. 181 ADVANCED **SE** Life Skills Activity Coping, p. 182 **TE** Reading Skill Builder Anticipation Guide, p. 182 BASIC **TE** Life Skill Builder Coping, p. 182 GENERAL **TE** Inclusion Strategies, p. 182 BASIC **CRF** Refusal Skills * GENERAL **CRF** Directed Reading * BASIC	**SE** Lesson Review, p. 183 **TE** Reteaching, Quiz, p. 183 **CRF** Concept Mapping * GENERAL **CRF** Lesson Quiz * ■ GENERAL	1.4, 1.6, 3.1, 3.3, 3.4, 3.6, 4.4, 5.1, 5.2, 5.3, 5.4, 5.5, 7.3, 7.4, 7.5
SE Study Tip Compare and Contrast, p. 184 **CRF** Cross-Disciplinary * GENERAL **CRF** Directed Reading * BASIC	**SE** Lesson Review, p. 185 **TE** Reteaching, Quiz, p. 185 **CRF** Lesson Quiz * ■ GENERAL	1.4, 3.1, 3.3, 3.4, 4.4, 5.2, 5.3, 5.4, 5.5, 7.3, 7.4, 7.5
SE Life Skills Activity Making Good Decisions, p. 187 **TE** Life Skill Builder Communicating Effectively, p. 188 ADVANCED **CRF** Directed Reading * BASIC	**SE** Lesson Review, p. 189 **TE** Reteaching, Quiz, p. 189 **CRF** Concept Mapping * GENERAL **CRF** Lesson Quiz * ■ GENERAL	1.4, 1.6, 3.1, 3.3, 3.4, 3.6, 4.4, 5.1, 5.2, 5.3, 5.4, 5.5, 5.6, 7.3, 7.4
TE Life Skill Builder Communicating Effectively, p. 190 GENERAL **CRF** Decision-Making * GENERAL **CRF** Refusal Skills * GENERAL **CRF** Directed Reading * BASIC	**SE** Lesson Review, p. 191 **TE** Reteaching, Quiz, p. 191 **CRF** Lesson Quiz * ■ GENERAL	1.4, 1.6, 1.7, 3.1, 3.3, 3.4, 3.6, 4.4, 5.1, 5.2, 5.3, 5.4, 5.5, 5.6, 6.3, 6.4, 7.4

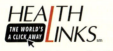

Topic: Abuse and Violence
HealthLinks code: HD4003
Topic: Abstinence
HealthLinks code: HD4002

www.scilinks.org/health

Maintained by the **National Science Teachers Association**

Technology Resources

One-Stop Planner
All of your printable resources and the Test Generator are on this convenient CD-ROM.

Guided Reading Audio CDs

VIDEO SELECT
For information about videos related to this chapter, go to go.hrw.com and type in the keyword **HD4RL7V**.

Chapter 9 • Chapter Planning Guide

CHAPTER 9

Encouraging Healthy Relationships
Chapter Resources

Teacher Resources

TEACHING TRANSPARENCIES
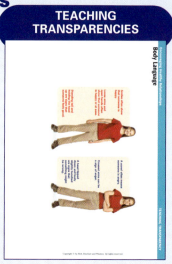

BELLRINGER TRANSPARENCIES
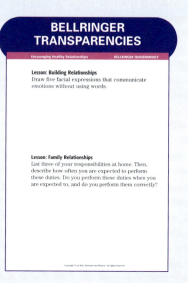

LESSON PLANS

PARENT LETTER
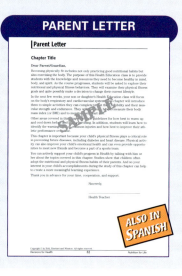

TEST ITEM LISTING
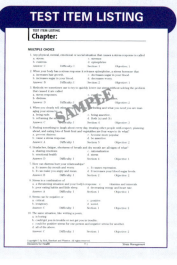

Meeting Individual Needs

DIRECTED READING
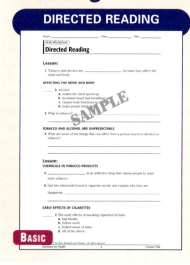

CONCEPT MAPPING
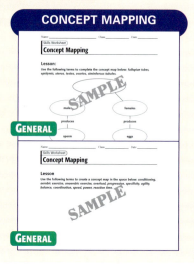

CONCEPT REVIEW
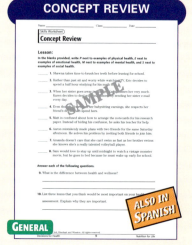

ENRICHMENT ACTIVITIES
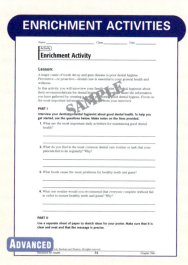

Resources

These worksheet pages can be found in the Chapter Resource File and the One-Stop Planner. The transparencies can be found in the Teaching Transparencies binder and on the One-Stop Planner.

Activities

LIFE SKILLS ACTIVITIES
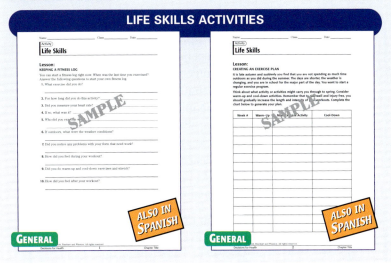

AT-HOME ACTIVITY
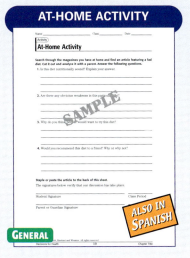

DATASHEETS FOR IN-TEXT ACTIVITIES
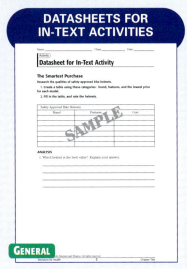

Applications

DECISION-MAKING
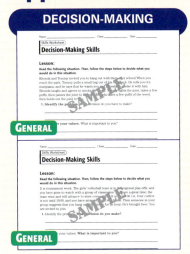

REFUSAL SKILLS
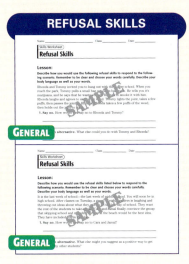

CROSS-DISCIPLINARY
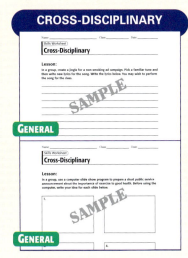

HEALTH BEHAVIOR CONTRACT
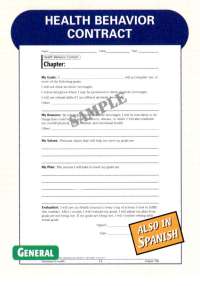

Assessments

HEALTH INVENTORY
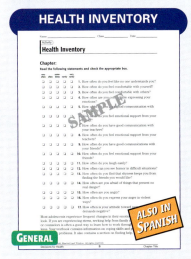

LESSON QUIZZES
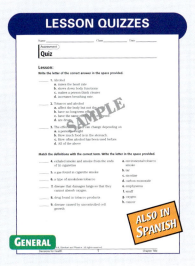

CHAPTER TEST
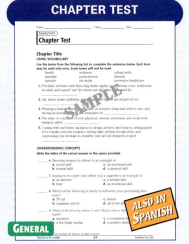

PERFORMANCE-BASED ASSESSMENT
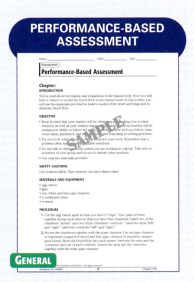

Chapter 9 • Chapter Resources and Worksheets   173D

CHAPTER 9: Background Information

The following information focuses on assertive behavior and how to use it in daily life. This material will help prepare you for teaching the concepts in this chapter.

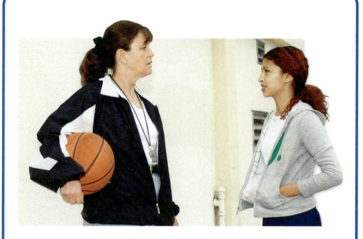

Behavior

- Behavior is how people choose to act or respond to a situation. There are three basic choices people can make. People can chose to be passive, aggressive, or assertive.

- Passiveness is behavior in which people choose not to act on their own behalf or according to their own values. People behaving passively are probably not pursuing what they want or doing what is in their best interest. They may do what others want, even if what others want is unhealthy or dangerous. Passive behavior seldom helps people achieve their goals.

- Aggressiveness is behavior in which people act on their own behalf without regard to the rights, wishes, or feelings of others. Aggressive behavior is often active, intimidating, and disrespectful. It is sometimes violent. People using aggressive behavior may achieve goals, but they often do so at the expense of others.

- Assertiveness is behavior in which people act on their own behalf, in accordance with their values, in a responsible, respectful way. Assertive behavior helps people achieve goals in healthy ways. Many people think that assertive behavior is always physically active, but assertive behavior can also be physically inactive. Learning to ski can be an assertive behavior. But a father who chooses to watch motionless as a child falls while learning to walk is also choosing assertive behavior.

Choosing Assertive Behavior

- People hold many misconceptions about assertive behavior. Some people think that assertiveness is rude. Some people think that assertiveness is a personality trait that some people are born with and that others can never have. But assertive behavior is not rude. And assertiveness is a healthy behavior that people can practice, learn, and choose. Choosing assertive behavior can help people keep themselves and those around them healthy.

- Relationships benefit from assertive behavior. When a person in a relationship acts assertively, he or she honestly expresses what he or she wants, feels, and needs. If these things are expressed assertively, then the person expressing them is not demanding that other people take care of his or her wants and needs. Rather, a person behaving assertively assumes responsibility for taking care of his or her own wants and needs and helps others to do the same.

- Behaving assertively in the face of pressure can be difficult. Here are some tips that can help.

  - Don't rush decisions. Think about what you really want so that when you express your thoughts and feelings, you can stand behind them.

  - Ask questions when you don't understand. Give people the chance to be clear so that you can answer them honestly.

  - Use brief, concise language. Say, "No" when you mean no. Don't hedge.

  - Repeat your response as often as needed.

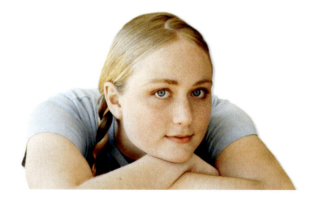

For background information about teaching strategies and issues, refer to the *Professional Reference for Teachers*.

ACTIVITIES

CHAPTER 9

Consider using the activities on this page as students explore the lessons of this chapter. Look for other activities throughout the Student Edition chapter.

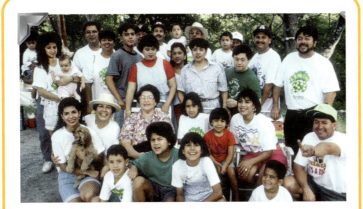

Considering Relationships

Procedure Give each student a pencil and either a paper plate or a piece of paper. Have each student draw five, evenly-spaced concentric circles on the paper or plate and write his or her name in the center circle. Write the following list on the board: mother, father, complete strangers, brother(s), sister(s), acquaintances, good friends, teacher, grandparents, closest friends, aunts, uncles, first cousins, second cousins, stepmother or stepfather, half brother, and half sister. Ask students to think about each relationship on the list. If they have a relationship described by one of the terms, have them write the term in one of the rings. Instruct the students to write the term nearer or farther from the center, depending on how close they feel to that person.

Analysis After students have filled in their circles, ask students to write answers to the following questions:

- How frequently do you see each person? (Answers may vary.)
- Do you share your private thoughts and feelings with all of these people? Explain why or why not. (Sample answer: No, not all relationships should include the sharing of personal information.)
- What determines how close you feel to people? (Answers may vary.)
- What is one thing you could do to improve the relationships you have with the family members you listed? (Answers may vary but may include spending more time with those family members.)

Librarian

Procedure Organize students into groups of three. Designate one student in each group to be a librarian. Hand other group members a slip of paper. One slip should read, "Ask: 'May I borrow this book for 2 minutes?' (Without explaining why it is late, return the book in 4 minutes.)" The other slip should read "After the other person has borrowed the book, ask: 'May I borrow this book 2 minutes from now when it is returned?'" Ask students to read their instructions silently and then follow the instructions. Tell the students who borrow the book that their assignment is to write down on a piece of paper everything they can find in the book about "personal responsibility." Students must use only the textbook the librarian handed them. Tell them that this assignment is due in 5 minutes.

Analysis Ask the following questions:

- To the first borrower in each group: "How did you react when the book was overdue? In real life, what would have been the responsible way to borrow and return the book?" (The first borrower could have returned the book on time or apologized for being late.)
- To the second borrower in each group: "How did you respond when the book was overdue?" (Sample answer: I became angry.) "How did you respond when you got the book with only 1 minute left to do the assignment?" (Sample answer: I became angry.)

Pen Pals

You may wish to start up a pen pal program in which students write letters to other students around the world. Pairing students up with students from other countries is an excellent way to encourage tolerance because students learn firsthand how different perspectives can influence them in a positive way.

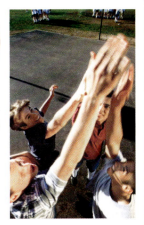

Chapter 9 • Activities   173F

CHAPTER 9

Overview
Tell students that this chapter will help them learn how to build healthy relationships, understand their role in the family, and address and solve problems in family relationships. This chapter describes the characteristics of healthy communities, how to identify and cope with unhealthy relationships, and offers strategies for maintaining abstinence.

Assessing Prior Knowledge
Students should be familiar with the following topics:
- decision making
- refusal skills

Question Box
Students may feel more comfortable asking questions if you set up a Question Box to collect their questions. Have students write and anonymously submit their questions about relationships, such as ideas for showing affection, maintaining sexual abstinence, or identifying abusive or neglectful relationships. Address these questions during class, or use these questions to introduce lessons that cover related topics.

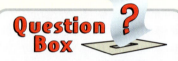

Check out *Current Health* articles and activities related to this chapter by visiting the HRW Web site at **go.hrw.com**. Just type in the keyword **HD4CH24T**.

Chapter Resource File
- Directed Reading **BASIC**
- Health Inventory **GENERAL**
- Parent Letter

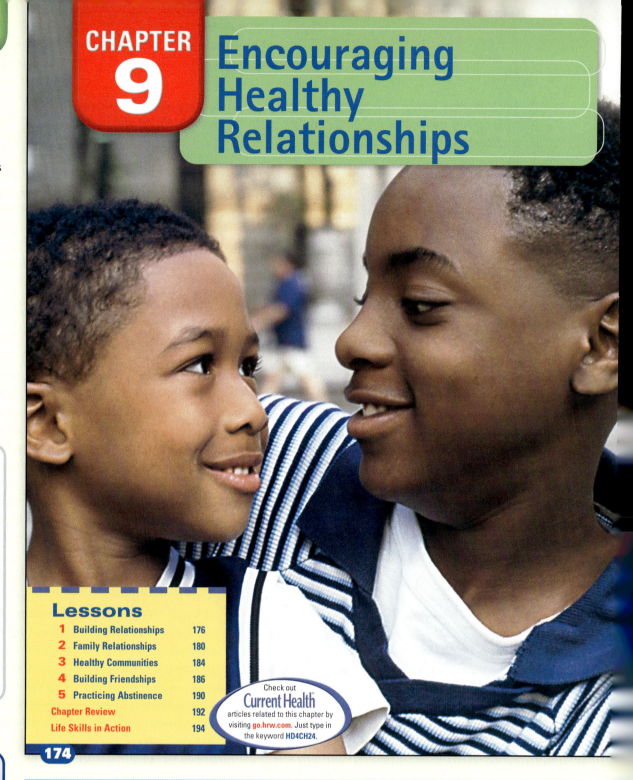

CHAPTER 9 Encouraging Healthy Relationships

Lessons
1	Building Relationships	176
2	Family Relationships	180
3	Healthy Communities	184
4	Building Friendships	186
5	Practicing Abstinence	190
Chapter Review		192
Life Skills in Action		194

Check out **Current Health** articles related to this chapter by visiting **go.hrw.com**. Just type in the keyword **HD4CH24**.

Standards Correlations

National Health Education Standards

1.4 Describe how family and peers influence the health of adolescents. (Lessons 1–5)

1.6 Describe ways to reduce risks related to adolescent health problems. (Lessons 1–2 and 4–5)

1.7 Explain how appropriate healthcare can prevent premature death and disability. (Lesson 5)

3.1 Explain the importance of assuming responsibility for personal health behaviors. (Lessons 1–5)

3.3 Distinguish between safe and risky or harmful behaviors in relationships. (Lessons 2–5)

3.4 Demonstrate strategies to improve or maintain personal and family health. (Lessons 1–5)

3.6 Demonstrate ways to avoid and reduce threatening situations. (Lessons 1–2 and 4–5)

4.4 Analyze how information from peers influences health. (Lessons 1–5)

5.1 Demonstrate effective verbal and non-verbal communication skills to enhance health. (Lessons 1–2 and 4–5)

5.2 Describe how the behavior of family and peers affects interpersonal communication. (Lessons 1–5)

> "My little brother, Ray, was **born deaf**. I'd be **careful** when watching any kid, but I have to be **really careful** when I watch him. He can't hear things like cars and dogs. When we play in the yard, I listen for both of us."

Health IQ

PRE-READING
Answer the following multiple-choice questions to find out what you already know about relationships. When you've finished this chapter, you'll have the opportunity to change your answers based on what you've learned.

1. **Body language**
   a. is a way of talking to your body.
   b. communicates information and feelings without words.
   c. is rarely helpful in communication.
   d. All of the above

2. **Personal responsibility is**
   a. doing your part.
   b. keeping promises.
   c. accepting the consequences of your actions.
   d. All of the above

3. **Abuse is**
   a. sometimes the victim's fault.
   b. always the victim's fault.
   c. never the victim's fault.
   d. All of the above

4. **The best way to cope with neglect is to**
   a. tell a trusted adult as soon as possible.
   b. ask your peers for advice.
   c. wait until someone asks about it.
   d. keep it a secret.

5. **A community is made stronger through**
   a. tolerance.
   b. neglect.
   c. aggressive behavior.
   d. None of the above

6. **Sexual abstinence**
   a. shows that you care about yourself and others.
   b. prevents many complications in your life.
   c. prevents pregnancy.
   d. All of the above

ANSWERS: 1. b; 2. d; 3. c; 4. a; 5. a; 6. d

Using the Health IQ

Misconception Alert
Answers to the Health IQ questions may help you identify students' misconceptions.

Question 3: Students may consider a victim to be at fault if they think a victim antagonized the abuser by saying or doing something to goad the abuser. Point out that nothing justifies abusive behavior. Abuse is never the victim's fault.

Question 4: Students may be used to seeking advice from their friends and select that answer to this question. Point out that peers may not be able provide informed, helpful advice about serious problems. Tell students that serious problems, such as neglect, should be reported to a trusted adult.

Question 6: Some students may not think that abstinence demonstrates caring. Point out that abstinence does demonstrate caring because it keeps teens healthy.

Answers
1. b
2. d
3. c
4. a
5. a
6. d

5.3 Demonstrate healthy ways to express needs, wants, and feelings. (Lessons 1–5)

5.4 Demonstrate ways to communicate care, consideration, and respect for self and others. (Lessons 1–5)

5.5 Demonstrate communication skills to build and maintain healthy relationships. (Lessons 1–5)

5.6 (partial) Demonstrate refusal and negotiation skills to enhance health. (Lessons 4–5)

6.3 Predict how decisions regarding health behaviors have consequences for self and others. (Lessons 1 and 5)

6.4 Apply strategies and skills needed to attain personal health goals. (Lesson 5)

7.3 (partial) Identify barriers to effective communication of information, ideas, feelings, and opinions about health issues. (Lessons 2–4)

7.4 Demonstrate the ability to influence and support others in making positive health choices. (Lessons 1–5)

7.5 Demonstrate the ability to work cooperatively when advocating for healthy individuals, families, and schools. (Lessons 1–3)

VIDEO SELECT
For information about videos related to this chapter, go to **go.hrw.com** and type in the keyword **HD4RL7V**.

Chapter 9 • Encouraging Healthy Relationships

Lesson 1 Focus

Overview
Before beginning this lesson, review with your students the objectives listed under the What You'll Do head in the Student Edition. In this lesson, students will investigate why relationships are important and what it means to demonstrate personal responsibility. Students will explore forms of communication and the benefits of assertive behavior.

🔔 Bellringer
Ask students to draw five facial expressions that communicate without words. Have students share their drawings and have the class guess what message is being sent by each drawing. **English Language Learners**
LS Visual

Answer to Start Off Write
Accept all reasonable answers. Sample answer: I let people know how I feel by the words I say, the way I stand, the expression on my face, and how I behave.

Motivate

Activity — GENERAL
Communicating Effectively
Whisper a phrase once to students at the front of each row of desks. Have those students whisper it once to the person behind them. Ask students at the end of each row to say aloud what they heard. Compare the phrases heard at the beginnings and ends of each row.
LS Auditory

Lesson 1

What You'll Do
- **Explain** how relationships can help you stay healthy.
- **Explain** how healthy relationships are like teams.
- **Explain** how people communicate by using words and body language.
- **Identify** how assertive behavior can help you learn and grow.

Terms to Learn
- relationship
- personal responsibility
- body language
- behavior

Start Off Write
How do you let people know how you feel?

Building Relationships

You have relationships with many people. Relationships take work to keep them healthy. When you work on your relationships, you improve your social health.

A **relationship** is an emotional or social connection between two or more people. You have relationships with your family, your friends, and your neighbors. All of these connections affect you. Many of these relationships are different, but similar skills are used to keep all relationships healthy.

Keeping You Healthy

When people in relationships are good to each other, they can help keep each other safe and healthy. People in healthy relationships look out for each other and help each other make good choices. They don't put each other in danger. You can have healthy relationships with your family and friends. Listen carefully, cooperate, and let people know what you need. Keeping your relationships healthy takes work, skill, and responsibility.

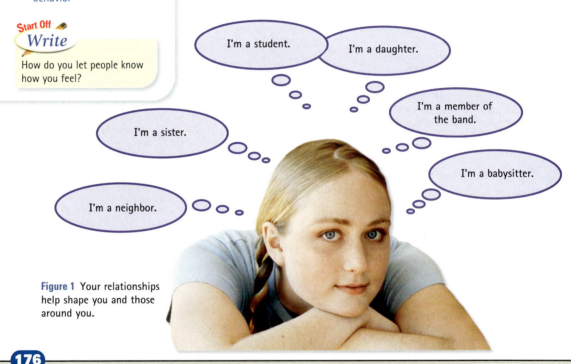

Figure 1 Your relationships help shape you and those around you.

Sensitivity ALERT
Discussing relationships may be difficult for many students. For example, students in a family crisis may feel awkward about discussing the importance of close family relationships. Students who are having a difficult time making or keeping friends may struggle to discuss the importance of helping friends. Be careful not to put students on the spot. Refer students who need help to appropriate professionals.

Chapter Resource File
- Directed Reading BASIC
- Lesson Plan
- Lesson Quiz GENERAL

Transparencies
TT Bellringer
TT Body Language

176 Chapter 9 • Encouraging Healthy Relationships

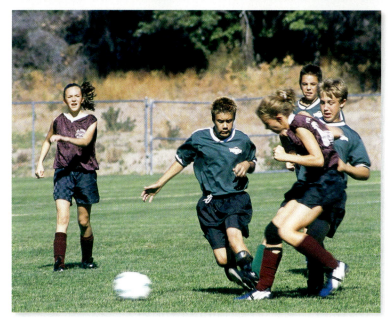

Figure 2 For a team to be effective, each player has to be responsible for his or her actions. For a relationship to thrive, each person has to take responsibility for himself or herself.

Teamwork

For relationships to be healthy, everybody in the relationship has to take personal responsibility. **Personal responsibility** is doing your part, keeping promises, and accepting the consequences of your actions. Taking personal responsibility shows that you are reliable and caring. You know what is expected of you. You let people know what you need, and you do your best to help others. When you are responsible, you correct your mistakes and learn from them. Everybody makes mistakes. When responsible people make a mistake, they don't blame anyone else. They apologize, fix the problem as well as they can, and learn how to keep from making the same mistake again.

Being responsible in a relationship is like being on a team. On a sports team, every player's position matters. For the team to be successful, all of the players have to work hard at their individual positions. And if one player struggles in his or her position, the other players help out.

You can show responsibility and teamwork every day at home by doing chores, being on time, and helping your brothers and sisters. Taking care of small problems that you see around you shows that you care about your role in your family. If you see trash in the yard, pick it up. If you are having an argument with a brother or sister, settle it calmly. Taking responsibility at home helps you learn to be responsible in all of your relationships.

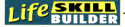 — GENERAL

Setting Goals Ask students how they have shown responsibility in school in the last week. (Sample answers: on-time attendance, turned in homework on time, studied for an exam) Ask students to list five ways they can take responsibility this week. (Answers may vary.) **LS** Intrapersonal

Teach

Discussion — GENERAL

Correcting Mistakes Ask students how they respond when they realize that they have made a mistake that affects other people. (Sample answer: I get angry that I have caused a problem and fearful that other people may respond in anger.) Correcting mistakes that involve others may involve only you, or it may require you and other people to respond responsibly. Ask students to consider the following situations:

- Your mother gives you money to walk to the corner store and buy bread and milk. You don't go straight to the store. You walk to a friend's house and play video games and then play a game of catch in his yard. You finally decide to go to the store. You get to the store and reach into your pocket and the money is gone. You look everywhere, but you can't find it. What can you do? (Sample answer: You can walk home, tell your mother that you lost the money, apologize for not doing as she asked, and offer to pay the money back by doing chores.)

- A friend asked you to teach him how to solve a math problem. You show him as best you can. During the quiz the next day, you realize that you showed him incorrectly. How can you and your friend show personal responsibility? (Sample answer: You can apologize and show him the correct way to solve the problem. Your friend can show responsibility by accepting your apology and trying to learn the correct way to solve the problem. He should also talk to his teacher about the trouble he is having.)

LS Interpersonal

Teach, continued

Life SKILL BUILDER — ADVANCED

Communicating Effectively Ask students to describe what happens to communication when people stand too far away from each other. (Sample answer: Communication is difficult because of the distance.) Ask what happens when one person stands too close. (Sample answer: One person may feel awkward or distracted if the other person stands too close.) Tell students that standing a respectful distance away from people when you talk is a kind of body language, too. It communicates respect. Students can practice finding this distance by standing up and walking toward each other as they talk. Have them stop when they both feel comfortable and can communicate clearly. LS **Kinesthetic**

Activity — GENERAL

Charades Organize students into groups of three to five. Hand out index cards describing different postures to each student in the group. (Sample ideas: cross your arms, hold your head with your hands, put your face in your hands, slouch your shoulders and look at the ground, put both your hands on your hips, smile with outstretched arms) Have students silently demonstrate the body language on the cards. Have other students write what they think the message is. (Sample answers: The person with crossed arms feels defensive. The person holding his head is nervous or has a headache. The person slouching may be sad, frustrated, or not feeling well. The person with her hands on her hips feels authoritative or bossy. The smiling person is happy to greet someone.)
LS **Kinesthetic**   **English Language Learners**

LANGUAGE ARTS ACTIVITY

Good speaking and listening skills do more than help us get along. They can save lives. Write a story about someone who uses good communication skills to help someone else who is in danger.

Figure 3 Reading body language is a skill. Body language uses the face, hands, and body position.

INCLUSION Strategies — BASIC

• **Visually Impaired**
Help students with visual impairments understand the concept of body language by asking other students to volunteer to demonstrate examples of facial expressions that communicate anger, happiness, surprise, disgust, and pain. Have students with visual impairments gently feel the volunteers' faces and describe the traits of the different expressions.   **English Language Learners**
LS **Kinesthetic**

Communicating Clearly

Healthy relationships are impossible if people do not understand each other. So, another important skill in healthy relationships is the ability to communicate clearly. Using good communication skills helps people share thoughts and feelings.

Good communication begins with speaking clearly. Think about what you are going to say before you speak. Face your listeners. Ask questions to make sure you are being understood.

You should also use good listening skills. Look at the person who is speaking. Make eye contact. Nod to let him or her know that you understand. If you are not sure what someone is saying, politely ask the person to clarify the message.

Using Body Language

Communication is more than expressing ideas and feelings with words. It is also understanding body language. **Body language** is a way of communicating by using the look on your face, the way you hold your hands, and the way you stand. The figure below identifies some common body language messages. Sending the same message clearly through both your words and your body language helps get your message across.

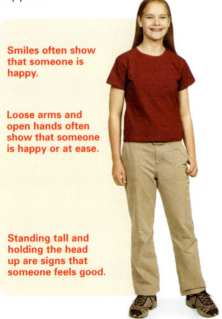

Smiles often show that someone is happy.

Loose arms and open hands often show that someone is happy or at ease.

Standing tall and holding the head up are signs that someone feels good.

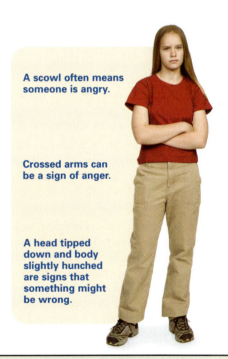

A scowl often means someone is angry.

Crossed arms can be a sign of anger.

A head tipped down and body slightly hunched are signs that something might be wrong.

Answer to Language Arts Activity

Accept all reasonable answers. Answers should reflect a clear understanding of good communication skills, including body language, good speaking, and keen listening.

Chapter 9 • Encouraging Healthy Relationships

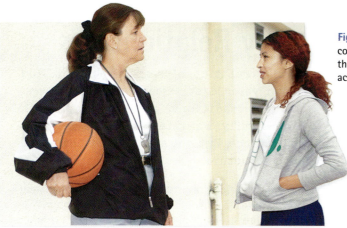

Figure 4 Politely asking a coach why you did not make the team is one example of acting assertively.

Choosing Behavior

You communicate by using words and body language, but you also communicate through your behavior. **Behavior** is the way you choose to act or respond. Acting on your thoughts and feelings in a way that respects the thoughts and feelings of others is being *assertive*.

What does acting assertively look like? Here's an example: If you tried out for a team and were not chosen, you may feel sad and angry. But how would you choose to behave? You could do nothing. You could blame others. Or you could be assertive. You could respectfully speak to the coach. You could ask why you didn't make the team. You could ask for tips on how to improve so that you could make the team next time. When you choose to be assertive, you take responsibility for what happened and help yourself succeed.

Myth & Fact

Myth: It is rude to be assertive.

Fact: Real assertiveness is respectful and sincere. It is not rude.

Lesson Review

Using Vocabulary
1. Define *relationship*, and explain how relationships help you stay healthy.

Understanding Concepts
2. Explain how understanding body language and using good speaking and listening skills help communication.

3. Explain how taking personal responsibility in a relationship is like being on a team.

Critical Thinking
4. **Applying Concepts** Ken wants to try out for a role in a play, but he has never acted before. How can Ken behave assertively to help him get a part?

Lesson 2

Focus

Overview
Before beginning this lesson, review with your students the objectives listed under the What You'll Do head in the Student Edition. This lesson explains why there are roles in a family and how family members nurture one another. Students will learn different ways to show respect, work through small family problems, and identify and deal with serious family problems.

🔔 Bellringer
Have students list three of their duties at home and describe how often they are expected to perform these duties. Ask students to explain whether they consistently meet their parents' expectations.
LS Verbal

Answer to Start Off Write
Accept all reasonable answers. Sample answer: Respect helps family members trust each other.

Motivate

Activity — GENERAL
Assigning Roles Ask students for a list of household duties, and write the list on the board. (Sample duties: paying bills, washing dishes, picking up the yard, preparing meals, earning money, feeding the pets, walking the dog, doing laundry) Ask students which duties on the list a middle school student could do if no one else in the home could do it. (Sample answers: washing dishes, preparing a simple meal) Ask which roles could not be filled by a middle school student. (Sample answer: earn enough to pay bills)

Lesson 2

What You'll Do
- **Explain** why there are a lot of family roles.
- **Describe** four ways that families nurture.
- **Describe** five ways to show respect.
- **Describe** two ways you can work through small family problems.
- **Identify** four serious problems and a way to deal with them.

Terms to Learn
- nurturing
- neglect
- abuse

Start Off Write
Why is respect important in all family relationships?

Family Relationships

Family relationships are important. You learn your first lessons about language, values, traditions, and cooperation in your family. Families are alike in their importance. But not all families have the same structure.

Families have different forms. You may live with two parents, or you may live with only your mom or your dad. You may live in a *blended family*, which is made when two families combine, or with an extended family. Your *extended family* can include grandparents, aunts, uncles, and cousins. Sometimes, extended families, such as the family in the figure below, get together for reunions. Yet no matter what your family looks like, everyone plays an important role.

Roles for Everybody

Being a family is a lot of work. Food must be cooked, dishes must be cleaned, and laundry must be washed. If you have a yard or pet, those things will also need care. There is enough work for everyone to have a role. Your role depends on what your family needs. Different families have different roles to fill. Your parents have probably told you what they expect of you. You may have chores to do and a room to keep clean. For your family to function smoothly, everyone must do his or her part.

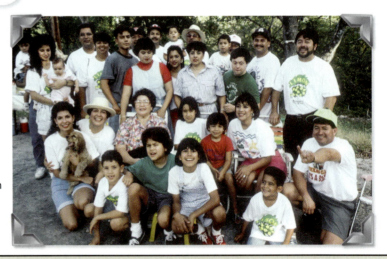

Figure 5 The Limon family gets together for a reunion every year.

Sensitivity ALERT
Students may be sensitive about their family structure or be concerned about how their family fits into the descriptions listed on the page. Be aware that adopted students may have questions about their adoption, and foster children may have been part of several families, each structured differently.

Chapter Resource File
- Directed Reading **BASIC**
- Lesson Plan
- Lesson Quiz **GENERAL**

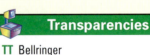
Transparencies
TT Bellringer

---

180 Chapter 9 • Encouraging Healthy Relationships

Nurturing

All of the roles in a family have the same basic purpose: to nurture. **Nurturing** (NUR chuhr ing) is providing the things that people need in order to live and grow. People in families nurture by providing

- love and acceptance
- the things needed for survival, such as food, clothing, and housing
- protection from danger and rules to keep everyone safe
- instruction in skills and values

Adults are usually responsible for most of the nurturing in a family. But you can help nurture, too. Help your brothers and sisters by being a good role model and by showing them love and acceptance.

Respect

Healthy relationships are based on respect. To respect people is to be considerate of them and to let them know they are important. When you show respect to the members of your family, you send the message that you care about their thoughts and feelings. Showing respect helps you trust each other and strengthens your relationships. Here are some ways to show respect for your family:

- Follow family rules.
- Keep your word.
- Discuss disagreements respectfully.
- Treat family members' property and rooms as you would like yours to be treated.
- Listen carefully when people speak to you, and respond politely.

Respecting your family members helps you trust and rely on each other. Being able to trust and rely on each other makes living together more pleasant. And getting through hard times is easier if you have the help of people who care about you.

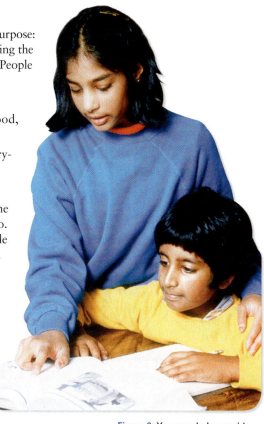

Figure 6 You can help provide nurturing by taking care of your brothers and sisters.

BIOLOGY CONNECTION — GENERAL

Nurturing Animals Ask students to choose a mammal and do some research on its behavior. Have students write a paragraph explaining how this mammal nurtures its young. (Students should draw clear parallels to the four characteristics of the term *nurture* given in the chapter. Sample answer: A wolf provides her pup with milk and hunts for food. She provides a den for her pups to be safe while she hunts. She provides warmth by snuggling her pups into her fur. She protects her pups from danger with her sharp teeth and claws and her keen sense of smell. She licks and plays with her pups and does not harm them if they get too rough while playing. As her pups grow older, she teaches them how to hunt.) **LS** Verbal

Teach

Life SKILL BUILDER — BASIC

Practicing Wellness Remind students that, if possible, staying in touch with grandparents and other extended family members is a great way to keep family ties strong. Have interested students write a letter or card to an extended family member. **LS** Verbal

Group Activity — GENERAL

Family Instruction Manual Have students write a general instruction manual for a family. Have students include as many chores, jobs and ways to show nurturing and respect as they can. Have volunteers present their manuals to the class. **LS** Verbal/Visual

Cultural Awareness — BASIC

Showing Respect Many languages, such as Spanish and French, have a specific verb tense to show respect to the elderly and authority figures. Ask students to list English phrases and titles that are used to show respect. (Sample answer: titles such as Mr., Mrs., Dr., Officer, Colonel, President, Pastor, and Rabbi; phrases include "Yes, Sir," and "Yes, Ma'am," and courtesies such as "please" and "thank you") **LS** Verbal

Life SKILL BUILDER — ADVANCED

Communicating Effectively Ask students to list ways that a child might NOT show respect to other family members in a column on a piece of paper. Then, beside the first column, have students list an opposite action. (Students may list pairs of actions such as the following: yelling/speaking softly and throwing other people's belongings on the ground/treating things with care.) **LS** Verbal

Lesson 2 • Family Relationships **181**

Teach, continued

READING SKILL BUILDER — BASIC

Anticipation Guide Before students read this page, ask them to describe the difference between neglect and abuse. Then, ask students to read the page to find out if their predictions were accurate.
LS Verbal

LIFE SKILLS ACTIVITY

Answer
Student answers may vary but should reflect a compromise in which both Beth and her brother benefit. Sample solution: One show could be taped on a VCR while the other person watches his or her show.

Life SKILL BUILDER — GENERAL

Coping Serious problems, such as abuse and neglect, are often very difficult subjects for people to discuss. Victims of abuse and neglect have many fears and concerns, often about their own safety or the safety of other family members, including the person who is hurting them. Tell students that the best way to address a serious problem is to talk about it with people who can help. Tell students that after a victim has identified an adult who can help, the victim can say to him or her something simple, such as, "I need to talk to someone." Most responsible adults will know how to guide the conversation from there. **LS** Interpersonal

LIFE SKILLS ACTIVITY

COPING

In small groups, role-play the following scenario:

Beth and her brother argue every night about which TV shows to watch.

How can Beth and her brother settle this problem? Try to find three solutions. When you are finished, have each group share solutions. Make a list of all the different solutions you find.

Minor Problems

Learning to work through everyday problems is a skill everybody needs to learn. When you have a minor problem, you can often resolve it yourself. Problems such as arguments between brothers and sisters can usually be solved if the people involved listen to each other, work together, and look for a solution that works for everyone.

One way to work on problems as a family is to hold regular family meetings. At a family meeting, the whole household meets to talk openly about everyone's thoughts and feelings. Everyone gets a chance to speak, and everyone listens carefully. By treating everyone's concerns respectfully, people can take care of minor problems before they grow into major problems.

Serious Problems

Not all problems are easy to handle. Some problems are more serious. Serious problems include neglect (ni GLECKT) and abuse (uh BYOOS). **Neglect** is the failure of a parent or responsible adult to provide for a child's basic needs, such as food, clothing, and shelter. **Abuse** is treating someone in a harmful or offensive way. Some forms of abuse are described in the table below. All forms of abuse and neglect are wrong.

Anybody can become a victim of abuse or neglect. Abuse and neglect can hurt a person physically and emotionally. Victims can have injuries to their bodies. They can feel worthless and powerless. But victims are valuable people who deserve to live safe, healthy lives. Help is available, and all victims should get help. If you know of anyone being abused or neglected, help that person by reporting the problem as soon as you can.

TABLE 1 Identifying Forms of Abuse

Problem	Description
Physical abuse	harmful treatment that causes injury to the body; sometimes results in cuts, burns, and broken bones
Emotional abuse	the repeated use of harsh words or threatening actions to control another person; treating a person as though he or she is worthless
Sexual abuse	any forced sexual contact or any sexual contact with a child

INCLUSION Strategies — BASIC

• **Developmentally Delayed**

Students with developmental delays sometimes have difficulty differentiating between major and minor problems. Help students understand that any problem that could cause a person to be seriously hurt is a major problem. Remind students to tell a trusted adult about any problems they have in which someone could get hurt. **LS** Interpersonal

Chapter 9 • Encouraging Healthy Relationships

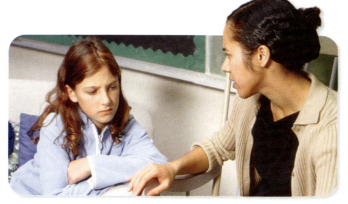

Figure 7 Talking to a counselor can help you solve many problems.

Help

Talking about serious problems is difficult. Many people who have been abused are afraid or ashamed. But there is nothing shameful about being abused or neglected. Abuse or neglect can happen to anyone and is never the victim's fault. Where can people who have been abused or neglected get help? The first step is to talk to a trusted adult, such as

- an adult family member (a parent, a grandparent, an aunt, or an uncle)
- someone at school (a teacher, a school nurse, a coach, or a counselor)
- a police officer or a firefighter

Any of these people will know how to help and should help. But if the first adult told about the abuse does not help, the victim should keep telling adults until the abuse stops.

Health Journal

If you had a friend with a serious problem, whom could you tell? In your Health Journal, make a list of trusted adults in your life. What do these people have in common?

Lesson Review

Using Vocabulary
1. What does *nurturing* mean?

Understanding Concepts
2. What are four ways that families nurture?
3. Define four serious family problems, and describe what should be done about them.
4. Explain why there are a lot of family roles.
5. Describe five ways of showing respect to your family.

Critical Thinking
6. **Making Good Decisions** Rosa and her brother both think that the other does not help enough around the house. Describe two ways they could work on their problem.

internet connect
www.scilinks.org/health
Topic: Abuse and Violence
HealthLinks code: HD4003
HEALTH LINKS. Maintained by the National Science Teachers Association

Lesson 3 Focus

Overview
Before beginning this lesson, review with your students the objectives listed under the What You'll Do head in the Student Edition. This lesson explains why tolerance is needed for healthy communities and how students can help keep a community healthy.

Bellringer
Ask students to list three characteristics of a community. (Communities are made up of people with a common background, location, or who share interests, beliefs, or goals.)
LS Verbal

Answer to Start Off Write
Accept all reasonable answers. Sample answer: My neighbors and I live in the same area, shop at the same stores, and have dogs.

Motivate

Group Activity —— GENERAL
Choosing Sides Collect newspaper articles on conflicts within communities. Give each article to two small student groups. Have students read the article. Assign each group to pretend that they are one of the groups in the article. Have them each summarize the conflict. Possible questions to ask each group: "How would you describe your own behavior? How would you describe the behavior of the other group? How do you feel about the other group?" You may wish to add more questions, depending on the article and the time available. Repeat with another pair of groups and a different article.
LS Interpersonal Co-op Learning

Lesson 3

What You'll Do
- **Explain** why tolerance is needed in communities.
- **List** five ways to keep a community healthy.

Terms to Learn
- community
- tolerance

Start Off Write
What do you have in common with your neighbors?

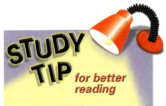

STUDY TIP for better reading

Compare and Contrast
How are healthy communities like healthy families? How are they different? Make a chart that compares and contrasts families and communities.

Figure 8 Healthy communities work together and use everybody's strengths. People of all ages can help make a community garden.

Answer to Study Tip
Accept all reasonable answers. Both healthy families and healthy communities work together and accept people for who they are. However, communities are often much larger than families.

Healthy Communities

Scott and his friends walk by a vacant lot every day on their way to school. The lot is filling with trash. Scott and his friends want to make the lot cleaner and safer. They'd like to plant a community garden.

Scott and his friends are part of a neighborhood community. A **community** is made up of people of who have a common background or location or who share similar interests, beliefs, or goals. Neighborhoods, schools, and teams are examples of communities.

Practicing Tolerance

Members of a community share some common interests. But in every community, people have differences. Because of differences, tolerance (TAHL urh uhns) is needed to keep communities healthy. **Tolerance** is the ability to respect differences in people and to accept people for who they are. By respecting differences in each other, people in a community can learn from each other. Tolerance also strengthens a community. People with different backgrounds and talents help the community solve problems in different ways. When you have more ways to solve problems, you are more likely to find good solutions.

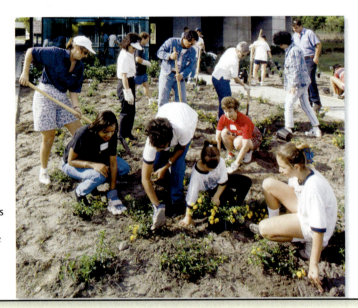

Chapter Resource File
- Directed Reading BASIC
- Lesson Plan
- Lesson Quiz GENERAL

Transparencies
TT Bellringer

184 Chapter 9 • Encouraging Healthy Relationships

Living in Communities

You are a member of many communities, including your neighborhood and your school. Doing your part helps keep these communities healthy. You help when you

- obey rules and laws
- practice tolerance
- take part in community activities
- respectfully point out problems
- work with others to find solutions to community problems

Being part of a community can also be fun. For example, being a member of a band and having a role in a play are ways to spend time with people who like to do the things you like to do.

Myth & Fact

Myth: Members of healthy communities always agree with each other.

Fact: Members of healthy communities often disagree. Learning to accept each other in spite of differences helps strengthen communities.

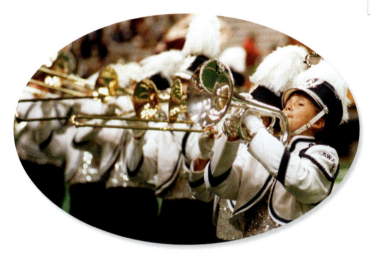

Figure 9 A marching band is a community made of individuals who like to play music. The band plays music best when all members of this community work together.

Lesson Review

Using Vocabulary

1. What is tolerance?
2. Define *community*, and give three examples of communities.

Understanding Concepts

3. How do communities benefit from tolerance?

4. List five ways you can be a responsible member of a community.

Critical Thinking

5. **Identifying Relationships** Larone is in the school band, which plays at school concerts, at football games, and in town parades. How does Larone's role in one community help the other communities he is a part of?

Answers to Lesson Review

1. Tolerance is the ability to respect differences in people and accept them for who they are.
2. Sample answer: A community is made up of people who have a common background or location or who share interests, beliefs, or goals. Neighborhoods, schools, and teams are three kinds of communities.
3. Sample answer: Communities benefit from tolerance because people from different backgrounds and talents help the community tackle problems in lots of different ways.
4. Sample answer: To be a responsible member of my community, I can obey rules and laws, practice tolerance, take part in community activities, respectfully point out problems, and work with others to find solutions to community problems.
5. Accept all reasonable answers. Sample answer: By playing in the band, Larone is an active member of the band community. His community helps provide music that enriches other communities, such as the school, the football team, and the town.

Teach

Discussion — GENERAL

Comprehension Check Ask students to identify roles within their school community. Students who have difficulty with this should fill in the blanks of the following sentence: A <u>student's</u> job in a school community is to <u>learn</u>. (Sample answers: students learn; teachers teach and assess; principals manage a school; nurses monitor the students' health)

Close

Reteaching — BASIC

Ways to Remember Ask students to create a mnemonic device for remembering ways to keep communities healthy. Have students share their devices with the class. (Sample answer: Using the first letter of every action in the list: o, p, t, r, w, students could write the sentence: Owen practices talking respectfully to Wendy.)

Quiz — GENERAL

1. Are people who take part in a recycling program part of a community? Explain your answer. (Yes, these people share the goal of promoting recycling.)
2. When Ian and Phil agree to overlook differences and work on a project together, they are practicing ____. (tolerance)
3. How does showing tolerance for people of all ages help provide more ways of solving problems? (Sample answer: People of all ages might look at problems differently and have many ways to solve them. Tolerance helps us take everyone's ideas seriously.)

Lesson 3 • Healthy Communities

Lesson 4

Focus

Overview
Before beginning this lesson, review with your students the objectives listed under the What You'll Do head in the Student Edition. This lesson describes what friends do and how supporting friends can help friends stay healthy. Students will explore how healthy forms of affection send positive messages to friends. In addition, students will learn how to identify and cope with an unhealthy relationship.

Bellringer
Have students list four personality traits that their friends have. (Sample answers: fun, encouraging, respectful, motivating) **LS Verbal**

Answer to Start Off Write
Accept all reasonable answers. Sample answer: I should support my friends because by supporting each other, we help each other succeed and stay healthy.

Motivate

Discussion — GENERAL

Lies and Friendship Ask students why it is harmful to befriend peers who encourage them to lie to other friends. (Sample answer: Lying is wrong. People who encourage lying will probably lie to me.) Ask students why a peer who encourages them to lie to parents is not behaving as a friend should. (Sample answer: A friend would respect me, my values, and the values of my family.) **LS Interpersonal**

Lesson 4 — Building Friendships

What You'll Do
- **Explain** why healthy friendships are important.
- **Describe** how supporting your friends can help them stay healthy.
- **Describe** three messages sent by healthy forms of affection.
- **Describe** how to identify and resolve an unhealthy relationship.

Terms to Learn
- friendship

Start Off Write
Why should you support your friends?

Miriam has been thinking about helping dogs at the animal shelter. She called the shelter and found out that the shelter needs volunteers to walk dogs. She mentioned her idea to her friend Leah, who said she would help, too. Miriam was glad to start her new project with a friend.

Doing projects together can build a friendship. A **friendship** is a relationship between people who enjoy being together, who care about each other, and who have similar interests. Good friends help each other by demonstrating and encouraging good character. Good character helps you maintain healthy friendships.

Identifying Healthy Friendships

Your friends do more than hang around with you and make you laugh. They help you make decisions that are good for you. They support your goals and help you do your best work in school.

Friends also respect your beliefs and values. Good friends would never ask you to do anything that would go against your values or the values of your family. The number of friends you have does not matter. What does matter is making sure that the friends you do have are caring and respectful.

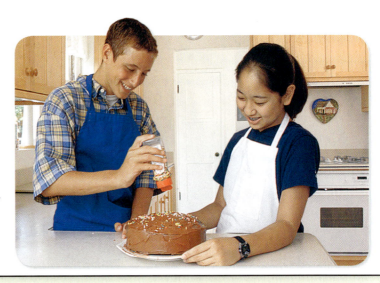
Figure 10 Friends enjoy being together, care about each other, and have similar interests.

MISCONCEPTION ALERT
Some students may have trouble distinguishing between friends and peers. Explain that peers are people their own age. But friends enjoy being together and care about each other. Most friends are probably peers, but not all peers are friends.

Chapter Resource File
- Directed Reading BASIC
- Lesson Plan
- Lesson Quiz GENERAL

Transparencies
TT Bellringer

186 Chapter 9 • Encouraging Healthy Relationships

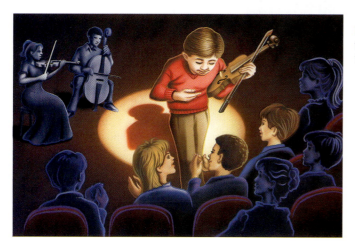

Figure 11 You can support your friends by cheering for them at a performance.

Supporting Each Other

One of the most important benefits of friendship is the support you give each other. Supporting your friends in healthy ways shows your commitment to helping them succeed. You can support your friends by

- helping them reach healthy goals
- cheering for them at a game or performance
- helping them with a project or chores
- studying or exercising together
- standing by them when they say no to unhealthy choices

You are always responsible for choosing your own behavior. Your friends are responsible for theirs, too. But you can help each other by supporting healthy choices.

Speaking Up

Supporting your friends does not mean agreeing with every choice they make. If you think a friend is making an unhealthy choice, say so. Sometimes changing someone's mind takes only one person's voice or actions. Stating your honest opinion about a friend's decision can be hard to do. But being honest with each other is an important part of friendship.

When friends support each other, they influence each other. Influencing friends to make good decisions is *positive peer pressure*. It can be hard to make a healthy choice by yourself. People who see friends making good decisions will often have the courage to make good decisions themselves.

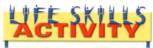

Myth: You are responsible for your friends' decisions.

Fact: Supporting your friends is important, but each person is responsible for his or her own decisions.

LIFE SKILLS ACTIVITY

MAKING GOOD DECISIONS

In pairs or groups, discuss how you could use positive peer pressure to help in the following scenario: Two peers are asking your friend to help them cheat on a quiz.

LIFE SKILLS ACTIVITY

Answer
Answers may vary but should reflect the ideas listed on this page. Sample answer: I would tell my friends not to cheat because cheating is wrong. I would also remind them that if they got caught, they would all be in trouble. I would point out to my friends that everyone should have studied for the quiz and that no one should get credit for another person's work.

Teach

Activity —— GENERAL

Poster Project Ask students to make a poster or a collage using magazine clippings showing ways that their friends show support. **English Language Learners**
LS **Visual**

Group Activity —— GENERAL

Using Positive Peer Pressure Organize the class into groups. Have each group select one person to go to the front of the classroom. Hold a contest to see who can balance on one leg for the longest time. Tell the class to be silent the first time but record the amount of time their teammate kept his or her balance. Then, repeat the contest, but this time allow each team to encourage their teammate to win. Have each group compare the times. After the activity, ask students the following questions:

- Did your teammate perform better when you used positive peer pressure? (Answers may vary but should be consistent with the recorded times.)
- How did you feel when you were not allowed to cheer for your teammate? (Answers may vary.)
- How did you feel when you were allowed to encourage your teammate? (Answers may vary.)
- How did you feel when your team cheered you on? (Answers may vary, but students generally feel better when they have been encouraged by their peers.)
- Which did you prefer, silence or the encouragement of your peers? (Answers may vary, but students generally prefer encouragement.) **English Language Learners**
LS **Kinesthetic**

Teach, continued

Using the Table —— BASIC

Showing Affection Explain that physical ways to show affection include touching the person for whom you feel affection and that nonphysical ways of showing affection include expressing affection without touching. Have students rewrite the list in the table, but divide it into two columns titled "Physical" and "Nonphysical." (Under "Physical," students could put giving a high-five and patting someone on the back; and under "Nonphysical," students could put saying kind words, offering a smile or a laugh, writing a letter or a card, and being understanding.) Ask students the following question: "What are more ways to show affection nonphysically?" (Sample answers: sending an e-mail message, giving a small gift, and supporting a difficult decision) **LS** Verbal

MISCONCEPTION ALERT

Students may think that because they mean to express affection, any message intended to show affection will be well-received. Make sure that students know that their message may not be received as it was intended. Tell students that if they express affection to someone who is upset by what they say or do, they should stop expressing affection in this way to this person immediately.

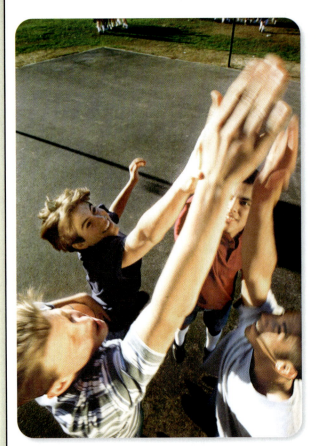

Figure 12 Friends can show affection by giving a high-five.

Showing Affection

Healthy relationships are strengthened when people show affection. Showing affection lets people know that you like them. Your affection shows your friends you think they are valuable. Knowing that someone thinks that they are valuable helps your friends feel good about themselves. This may help your friends make decisions that are good for them. Giving affection also shows your friends that they are not alone, even during difficult times.

Some forms of affection are simpler than others. A smile is usually easy and says a lot. Writing a letter or card can be more difficult. Sometimes expressing affection in words is easier if you first plan what you want to say.

Not everybody likes or appreciates the same forms of affection. Never show affection in a way that is unwelcome. For example, some people don't like to be touched. Don't touch them. And be sure to tell people if they are showing you affection in a way that you do not like. Once you tell them to stop, they should stop. If they do not, tell a parent or another trusted adult.

Health Journal
What are some of the qualities you really like in your good friends? In your Health Journal, write a list of some of your friends, and list some of the qualities you admire in each of them.

TABLE 2 Six Healthy Ways to Show Affection
saying kind words
offering a smile or a laugh
giving a high-five
writing a card or letter
patting someone on the back
being understanding, especially during hard times

Answer to Health Journal

Answers may vary. Sample answer: I like my friend's discipline and good nature. I admire her infectious laugh and her good exercise and study habits. Although we don't always agree, my friend listens to me and offers good advice when it is needed most.

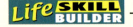 —— ADVANCED

Communicating Effectively Have students write a story about two friends who are having an argument. Then, ask students to trade stories. Have students analyze the behavior of the characters in the stories. Ask questions such as the following: "Could the characters have been calmer, listened more, or said something different that might have changed the outcome?" Students should summarize what the characters could have done differently. **LS** Interpersonal

Unhealthy Relationships

People change, and sometimes friendships turn bad. If you are in a relationship with someone who hurts you, threatens you, or encourages you to ignore your values, that relationship is unhealthy. In some unhealthy relationships, one person tries to control the actions of another person or to keep the other person away from other friends. Any unhealthy relationship can cause problems for you. An unhealthy relationship can also cause problems in your other relationships. If you or your parents are worried about any of your relationships, take a close look at how that relationship is affecting your life.

Resolving Unhealthy Relationships

If you are in an unhealthy relationship, first talk to your parents about resolving it. Sometimes, talking with the other person in the unhealthy relationship can also help. First, say why you are upset. For example, you could say, "I don't like to spend as much time with you anymore because you say mean things about my other friends." Next, say how you feel. For example, you could say, "When you make fun of my other friends, I get upset because I really like them." If the person continues to do things you find upsetting, you may need to say goodbye. You could say, "I don't think we can be friends anymore. I want the people around me to be good to all my friends." Honesty takes courage. But resolving unhealthy relationships gives you more time and energy for healthy ones.

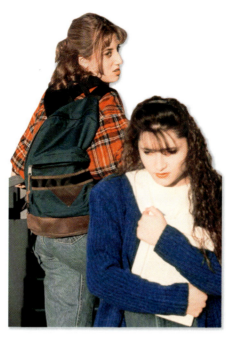

Figure 13 Sometimes, a relationship is unhealthy enough that you need to walk away.

Lesson Review

Using Vocabulary
1. Define *friendship*, and explain why healthy friendships are important.

Understanding Concepts
2. What is an unhealthy relationship? What is the first thing you should do if you find yourself in an unhealthy relationship?

3. What three messages does showing healthy affection send to your friends?

Critical Thinking
4. **Applying Concepts** Maria wants to run for class treasurer. She is very smart, good at math, and organized. But she is afraid to give speeches. What can her friends do to support her decision to run for office?

Answers to Lesson Review
1. Sample answer: Friendship is a relationship between people who enjoy being together, who care about each other, and who have similar interests. Healthy friendships keep people safe.
2. An unhealthy relationship in one in which someone hurts you, threatens you, or encourages you to ignore your values. Students in unhealthy relationships should talk with their parents right away.
3. Showing healthy affection tells friends that I like them, that they are valuable, and that they are not alone.
4. Sample answer: Maria's friends can help her write her speeches, allow her to practice in front of them, and provide helpful suggestions on how not to be nervous in front of a crowd.

Close

Reteaching — BASIC
Peer Pressure Students may think that positive peer pressure has to be a major event. Tell students that positive peer pressure may involve a very small, everyday act, or a series of small acts. Reminding a friend not to cross a busy road until the crossing light indicates that it's safe or congratulating a friend on a good grade are both examples of positive peer pressure. Have students list other small ways to show positive peer pressure. **LS Interpersonal**

Quiz — GENERAL
1. List three appropriate ways to show affection to your friends. (Answers may vary. Sample answers: saying kind words, smiling, writing a card or a letter, patting on the back, or giving a high-five)
2. Your friend is trying to eat fewer sweets and has just refused some chocolate cake. However, another student keeps coaxing her to try it. What could you do to be a supportive friend? (Answers may vary but should reflect an attempt to support a friend in making a healthy choice.)
3. How could ending an unhealthy relationship be good for you? (Sample answer: Walking away from an unhealthy relationship gives me more time and energy for good relationships.)

Lesson 5

Focus

Overview
Before beginning this lesson, review with your students the objectives listed under the What You'll Do head in the Student Edition. This lesson explains how abstinence shows that you care about yourself and others.

🔔 **Bellringer**
Have students list two risks of sexual activity. (Answers may vary. Sample answers: pregnancy and disease) **LS Verbal**

Answer to Start Off Write
Accept all reasonable answers. Sample answer: I can tell someone cares about me by the way that he or she treats me. A person who looks out for my health and safety cares about me.

Motivate

Activity — GENERAL
Goals Ask students to name five goals that would be more difficult to meet if they had to care for a baby at the same time. (Sample answer: playing on a sports team, saving money for college, going to college, studying, and supporting my friends) Ask why those goals are often more difficult to reach while also caring for a baby. (Sample answers: I would have less money, time, and energy.) **LS Logical**

Lesson 5 — Practicing Abstinence

What You'll Do
- **Explain** how abstinence is a way to show that you care about yourself and others.
- **Describe** how refusal skills can help you maintain abstinence.
- **Identify** a sure way to prevent pregnancy and some diseases.

Terms to Learn
- sexual abstinence

Start Off Write
How can you tell that someone cares about you?

You are responsible for your own behavior. Decisions about your behavior affect your health and your relationships. Choosing sexual abstinence is one way to help protect yourself and others.

Risky or harmful behavior puts you in danger. Refusing risky behavior helps keep you safe. For example, refusing to smoke helps you to stay healthy. Sexual activity is risky and harmful for teens, too. Sexual activity can lead to pregnancy and can expose you to deadly diseases. Refusing to take part in sexual activity is called **sexual abstinence** (SEK shoo uhl AB stuh nuhns). Practicing sexual abstinence is the best choice for teens.

Caring

Peer pressure to become sexually active can be very strong. People who pressure you to become sexually active are not looking out for your health or showing that they care about you. Choosing abstinence shows that you care about yourself and your future. It also shows that you care about the people around you. It shows that you want them to be safe from pregnancy and diseases. Maintaining abstinence in a relationship shows one of the highest levels of respect and love for someone.

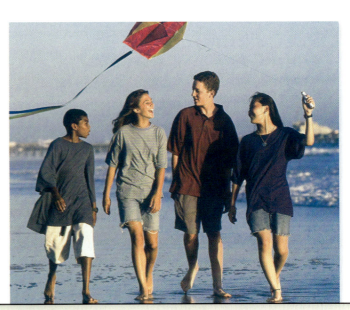
Figure 14 Friends have fun and take care of each other. Good friends never pressure you to risk your health.

190

 Life SKILL BUILDER — GENERAL

Communicating Effectively Sometimes strong emotions can get in the way of demonstrating care, even for the best of friends. Ask students why anger, fear, or jealousy could keep someone from showing a friend that he or she cares. Remind students that no matter what they are feeling, honest communication is the best way to keep friendships strong and healthy. **LS Interpersonal**

Chapter Resource File
- Directed Reading **BASIC**
- Lesson Plan
- Lesson Quiz **GENERAL**

Transparencies
TT Bellringer

---

190 Chapter 9 • Encouraging Healthy Relationships

Refusal Skills

Maintaining abstinence is easier when you are in healthy relationships. Good friends don't pressure you to change your values or risk your health. Refusal skills can also help. Try not to put yourself in risky situations. Say no whenever you need to. Stating your values can stop others from pressuring you. Remember: You always have the right to say no.

Risks

Teens who become sexually active risk harming themselves physically and emotionally. Sexually active teens risk pregnancy. They also risk getting diseases that are spread by sexual activity. Sexual abstinence prevents pregnancy and exposure to these diseases. Sexually active teens also risk feeling guilty and losing self-respect. Sexual abstinence helps avoid these problems, too. Being a teen is complicated enough without having the additional problems related to sexual activity. Teens who choose abstinence make their lives safer, healthier, and simpler.

Health Journal
During the next week, keep a record of how someone special to you has shown you affection in nonphysical ways. Keep a list of how you have demonstrated nonphysical affection to others.

TABLE 3 Six Benefits of Sexual Abstinence

preventing pregnancy with 100 percent certainty
avoiding exposure to diseases
knowing you made a healthy choice
avoiding emotional scars from being sexually active
keeping your self-respect
making your life less complicated

Lesson Review

Using Vocabulary

1. Define *sexual abstinence*, and identify two benefits of sexual abstinence.

Understanding Concepts

2. How does abstinence show that you care for yourself and others?

Critical Thinking

3. **Identifying Relationships** Alcohol and drugs hurt your ability to make decisions. How does avoiding drugs and alcohol help you maintain sexual abstinence?

internet connect
www.scilinks.org/health
Topic: Abstinence
HealthLinks code: HD4002
HEALTH LINKS. Maintained by the National Science Teachers Association

---

Teach

Discussion — GENERAL

Emotional Connections Students may be surprised to learn that sexual abstinence has emotional as well as physical benefits. Explain that their mind develops as their body changes. Practicing abstinence as a teen allows students time to discover what they enjoy doing most and to prepare for life as an adult. Ask students, "How can you spend time working on your future?" (Sample answers: by setting goals and making plans to achieve them) **LS Interpersonal**

Answer to Health Journal
Answers may vary. This Health Journal may be a good way to close the lesson.

Close

Reteaching — BASIC

Refusal Skills Have students write down one refusal skill from the page. Then, have students write a specific way to use that refusal skill if someone pressures them to begin sexual activity. (Sample answer: Stating my values: "I value my health. I'm taking care of myself by choosing sexual abstinence.") **LS Verbal**

Quiz — GENERAL

1. How does sexual abstinence make your life less complicated? (Sample answers: I do not risk pregnancy, sexually-transmitted diseases, or the emotional scars that come from taking part in sexual activity.)

2. If a person pressures you to be sexually active, what messages is he or she sending you? (Answers may vary. Students should indicate that such pressure demonstrates a lack of respect for their health and values.)

Answers to Lesson Review

1. Sexual abstinence is refusing to take part in sexual activity. Sexual abstinence prevents pregnancy and some diseases.

2. Maintaining abstinence in a relationship shows that you want to keep yourself and others safe from pregnancy and diseases.

3. Sample answer: The effects of drugs and alcohol can cause you to make choices that you would not otherwise make. Abstaining from drugs and alcohol helps you maintain sexual abstinence because it strengthens your ability to use your refusal skills and keeps you thinking clearly.

9 CHAPTER REVIEW

Assignment Guide

Lesson	Review Questions
1	2, 10–11, 19–20, 23
2	4–5, 9, 12, 16, 21
3	6–7
4	8, 14, 18, 22, 24
5	3, 13, 15, 17
1 and 3	1

ANSWERS

Using Vocabulary

1. Sample answers: People who are socially or emotionally connected to each other have a relationship. Body language is a form of communication. Tolerance is the ability to respect differences in people and accept them for who they are.
2. behavior
3. Sexual abstinence
4. nurturing
5. abuse
6. community
7. tolerance
8. friendship

Understanding Concepts

9. Sample answer: An extended family includes grandparents, aunts, uncles, and cousins.
10. Sample answer: Thoughts and feelings can be shared by speaking clearly and having appropriate hand movements or expressions on your face. For example, a smile and a cheerful greeting could let people know that you are happy to see them.
11. Sample answer: By using assertive behavior, a person can find out what he or she can do to improve his or her skills. For example, a person cut from a team can ask a coach how to improve enough to make the team next time.
12. Sample answer: You can solve a minor family problem by listening to each other, working together, and looking for solutions that work for everyone. You could also work on problems by holding regular family meetings.

Chapter Summary

- Healthy relationships require good communication skills, healthy behavior, and work.
- Working together as a family requires taking roles seriously and supporting each member with nurture and respect.
- When the family has problems, the family should work on those problems.
- More serious problems, such as abuse and neglect, should be reported to a trusted adult as soon as possible.
- Communities are made up of people who have something in common. Healthy communities also tolerate differences.
- Friendships are healthy relationships between people who have similar interests and values. Friends support and care for each other.
- Unhealthy relationships are risky.
- Sexual abstinence prevents pregnancy and some diseases.

Using Vocabulary

1. Use each of the following terms in a separate sentence: *relationship*, *body language*, and *tolerance*.

For each sentence, fill in the blank with the proper word from the word bank provided below.

sexual abstinence	personal responsibility
community	behavior
friendship	nurturing
abuse	tolerance
neglect	body language

2. The way you choose to act or respond is called your ___.
3. ___ means not taking part in sexual activity.
4. Providing the things that people need in order to grow is called ___.
5. Treating someone in a harmful or offensive way is called ___.
6. People who have a common background or location or similar goals make up a(n) ___.
7. When you overlook differences and accept people as they are, you are showing ___.
8. A(n) ___ is a relationship between people who like and care for each other.

Understanding Concepts

9. Who makes up an extended family?
10. Explain how people communicate by using words and body language.
11. Explain how assertive behavior can help you learn and grow.
12. Describe two ways you can work through small family problems.
13. Describe the benefits of abstinence from sexual activity.
14. Describe three healthy ways to show affection to a friend.
15. What is a sure way to prevent pregnancy and other risks related to sexual activity?
16. Describe a way to cope with a serious problem, such as abuse or neglect.
17. Describe how refusal skills can help you maintain abstinence.
18. Describe how to identify and cope with an unhealthy relationship.

Chapter Resource File

- Concept Review GENERAL
- Concept Mapping GENERAL
- Performance-Based Assessment GENERAL
- Chapter Test GENERAL

Critical Thinking

Applying Concepts

19. Teresa was dribbling a basketball in the house after her mother had asked her to stop. The ball took a bad bounce and knocked over a lamp. The lamp broke. How can Teresa respond in a way that shows personal responsibility?

20. Max wants to be a lifeguard when he is in high school. He knows how to swim, but he needs to learn rescue skills. How can Max use assertive behavior to learn what he needs to know to become a lifeguard?

21. Brianna's parents have asked Brianna to call home when she arrives at her friends' houses so that they know that Brianna has arrived safely. Most of the time, Brianna's friends understand. But Dominique teases Brianna and tells Brianna not to bother calling. This upsets Brianna and her parents. How could Brianna handle this relationship?

Making Good Decisions

22. You and your friend stop by a local store on your way home from school. You both buy a few things to eat and then leave the store. Your friend tells you that he shoplifted some candy. What would you do?

23. Brian borrowed Paul's guitar and broke a string. Brian dropped off the guitar at Paul's house while Paul was at soccer practice. Brian didn't tell Paul that the string was broken. When Paul asked Brian about the string, Brian said that it was no big deal and the guitar wasn't that nice anyway. How should Paul respond?

24. Lately, Clara has been lying to her friends a lot. Clara's friend, Denise, is angry with Clara and told her so. Clara thinks this criticism makes Denise a bad friend. Is Denise a bad friend? Explain your answer.

25. Use what you have learned in this chapter to set a personal goal. Write your goal, and make an action plan by using the Health Behavior Contract for your relationship skills. You can find the Health Behavior Contract at go.hrw.com. Just type in the keyword HD4HBC07.

Reading Checkup

Take a minute to review your answers to the Health IQ questions at the beginning of this chapter. How has reading this chapter improved your Health IQ?

---

13. Sample answer: Abstinence from sexual activity prevents pregnancy and certain diseases.
14. Sample answer: Writing a letter, smiling, and giving a high-five are healthy ways to show affection to a friend.
15. A sure way to prevent pregnancy and other risks related to sexual activity is to practice sexual abstinence.
16. Sample answer: The best way to cope with abuse or neglect is to talk to a trusted adult.
17. Sample answer: Refusal skills can help you maintain abstinence because refusal skills help you say no to dangerous or risky behavior.
18. Sample answer: Unhealthy relationships are relationships that can hurt a person, threaten a person, or cause a person to ignore their values. People in unhealthy relationships should talk to a parent or another trusted adult as soon as possible.

Critical Thinking

Applying Concepts

19. Sample answer: Teresa should tell her mother how the lamp was broken, apologize, clean up the mess, and either repair or replace the lamp.
20. Sample answer: Max could ask a lifeguard or coach how he can learn rescue skills. He needs to take classes to become a certified lifeguard.
21. Sample answer: Brianna should tell her parents that she is feeling pressure to disobey them. She should also tell Dominique that pressuring her to disobey her parents is disrespectful and may result in their friendship ending.

Making Good Decisions

22. Sample answer: I would tell my friend that I am upset because his shoplifting is wrong and could get us both in trouble, and I would not go into stores with him until he paid for the candy he stole.
23. Sample answer: Paul should ask Brian to fix the string he broke. If Brian does not agree to fix the string, Paul should refuse to lend Brian anything else.
24. Sample answer: No, Denise is a good friend. She is trying to help Clara by being honest with her.
25. Accept all reasonable responses. Note: A Health Behavior Contract for each chapter can be found in the Chapter Resource File and at the HRW Web site, go.hrw.com.

Chapter 9 • Chapter Review

Model

Introduce this activity by reminding students that using this Life Skill will help them take personal responsibility for their behavior. Then, review the scenario with the class.

Prepare students for this activity by modeling each of the steps of the skill. Make sure students understand each step before you move on to the next one.

Guided Practice: Practice with a Friend

Guided Practice is the stage in which you and the students analyze their approach to solving the problem given in the scenario and analyze their ability to evaluate media messages. Have students read Act 1. Discuss with the class the situation described and the way students are to act it out. Organize the class into groups of three. In each group, one person plays the role of Elisa, another person plays Brett, and the third person is the observer.

Proper pacing during the Guided Practice is important. The suggestions listed below will help you control the pace.

1. Stop after completing each step of evaluating media messages.
2. Discuss with each group the observer's comments.
3. Ask the other members of each group to listen to the observer's suggestions and to suggest ways to improve the way they evaluate media messages.
4. Instruct students to repeat the steps that need improvement and to include their modifications.

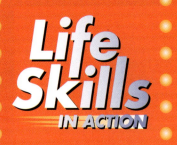

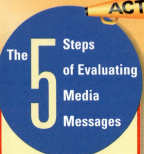

The 5 Steps of Evaluating Media Messages

1. Examine the appeal of the message.
2. Identify the values projected by the message.
3. Consider what the source has to gain by getting you to believe the message.
4. Try to determine the reliability of the source.
5. Based on the information you gather, evaluate the message.

194

Evaluating Media Messages

You receive media messages every day. These messages are on TV, the Internet, the radio, and in newspapers and magazines. With so many messages, it is important to know how to evaluate them. Evaluating media messages means being able to judge the accuracy of a message. Complete the following activity to improve your skills in evaluating media messages.

Happy Family?

Setting the Scene

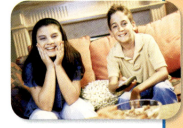

Elisa and her brother Brett love watching the TV show *Happy Family*. The two teenage characters on the show get into trouble a lot, and their parents are always yelling at them. Elisa and Brett think it is very funny when this happens. The best part of the show is when the teens talk their parents out of the punishment. In spite of all the trouble the teens cause, the show always ends with everyone being happy and laughing. Elisa and Brett wish that their family was like the family on the show.

Guided Practice

Practice with a Friend

Form a group of three. Have one person play the role of Elisa and another person play the role of Brett. Have the third person be an observer. Walking through each of the five steps of evaluating media messages, role-play Elisa and Brett analyzing the *Happy Family* TV show. They should consider whether the interactions between the characters are realistic. The observer will take notes, which will include observations about what the people playing Elisa and Brett did well and suggestions of ways to improve. Stop after each step to evaluate the process.

5. Check to make sure that students understand each step before they move on to the next step.
6. If time permits, repeat the exercise three times, switching roles each time. Each student should have the opportunity to play each role. Co-op Learning

Independent Practice

Check Yourself

After you have completed the guided practice, go through Act 1 again without stopping at each step. Answer the questions below to review what you did.

1. What audience is *Happy Family* trying to appeal to?
2. What values are projected by the behavior of the characters on *Happy Family*?
3. How realistic are the interactions between the characters on *Happy Family*?
4. Think about a TV show you like to watch. How do the characters on the show behave toward each other? Is their behavior similar to the behavior of people around you? Explain your answer.

On Your Own

While watching *Happy Family* one evening, Elisa and Brett see a commercial for a new video game. Brett tells Elisa that he wants to buy that video game. Elisa tells Brett that one of the video games he already owns looks very similar to the new one. But Brett points out that the commercial says that the new video game is a big improvement over the one that he has. Make an outline showing how Brett could use the five steps of evaluating media messages to analyze the commercial for the video game.

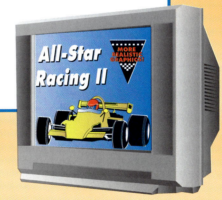

Act 2: On Your Own

This additional scenario gives students an opportunity to apply what they have learned in both the Guided Practice and the Independent Practice to a new situation.

Suggest to students that they use the Check Yourself questions as a starting point for evaluating media messages in the new situation. Encourage students to be creative and to think of ways to improve their ability to evaluate media messages.

Assessment

Review the outlines that students have written as part of the On Your Own activity. The outlines should show that the students followed the steps of evaluating media messages in a realistic and effective manner. If time permits, ask student volunteers to write one or more of their outlines on the blackboard. Discuss the outlines and the way the students used the steps of evaluating media messages.

Independent Practice: Check Yourself

Instruct students to repeat Act 1 without stopping at each step. Remind students to apply what they learned in the Guided Practice to the Independent Practice.

Encourage students to use the Check Yourself questions as a starting point for reviewing and analyzing their Independent Practice. Remind students that as they change roles, the answers to these questions may change for each actor. Encourage students to create additional questions for checking their ability to evaluate media messages. When students have finished the Independent Practice, have them answer the Check Yourself questions in writing. Use their answers to assess their understanding of the steps of evaluating media messages and to assess their use of the steps to solve a problem.

Check Yourself Answers

1. Sample answer: *Happy Family* is trying to appeal to teens by showing teens talking their way out of trouble.
2. Sample answer: The show tells people that it is okay to cause problems and to get into trouble because you can always get out of it.
3. Sample answer: The interactions on *Happy Family* are not realistic because most parents won't let their teens talk them out of punishments.
4. Sample answer: The characters on a TV show that I like to watch always play jokes on each other. People around me don't behave this way because other people would probably be very angry with them if they were always playing jokes.

CHAPTER 10: Conflict and Violence
Chapter Planning Guide

PACING	CLASSROOM RESOURCES	ACTIVITIES AND DEMONSTRATIONS
BLOCK 1 • 45 min pp. 196–201 **Chapter Opener**	CRF Health Inventory * ■ GENERAL CRF Parent Letter * ■	SE Health IQ, p. 197 CRF At-Home Activity * ■
Lesson 1 What Is Conflict?	CRF Lesson Plan * TT Bellringer *	TE Activity Exploring Values, p. 199 GENERAL TE Activity Illustrating Conflicts, p. 200 BASIC TE Group Activity Conflicts at School, p. 201 GENERAL CRF Enrichment Activity * ADVANCED
BLOCK 2 • 45 min pp. 202–207 **Lesson 2** Communicating During Conflicts	CRF Lesson Plan * TT Bellringer * TT Conflict Flowchart *	TE Activities Practicing Negotiation, p. 195F TE Group Activity Skit, p. 202 GENERAL SE Hands-on Activity, p. 203 CRF Datasheets for In-Text Activities * GENERAL TE Activity Sending Messages, p. 203 ♦ GENERAL TE Group Activity Developing Listening Skills, p. 204 GENERAL CRF Life Skills Activity * ■ GENERAL CRF Enrichment Activity * ADVANCED
Lesson 3 Getting Help for Conflicts	CRF Lesson Plan * TT Bellringer * TT Signs That a Conflict Is Out of Control *	TE Activity Conflict in the News, p. 206 ♦ GENERAL SE Language Arts Activity, p. 207 CRF Enrichment Activity * ADVANCED
BLOCK 3 • 45 min pp. 208–213 **Lesson 4** Violence: When Conflict Becomes Dangerous	CRF Lesson Plan * TT Bellringer *	TE Activities Measuring Exposure to TV Violence, p. 195F TE Activity Poster Project, p. 209 ♦ GENERAL SE Life Skills in Action Communicating Effectively, pp. 216–217 CRF Life Skills Activity * ■ GENERAL CRF Enrichment Activity * ADVANCED
Lesson 5 Preventing Violence	CRF Lesson Plan * TT Bellringer *	CRF Enrichment Activity * ADVANCED

BLOCKS 4 & 5 • 90 min — Chapter Review and Assessment Resources

- SE Chapter Review, pp. 214–215
- CRF Concept Review * ■ GENERAL
- CRF Health Behavior Contract * ■ GENERAL
- CRF Chapter Test * ■ GENERAL
- CRF Performance-Based Assessment * GENERAL
- OSP Test Generator
- CRF Test Item Listing *

Online Resources

Visit **go.hrw.com** for a variety of free resources related to this textbook. Enter the keyword **HD4CV7**.

Students can access interactive problem solving help and active visual concept development with the *Decisions for Health* Online Edition available at **www.hrw.com**.

CNN Student News — cnnstudentnews.com
Find the latest health news, lesson plans, and activities related to important scientific events.

Compression guide:
To shorten your instruction because of time limitations, omit Lesson 3.

KEY

TE Teacher Edition	**CRF** Chapter Resource File	* Also on One-Stop Planner
SE Student Edition	**TT** Teaching Transparency	■ Also Available in Spanish
OSP One-Stop Planner		♦ Requires Advance Prep

SKILLS DEVELOPMENT RESOURCES	LESSON REVIEW AND ASSESSMENT	STANDARDS CORRELATION
		National Health Education Standards
TE Life Skill Builder Coping, p. 198 GENERAL TE Reading Skill Builder Reading Organizer, p. 199 BASIC TE Life Skill Builder Making Good Decisions, p. 200 GENERAL TE Inclusion Strategies, p. 200 ♦ GENERAL CRF Decision-Making * GENERAL CRF Directed Reading * BASIC	SE Lesson Review, p. 201 TE Reteaching, Quiz, p. 201 CRF Concept Mapping * GENERAL CRF Lesson Quiz * ■ GENERAL	5.7
TE Life Skill Builder Communicating Effectively, p. 202 BASIC SE Life Skills Activity Communicating Effectively, p. 204 TE Reading Skill Builder Anticipation Guide, p. 204 BASIC SE Study Tip Reviewing Information, p. 205 CRF Refusal Skills * GENERAL CRF Cross-Disciplinary * GENERAL CRF Directed Reading * BASIC	SE Lesson Review, p. 205 TE Reteaching, Quiz, p. 205 TE Alternative Assessment, p. 205 GENERAL CRF Concept Mapping * GENERAL CRF Lesson Quiz * ■ GENERAL	5.1, 5.3, 5.5, 5.6, 5.8
TE Inclusion Strategies, p. 206 BASIC CRF Decision-Making * GENERAL CRF Directed Reading * BASIC	SE Lesson Review, p. 207 TE Reteaching, Quiz, p. 207 CRF Lesson Quiz * ■ GENERAL	3.6, 5.8
TE Life Skill Builder Using Refusal Skills, p. 209 BASIC SE Life Skills Activity Making Good Decisions, p. 210 TE Reading Skill Builder Paired Summarizing, p. 210 BASIC TE Life Skill Builder Making Good Decisions, p. 210 GENERAL CRF Cross-Disciplinary * GENERAL CRF Directed Reading * BASIC	SE Lesson Review, p. 211 TE Reteaching, Quiz, p. 211 TE Alternative Assessment, p. 211 GENERAL CRF Lesson Quiz * ■ GENERAL	3.6
TE Life Skill Builder Practicing Wellness, p. 213 BASIC CRF Refusal Skills * GENERAL CRF Directed Reading * BASIC	SE Lesson Review, p. 213 TE Reteaching, Quiz, p. 213 CRF Lesson Quiz * ■ GENERAL	3.6

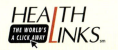

Topic: Emotions
HealthLinks code: HD4035

Topic: Communication Skills
HealthLinks code: HD4022

www.scilinks.org/health
Maintained by the **National Science Teachers Association**

Technology Resources

 One-Stop Planner
All of your printable resources and the Test Generator are on this convenient CD-ROM.

 Guided Reading Audio CDs

VIDEO SELECT
For information about videos related to this chapter, go to **go.hrw.com** and type in the keyword **HD4CV7V**.

Chapter 10 • Chapter Planning Guide   **195B**

CHAPTER 10
Conflict and Violence
Chapter Resources

Teacher Resources

TEACHING TRANSPARENCIES

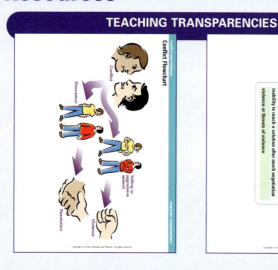
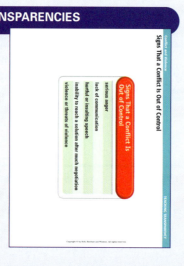

BELLRINGER TRANSPARENCIES

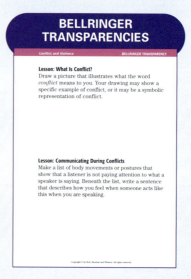

LESSON PLANS
PARENT LETTER
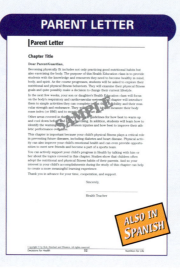

TEST ITEM LISTING
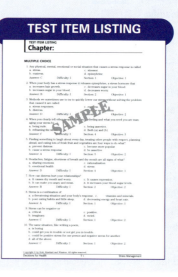

Meeting Individual Needs

DIRECTED READING
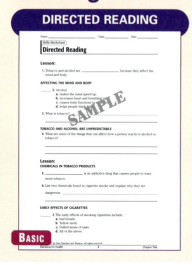

CONCEPT MAPPING
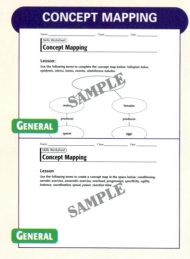

CONCEPT REVIEW
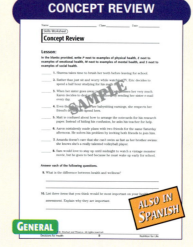

ENRICHMENT ACTIVITIES
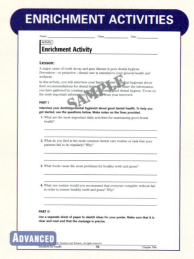

195C   Chapter 10 • Conflict and Violence

Resources

These worksheet pages can be found in the Chapter Resource File and the One-Stop Planner. The transparencies can be found in the Teaching Transparencies binder and on the One-Stop Planner.

Activities

LIFE SKILLS ACTIVITIES
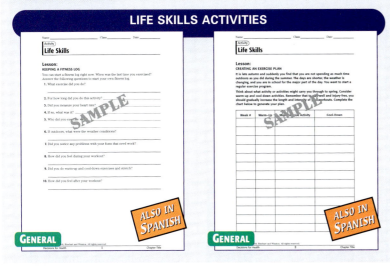

AT-HOME ACTIVITY
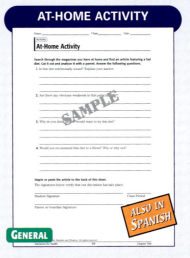

DATASHEETS FOR IN-TEXT ACTIVITIES
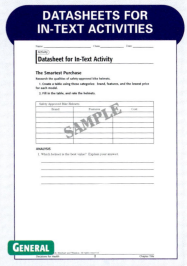

Applications

DECISION-MAKING
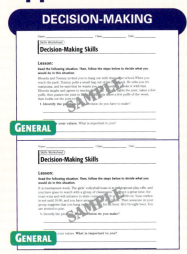

REFUSAL SKILLS
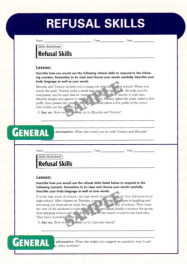

CROSS-DISCIPLINARY
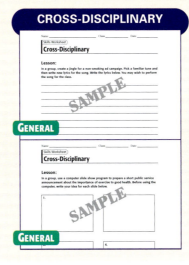

HEALTH BEHAVIOR CONTRACT
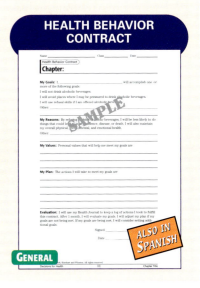

Assessments

HEALTH INVENTORY
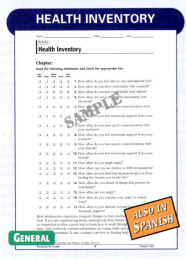

LESSON QUIZZES
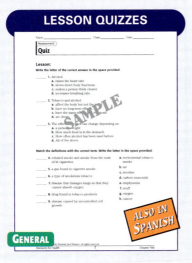

CHAPTER TEST
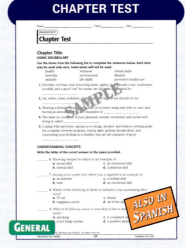

PERFORMANCE-BASED ASSESSMENT
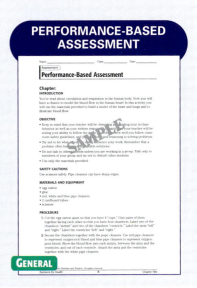

Chapter 10 • Chapter Resources and Worksheets   **195D**

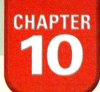

CHAPTER 10

Background Information

The following information focuses on adolescent violence and anger. This material will help prepare you for teaching the concepts in this chapter.

Adolescent Violence

- Violence affects adolescents and young adults more than any other age group. According to a national survey, juveniles between the ages 12 and 17 and young adults between the ages 18 and 24 are twice as likely to be victims of crime than adults between the ages of 25 and 34 are. Furthermore, juveniles and young adults are five times more likely to be crime victims than adults over the age of 35 are.

- Gang violence, robbery, and dating violence are the most common forms of violence in which adolescents participate. Adolescents often commit these acts of violence to fulfill an age-specific need. For example, young males usually participate in gang violence to attain high status and social identity. Adolescents usually commit robbery to satisfy their material needs. Finally, teens often use dating violence to fulfill a need for power and social control. All three forms of violence are acts that defy authority, which is another objective of some adolescents.

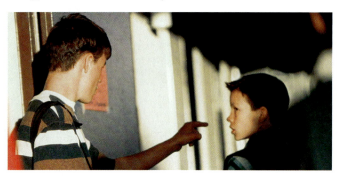

The Effect of Violence on Teen Girls

- Researchers at the University of Texas at Galveston studied the effect of violence on the health behaviors of teen girls. Over 500 girls participated in the study. Of the participants, 20 percent reported being only a witness to violence, 14 percent reported being only a victim of violence, and 13 percent reported being both a witness and a victim of violence.

- Compared to teen girls who were neither witnesses or victims of violence, girls who were witnesses were two to three times more likely to use tobacco and drugs and to engage in risky sexual behavior.

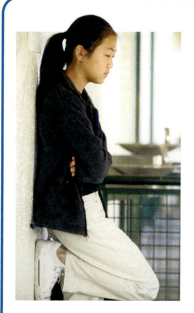

- Girls who were victims of violence were more likely to engage in risky sexual behaviors and more likely to have a sexually transmitted disease. Girls who were both witnesses and victims of violence were three to six times more likely to have considered suicide, to have attempted suicide, or to have intentionally injured themselves.

Anger

- Anger is defined as an emotional state that varies in intensity from irritation to rage. Anger is accompanied by physiological and biological changes, such as increased heart rate and elevated levels of epinephrine and other hormones.

- Both external and internal events can trigger feelings of anger. External events that can trigger anger include situations—such as a traffic jam—and interactions with specific individuals—such as a fight with a friend. Internal events that can trigger anger include reactions to failure and disappointment. Regardless of what triggers anger, people appear to have a natural inclination to express anger in an aggressive manner.

- Two common methods of dealing with anger are expressing and suppressing. Expressing refers to releasing angry feelings outward. This is healthy when the feelings are expressed in a manner that is not harmful to anyone or anything. Suppressing refers to holding angry feelings within oneself. Suppressing anger can be healthy if a person converts his or her suppressed anger into constructive, nonviolent behavior. However, if a person does not do this, the anger remains contained, and hypertension, high blood pressure, or depression may result.

For background information about teaching strategies and issues, refer to the *Professional Reference for Teachers*.

ACTIVITIES

CHAPTER 10

Consider using the activities on this page as students explore the lessons of this chapter. Look for other activities throughout the Student Edition chapter.

Practicing Negotiation

Hands on

Procedure Organize students into four groups. Assign a color to each group: red, blue, green, and yellow. Have each group stand in a different corner of the classroom and divide the room into four areas. Tell students that the area around their corner is their group's territory and that members of the other groups are not allowed to enter their territory. Have each group make a list of at least five actions they can no longer do because of the way the classroom is divided. For example, the people in the red group cannot sharpen their pencils because the pencil sharpener is in the blue group's territory. After the groups make their lists, have members of different groups negotiate compromises or collaborations that allow each group to do three of the actions on its list. For example, the blue group might agree to let the red group use the pencil sharpener if the red group lets the blue group have access to the dictionary.

Analysis Ask students the following questions:

- Which actions on your list were most important to your group? Why? (Sample answer: It was most important that we have access to the door so we could go in and out of the room.)

- Which actions were least important? (Sample answer: We didn't think it was important to be able to write on the blackboard.)

- Did you find it easy or difficult to negotiate solutions? Explain. (Answers may vary.)

- Were your agreements compromises, collaborations, or both? Explain. (Answers may vary.)

- What was the most difficult part of your negotiations? (Answers may vary.)

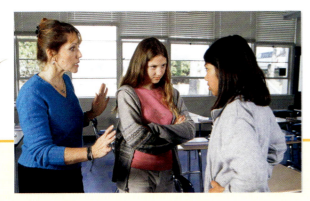

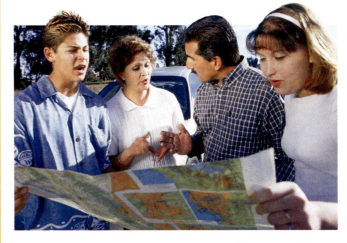

Measuring Exposure to TV Violence

Hands on

Procedure Help students construct a chart that they can use to keep track of all the violent acts they see on TV. The chart should have places where students can enter the time they saw the violent act, the name of the show that contained the act, and a brief description of the act. Tell students to keep this chart with them whenever they watch TV for one week. Remind students to record all acts of violence including "funny" cartoon violence and descriptions of violence in news reports. After students finish collecting their data, have them group the violent acts into 4 to 5 categories. The categories may include acted violence, cartoon violence, real violence resulting in injury, and real violence resulting in death. Have students construct a bar graph using their data.

Analysis Ask students the following questions:

- Which category of violence did you see most frequently? (Answers may vary. Sample answer: I saw acted violence most frequently.)

- What kind of shows had the most acts of violence? (Answers may vary. Sample answer: TV shows about police officers had the most acts of violence.)

- How did you feel after seeing the acts of violence? (Answers may vary. Sample answer: Some acts of violence made me unhappy and uncomfortable, but the cartoon acts of violence made me laugh.)

Chapter 10 • Activities   195F

CHAPTER 10

Overview
Tell students that this chapter will help them understand the nature of conflict and violence. Students will learn to recognize conflict and will learn that good communication helps resolve conflicts. Students will understand that mediators are sometimes needed to resolve conflicts. Students will also learn how conflict can turn to violence and learn ways to control their anger and avoid violence.

Assessing Prior Knowledge
Students should be familiar with the following topics:
- refusal skills
- communication skills
- decision-making skills
- coping

Question Box
Students may feel more comfortable asking questions if you set up a Question Box to collect their questions. Have students write and anonymously submit their questions about conflict and violence. Address these questions during class, or use these questions to introduce lessons that cover related topics.

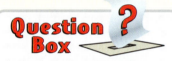

Check out *Current Health* articles and activities related to this chapter by visiting the HRW Web site at **go.hrw.com.** Just type in the keyword **HD4CH25T.**

Chapter Resource File
- Directed Reading BASIC
- Health Inventory GENERAL
- Parent Letter

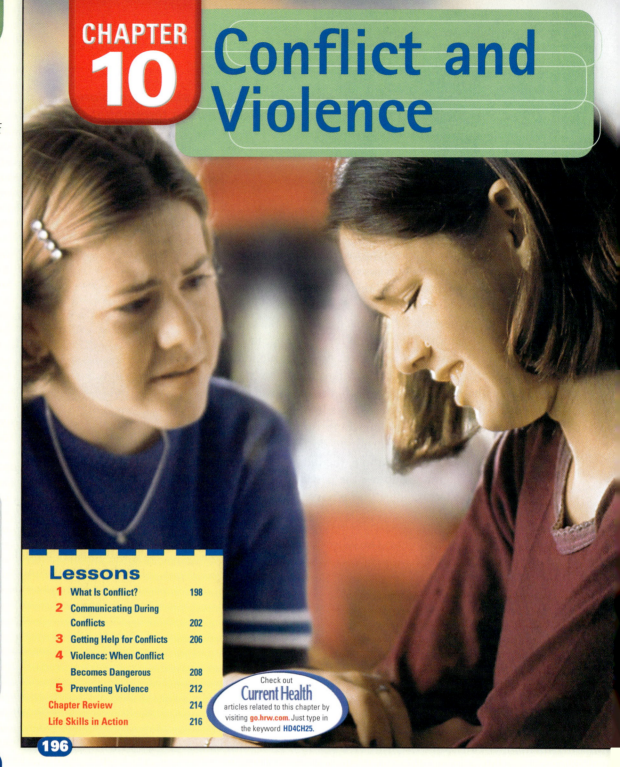

CHAPTER 10 Conflict and Violence

Lessons
1. What Is Conflict? 198
2. Communicating During Conflicts 202
3. Getting Help for Conflicts 206
4. Violence: When Conflict Becomes Dangerous 208
5. Preventing Violence 212

Chapter Review 214
Life Skills in Action 216

Check out **Current Health** articles related to this chapter by visiting **go.hrw.com.** Just type in the keyword **HD4CH25.**

Standards Correlations

National Health Education Standards

3.6 Demonstrate ways to avoid and reduce threatening situations. (Lessons 3–5)

5.1 Demonstrate effective verbal and nonverbal communication skills to enhance health. (Lesson 2)

5.3 Demonstrate healthy ways to express needs, wants and feelings. (Lesson 2)

5.5 Demonstrate communication skills to build and maintain healthy relationships. (Lesson 2)

5.6 (partial) Demonstrate refusal and negotiation skills to enhance health. (Lesson 2)

5.7 Analyze the possible causes of conflicts among youth in schools. (Lesson 1)

5.8 Demonstrate strategies to manage conflict in healthy ways. (Lessons 2 and 3)

> "I got into a huge **fight** with my **mother** over my **curfew**. I got very angry and said some **terrible** things that I really didn't mean. My mother was upset. I think I hurt her feelings. I wish I could take it all back."

Health IQ

PRE-READING

Answer the following true/false questions to find out what you already know about conflict and violence. When you've finished this chapter, you'll have the opportunity to change your answers based on what you've learned.

1. Violence appears in many places in our society.
2. Conflict does not happen in close relationships.
3. Bullies usually pick on people smaller than they are.
4. Body language is not a real form of communication.
5. People who tease others usually like to do so in front of an audience.
6. If a conflict gets out of control, the best thing to do is to keep working on the conflict until it is better.
7. To compromise is to give into another person's demands.
8. Anyone who is not part of a conflict can help to mediate that conflict.
9. Drinking or using drugs increases the chances that a person will become violent.
10. Violence and aggression are the same thing.
11. It is unnecessary to report threats of violence that sound like jokes.
12. The way you express yourself during conflict determines how a conflict ends.

ANSWERS: 1. true; 2. false; 3. true; 4. false; 5. true; 6. false; 7. false; 8. false; 9. true; 10. false; 11. false; 12. true

Using the Health IQ

Misconception Alert
Answers to the Health IQ questions may help you identify students' misconceptions.

Question 8: Some students may believe that anyone who is not involved in a conflict can effectively mediate the situation. Explain that a mediator is a trained individual who uses certain skills to resolve a conflict. For example, a mediator sets ground rules for the negotiation, does not take sides, and offers solutions to the conflict. If an untrained person tries to mediate a conflict, he or she could make the conflict worse.

Question 10: Students may think that violence and aggression are the same. Explain that aggression is any hostile or threatening action against another person. Violence is the use of physical force to harm someone or something. Aggression is often a warning that violence may occur.

Answers
1. true
2. false
3. true
4. false
5. true
6. false
7. false
8. false
9. true
10. false
11. false
12. true

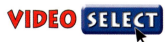

For information about videos related to this chapter, go to **go.hrw.com** and type in the keyword **HD4CV7V**.

Lesson 1

Focus

Overview
Before beginning this lesson, review with your students the objectives listed under the What You'll Do head in the Student Edition. In this lesson, students learn to recognize signs that conflict is about to happen. Students also learn why conflicts occur at home, with peers, and at school.

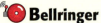**Bellringer**
Ask students to draw a picture that illustrates what the term *conflict* means to them. Tell students that their drawing may show a specific example of conflict or may be a symbolic representation of conflict. **LS Visual** *English Language Learners*

Answer to Start Off Write
Accept all reasonable answers. Sample answer: Teasing is making fun of another person. Bullying is using threats or physical force to scare or control another person.

Motivate

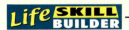 — **GENERAL**

Coping Ask students to raise their hands if they have ever experienced conflict with another person. *(Expect all students to raise their hands.)* Explain that this quick survey shows that everyone experiences conflict from time to time. Invite volunteers to describe how they cope with conflict in their lives. **LS Intrapersonal**

Lesson 1 — What Is Conflict?

What You'll Do
- **Describe** three signs that a conflict is happening or is about to happen.
- **Identify** three reasons that conflicts happen.
- **Describe** how conflicts can happen at home, with peers, and at school.

Terms to Learn
- conflict
- bullying

Start Off Write
What is the difference between teasing and bullying?

Have you ever disagreed with somebody? Maybe you and your brother or sister wanted to watch different TV shows. Maybe your parents wanted you to do homework, but you wanted to go out with friends.

If you have had these types of disagreements, then you have experienced conflict. **Conflict** is any clash of ideas or interests. Everybody experiences conflict in his or her life. Conflict happens even in the closest relationships.

Recognizing Conflict
The first step toward solving any conflict is to recognize when conflict is happening or when conflict is about to happen. The following signs can tell you that a conflict is occurring or that a conflict is about to occur:

- **Disagreement** Every conflict starts with disagreement over an issue.
- **Emotions** If you find that a disagreement is causing emotions, such as anger or jealousy, the disagreement is becoming a conflict.
- **Other People's Behavior** If the other person or people in a disagreement begin ignoring you, raising their voices, or crossing their arms, a conflict is happening.

Figure 1 Conflict can arise anywhere, even when you are doing something fun, such as going on a vacation.

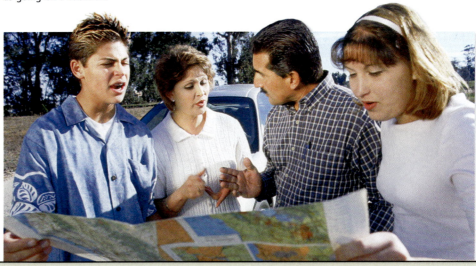

MISCONCEPTION ALERT
Some students may believe that all conflict is bad and should be avoided. Explain to students that conflicts often are opportunities to learn and grow. Further explain that people must use good communication skills to effectively benefit from conflict.

Chapter Resource File
- Directed Reading **BASIC**
- Lesson Plan
- Lesson Quiz **GENERAL**

Transparencies
TT Bellringer

198 Chapter 10 • Conflict and Violence

Why Does Conflict Happen?

Although conflict can happen over almost any issue, it usually happens for one of three reasons:

- **Resources** Conflicts can happen when two or more people want the same thing, but not all of them can have it.
- **Values and Expectations** Different things are important to different people. Many conflicts happen because people have different ideas about what is important or how things should be done.
- **Emotions** Conflicts can happen because people feel hurt or angry at the behavior of others.

Conflicts at Home

You and your family members usually spend a lot of time together. Because of this, there are many chances for conflict to arise at home. Conflicts can happen between you and your parents or caregivers because each of you has different expectations. For example, your parents may expect you to do certain chores, and you may feel that you shouldn't have to do as many chores. Conflict can also happen between you and your parents or caregivers because you disagree with their opinions or their rules for you.

You may also have conflicts with a brother or sister. For example, you may feel that you are asked to do more than your brother or sister. Or you may have conflict with a brother or sister over resources, such as the telephone or the computer. You may even feel that your brother or sister gets more attention than you do.

Conflicts in the home affect everyone in the family. For example, an unresolved conflict with your brother or sister may make your parents unhappy. When you have conflicts with members of your family or household, it is important to solve them quickly. Allowing conflicts at home to go on for too long can create a very difficult living situation.

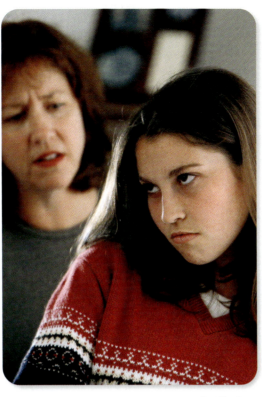

Figure 2 Conflict between you and your parents often occurs because they have different expectations than you do.

Myth: Conflict is bad, and it should always be avoided.

Fact: Conflict is a natural result of being around other people. Conflict itself is not bad, but the way in which people deal with conflict can be healthy or unhealthy.

LANGUAGE ARTS CONNECTION — ADVANCED

Conflict in Literature In literature, conflict is often classified into three main categories. *Person versus himself* refers to a conflict in which a character is struggling to make a decision. *Person versus person* refers to a conflict between two characters or between a character and a group of characters. *Person versus nature* refers to a conflict in which a character must overcome some aspect of the natural world. Have interested students read five short stories and determine the category of conflict used in each story. **LS Verbal**

Teach

READING SKILL BUILDER — BASIC

Reading Organizer Have students make an outline of this lesson as they read through it. Students should use the headings and boldface words to help them construct their outline. Tell students that their outlines may be used to study for the lesson quiz and the chapter review. **LS Logical**

Discussion — BASIC

Comprehension Check Ask students to define the term *conflict*. (Conflict is any clash of ideas or interests.) Ask students to explain why conflict is part of everyone's life. (Sample answer: Everyone has a different view of the world. As a result, people occasionally have opinions that clash.) Have volunteers describe three signs that conflict is occurring or about to occur. (The three signs are disagreement over an issue, emotions—such as anger or jealousy—and behavior—such as raised voices or crossed arms.) **LS Verbal**

Activity — GENERAL

Exploring Values Tell students that values are beliefs that a person considers to be of great importance. Explain that truthfulness and honesty are two examples of values. Then, have each student make a list of his or her own personal values. Allow students a few minutes to compare their lists with those of classmates to determine whether any of the lists are exactly the same. (Although several items on the lists may be similar, few students will have identical lists.) Guide students to understand that people have different values and these differences can sometimes lead to conflict. **LS Interpersonal**

Lesson 1 • What Is Conflict?

Teach, continued

Answer to Health Journal
Answers may vary. This Health Journal can be used to begin a class discussion on conflict with peers. Remember that some students may be uncomfortable sharing personal information.

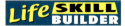 ——— GENERAL

Making Good Decisions Have students apply their decision-making skills to the following scenario: "When you enter the school lunchroom, you find a classmate bullying some younger students into giving him their loose change. When one boy says no to your classmate, the classmate spills the boy's milk onto his lunch tray. What would you do?" **LS** Interpersonal

REAL-LIFE CONNECTION — ADVANCED

Bullying Have interested students interview a guidance counselor or member of the administration to learn about your school's policy on bullying. Encourage the interviewers to determine what actions a student should take if being bullied by a classmate. Allow the interviewers to share their findings with the class. **LS** Verbal

Activity — BASIC

Illustrating Conflicts Have students draw a comic strip about a conflict between two friends. The comic strip should show the cause of the conflict and how the friends resolved it. Students fluent in another language can write the dialog bubbles in both English and their other language. 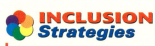 **LS** Visual

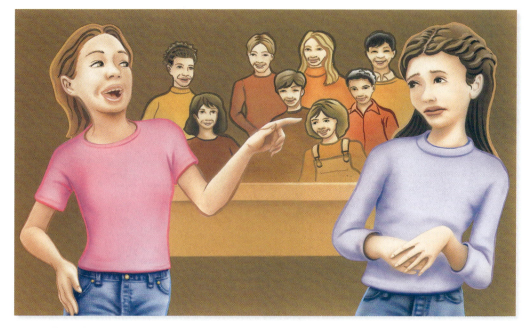

Figure 3 People who tease others often do so in front of an audience. Having an audience makes people who tease feel better about themselves.

Health Journal
Has anyone ever teased you? What happened? How did the teasing make you feel? Write about your experience in your Health Journal.

Conflicts with Peers

Often, conflicts happen with your peers. Your *peers* are people who are close to your own age with whom you interact. Many kinds of conflict can happen between peers. Some of these types of conflict are described below.

- **Conflicts with Friends** Even close friendships can face conflict. You and your friends may argue over what you want to do for fun. Or you may argue because you are jealous of other friendships. Whatever the reason for conflict between friends, these conflicts should be solved quickly before they destroy the friendship.

- **Teasing** You probably have been teased or have teased someone else before. It is important to realize that teasing can result in hurt feelings and emotional problems. Usually, people tease others in front of an audience to make themselves look better. You can deal with teasing by ignoring it, making a joke about it, or by confronting the teaser.

- **Bullying** Scaring or controlling another person by using threats or physical force is called **bullying**. Bullies almost always pick on people who are younger or smaller than they are. If a bully won't leave you alone or if any violence occurs, report the bully to an authority figure, such as a parent or teacher.

Background
Bullies and Their Victims Research shows that most bullies are outgoing individuals who are concerned with their own pleasure. Most are willing to break rules and exert power over others in order to achieve their goals. Bullies tend to prey on victims who are shy, sensitive, and somewhat anxious.

INCLUSION Strategies — GENERAL
• Attention Deficit Disorder • Learning Disabled

Use a TV show as an alternate input mode to help students recognize the reasons why conflict occurs. In class, watch a sitcom that has various examples of conflicts. Have students take notes on each example as they watch. When the show is over, ask students to describe the conflicts in the show and to identify the reason why each conflict occurred. (Students should identify the reasons as being resources, values and expectations, or emotions.) **LS** Visual

Conflicts at School

You spend a lot of time at school. While you are at school, you deal with different people, including friends, classmates, teachers, and other school authorities. Your relationships with these people are important for your social and mental development. But these relationships can also be sources of conflict. Some of the conflicts that can occur at school are listed below.

- **Conflicts with Peers** All of the conflicts with peers listed on the previous page can happen at school. In fact, these types of conflicts are the most common conflicts at school.
- **Competition with Classmates** Students often compete with one another in schoolwork or in sports. Some competition can be healthy, but if the competition begins to cause anger or hurt feelings, it may become a problem.
- **Conflicts with Teachers or Other School Authorities** Conflict can arise with teachers for many reasons. Sometimes, you may feel that a teacher is being too strict or unfair. A teacher may feel that you are causing trouble or are not doing your best.

Remember that you are at school to learn. It is very important to solve conflicts at school before they interfere with your education. If you need help with a conflict at school, you can ask a trusted adult, such as a parent, teacher, or counselor, for help.

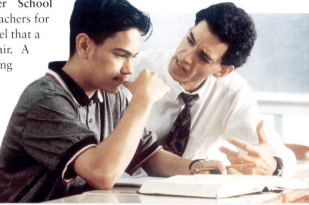

Figure 4 Conflict at school sometimes happens with school authorities. It is important to recognize and solve these conflicts quickly.

Lesson Review

Using Vocabulary
1. What is conflict?

Understanding Concepts
2. Describe three signs that a conflict is happening or is about to happen.
3. List three reasons that conflict happens.
4. Describe three types of conflict with peers.
5. What are three types of conflict that may occur at school?

Critical Thinking
6. **Making Inferences** Howard and his sister wanted to use the computer at the same time. Howard became angry and called his sister a hurtful name. Howard's sister became very angry, and Howard and his sister started fighting. Why did this conflict happen?

internet connect
www.scilinks.org/health
Topic: Emotions
HealthLinks code: HD4035
HEALTH LINKS. Maintained by the National Science Teachers Association

Lesson 2 Focus

Overview
Before beginning this lesson, review with your students the objectives listed under the What You'll Do head in the Student Edition. In this lesson, students learn the importance of good communication in a conflict. Students also learn why body language is important in communication. Finally, students learn good listening skills and methods of resolving conflicts.

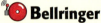 **Bellringer**
Have students make a list of body actions that show a listener is not paying attention to what the speaker is saying. Beneath the list, students should write a sentence describing how they feel when their listeners act in this manner.
LS Interpersonal

Answer to Start Off Write
Accept all reasonable answers. Sample answer: Speaking calmly and clearly is a positive way to express yourself during a conflict.

Motivate

Group Activity —— GENERAL
Skit Organize students into groups. Have each group write and perform a skit about a conflict. Each skit should have two endings. One ending should show how healthy communication led to a positive outcome and the other ending should show how unhealthy communication led to a negative outcome. Explain to students that they should always try to use healthy communication when in a conflict. **LS** Verbal

---

Lesson 2 Communicating During Conflicts

What You'll Do
- **Describe** the importance of good communication.
- **Describe** body language and its importance.
- **Identify** five skills for good listening.
- **Describe** negotiation, compromise, and collaboration.

Terms to Learn
- body language
- negotiation
- compromise
- collaboration

Start Off Write
What is a positive way to express yourself during a conflict?

Pilar's sister was always using the phone. Pilar told her sister that she wanted to be able to use the phone, too. Pilar and her sister talked about the problem and worked out a schedule for using the phone.

Most conflicts can be solved easily by using good communication skills. By telling her sister how she felt and by working with her sister to solve the problem, Pilar was able to use the phone and to avoid fighting with her sister.

Expressing Yourself
The way you choose to express your emotions during a conflict will often determine whether the conflict is solved in a positive way or a negative way. When you are in a conflict, it is important to communicate honestly and openly. You must also avoid communicating in an angry or threatening way. Anger or threats almost always cause a conflict to end poorly. For example, in the situation above, if Pilar had started yelling at her sister or calling her sister names, the conflict would have ended differently. Pilar's sister could have become angry too, and the conflict may have ended in a screaming fight instead of a productive solution.

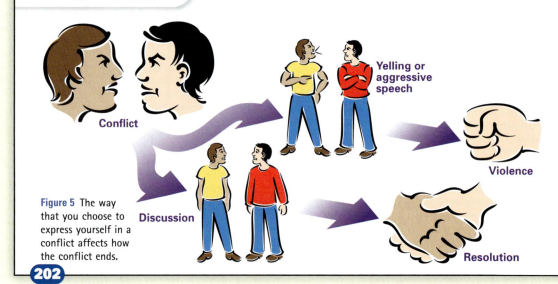

Figure 5 The way that you choose to express yourself in a conflict affects how the conflict ends.

 BASIC

Communicating Effectively Use the figure on this page of the Student Edition to emphasize the idea that conflicts have two possible outcomes. One possible outcome is resolution and another possible outcome is violence. Tell students that the difference between the two outcomes is the type of communication between the parties involved in the conflict.
LS Visual

Chapter Resource File
- Directed Reading **BASIC**
- Lesson Plan
- Datasheets for In-Text Activities **GENERAL**
- Lesson Quiz **GENERAL**

Transparencies
TT Bellringer
TT Conflict Flowchart

202 Chapter 10 • Conflict and Violence

Choosing the Right Words

When you talk to another person during a conflict, choosing your words carefully is important. The words you choose should clearly describe how you feel in a way that is not hurtful, angry, or threatening. Do not call the other person names or make fun of his or her ideas. Instead, choose statements that accurately express your expectations and feelings about the situation. If possible, plan what you want to say ahead of time. By choosing the right words, you can make sure that the other person knows exactly how you feel. This understanding makes it possible to begin working on a solution to the conflict.

Body Language

Words are not the only way that you communicate your feelings to others. Your body often tells others a lot about how you feel. Communication that is done by the body rather than by words is called **body language.** You communicate with your body during a conflict in several ways.

- Facial expressions, such as frowns or smiles, communicate a lot about how you feel. In a conflict, make sure that the expression on your face is calm rather than angry or threatening.
- Gestures, such as pointing your finger at someone or shaking your fist at someone, can be very threatening or insulting. Avoid making these types of gestures in a conflict.
- Posture is very important in a conflict. Folding your arms tells the other person that you are not interested in what he or she is saying. Standing too close to someone can be very threatening. Try to keep a relaxed and open posture.

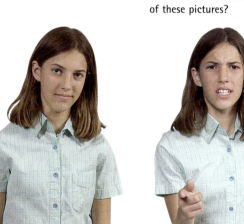

Hands-on ACTIVITY

BODY LANGUAGE ON TV

1. The next time you watch your favorite TV show, turn off the sound for 5 minutes.
2. Write down what you think the characters are talking about. Are they arguing? Are they joking? How can you tell?

Analysis
1. What body language made you think that the actors were saying what you thought they were saying? Explain.
2. By watching the rest of the show, can you tell what the actors were really talking about? Was your guess right?

Figure 6 Body language can tell you a lot about how somebody feels. Can you tell how this teen feels in each of these pictures?

LANGUAGE ARTS CONNECTION — ADVANCED

Connotations of Words Tell students that connotation refers to the overall feeling a word conveys. Explain that two words may share the same meaning yet convey different connotations. Reinforce this concept by asking students to identify the common meaning and different connotations of these word pairs: *cheap/thrifty, stubborn/determined, fat/plump,* and *concerned/worried*. Guide students in recognizing that a good communicator uses words with a positive connotation to send messages. **LS Verbal**

Teach

Hands-on ACTIVITY

Answers
1. Accept all reasonable answers. Sample answer: A smile showed affection, a nod showed agreement, and a look of surprise showed disbelief.
2. Answers may vary. It is likely that students will be able to infer what was said after watching the remainder of the program.

Cultural Awareness

Gestures The meaning associated with a specific body gesture may vary among cultures. For example, in the United States, you send the message "go away from me" by extending your arm outward and moving your fingers away from your body and toward the person. In Japan, this gesture means "come here." Also, in the United States you can ask the question, "Me?" by pointing toward your chest. In Japan, you can ask this same question by pointing to the tip of your nose.

Activity — GENERAL

Sending Messages Write the following messages on slips of paper: "I love you; I'm angry with you; I think you are funny; I'm insulted by that; I don't believe you; I'm afraid of you; You can trust me; I'm sad about that; I am proud of you." Place all slips in a paper bag. Have volunteers draw slips from the bag and use body language to convey the message on their slips. Have observers identify the message they receive from the body language displayed. **LS Kinesthetic**

Lesson 2 • Communicating During Conflicts 203

Teach, continued

READING SKILL BUILDER — BASIC

Anticipation Guide Before students read the next two pages in the Student Edition, have them answer the following true/false questions.

- It is okay to interrupt someone if you disagree with them. (false)
- You should try to repeat what a person says if you don't understand him or her. (true)
- You can reach a solution to a conflict through negotiation. (true)
- There is no difference between compromise and collaboration. (false)

Give students a chance to review and change their answers after reading the rest of the lesson.
LS Verbal

Group Activity — GENERAL

Developing Listening Skills
Organize students into groups of three. Have one student be a speaker, one student be a listener, and one student be an observer. Have the speaker describe what he or she did over the weekend to the listener. The listener should use the listening skills described in the Student Edition. The observer should take notes on what the listener did well and should give suggestions on ways that he or she could improve.
LS Interpersonal   Co-op Learning

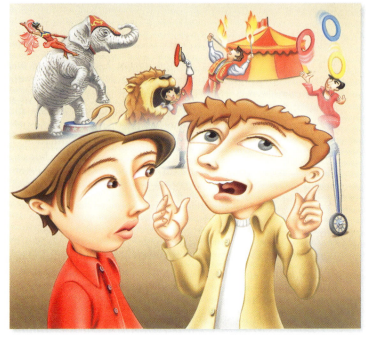

Figure 7 Good listening means focusing on the person who is talking, even if there are distractions.

LIFE SKILLS ACTIVITY

COMMUNICATING EFFECTIVELY

Think of an imaginary conflict between you and one of your friends. Write your idea on an index card. After all of the cards have been collected, your teacher will pick two members of your class to come to the front of the room. They will choose one of the cards and will then act out the conflict written on it. When they are done, the class will describe the ways in which the actors communicated well and the ways in which the actors could have communicated better.

Listening

When you are working to solve a conflict, good listening skills are just as important as good communication skills. By listening carefully to the other person's opinions, you can help to find a solution to the conflict that makes both sides happy. When you listen to another person, make eye contact. Do not become distracted by things that are going on around you. Keep your body relaxed and open. If you are unsure of what the other person said, repeat it to make sure you understand. Do not interrupt the person even if you disagree with him or her. Following these listening tips will let the other person know that you value his or her feelings. In addition, you will better understand the other person's opinions. When you understand the other person's opinions, solving the conflict will be much easier.

Negotiation

The most important tool for solving conflicts is negotiation. **Negotiation** is a discussion to reach a solution to a conflict. For negotiation to work, both sides must be willing to discuss their feelings and their needs openly and honestly. They must also be willing to listen carefully to the other person. Negotiation usually requires both sides to be willing to make sacrifices to reach a solution. If negotiation is used properly, it can solve conflicts positively and often quickly.

SOCIAL STUDIES CONNECTION — ADVANCED

Negotiation Tell students that negotiation is often used to resolve conflicts between countries and political groups. Encourage interested students to study historical examples of negotiation and to determine if the resolution of each example involved compromise or collaboration. Have students present their findings in a poster or an oral report.
LS Verbal

LIFE SKILLS ACTIVITY

Answer
Answers may vary.
Extension: Ask students to describe how the conflict presented could be resolved through compromise or collaboration.

Chapter 10 • Conflict and Violence

Compromise and Collaboration

Compromise and collaboration are two types of solutions to conflicts. **Compromise** is a solution in which each person gives up something to reach a solution that pleases everyone. For example, if you want to go to the park and your friend wants to go eat, you could compromise by going out to eat today and going to the park tomorrow. But an even better solution to conflict is collaboration. **Collaboration** is a solution to a conflict in which neither side has to give up anything to reach a solution that pleases everyone. Imagine again that your friend wants to eat, but you want to go to the park. Collaboration in this situation would be to have a picnic in the park. Unfortunately, not every conflict can be solved through collaboration. Most conflicts are solved by making sacrifices.

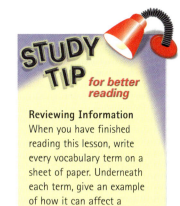

STUDY TIP *for better reading*

Reviewing Information When you have finished reading this lesson, write every vocabulary term on a sheet of paper. Underneath each term, give an example of how it can affect a conflict.

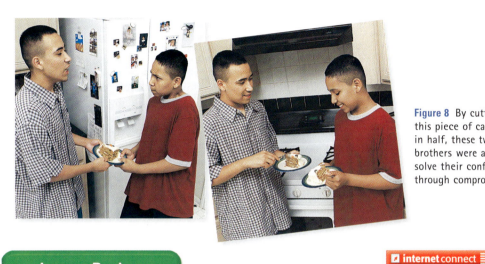

Figure 8 By cutting this piece of cake in half, these two brothers were able to solve their conflict through compromise.

Lesson Review

Using Vocabulary
1. What is body language and why is it important?
2. What is the difference between compromise and collaboration?

Understanding Concepts
3. Why is it important to use good communication skills in a conflict?
4. Name five things that you can do to be a good listener.
5. How can negotiation, compromise, and collaboration be used in a conflict?

Critical Thinking
6. **Applying Concepts** How can body language help you avoid a potential conflict? Explain.

internet connect
www.scilinks.org/health
Topic: Communication Skills
HealthLinks code: HD4022
HEALTH LINKS. Maintained by the National Science Teachers Association

---

Close

Reteaching — BASIC
Compromise and Collaboration
Tell students the following scenario: "Alec and Kim have plans to see a movie Friday night. Friday afternoon, a neighbor asks Kim to babysit so that the neighbor can visit a sick relative. Kim does not want to disappoint Alec, yet she wants to help her neighbor out, too." Then, ask students to determine which of the following solutions is a compromise and which one is a collaboration: "Alec and Kim rent a movie to watch while Kim is babysitting." (collaboration) "Kim babysits on Friday night and then goes to the movies with Alec on Saturday night." (compromise)
LS Logical

Quiz — GENERAL
1. How does careful word selection help resolve a conflict? (Carefully choosing the right words will help insure that other people know how you feel. This makes it possible to work on a solution to the conflict.)
2. What type of facial gestures should be avoided when attempting to resolve a conflict? (Accept all reasonable answers. Sample answers: frowns, smirks, and other expressions that show anger or disrespect for the other person)
3. What must both parties do in a negotiation for it to be successful? (Both parties must be willing to discuss their feelings openly and honestly, must listen to the other party, and must be willing to make sacrifices.)

Alternative Assessment — GENERAL
Pamphlet Have students work in small groups to design and write a pamphlet that explains how to be a good listener. Students fluent in another language can write the pamphlet in both English and their other language. **English Language Learners**
LS Verbal

Answers to Lesson Review
1. Body language is communication that is done by the body rather than by words. Body language is important because it can tell others how you feel.
2. Compromise is a solution in which each person gives up something in order to reach a solution. Collaboration is a solution in which neither side has to give up anything in order to reach a solution.
3. It is important to use good communication skills so that the conflict can be resolved in a positive way.
4. Five things you can do to be a good listener include: making eye contact, not being distracted, having open body language, repeating the speaker's words, and not interrupting.
5. Negotiation is a discussion in which both parties involved in a conflict communicate in a healthy way in order to reach a resolution. Some resolutions are compromises and others are collaborations.
6. If you maintain open body language, other people are less likely to become angry with you.

Lesson 2 • Communicating During Conflicts

Lesson 3

Focus

Overview
Before beginning this lesson, review with your students the objectives listed under the What You'll Do head in the Student Edition. In this lesson, students learn five warning signs that a conflict may be out of control. Students also learn how mediation can help resolve a conflict and learn the seven skills of a trained mediator.

Bellringer
Have students think about a time when they saw a conflict get out of control. Ask them to make a list of the actions they observed. Beneath the list, have students write a paragraph describing how they felt upon witnessing the event. **LS Verbal**

Answer to Start Off Write
Accept all reasonable answers. Sample answer: You should get help to solve a conflict if it is out of control.

Motivate

Activity — GENERAL
Conflict in the News Newspapers often have articles about conflicts that have grown out of control. Have students scan newspapers to find examples of such articles. Ask students to present an oral summary of the articles they found. For each summary, ask the class: "What signs indicated that the conflict was out of control?" (Sample answers: anger, lack of communication, hurtful or insulting speech, inability to reach a solution, and violence or threats of violence) **LS Verbal**

Lesson 3 — Getting Help for Conflicts

What You'll Do
- **Identify** five warning signs that a conflict may be out of control.
- **Describe** the use of mediation for solving out-of-control conflicts.
- **Identify** seven skills of a trained mediator.

Terms to Learn
- mediation

Start Off Write
How do you know when to get help to solve a conflict?

Health Journal
Describe a time when you were in a conflict that you couldn't solve without help from another person. What did that person do to help solve the conflict?

Elena and her friend Toni were having an argument. Toni got so angry that she decided to stop talking to Elena. Elena can't solve the conflict now because Toni won't talk to her. Is there anything Elena can do?

Sometimes, a conflict gets to a point that the people cannot solve the conflict by themselves. When Toni stopped talking to Elena, she made it impossible for them to solve the conflict. With a little help, however, this conflict can be solved.

When Is a Conflict Out of Control?
There are many ways that a conflict can get out of control. By identifying the warning signs that a conflict is out of control, you can take steps to calm down and work toward a solution. A conflict may be out of control when communication becomes insulting or hurtful or when either person becomes very angry. If violence or threats are used, a conflict is definitely out of control. Sometimes, people in a conflict stop communicating, or they negotiate for a long time but cannot reach a solution. In these cases, the conflict is out of control because the people in the conflict cannot solve it. If a conflict that you are in gets out of control, take a break and return to the conflict later. The break will give you and the other person a chance to calm down. During the break, think about what you want from the conflict and what you are willing to give up. If you still cannot solve the conflict, you may need to talk to another person who is not part of the conflict.

TABLE 1 Signs That a Conflict Is Out of Control
Serious anger
Lack of communication
Hurtful or insulting speech
Inability to reach a solution after much negotiation
Violence or threats of violence

INCLUSION Strategies — BASIC
- Developmentally Delayed
- Behavior Control Issues

Some students may not know who they can turn to for help solving a conflict. Ask students to list the names of people in each of the following categories: family members, friends, neighbors, and teachers. Have students put stars next to the names of people on their lists that they feel comfortable talking to about problems. Tell students that they know many people who can help when the students are in a conflict. **LS Interpersonal**

Chapter Resource File
- Directed Reading **BASIC**
- Lesson Plan
- Lesson Quiz **GENERAL**

Transparencies
- TT Bellringer
- TT Signs That a Conflict Is Out of Control

---

206   Chapter 10 • Conflict and Violence

Mediation

The best way to solve a conflict that is out of control is to seek the help of somebody who is not part of the conflict. A third person can often think of solutions that neither side has considered. A third person can also help lower the level of anger in a conflict and can keep the discussion on track. This third party is called a *mediator*. A mediator is an uninvolved person who helps solve a conflict between other people. The process of using a mediator to solve a conflict is called mediation.

Not everyone can be a mediator. When selecting a mediator, you should select somebody who has special training in mediation. A person who is not trained in mediation can make a conflict worse or can become a part of the conflict. A good mediator

- sets ground rules, such as no name calling and no interrupting, and makes sure that everyone follows the rules
- keeps the conflict focused on finding a solution
- does not take sides
- listens carefully to both sides
- asks questions
- offers solutions
- does not allow the conversation to become angry

If you need to find a trained mediator to help solve a conflict, talk to a parent, teacher, or other trusted adult. He or she can help you find a trained mediator.

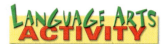

Write a short story about two teens who seek the help of a mediator to solve a conflict.

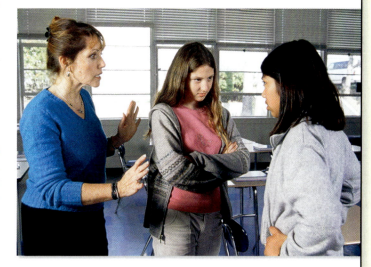

Figure 9 These two teens are using a mediator to help them solve a conflict that they could not solve on their own.

Lesson Review

Using Vocabulary

1. Define *mediation*, and give an example of when it may be used to solve a conflict.

Understanding Concepts

2. List five signs that a conflict may be getting out of control.

3. Why is it important for a mediator to have special training?

4. List seven skills of a trained mediator.

Critical Thinking

5. **Applying Concepts** Think of three rules not listed in the text that a mediator may set.

Answers to Lesson Review

1. Mediation is a process in which an uninvolved party helps others resolve a conflict. Sample answer: Mediation can be used to resolve a conflict between friends who have stopped talking to one another.
2. Five signs that a conflict may be out of control are anger, a lack of communication, hurtful or insulting speech, the inability to reach a solution after much negotiation, and violence or threats of violence.
3. A mediator who lacks special training can make a conflict worse or can become part of the conflict.
4. A trained mediator sets rules and makes sure they are followed, keeps the conflict focused on finding a solution, does not take sides, listens carefully to both sides, asks questions, offers solutions, and does not allow the conversation to become angry.
5. Accept all reasonable answers. Sample answer: Some rules may include keeping the discussion confidential, remaining seated during discussions, and only using facts to support an argument.

Teach

Using the Figure — GENERAL

Recognizing Signs Ask students to read the table on the previous page of the Student Edition. Organize the students into five groups and assign each group an entry from the table. Ask the groups to write and perform a skit that shows how the assigned entry indicates that conflict has gotten out of control. **LS** Verbal

Close

Reteaching — BASIC

Writing Questions Pair each student with a partner. Have the student pairs write five short-answer questions about this lesson. After they write their questions, students should write answers to the questions in complete sentences. **LS** Verbal

Quiz — GENERAL

1. How can an uninvolved person help resolve a conflict? (An uninvolved person can think of solutions that neither side has considered. The person can also help lower the anger level of the conflict and keep the discussion on track.)
2. Why is it important to be able to identify the signs that a conflict is out of control? (If you can recognize when a conflict is out of control, you can take steps to calm down and work toward a solution.)
3. Suppose you feel that a mediator is needed to resolve a conflict with a peer. How can you find a mediator? (You should ask a trusted adult, such as a parent, teacher, or counselor, to help you find a mediator.)

Lesson 3 • Getting Help for Conflicts

Lesson 4

Focus

Overview
Before beginning this lesson, review with your students the objectives listed under the What You'll Do head in the Student Edition. In this lesson, students learn how conflicts turn to violence and learn to identify signs that a conflict may become violent. Students also learn the importance of reporting all threats of violence.

🔔 Bellringer
Have students write the word *VIOLENCE* vertically down the side of a paper. Next to each letter, have them write a word or phrase that they associate with this term. For example, the word *Victim* might be placed next to the letter *V*.
LS Verbal

Answer to Start Off Write
Accept all reasonable answers. Sample answer: You can tell that a conflict is about to become violent if you hear threats and angry speech.

Motivate

Discussion —— GENERAL
Signs of Violence Tell students that it is common for young siblings to get into fights with one another. Have students think about a time when they got into a fight with their siblings. Ask students to describe what occurred before the fight started. (Sample answers: We called each other names, we started yelling at each other, and we become very angry.) Tell students their answers also describe what happens before violence occurs between people of all ages.
LS Verbal

Lesson 4

Violence: When Conflict Becomes Dangerous

What You'll Do
- **Describe** how a conflict becomes violent.
- **Identify** four signs that a conflict may become violent.
- **Explain** the importance of reporting all threats of violence.

Terms to Learn
- violence
- aggression

Start Off Write
How can you tell if a conflict is about to become violent?

Figure 10 You may often read about violent events in the newspaper. Unfortunately, violence is common in our world.

Tom got in a fight at school. He was arguing with a classmate named Arman during lunch. The two teens got angrier and angrier until Arman hit Tom. Why did this conflict become violent? Could Tom have seen the violence coming?

Most conflicts will not become violent. However, if a conflict is handled poorly or is allowed to get out of control, it can become violent. Fortunately, there are signs that can warn you of violence before it happens. If Tom had known what signs to look for, he probably could have avoided violence.

What Is Violence?
You probably have an idea of what violence is. You may even have experienced violence. But what exactly is violence? **Violence** is the use of physical force to harm someone or something. Unfortunately, violence exists in many places in society. Movies and TV shows often include violence. Newspapers and news broadcasts report many stories of violence throughout the world. By knowing how and why conflicts become violent, you can avoid becoming a victim of violence.

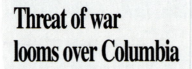

Attention Grabber
Tell students the following statistic to illustrate how common violence is among teens: A national survey taken in 1999 showed that one in three high school students had been in a fight during the previous twelve months.

Chapter Resource File
- Directed Reading **BASIC**
- Lesson Plan
- Lesson Quiz **GENERAL**

Transparencies
TT Bellringer

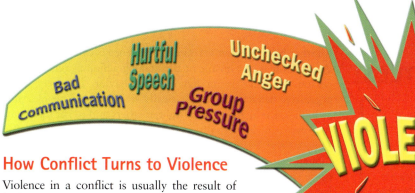

How Conflict Turns to Violence

Violence in a conflict is usually the result of bad communication. When people in a conflict use language that is hurtful or insulting or use body language that is threatening, anger increases. If anger continues to increase, the result can be violence. By knowing the signs to watch for, you can tell when violence is about to happen. If you see signs that a conflict is about to become violent, walk away. Walking away will give you and the other person a chance to calm down. Hopefully, you can solve the conflict later and can avoid a violent situation.

Figure 11 Several things, such as bad communication, anger, and group pressure, can cause a conflict to turn violent.

Watch for the Signs

Violence can happen quickly in a conflict. There are several signs that violence may happen. Recognizing these signs will help you avoid and prevent violent situations. The following signs can tell you that a conflict may become violent.

- **Bad Communication** When people in a conflict communicate in a negative way, violence can result. Bad communication can be hurtful speech—such as shouting, insults, and profanity—or can be refusal to listen to the other side.
- **Body Language** A person's body language can be a very good sign that the person is about to become violent. Examples of threatening body language include having clenched fists, standing too close, or having a clenched jaw.
- **Anger** People in a conflict often get angry. Anger is a normal emotion and can be expressed in positive and negative ways. If people are using negative expressions of anger, a conflict can turn to violence.
- **Group Pressure** People are more likely to become violent when other people are watching them. The group may be encouraging them, or they may want to look powerful in front of the group. Either way, be careful in conflicts that happen in front of an audience.

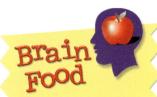

Brain Food

When a person is under a lot of stress, he or she is more likely to show violent behavior. Studies have shown that regular exercise can reduce stress significantly.

MISCONCEPTION ALERT

TV Violence Students may believe that violence that they see on TV does not affect them. However, research has identified three major effects of viewing violence on TV. The effects are that people become less sensitive to the suffering of others, people are more fearful of the world around them, and people are more likely to behave in aggressive ways toward others. This is even true for "fake" violence such as violence seen in some cartoon shows. Children who watch violent cartoons are more likely to hit others, argue, and disobey rules.

Teach

Life SKILL BUILDER — BASIC

Using Refusal Skills Remind students that the five refusal skills are avoiding dangerous situations, saying no, standing your ground, staying focused on the issue, and walking away. Ask students to describe how each refusal skill can be used when a conflict begins to turn toward violence. **LS** Verbal

Activity — GENERAL

Poster Project Organize students into groups of three. Have each group design and construct a poster that describes the signs that violence may occur in a conflict. Students may illustrate their posters with original drawings or photos cut from magazines and newspapers. The posters should also describe how a teen could avoid being caught in a violent situation. In each group, one student should create or gather the images, one student should write the text, and one student should be in charge of leading an oral presentation of the poster. **LS** Visual Co-op Learning

Sensitivity ALERT

Desensitization to Violence Some of your students may come from homes with abusive people. Such students may be desensitized to the signs that violence may occur. Because they may be exposed to these signs every day, they may consider them to be normal. As a result, they may demonstrate the signs more frequently than other students and have more difficulties resolving conflicts. If you suspect that a student is being abused, report your suspicions to your school's counselors.

Teach, continued

LIFE SKILLS ACTIVITY

Answer
Accept all reasonable answers. Sample answer: I would talk to the teacher in private and tell her about the cheating and Michelle's threat.

READING SKILL BUILDER — BASIC

Paired Summarizing Pair each student with a partner. Have students read this lesson silently. Tell students to mark passages they don't understand with a sticky note. After they finish reading, have the students help each other with the passages that one or both of them marked with a sticky note. Finally, have one student in each pair summarize the main ideas of the lesson. The other student should listen and point out any mistakes in the retelling. **LS Verbal**

Life SKILL BUILDER — GENERAL

Making Good Decisions Tell students the following scenario: "Manuel's friend Ian is furious because he was cut from the school basketball team. Ian tells Manuel, 'I'm going to make the coach sorry that he cut me from the team.' When Manuel asks Ian what he means, Ian tells him not to worry about it." Have students role-play the part of Manuel as he follows the six steps of making good decisions to determine what to do about Ian's threat. **LS Logical**

LIFE SKILLS ACTIVITY

MAKING GOOD DECISIONS
During a math test, Kara notices that Michelle is cheating. Before Kara lets the teacher know, Michelle tells Kara, "If you say anything, I will tell everyone that you are a tattletale. And no one will talk to you ever again." What would you do if you were Kara?

Aggression

Another behavior that is related to violence is called *aggression*. **Aggression** is any hostile or threatening action against another person. Violence is an aggressive behavior. However, most aggressive behavior is not physically violent. Some people, such as bullies, use aggression to frighten others and to get their way. A person can be verbally aggressive by teasing or humiliating someone else. Even a mean look can be a form of aggression. Even though aggression may not always cause physical harm, it can cause serious emotional damage. Aggression is also a good warning sign that violence may happen. A person who regularly uses aggression is likely to become violent in a conflict. If someone is being aggressive toward you, you should tell a trusted adult.

Threats

The most obvious sign that violence is about to happen is a threat. A *threat* is an expressed intention or plan to do harm to something or someone. Some threats are made in person. Other times, threats are sent in writing or are delivered by someone else. Sometimes, you may even hear someone threaten another person who is not present. People may use threats to get their own way, or threats may be a reaction to anger or other emotions. Whatever the reason for threats, all threats should be taken seriously. You cannot always tell whether a person is serious about a threat. Therefore, it is much better to be safe and to report the threat than to ignore the threat and find that the threat was real.

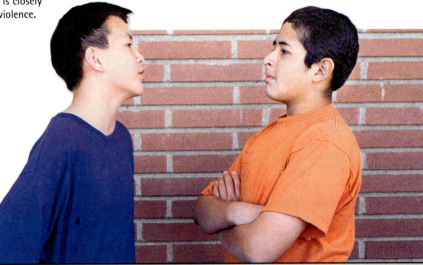

Figure 12 The teens in this picture are being aggressive toward each other. Aggression is closely related to violence.

PSYCHOLOGY CONNECTION — ADVANCED

Relational Aggression Psychologists have recently identified a type of aggression called relational aggression. It is characterized by meanness and attacks on another person's social status and relationships. Some forms of relational aggression include giving someone the silent treatment, excluding someone from a social group, and gossiping. The intent behind this type of aggression is to manipulate friendships and emotions to harm another person. Relational aggression is more commonly observed among girls than it is among boys. Have students study the use of relational aggression in your school and write a report on their findings. **LS Interpersonal**

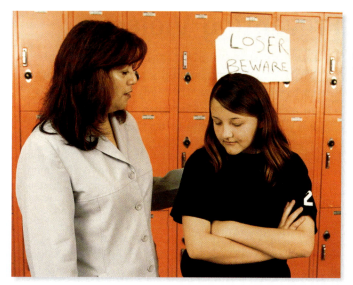

Figure 13 Report any threat to a trusted adult.

Reporting Threats of Violence

Reporting all threats of violence to a responsible adult is very important. If you know of a threat to yourself or to someone else, it is your responsibility to tell an authority or trusted adult of the danger. If you do not tell someone, violence that could have been avoided may happen. For example, many of the extremely violent events that have happened in schools recently could have been avoided if threats had been reported. In these cases, people heard threats but did not take them seriously. Even if you think that someone is joking, you must report any threat of violence. The possible consequences of not reporting threats are too great.

Health Journal
If you experienced acts or threats of violence, to whom could you report them? Make a list of 10 adults to whom you could report acts or threats of violence.

Lesson Review

Using Vocabulary
1. Define *violence*, and identify places where you might see violence.

Understanding Concepts
2. How does a conflict become violent?
3. Identify four signs that a conflict may become violent.
4. Why is it important to report all threats to a responsible adult?

Critical Thinking
5. **Identifying Relationships** Is all violence aggressive? Is all aggression violent? Explain your answers.
6. **Making Inferences** Do you need to report threats made against someone's property? Explain your answer.

Answers to Lesson Review
1. Violence is the use of physical force to harm someone or something. You might see violence in movies, television, newspapers, and news broadcasts.
2. A conflict may become violent when bad communication causes the people involved in the conflict to become angry.
3. Signs that a conflict may become violent are bad communication, anger, threatening body language, and group pressure.
4. It is important to report all threats so that violence can be avoided.
5. yes; Violence is an aggressive behavior. no; Aggression is not always physically violent.
6. yes; A threat against property should be reported. Harming or destroying someone's property is violence and should be prevented.

Answer to Health Journal
Answers may vary. This Health Journal may be a good way to close the lesson.

Close

Reteaching — BASIC
Outline Have students create an outline of this lesson using the lesson title and the subheads. Have students review the objectives under the What You'll Do head in the Student Edition to make sure that their outlines include information about each objective.
LS Logical

Quiz — GENERAL
1. Describe how a person may communicate in a conflict that is turning to violence. (A person may use angry or hurtful speech such as shouting, insults, or threats.)
2. What is a benefit of walking away from a conflict that is about to become violent? (Walking away will give you and the other person a chance to calm down. You can resolve the conflict later and avoid a violent situation.)
3. What is aggression? (Aggression is any hostile or threatening action against another person.)
4. Why do some people use threats? (People may use threats to get their own way or may use them to express anger or other emotions.)

Alternative Assessment — GENERAL
Skit Have students work in small groups to write and perform a skit that shows a student speaking with her guidance counselor about a threat that she overheard. **LS** Verbal

Lesson 4 • Violence: When Conflict Becomes Dangerous

Lesson 5 Focus

Overview
Before beginning this lesson, review with your students the objectives listed under the What You'll Do head in the Student Edition. In this lesson, students learn five ways to control their anger and learn five ways to protect themselves from violent situations.

🔔 Bellringer
Have students write a paragraph describing a time when they were angry. Students should explain why they were angry and describe how they controlled their anger. Invite volunteers to read their paragraphs aloud. **LS** Verbal

Answer to Start Off Write
Accept all reasonable answers. Sample answer: One way to protect yourself from violent situations is to walk away from conflicts that are out of control.

Motivate

Discussion — GENERAL
Anger Control Ask students to describe how they control their anger. (Sample answer: I play a sport or I watch TV to take my mind off my problems.) Explain to students that different methods of anger control work for different people—playing sports might work for some of them, but might not work for others. Ask students what might happen if they don't control their anger. (Sample answer: Conflicts may become violent and I may be hurt.) You may wish to close this discussion by sharing your method of controlling your anger with your students. **LS** Verbal

Lesson 5

What You'll Do
- **Identify** five ways to control anger.
- **Identify** five ways to protect yourself from violent situations.

Start Off Write
What can you do to protect yourself from violent situations?

Preventing Violence

> Luke got into a big fight with his little brother. Luke got so angry that he was about to hit his brother. Instead, Luke decided to go to his room to calm down. Later, Luke was very glad that he hadn't hit his brother.

Luke did the right thing by taking a break to control his anger. If Luke had hit his brother, the situation would have been much worse. Everybody has a responsibility to control his or her anger and to keep violence from happening.

Controlling Anger

Anger is like air filling a balloon. If the air is not allowed to escape, the balloon will eventually burst. To prevent anger from erupting into violence, use the following strategies:

- **Take a break.** Often, removing yourself from an angry situation for even a short time will allow you to calm down.
- **Focus on calming yourself.** Count to 10, and take deep, slow breaths.
- **Release your anger in a safe way.** Punching a pillow or a punching bag can allow you to release your anger without harming anyone or anything.
- **Exercise.** Physical activity can release anger and can allow you to focus on something else until you calm down.
- **Be creative.** Try drawing or writing in a journal. Creative activities can allow you to release your anger in a healthy and productive way. Some creative activities can also help you work through your problems.

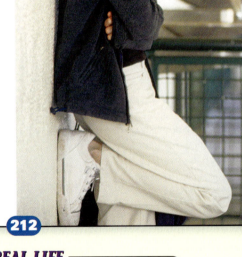

Figure 14 If you are getting too angry, take a break to calm down.

REAL-LIFE CONNECTION — ADVANCED
Anger Management Seminars Tell students that some community organizations conduct anger management seminars for people who have difficulties controlling their anger. Separate seminars are given for children, teens, and adults. Participants in these seminars learn healthy ways to express and control their anger. Encourage interested students to research a seminar designed for teens and report their findings to the class. **LS** Interpersonal

Chapter Resource File
- Directed Reading **BASIC**
- Lesson Plan
- Lesson Quiz **GENERAL**

Transparencies
TT Bellringer

212 Chapter 10 • Conflict and Violence

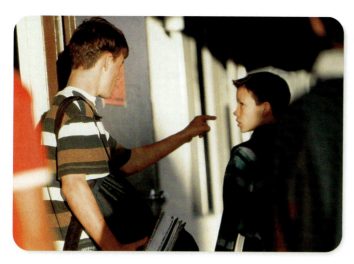

Figure 15 If you think a situation could become violent, walk away.

Protecting Yourself

Just as you have a responsibility to others to control your anger, you also have a responsibility to yourself to avoid violent situations. To lower your risk of becoming a victim of violence, do the following things:

- Pay attention to signs that violence might occur.
- Walk away from out-of-control conflicts.
- Take all threats seriously.
- Avoid people who carry weapons.
- Avoid conflict with people who have been drinking or using drugs. These behaviors increase the chance that a person will become violent.

Myth & Fact

Myth: If you avoid violent situations, you are a coward.

Fact: Violence does not solve anything. Avoiding violent situations is smart, not cowardly.

Lesson Review

Understanding Concepts

1. Name five things that you can do to control your anger.
2. Name five things that you can do to protect yourself from violent situations.
3. Why should you avoid conflict with people who have been drinking or using drugs?

Critical Thinking

4. **Applying Concepts** Steven is very angry at his brother, Eric. What is a positive way he can release his anger? What is a negative way he can release his anger? Explain.

CHAPTER 10 REVIEW

Assignment Guide

Lesson	Review Questions
1	9, 12, 19, 20
2	2, 4, 5, 11, 13, 14
3	6, 8, 10, 22
4	3, 7, 15–17, 21, 23
5	18, 24, 25
2 and 3	1

ANSWERS

Using Vocabulary

1. Negotiation is a discussion to reach a solution to a conflict. Mediation is the process of using an uninvolved third party to help resolve a conflict.
2. Compromise is a solution to a conflict in which each person gives up something to reach a solution that pleases everyone. Collaboration is a solution in which neither side has to give up anything to reach a solution that pleases everyone.
3. Aggression is any hostile or threatening action against another person. Violence is an aggressive behavior in which physical force is used to harm someone or something.
4. body language
5. Negotiation
6. mediator
7. threat

Understanding Concepts

8. Signs that a conflict is out of control are anger, lack of communication, hurtful or insulting speech, the inability to reach a solution after much negotiation, and violence or threats of violence.

Chapter Summary

- Conflict is any clash of ideas or interests. ■ Most conflicts happen at home, with peers, or at school. ■ The way that you communicate during a conflict can often determine whether the conflict ends positively or negatively. ■ Communication by the body is called *body language*. ■ Tools for resolving conflicts include negotiation, compromise, collaboration, and mediation. ■ Watch for the signs that a conflict is out of control, and seek help for out-of-control conflicts. ■ Uncontrolled anger can lead to violence. ■ Watch for the warning signs that a conflict may turn violent. Walk away from conflicts that may turn violent. ■ Report any threats to authorities. ■ Controlling anger and avoiding violent situations are two ways to prevent violence.

Using Vocabulary

For each pair of terms, describe how the meanings of the terms differ.

1. negotiation/mediation
2. compromise/collaboration
3. aggression/violence

For each sentence, fill in the blank with the proper word from the word bank provided below.

mediator	body language
negotiation	threat
aggression	compromise

4. Communication by the body is called ___.
5. ___ is a discussion to reach a solution to a conflict.
6. An uninvolved person who helps solve a conflict between other people is called a(n) ___.
7. An expressed intention or plan to do harm to something or someone is called a(n) ___.

Understanding Concepts

8. How can you tell if a conflict is out of control?
9. Describe two types of conflict that can happen at home.
10. Why must a mediator be uninvolved in a conflict?
11. What is needed for negotiation to work?
12. Why is it important to resolve conflicts at school?
13. Why is collaboration better than compromise?
14. Give three examples of body language. Describe how each one could be used positively and negatively in a conflict.
15. How can bad communication increase the chance of violence?
16. How can group pressure increase the chance of violence?
17. Why should all threats be taken seriously?
18. How can exercise help you control your anger?

---

9. Two types of conflict that can happen at home are conflicts between children and parents and conflicts between siblings.
10. A mediator must be uninvolved in a conflict so he or she can help solve the conflict without taking sides.
11. For negotiation to work, both sides must be willing to discuss their feelings openly and honestly, be willing to listen to the other side, and be willing to make sacrifices.
12. It is important to resolve conflicts at school because the conflicts may interfere with your education.
13. Collaboration is better than compromise because no one has to give up anything important to reach a solution.
14. Sample answer: Facial expressions—smiles are positive and frowns are negative. Gestures—open hands are positive and shaking a fist is negative. Posture—a relaxed posture is positive and standing with folded arms is negative.
15. Sample answer: Bad communication, such as shouting and insults, can lead to anger. Angry people are more likely to become violent.
16. Groups sometimes encourage people to be violent.

Critical Thinking

Making Inferences

19. How are bullies and people who tease others alike?

20. Even friends experience conflict with each other. In fact, in many cases, close friends experience more conflict than friends who aren't close. Why might close friends have more conflict?

21. Group pressure can cause a person to become violent in a situation in which he or she normally would not have become violent. Name two other situations in which group pressure may cause a person to do something that he or she normally would not do.

Making Good Decisions

22. Imagine that you are in a conflict with a classmate. After arguing for a while, you both realize that you need the help of a mediator. Your classmate says that her mother is a trained mediator and can help you solve the conflict. Is your classmate's mother a good selection for a mediator in this case? Explain.

23. Imagine that you have a friend who is very angry at another boy at school. Your friend tells you how much he hates this other boy and tells you that he plans to bring a knife to school to threaten the other boy. When you tell your friend that bringing a knife to school is a bad idea, he says that he was joking. What should you do in this situation?

24. Imagine that you are very angry about a conflict that you are having with a friend. What is one physical way that you could control your anger? What is one creative way that you could control your anger? Which way do you think would work best for you? Explain.

25. Use what you have learned in this chapter to set a personal goal. Write your goal, and make an action plan by using the Health Behavior Contract for preventing violence and controlling your anger. You can find the Health Behavior Contract at go.hrw.com. Just type in the keyword HD4HBC08.

Reading Checkup

Take a minute to review your answers to the Health IQ questions at the beginning of this chapter. How has reading this chapter improved your Health IQ?

Chapter Resource File

- Concept Review GENERAL
- Concept Mapping GENERAL
- Performance-Based Assessment GENERAL
- Chapter Test GENERAL

17. All threats must be taken seriously to prevent violence from occurring.

18. Exercise can release your anger and can allow you to focus on something else until you calm down.

Critical Thinking

Making Inferences

19. Bullies and people who tease act the way they do to make themselves look and feel powerful at another person's expense.

20. Close friends tend to spend a lot of time together. Spending time together increases the chances for conflicts to occur.

21. Accept all reasonable answers. Sample answers: A teen may try alcohol at a party because others are pressuring him or her to do so. A person might wear clothes he or she doesn't like in order to fit in to a group.

Making Good Decisions

22. no; The mother of your classmate would not be a good mediator because she might take her daughter's side.

23. You should take the threat seriously and report it to a trusted adult.

24. Accept all reasonable answers. Sample answer: A physical way to control anger is to play basketball or another sport. A creative way to control anger is to write in a journal. Answers about which way would work the best for a student may vary.

25. Accept all reasonable responses. Note: A Health Behavior Contract for each chapter can be found in the Chapter Resource File and at the HRW Web site, go.hrw.com.

Model

Introduce this activity by reminding students that using this Life Skill will help them take personal responsibility for their behavior. Then, review the scenario with the class.

Prepare students for this activity by modeling each of the steps of the skill. Make sure students understand each step before you move on to the next one.

Guided Practice: Practice with a Friend

Guided Practice is the stage in which you and the students analyze their approach to solving the problem given in the scenario and analyze their communication skills. Have students read Act 1. Discuss with the class the situation described and the way students are to act it out. Organize the class into groups of three. In each group, one person plays the role of Ramón, another person plays Jonas, and the third person is the observer.

Proper pacing during the Guided Practice is important. The suggestions listed below will help you control the pace.

1. Stop after completing each step of communicating effectively.
2. Discuss with each group the observer's comments.
3. Ask the other members of each group to listen to the observer's suggestions and to suggest ways to improve their communication skills.
4. Instruct students to repeat the steps that need improvement and to include their modifications.
5. Check to make sure that students understand each step before they move on to the next step.
6. If time permits, repeat the exercise three times, switching roles each time. Each student should have the opportunity to play each role. **Co-op Learning**

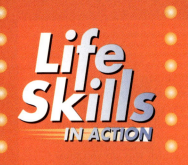

Life Skills IN ACTION

Communicating Effectively

Have you ever been in a bad situation that was made worse because of poor communication? Or maybe you have difficulty understanding others or being understood. You can avoid misunderstandings by expressing your feelings in a healthy way, which is communicating effectively. Complete the following activity to develop effective communication skills.

The Threat

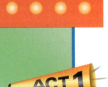

Setting the Scene

Ramón and his friend Jonas are joking around as they walk down a hallway in school. Jonas accidentally bumps into an older student named Kevin and causes Kevin's books and schoolwork to scatter across the hallway. Jonas apologizes and helps Kevin pick up his things, but Kevin is furious. "You're going to pay for this!" growls Kevin.

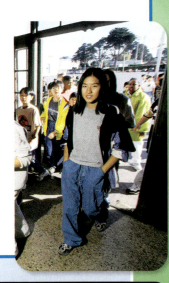

The 4 Steps of Communicating Effectively

1. Express yourself calmly and clearly.
2. Choose your words carefully.
3. Use open body language.
4. Use active listening.

Guided Practice

Practice with a Friend

Form a group of three. Have one person play the role of Ramón and another person play the role of Jonas. Have the third person be an observer. Walking through each of the four steps of communicating effectively, role-play Ramón and Jonas talking about the situation. In the conversation, Ramón should try to convince Jonas to report Kevin's threat. Jonas should explain why he doesn't want to report the threat. The observer will take notes, which will include observations about what the person playing Ramón did well and suggestions of ways to improve. Stop after each step to evaluate the process.

Independent Practice

Check Yourself

After you have completed the guided practice, go through Act 1 again without stopping at each step. Answer the questions below to review what you did.

1. Why should Ramón express himself calmly and clearly when talking to Jonas?
2. What should Ramón say to Jonas to convince him that it is important to report the threat?
3. Why is it important for Ramón to use active listening when Jonas is talking?
4. Why is it important to report all threats of violence?

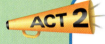

On Your Own

Over the next few days, Kevin threatens Jonas whenever he sees Jonas. Jonas is unhappy about the threats, and Ramón is finally able to convince Jonas to report them. Jonas goes to talk with one of his teachers about the threats. Draw a comic strip showing how Jonas could use the four steps of communicating effectively to tell his teacher about the threats.

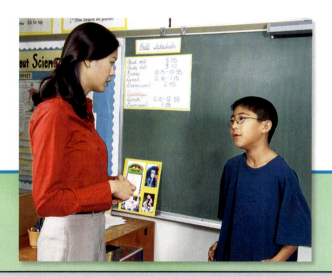

Independent Practice: Check Yourself

Instruct students to repeat Act 1 without stopping at each step. Remind students to apply what they learned in the Guided Practice to the Independent Practice. Students do not have to use the steps in the order listed to communicate effectively.

Encourage students to use the Check Yourself questions as a starting point for reviewing and analyzing their Independent Practice. Remind students that as they change roles, the answers to these questions may change for each actor. Encourage students to create additional questions for checking their communication skills. When students have finished the Independent Practice, have them answer the Check Yourself questions in writing. Use their answers to assess their understanding of the steps of communicating effectively and to assess their use of the steps to solve a problem.

Check Yourself Answers

1. Sample answer: Ramón should express himself calmly and clearly because he wants Jonas to understand that he is serious about reporting Kevin's threat.
2. Sample answer: Ramón should tell Jonas that Jonas may be seriously hurt if Kevin follows through with the threat.
3. Sample answer: Ramón should use active listening to show that he respects Jonas and that he is interested in what Jonas is saying.
4. Sample answer: You can help prevent violence from occurring if you report all threats.

Act 2: On Your Own

This additional scenario gives students an opportunity to apply what they have learned in both the Guided Practice and the Independent Practice to a new situation.

Suggest to students that they use the Check Yourself questions as a starting point for communicating effectively in the new situation. Encourage students to be creative and to think of ways to improve their communication skills.

Assessment

Review the comic strips that students have created as part of the On Your Own activity. The comic strips should show that the students used their communication skills in a realistic and effective manner. Display the comic strips around the room. If time permits, ask student volunteers to act out the dialogues of one or more of the comic strips. Discuss the comic strip's dialogue and the use of communication skills.

CHAPTER 11

Teens and Tobacco
Chapter Planning Guide

PACING	CLASSROOM RESOURCES	ACTIVITIES AND DEMONSTRATIONS
BLOCK 1 • 45 min pp. 218–223 **Chapter Opener**	CRF Health Inventory * ■ GENERAL CRF Parent Letter * ■	SE Health IQ, p. 219 CRF At-Home Activity * ■
Lesson 1 Tobacco: Dangerous from the Start	CRF Lesson Plan * TT Bellringer *	TE Activity Poster Project, p. 221 GENERAL TE Activity Consequences, p. 223 GENERAL SE Life Skills in Action Making Good Decisions, pp. 242–243 CRF Enrichment Activity ◆ ADVANCED
BLOCK 2 • 45 min pp. 224–229 **Lesson 2** Tobacco Products, Disease, and Death	CRF Lesson Plan * TT Bellringer *	SE Hands-on Activity, p. 225 ◆ CRF Datasheets for In-Text Activities * GENERAL TE Demonstration Modeling the Effect of Emphysema, p. 225 ◆ GENERAL CRF Life Skills Activity * ■ GENERAL CRF Enrichment Activity ◆ ADVANCED
Lesson 3 Social and Emotional Effects of Tobacco	CRF Lesson Plan * TT Bellringer *	TE Group Activity Social Strain, p. 228 GENERAL CRF Enrichment Activity ◆ ADVANCED
BLOCK 3 • 45 min pp. 230–233 **Lesson 4** Forming a Tobacco Addiction	CRF Lesson Plan * TT Bellringer * TT Nicotine Receptors *	CRF Enrichment Activity ◆ ADVANCED
Lesson 5 Why People Use Tobacco	CRF Lesson Plan * TT Bellringer *	TE Activities Scavenger Hunt, p. 217F CRF Life Skills Activity * ■ GENERAL CRF Enrichment Activity ◆ ADVANCED
BLOCK 4 • 45 min pp. 234–239 **Lesson 6** Quitting	CRF Lesson Plan * TT Bellringer *	TE Demonstration Relaxation Exercise, p. 236 GENERAL SE Math Activity, p. 237 CRF Enrichment Activity ◆ ADVANCED
Lesson 7 Choosing Not to Use Tobacco	CRF Lesson Plan * TT Bellringer * TT Refusing Cigarettes *	TE Activities Mock Trial, p. 217F TE Group Activity Peer Pressure, p. 238 GENERAL TE Activity Dealing with Pressure, p. 239 GENERAL CRF Enrichment Activity ◆ ADVANCED

BLOCKS 5 & 6 • 90 min **Chapter Review and Assessment Resources**

- SE Chapter Review, pp. 240–241
- CRF Concept Review * ■ GENERAL
- CRF Health Behavior Contract * ■ GENERAL
- CRF Chapter Test * ■ GENERAL
- CRF Performance-Based Assessment * GENERAL
- OSP Test Generator
- CRF Test Item Listing *

Online Resources

go.hrw.com — Visit go.hrw.com for a variety of free resources related to this textbook. Enter the keyword **HD4TO7**.

Holt Online Learning — Students can access interactive problem solving help and active visual concept development with the *Decisions for Health* Online Edition available at **www.hrw.com**.

CNN Student News — cnnstudentnews.com — Find the latest health news, lesson plans, and activities related to important scientific events.

217A Chapter 11 • Teens and Tobacco

Compression guide:
To shorten your instruction because of time limitations, omit Lessons 3 and 7.

KEY

- **TE** Teacher Edition
- **SE** Student Edition
- **OSP** One-Stop Planner
- **CRF** Chapter Resource File
- **TT** Teaching Transparency
- ***** Also on One-Stop Planner
- **■** Also Available in Spanish
- **♦** Requires Advance Prep

SKILLS DEVELOPMENT RESOURCES	LESSON REVIEW AND ASSESSMENT	STANDARDS CORRELATION
		National Health Education Standards
TE Reading Skill Builder Anticipation Guide, p. 221 BASIC CRF Directed Reading * BASIC	SE Lesson Review, p. 223 TE Reteaching, Quiz, p. 223 CRF Concept Mapping * GENERAL CRF Lesson Quiz * ■ GENERAL	1.1, 1.6
TE Reading Skill Builder Paired Summarizing, p. 226 BASIC CRF Directed Reading * BASIC	SE Lesson Review, p. 227 TE Reteaching, Quiz, p. 227 TE Alternative Assessment, p. 227 GENERAL CRF Lesson Quiz * ■ GENERAL	1.8
SE Study Tip Organizing Information, p. 228 TE Life Skill Builder Using Refusal Skills, p. 228 SE Life Skills Activity Assessing Your Health, p. 229 CRF Cross-Disciplinary * GENERAL CRF Directed Reading * BASIC	SE Lesson Review, p. 229 TE Reteaching, Quiz, p. 229 CRF Lesson Quiz * ■ GENERAL	6.3
TE Reading Skill Builder Discussion, p. 231 BASIC CRF Cross-Disciplinary * GENERAL CRF Directed Reading * BASIC	SE Lesson Review, p. 231 TE Reteaching, Quiz, p. 231 CRF Lesson Quiz * ■ GENERAL	
TE Inclusion Strategies, p. 232 ♦ BASIC CRF Decision-Making * GENERAL CRF Directed Reading * BASIC	SE Lesson Review, p. 233 TE Reteaching, Quiz, p. 233 CRF Lesson Quiz * ■ GENERAL	1.4, 4.2, 4.4, 6.2
TE Inclusion Strategies, p. 234 BASIC SE Life Skills Activity Refusal Skills, p. 236 CRF Refusal Skills * GENERAL CRF Directed Reading * BASIC	SE Lesson Review, p. 237 TE Reteaching, Quiz, p. 237 TE Alternative Assessment, p. 237 ♦ GENERAL CRF Concept Mapping * GENERAL CRF Lesson Quiz * ■ GENERAL	1.1
CRF Decision-Making * GENERAL CRF Refusal Skills * GENERAL CRF Directed Reading * BASIC	SE Lesson Review, p. 239 TE Reteaching, Quiz, p. 239 CRF Lesson Quiz * ■ GENERAL	1.6, 5.6

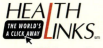

www.scilinks.org/health
Maintained by the **National Science Teachers Association**

Topic: Carbon Monoxide
HealthLinks code: HD4021
Topic: Lung Cancer
HealthLinks code: HD4063
Topic: Nicotine
HealthLinks code: HD4069

Topic: Tobacco
HealthLinks code: HD4101
Topic: Smoking and Health
HealthLinks code: HD4090

Technology Resources

 One-Stop Planner
All of your printable resources and the Test Generator are on this convenient CD-ROM.

Guided Reading Audio CDs

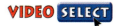
For information about videos related to this chapter, go to **go.hrw.com** and type in the keyword **HD4TO7V**.

Chapter 11 • Chapter Planning Guide

CHAPTER 11

Teens and Tobacco
Chapter Resources

Teacher Resources

TEACHING TRANSPARENCIES

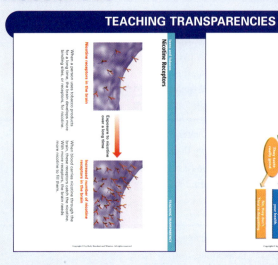
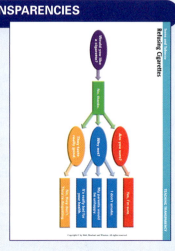

BELLRINGER TRANSPARENCIES

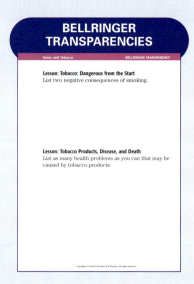

LESSON PLANS

PARENT LETTER

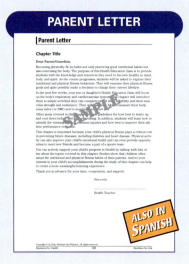

TEST ITEM LISTING

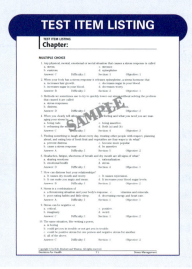

Meeting Individual Needs

DIRECTED READING
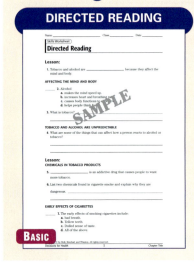

CONCEPT MAPPING
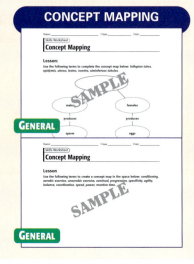

CONCEPT REVIEW
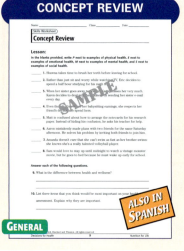

ENRICHMENT ACTIVITIES
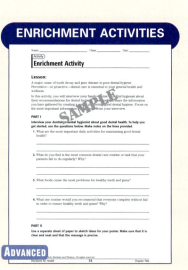

Resources

These worksheet pages can be found in the Chapter Resource File and the One-Stop Planner. The transparencies can be found in the Teaching Transparencies binder and on the One-Stop Planner.

Activities

LIFE SKILLS ACTIVITIES
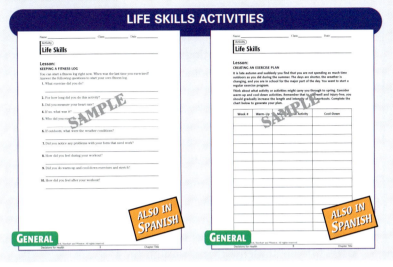

AT-HOME ACTIVITY
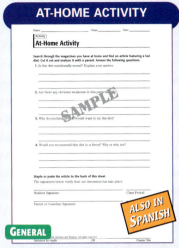

DATASHEETS FOR IN-TEXT ACTIVITIES
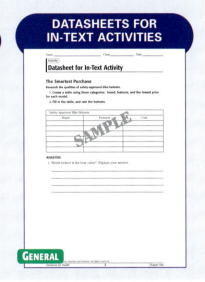

Applications

DECISION-MAKING
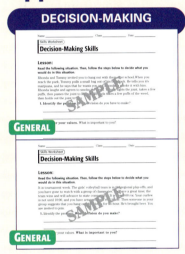

REFUSAL SKILLS
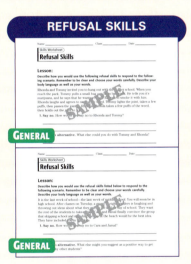

CROSS-DISCIPLINARY
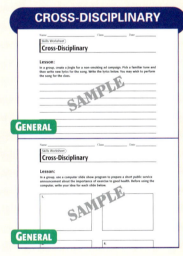

HEALTH BEHAVIOR CONTRACT
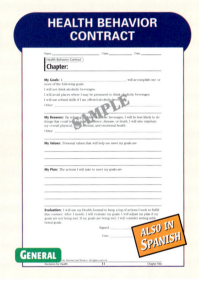

Assessments

HEALTH INVENTORY
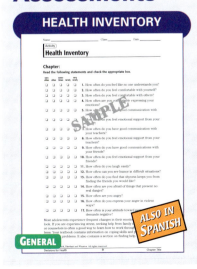

LESSON QUIZZES
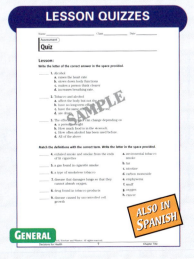

CHAPTER TEST
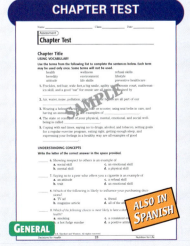

PERFORMANCE-BASED ASSESSMENT
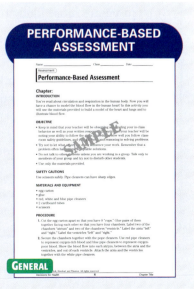

Chapter 11 • Chapter Resources and Worksheets

CHAPTER 11 | Background Information

The following information focuses on some of the key issues related to teens and tobacco use. This material will help prepare you for teaching the concepts in this chapter.

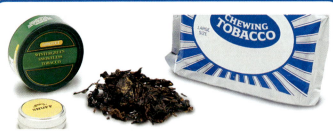

Prevalence of Adolescent Tobacco Use

- The information below is from a national survey that is conducted annually.

- Fewer teens are using tobacco today than 5 years ago. In 1996, 49.2 percent of 8th graders tried cigarettes, and 20.4 percent tried smokeless tobacco. By 2001, 36.6 percent of 8th graders had tried cigarettes, and 11.7 percent had tried smokeless tobacco.

- In 200l, 12.2 percent of 8th graders had smoked a cigarette in the past 30 days.

- In 2001, 5.5 percent of 8th graders were daily smokers.

Risk factors in Adolescent Tobacco Use

- Peers have consistently been shown to be powerful influences on adolescent tobacco use.

- Adolescents who associate with peers and adults who use tobacco products are more likely to use tobacco.

- While parents who smoke have not been shown to be as influential on teens as peers are, many studies do indicate that if a parent uses tobacco, his or her children are more likely to use tobacco.

- Adolescents from lower income households have been shown to be at greater risk of using tobacco products.

- How much an adolescent knows about the health risks of tobacco use does not seem to predict whether or not he or she will smoke cigarettes, but knowing the health risks of smokeless tobacco does appear to help adolescents decide not to use these products.

- Poor performance in school, lack of involvement in school, lack of skills to resist peer influence, and low self-esteem are factors in adolescent tobacco use.

Tobacco Marketing Strategies

- **Point-of-Purchase Promotions** The tobacco industry promotes its products at places that sell its products. These point-of-purchase promotions include the following: self-service cigarette displays, multipack discounts, free items such as counter mats, shopping baskets with tobacco advertising, and advertisements placed in windows and inside the store.

- **Product placement** Tell students that product placement—paying to have a product shown in a movie or on a television show—has become a popular way for companies to promote their products. Inform students that although the tobacco industry voluntarily agreed not to engage in product placement, one study indicated that more than three-fourths of the top 25 box-office films from 1988 to 1997 showed tobacco use, and 28 percent showed specific tobacco brands.

Effective Approaches to Tobacco Use Prevention

- The most effective school-based prevention programs are ones that help students develop the skills to resist social pressures to use tobacco products. These social pressures include the following: the misperception that everyone uses tobacco products, the positive image of smoking as seen in advertisements and movies, and peer pressure.

- Successful programs focus on both the positive and negative social consequences of smoking and encourage students to examine how tobacco products are marketed.

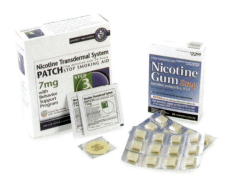

For background information about teaching strategies and issues, refer to the *Professional Reference for Teachers.*

ACTIVITIES

CHAPTER 11

Consider using the activities on this page as students explore the lessons of this chapter. Look for other activities throughout the Student Edition chapter.

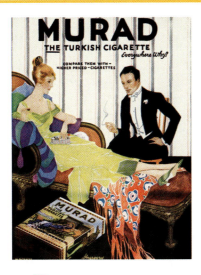

Scavenger Hunt

Procedure The purpose of this activity is to show the students how many pro-tobacco messages they see every day. Tell students that they will be looking for pro-tobacco messages in their everyday lives and will be tracking these messages for one week. Make a score sheet for the scavenger hunt. The score sheet should contain a list of items and places where the students can find advertisements for tobacco products. Examples of items and places include ashtrays, hats, key chains, buses, calendars, matchbooks, lighters, posters or signs, T-shirts, brochures, magazines and coupons. Draw a blank line next to each item so that the students can enter the number of times they saw that type of message. Use the score sheet at the end of the activity to tally each team's score. You may want to brainstorm with the students and have them make up a score sheet as part of the project.

Organize the class into teams of three or four students. Each student on the team should keep track of the following on a blank piece of notebook paper (save the score sheet for later):

- the time that the message was seen
- the location of the message (on the side of a taxi or bus, in a store, on a scoreboard, in a magazine, etc.)
- the length of the message (number of words) or size of the ad (on a billboard)
- the type and brand of tobacco being advertised (chewing tobacco, snuff, cigarettes, etc.)

Hands on

Analysis

- At the end of the hunt, have every student on each team fill out their score sheets. Tell students to use their notes to log in the total number of tobacco messages they found for each item or place. Also, have students make a list on the bottom of their score sheet of all of the brands of tobacco products they found.

- Students may want to write a short article about their findings and publish the findings in their school newspaper. Or students may place the information on the classroom bulletin board.

Activity

Mock Trial—Helping Prevent Tobacco Use Encourage students to take action to prevent tobacco use. Have students stage a mock trial. The defendant is an executive of a tobacco company charged with causing health diseases and death. Other roles include a judge, the jury, witnesses, the prosecuting attorneys, and the defense attorneys. The prosecuting attorneys will try to prove that cigarettes cause illness and death, and the defense attorneys will argue that people choose to smoke.

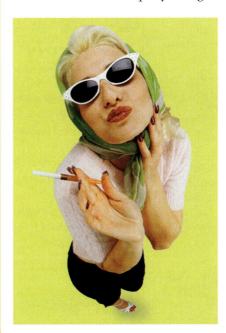

National Public Health Week

National Public Health Week helps focus attention on major health issues in our communities. During the first week of April, have students find out about events such as the American Cancer Society's Great American Smokeout and come up with ideas on how they can participate in or create their own event.

CHAPTER 11

Overview
Tell students that this chapter will help them learn how tobacco affects a person's health and wellness and why tobacco products are addictive. They will also learn about why people use tobacco, ways people can quit using tobacco, and how to remain tobacco free.

Assessing Prior Knowledge
Students should be familiar with the following topics:
- health and wellness
- decision making
- self-esteem
- physical fitness

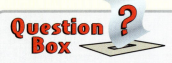

Students may feel more comfortable asking questions if you set up a Question Box to collect their questions. Have students write and anonymously submit their questions about tobacco use, how to help someone quit using tobacco, or how to handle negative peer pressure. Address these questions during class, or use these questions to introduce lessons that cover related topics.

Current Health
Check out *Current Health* articles and activities related to this chapter by visiting the HRW Web site at go.hrw.com. Just type in the keyword HD4CH26T.

Chapter Resource File
- Directed Reading Worksheet **BASIC**
- Health Inventory **GENERAL**
- Parent Letter

CHAPTER 11 Teens and Tobacco

Lessons
1	Tobacco: Dangerous from the Start	220
2	Tobacco Products, Disease, and Death	224
3	Social and Emotional Effects of Tobacco	228
4	Forming a Tobacco Addiction	230
5	Why People Use Tobacco	232
6	Quitting	234
7	Choosing Not to Use Tobacco	238
	Chapter Review	240
	Life Skills in Action	242

Check out **Current Health** articles related to this chapter by visiting go.hrw.com. Just type in the keyword HD4CH26.

Standards Correlations

National Health Education Standards

1.1 Explain the relationship between positive health behaviors and the prevention of injury, illness, disease, and premature death. (Lessons 1 and 6)

1.4 Describe how family and peers influence the health of adolescents. (Lesson 5)

1.6 Describe ways to reduce risks related to adolescent health problems. (Lessons 1 and 7)

1.8 Describe how lifestyle, pathogens, family history, and other risk factors are related to the cause or prevention of disease and other health problems. (Lesson 2)

4.2 Analyze how messages from media and other sources influence health behaviors. (Lesson 5)

4.4 Analyze how information from peers influences health. (Lesson 5)

5.6 (partial) Demonstrate refusal and negotiation skills to enhance health. (Lesson 7)

6.2 Analyze how health-related decisions are influenced by individuals, family, and community values. (Lesson 5)

6.3 Predict how decisions regarding health behaviors have consequences for self and others. (Lesson 3)

> " I promised both **my parents** and **myself** that I would **never try smoking.**
>
> There are a couple of kids that I hang out with who have just started smoking. And they have been bugging me lately to give it a try. I'm not going to start smoking, but I wish I knew how to get them to quit. "

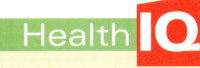

PRE-READING

Answer the following true/false questions to find out what you already know about tobacco. When you've finished this chapter, you'll have the opportunity to change your answers based on what you've learned.

1. As long as someone remains a light smoker, that person will not experience the harmful side effects of smoking.
2. You have to use tobacco products for many years before the tobacco has harmful effects on you.
3. The smoke that comes from the tip of a burning cigarette is not as dangerous to your health as the smoke that is inhaled by the smoker.
4. It is against the law to sell any form of tobacco product to someone under the age of 18.
5. Nicotine is a drug.
6. Young people do not get hooked on cigarettes as easily adults do.
7. Most people can quit smoking without any help.
8. Chewing tobacco does not cause cancer.
9. More women die from breast cancer than from lung cancer.
10. Cigarettes are as addictive as heroin and cocaine.
11. The only way to successfully quit smoking is to just go "cold turkey."
12. Cigar and pipe smoking are safer than cigarette smoking because people rarely inhale smoke from cigars and pipes.

ANSWERS: 1. false; 2. false; 3. false; 4. true; 5. true; 6. false; 7. false; 8. false; 9. false; 10. true; 11. false; 12. false

Using the Health IQ

Misconception Alert
Answers to the Health IQ questions may help you identify students' misconceptions.

Question 1: Students may not realize that someone who only occasionally smokes can experience negative effects, including shortness of breath and impaired sense of smell.

Question 5: The terms *drug* or *drug use* are generally used in relation to illegal drugs. Students might not realize that nicotine is a drug and that when a person smokes cigarettes, he or she is using a drug.

Question 8: Students may not realize that chewing tobacco can cause cancers of the mouth, head, and neck.

Answers
1. false
2. false
3. false
4. true
5. true
6. false
7. false
8. false
9. false
10. true
11. false
12. false

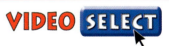

For information about videos related to this chapter, go to **go.hrw.com** and type in the keyword **HD4TO7V**.

Lesson 1

Focus

Overview
Before beginning this lesson, review with your students the objectives listed under the What You'll Do head in the Student Edition. In this lesson, students will learn about how tobacco affects their health. They will also be able to identify tobacco products other than cigarettes and will learn why environmental tobacco smoke is harmful.

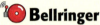

Have students write down two negative consequences of smoking.

Answer to Start Off Write
Accept all reasonable answers. Sample answer: lung cancer, mouth cancer, and heart disease

Motivate

Discussion — GENERAL
What Is Tobacco? Ask students to list different kinds of tobacco products. (Students should list cigarettes, cigars, pipe tobacco, chewing tobacco, and snuff.) Ask students what kinds of things tobacco products might contain other than tobacco and why? (Sample answers: agricultural chemicals from when the tobacco was grown; flavorings that enhance taste; chemical preservatives that lengthen shelf life and flavor; chemicals that keep a cigarette from going out) Help students understand that when a person uses tobacco, he or she is also consuming a wide variety of other substances. **LS Interpersonal**

Lesson 1 — Tobacco: Dangerous from the Start

What You'll Do
- **List** three chemicals that are produced when a cigarette is lit.
- **List** five effects of tobacco on your body that appear early in a cigarette habit.
- **Describe** health problems associated with smokeless tobacco use.
- **Identify** four types of tobacco products other than cigarettes.
- **Explain** why environmental tobacco smoke is harmful.

Terms to Learn
- additive
- nicotine
- environmental tobacco smoke (ETS)

What are some of the dangerous effects of tobacco?

`Approximately one in two people who smoke throughout their lifetime will die prematurely!`

Smoking has many harmful effects. Yet, many people continue to smoke and eventually become ill or die from a smoking-related illness. In this lesson, you will learn about the different types of tobacco products and how they affect your health.

What's in a Tobacco Product?
The tobacco plant has grown naturally in this country for centuries. But tobacco products are far from natural. When tobacco is processed, the leaves of the tobacco plant are combined with hundreds of other ingredients called additives. **Additives** are the chemicals that help keep the tobacco moist, help it to burn longer and taste better. One example of an additive is ammonia. Ammonia is also found in urine and in cleaning products.

When you light a cigarette, the burning tobacco produces smoke that contains thousands of chemicals. One of these chemicals is benzene, which is known to cause cancer. Other chemicals that are produced by the burning smoke are tar and carbon monoxide. Carbon monoxide is a gas that enters the bloodstream and starves your body of oxygen. Tar is a solid, sticky substance. When tar is inhaled, it coats the airways and lungs, blocking small air sacs. Chronic bronchitis, lung cancer, and other lung diseases can eventually result from smoking.

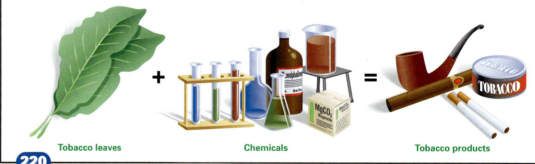

Figure 1 Cigarettes and other tobacco products contain many ingredients other than just tobacco.

Tobacco leaves + Chemicals = Tobacco products

Attention Grabber
Students may not realize how many deadly chemicals are in cigarettes. The following is a list of some of these chemicals and the products they can be found in:

- arsenic—rat poison
- acetone—nail-polish remover
- formaldehyde—embalming fluids
- nitrobenzene—gasoline
- hydrogen cyanide—the poison in gas chambers
- lead—some paints
- vinyl chloride—garbage bags

Chapter Resource File
- Directed Reading Worksheet **BASIC**
- Lesson Plan
- Lesson Quiz **GENERAL**

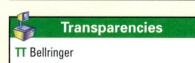

TT Bellringer

220 Chapter 11 • Teens and Tobacco

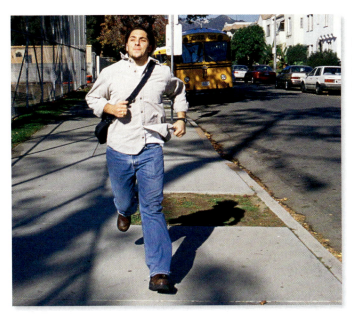

Figure 2 Even things as simple as running to get to school on time become difficult for people who smoke.

Cigarettes: Effects Appear Early

You do not have to be a heavy or lifelong smoker to feel the harmful effects of cigarettes. The harm begins with the first puff, when nicotine enters the lungs. **Nicotine** is a highly addictive drug that occurs naturally in the leaves of the tobacco plant. Some early effects of tobacco on your body are as follows:

- Nicotine travels from the lungs into the bloodstream and into the brain, where the nicotine raises the heart rate and blood pressure.
- Skin, breath, hair, and clothing will immediately smell of smoke. And other people usually notice the odor first.
- Most people feel nauseated and dizzy when they begin smoking because they are not used to the chemicals that enter their bloodstream and brain.
- Your senses of smell and taste usually suffer. As a result, foods no longer smell or taste the same.
- Even light smokers report shortness of breath and increased coughing. Smokers are unable to run as long or as fast as they did before they started smoking.
- Smokers are sick more frequently and stay sick longer.

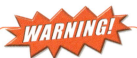

Contents of Smoke

Carbon monoxide is found in car exhaust fumes, tar is used to pave roads, and cyanide is found in rat poison. These chemicals are also found in tobacco smoke, and they enter your body when you smoke!

Teach, continued

Discussion —— GENERAL

Smokeless Tobacco Let students know that the largest smokeless tobacco manufacturer has a smokeless tobacco product that releases a low level of nicotine, is flavored with wintergreen, and comes in little individual serving-sized pouches. This product only has about 2 percent of the smokeless tobacco market. Meanwhile, the company's bestselling product has 42 percent of the market and releases a much higher level of nicotine.

Ask students the following questions:

- Which of these two products would most new tobacco users probably try first? (the product that is flavored with wintergreen)

- Why would most new users start out with a tobacco product that releases the least amount of nicotine? (This product would make the new tobacco user less nauseated and dizzy.)

- Why is the product that releases the greater amount of nicotine more popular than the smoother tasting, low-nicotine product? (The tobacco user soon develops a tolerance to nicotine and requires more nicotine to get the same effect.)

- Why would the manufacturer benefit from having a product that has only 2 percent of the market? (The product that has only 2 percent of the market is used to get the new tobacco user addicted to nicotine. The user then graduates to a stronger tobacco product, thus benefiting the manufacturer.)

LS Auditory

Smokeless Tobacco Products

Tobacco products are not always smoked or burned. *Smokeless tobacco* includes chewing tobacco and snuff. *Chewing tobacco* is coarsely chopped tobacco leaves that contain flavorings and additives much like the tobacco in cigarettes. Chewing tobacco is placed in the mouth and chewed. Nicotine enters the bloodstream through the lining of the mouth. Chewing creates brown-stained saliva that must be spit out often. *Snuff* is also put in the mouth, but it is a flavored powder. It is placed between the cheek and gum. Snuff doesn't need to be chewed for the nicotine to be absorbed into your body. If saliva from either chewing tobacco or snuff is swallowed, the user can become very sick. First-time users of these products often become nauseated and dizzy. Long-term effects include bad breath, yellowed teeth, and an increased risk of oral cancer.

Other Tobacco Products

Pipe tobacco, cigars, and clove cigarettes are other common tobacco products that are smoked. The way that tobacco in pipes and cigars is processed allows the nicotine to be absorbed more easily than the nicotine from cigarettes is. Cigars can contain seven times more tar and four times more nicotine than cigarettes do.

Bidis (BEE deez) are unfiltered cigarettes that are wrapped in tobacco leaves. Bidis are flavored to make them attractive to teens. But with their high levels of nicotine, tar, and carbon monoxide, bidis may be more dangerous to your health than cigarettes are.

Myth & Fact

Myth: If I don't inhale the smoke from my cigarette, it can't hurt me.

Fact: Even puffing smoke that you don't purposefully inhale can hurt you. It can give you bad breath, yellow teeth, and can put you at greater risk for mouth or throat cancer.

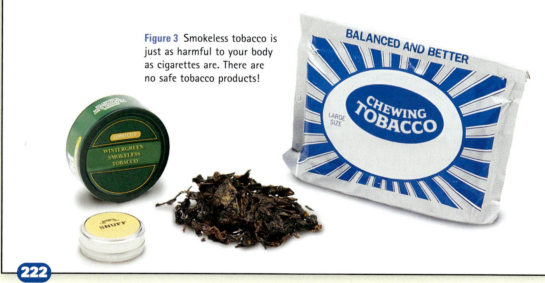

Figure 3 Smokeless tobacco is just as harmful to your body as cigarettes are. There are no safe tobacco products!

SOCIAL STUDIES CONNECTION —— ADVANCED

Writing Have students find out which laws related to environmental tobacco smoke exist in their state and communities. Have students turn in their answers to the following questions:

- When were ETS laws enacted?
- What are the penalties for breaking the law?
- What governmental department is responsible for investigating compliance? (For example, if a restaurant breaks the law by failing to provide a nonsmoking section, whom should a citizen contact?) **Verbal**

MISCONCEPTION ALERT

Some smokers may think that using smokeless tobacco is a good way to quit smoking. But smokeless tobacco contains much more nicotine than cigarettes do, which makes smokeless tobacco just as addictive and dangerous to your health as cigarettes are. And smokeless tobacco users quadruple their risk for oral cancer.

Environmental Tobacco Smoke

Smokers are not the only ones who are exposed to the dangerous chemicals found in tobacco products. Smoke that comes from the tip of a lit cigarette and the smoke that is exhaled from a smokers' mouth are called **environmental tobacco smoke**, or **ETS**. ETS is also called secondhand smoke. People who are around smokers breathe second-hand smoke and are sometimes called *passive smokers*. The same chemicals that are found in the smoke inhaled by smokers are also found in ETS—sometimes in higher concentrations. Therefore, it is harmful to be near a person who is smoking even if you are not smoking.

Until recently, smoking was allowed in most public places, which exposed nonsmokers to ETS. More laws are now in place to protect nonsmokers. These laws may differ from state to state. Some states have stricter laws than other states do. For example, some states have laws that require a nonsmoking section in restaurants. But this area of the restaurant is not protected from ETS unless it is in a completely separate room. Other cities forbid smoking anywhere in restaurants.

Nonsmokers who breathe ETS are at risk for the same health problems that smokers are. And many of these nonsmokers will die each year from smoking-related illnesses.

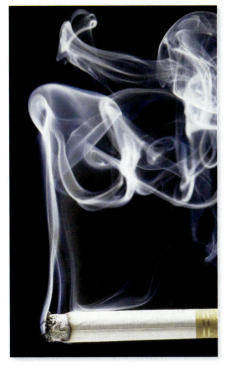

Figure 4 Smoke from a cigarette tip may contain a higher concentration of chemicals than inhaled smoke does because the filter traps a small portion of the chemicals.

Lesson Review

Using Vocabulary
1. Define *additive*.
2. What is nicotine?
3. Define *ETS*, and explain why it is dangerous.

Understanding Concepts
4. What are three chemicals produced by a burning cigarette?
5. What are five health problems that occur early in a smoking habit?
6. What are three long-term effects of smokeless tobacco?
7. What are four forms of tobacco other than cigarettes and smokeless tobacco?

Critical Thinking
8. **Making Inferences** What is one way that you think advertisers make smoking appealing to kids?

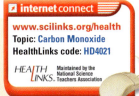

Topic: Carbon Monoxide
HealthLinks code: HD4021
HEALTH LINKS — Maintained by the National Science Teachers Association

---

Activity — GENERAL

Consequences Have students make two columns on their paper. One column should be titled "Short-term consequences," and the other column should be titled "Long-term consequences." Ask students to write examples of short-term consequences of not brushing their teeth for a week. (Students might say having bad breath and having yellow teeth.) Ask students to list examples of long-term consequences of not brushing their teeth. (Students might list tooth decay or gum disease.) Instruct students to write a short-term consequence of using tobacco and a long-term consequence. (Short-term consequenses of using tobacco include bad breath and clothes that smell like smoke. Examples of long-term consequences are lung cancer, mouth cancer, respiratory disease, and heart problems.) **LS Verbal**

Close

Reteaching — BASIC

Outlining Instruct students to write down each of the heads in this lesson. Have the students read the material under each head and make an outline of what they have read. **LS Verbal**

Quiz — GENERAL

1. What is one chemical found in cigarette smoke that is known to cause cancer? (benzene)
2. Why does smoking affect the way food tastes to the smoker? (Smoking can affect a person's sense of smell, and smell is very important to the way food tastes.)
3. Why would people who never smoked die from smoking-related illnesses? (People who are exposed to ETS are exposed to the same dangerous chemicals found in tobacco products.)

Answer to Lesson Review
1. Additives are chemicals that help tobacco stay moist, burn longer, and taste better.
2. Nicotine is a highly addictive drug found in the leaves of the tobacco plant.
3. Environmental tobacco smoke comes from the tip of a lit cigarette or from a smoker's mouth. ETS contains the same chemicals that are found in the smoke inhaled by smokers.
4. Carbon monoxide, tar, and benzene are produced when a cigarette is burning.
5. Sample answer: Early effects of smoking include nausea, impaired senses of smell and taste, shortness of breath, coughing, and an increased number of illnesses.
6. Three long-term effects of smokeless tobacco are bad breath, yellow teeth, and an increased risk of oral cancer.
7. Other forms of tobacco include pipe tobacco, cigars, clove cigarettes, and bidis.
8. Sample answer: Advertisements that show well-dressed, popular people smoking often appeal to kids.

Lesson 1 • Tobacco: Dangerous from the Start

Lesson 2

Focus

Overview
Before beginning this lesson, review with your students the objectives listed under the What You'll Do head in the Student Edition. This lesson describes respiratory diseases associated with smoking and explains how smoking affects the cardiovascular system. Students will also learn about the relationship between smoking and cancer.

Bellringer
Ask students to list health problems caused by tobacco use. (Students may list cancer, heart disease, gum disease, and emphysema.)

Answer to Start Off Write
Sample answer: Smoking can cause lung diseases, such as emphysema or lung cancer.

Motivate

Discussion —— GENERAL
Chronic Smoking-Related Illnesses Have students describe how being sick affects their social life. Ask students if they ever had to miss something they wanted to attend because they were sick, or had a bad time at an event because they weren't feeling very well. Have students imagine what it might be like to have a lung disease that made breathing very difficult. This disease would limit their ability to enjoy most of the fun things they like to do. Tell students that tobacco use usually leads to a chronic illness long before it kills a person. A chronic illness forces a person to live his or her life with many limitations. **LS Auditory**

Lesson 2

What You'll Do
- **Describe** two respiratory diseases associated with smoking.
- **Explain** how smoking affects the cardiovascular system.
- **Describe** the relationship between smoking and cancer.
- **Identify** five other health problems associated with using tobacco products.

Terms to Learn
- chronic bronchitis
- emphysema
- cardiovascular disease

Start Off Write
How can smoking affect your respiratory system?

Tobacco Products, Disease, and Death

Bradley was worried about his mother because she had smoked cigarettes for a long time. And Bradley knew that smoking could cause terrible diseases and even death. Bradley was hoping that his mom would quit smoking soon.

It's never too late to quit smoking. Many of the effects of smoking can be reversed after a person quits. In this lesson, you will learn about the diseases that are caused by smoking. You will also learn why it is so important to never start smoking.

Respiratory Problems

Shortness of breath and coughing are common signs of chronic respiratory disease which affects most smokers. A *chronic disease* is a disease that, once developed, is always present and will not go away. Two chronic respiratory diseases are chronic bronchitis and emphysema. **Chronic bronchitis** is a disease that causes the airways of the lungs to become irritated and swollen. This irritation causes the person to produce a lot of mucus in the lungs. As a result, the person coughs a lot. **Emphysema** destroys the tiny air sacs and the walls of the lung. The holes in the air sacs cannot heal. Eventually, the lung tissue dies, and the lungs can no longer work.

Cigarette smoke causes more than 80 percent of all cases of chronic bronchitis and emphysema. Death from heart failure follows. Usually, the more cigarettes people smoke each day, the more serious the respiratory disease is.

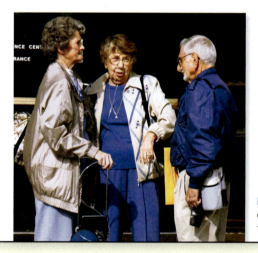

Figure 5 People who have emphysema often have to carry oxygen tanks with them so they can breathe.

Sensitivity ALERT
Be aware that some students may have family members who have a chronic illness related to smoking or a family member who has died from a smoking-related illness. Also be aware that some students may have a chronic illness that is not related to smoking but may also limit their ability to participate in many activities.

Chapter Resource File
- Directed Reading BASIC
- Lesson Plan
- Lesson Quiz GENERAL

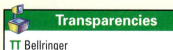
Transparencies
TT Bellringer

---

224   Chapter 11 • Teens and Tobacco

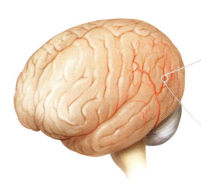
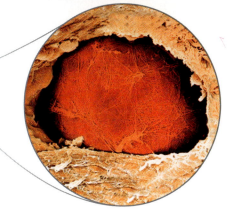

Figure 6 Blood clots in the brain can block the flow of blood through a blood vessel. This blockage can cause a stroke.

Cardiovascular Disease

Scientific research has shown a direct link between smoking and cardiovascular disease. A **cardiovascular disease** is a disorder of the circulatory system. This type of disorder includes high blood pressure, heart disease, and stroke. These diseases prevent organs and limbs from getting the amount of blood they need. Cardiovascular disease is the leading cause of death for adults in the United States.

Smoking also damages the inside lining of the arteries. This damage allows solid material to build up inside the artery. Eventually, the artery becomes blocked. When the arteries that supply oxygen to the heart become blocked, a heart attack results. A stroke results when the arteries that supply blood to the brain become blocked. Blocked arteries that supply blood to limbs of the body can cause severe pain. Sometimes, the need for an amputation, which is the surgical removal of an arm or leg, can result from blocked arteries that can no longer supply blood to the arms or legs. The younger people are when they start smoking and the more they smoke, the higher their risk for stroke and heart attack.

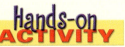

HOW MUCH TAR?

1. The teacher will pass out the outer paper wrappings of cigarettes that have been laminated. These papers are from regular and low-tar brands of cigarettes.
2. Compare the paper wrapper from a regular brand of cigarettes to the low-tar wrapper by holding the papers up to the light. Count the number of holes in each paper wrapper.

Analysis
1. Which paper had more holes? Why do you think the holes are present in the wrapping papers? Do you think the holes in the cigarette papers do what they are intended to do? Explain your answer.
2. Do these increased number of holes make low-tar cigarettes safer than regular cigarettes? Explain your answer.

Teach

Demonstration —— GENERAL

Modeling the Effect of Emphysema Bring enough cocktail straws for everyone in the class to have one. Let students know that emphysema is a disease resulting from damage to the lungs caused by smoking and that people with emphysema have difficulty exhaling. Hand out the straws to all the students. Ask the students to breathe in through their mouth or nose and exhale through the straw for 20 seconds. Ask the students what it was like to have their breathing restricted during the exercise. (Students will probably say that it was difficult and took a while to exhale through the straw.) Let them know that people who suffer from emphysema have their breathing restricted all the time. Explain to students that it is very difficult for people with emphysema to exhale. Ask students how having emphysema might affect their daily lives. (Possible answers are that emphysema restricts your ability to play sports, to be in the band, or to exercise.) **LS Kinesthetic**

Sensitivity ALERT

For students with asthma, this activity may be inappropriate. To avoid having a student with asthma feel left out of the activity, you might ask him or her to help you by keeping track of the time.

Hands-on ACTIVITY

Answer
1. Papers from the low-tar brands have more holes in them. The holes allow air to enter the cigarette filter and to mix with the nicotine and tar in the cigarette. This limits the amount of nicotine and other chemicals that enters the lungs. Because the mouth and/or fingers cover many of the holes, the air is prevented from entering the cigarette. Therefore, the holes in the paper do not do what they were intended to do.
2. Low-tar brands of cigarettes are just as dangerous as regular brands because smokers compensate by either smoking more cigarettes, inhaling more deeply, or covering the holes in the filter paper with their fingers.

Lesson 2 • Tobacco Products, Disease, and Death 225

Teach, continued

READING SKILL BUILDER — BASIC

Paired Summarizing Have students get in pairs and read this page and the next page silently. Students should then take turns summarizing what they read. Have students describe to each other one negative consequence of smoking listed in this lesson that they didn't already know about. **LS** Verbal

Debate — ADVANCED

Who Is Responsible? Have interested students research the various lawsuits brought against the tobacco industry. Some of these lawsuits were filed by smokers, while others were filed by different state governments. Have students debate whether the tobacco industry should be held financially responsible for damages caused by tobacco products. **LS** Verbal/Auditory

Discussion — GENERAL

Smoking Issues Ask students which of the many problems that are caused by smoking and described in this lesson would concern people their age and which problems would not concern them. Have students discuss why their peers might care more about some problems than others. Have willing students offer their own reasons for not using tobacco. Ask students to describe what they tell younger siblings, nieces, or nephews to discourage them from smoking. **LS** Auditory

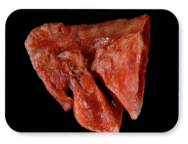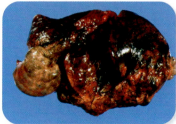

Figure 7 A normal, healthy lung is shown in the left photo. The right photo shows a lung that has been damaged from cigarette smoke.

Lung Cancer

Smoking causes cancer. *Cancer* is a disease in which damaged cells grow out of control. All tobacco products contain chemicals that cause cancer. Smoking can cause cancer of the bladder, kidneys, throat, mouth, and lung. But lung cancer is the leading cause of cancer deaths among both men and women who smoke. Finding lung cancer early is difficult because it spreads very quickly. Also, symptoms usually don't appear until the disease is advanced. If a smoker quits, then the risk of cancer decreases. But it usually does not decrease to the level of someone who has never smoked.

Surprisingly, the risk of lung cancer is just as high for people who smoke light and low-tar cigarettes as it is for those who smoke regular brands. Because smoke from light cigarettes is made to feel smoother, smoke is usually inhaled more deeply into the lungs. This increases the damage done to the lungs.

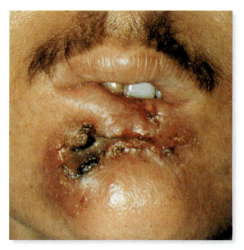

Figure 8 Smokeless tobacco can cause the formation of lesions, which can become cancerous.

Mouth Cancer

Smokeless tobacco causes cancers of the mouth, head, and neck. In fact, a person that uses smokeless tobacco has a higher risk of getting mouth cancer than a cigarette smoker does. Sores form in the mouth of one-half to three-quarters of smokeless tobacco users. These sores may develop into cancer. When the user quits, these sores can disappear. The risk of oral, or mouth cancer depends on how long and how much smokeless tobacco was used. Quitting smokeless tobacco lowers the risk of getting oral cancer. And if a person does get oral cancer, he or she has a better chance of surviving if he or she has quit using smokeless tobacco.

SPORTS CONNECTION — GENERAL

Smoking and Athletics Ask students to think about how smoking cigarettes would affect a person's ability to play sports. Have interested students interview school coaches. Have the students ask the coaches their opinion about how smoking affects athletes. Instruct students to write a short story about a student athlete who began smoking and how his or her performance changed over time. A student who is fluent in another language may want to write this story in English and in his or her other language. **LS** Interpersonal/Verbal **English Language Learners**

Other Health Problems

Not surprisingly, the ingredients and additives in tobacco can lead to many different illnesses. The following list contains more reasons to avoid tobacco products.

- Cigarette smokers catch the flu and colds more often. And they do not recover from them as quickly as nonsmokers do.
- Smokers take longer to heal from wounds and surgeries than nonsmokers do.
- All tobacco products increase the risk for gum and dental diseases.
- Cigarette smoking has been associated with many eye diseases.
- Smoking can cause premature signs of aging. Smoke has negative effects on certain tissues in the skin, which causes premature wrinkling.
- Smoking is harmful to a fetus. When a pregnant woman smokes, she is more likely to have a miscarriage.
- Babies born of mothers who smoked during pregnancy are often smaller and may suffer from health complications as well. These babies are also at a higher risk for sudden infant death syndrome, or SIDS.

The list could go on and on. There are NO good effects of smoking.

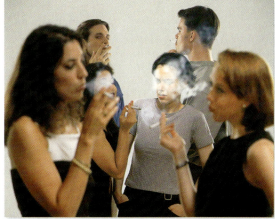

Figure 9 Smoke does more than just harm the person who is smoking; it has negative effects on other people, too.

Lesson Review

Using Vocabulary
1. Define *chronic bronchitis*.
2. Define *emphysema*.

Understanding Concepts
3. Describe four health problems other than respiratory problems, cardiovascular problems, and cancer that are caused by tobacco use.
4. Explain how smoking affects the cardiovascular system.
5. What is the relationship between smoking and cancer?

Critical Thinking
6. **Making Inferences** Explain why a person who has a respiratory disease, such as asthma, should not be around people who are smoking.
7. **Analyzing Ideas** Explain whether you agree or disagree with the following statement: If a smoker already has chronic bronchitis, it's too late to quit smoking.

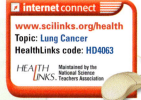

internet connect
www.scilinks.org/health
Topic: Lung Cancer
HealthLinks code: HD4063
HEALTH LINKS. Maintained by the National Science Teachers Association

Answers to Lesson Review
1. Chronic bronchitis causes the airways of the lungs to become irritated and swollen.
2. Emphysema is a disease that destroys the air sacs and walls of the lungs.
3. Sample answer: Tobacco use can cause eye disease, gum and dental problems, premature wrinkles, and harm to an unborn baby.
4. Smoking damages the inside lining of the arteries, so plaques can form inside the arteries and can eventually block the artery.
5. Smoke from cigarettes contains chemicals that cause cancer.
6. People who have asthma should not be around cigarette smoke because they will breathe in the same chemicals that a smoker inhales. People with asthma already have respiratory problems, and ETS further damages an asthmatic's air passages and lungs.
7. Sample answer: If a person stops smoking, many of the negative effects of smoking can be reversed. (Symptoms of chronic bronchitis become milder if the person quits smoking. However, chronic bronchitis can eventually lead to emphysema if the person continues to smoke, and emphysema is non-reversible.)

Close

Reteaching — BASIC
Harmful Effects Have students go through the lesson and identify all of the parts of the body that are negatively affected by tobacco use. Help students see that nicotine is a poison that causes damage to their bodies. Remind students that people who use tobacco while they are pregnant risk harm to their unborn baby. **LS Verbal**

Quiz — GENERAL
1. What is a chronic disease? (A chronic disease is one that is always present and will not go away.)
2. What is cardiovascular disease? (Cardiovascular disease is a disorder of the circulatory system.)
3. How could cigarette smoking lead to the amputation of an arm or leg? (If arteries that supply blood to a limb become blocked, the limb may need to be amputated.)
4. Why is treating lung cancer early so difficult? (Symptoms usually don't appear until the disease is advanced.)

Alternative Assessment — GENERAL
Writing Have students write a story about someone who began smoking when he or she was a teen and continued to smoke throughout his or her life. Instruct students to describe the effects of smoking on this person. Tell students that this person now has more than one smoking-related disease, and ask students to describe each disease. **LS Verbal**

Lesson 2 • Tobacco Products, Disease, and Death

Lesson 3

Focus

Overview
Before beginning this lesson, review with your students the objectives listed under the What You'll Do head in the Student Edition. This lesson describes the laws and school policies regarding teen tobacco use, and explains how using tobacco can lead to social strain.

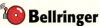**Bellringer**
Ask students to write down any city or state laws they know that are related to tobacco sales, advertising, and consumption.

Answer to Start Off Write
Accept all reasonable answers. Sample answer: Underage smoking can cause strain within the family when the teen gets caught smoking or lying about smoking.

Motivate

Group Activity — GENERAL

Social Strain Have students work in small groups. Instruct students to brainstorm negative and positive ways in which smoking might affect their social lives. (Students will determine that negative consequences outweigh positive ones.) Have students include how other people, such as friends and family members, might react to their smoking. Instruct students to think of all of the consequences that could result from getting caught smoking. Ask one student from each group to volunteer to speak to the class about his or her group's discussion.
LS Interpersonal

Lesson 3 — Social and Emotional Effects of Tobacco

What You'll Do
- **Describe** laws and school policies regarding teen tobacco use.
- **Explain** how using tobacco can lead to social strain.

Terms to Learn
- social strain

Start Off Write
How can underage smoking lead to strain within the family?

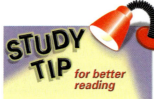
Organizing Information Make a chart that has two columns. Title one column "Breaking rules" and the other column "Social strain." List as many rules about smoking as you can think of in the first column. In the second column, list social problems caused by smoking.

Greg felt guilty about avoiding his father lately. But he didn't want his father to smell the cigarette smoke on his clothes or breath. Now, whenever Greg comes home, he goes directly to his room.

There are other consequences for smoking than health problems. For example, lying to family or friends, feeling weak about giving in to peer pressure, and sneaking around to avoid getting caught are just a few of the problems that teen smokers face.

Breaking Rules

As the public learned about the dangers of tobacco products, more laws were developed to decrease the use of tobacco. Governments want to reduce the number of people who get sick and die because of tobacco use. So, many states are writing new policies about tobacco use. For example, it is against the law to sell tobacco products to anyone under the age of 18. Schools forbid smoking on school grounds and at school events. And most parents have their own rules regarding tobacco products. So, deciding to smoke means breaking rules on many different levels. Smoking also means hiding tobacco use from others, which is not always an easy thing to do. Cigarette smoke makes your skin, hair, and clothing smell bad. And tobacco products give you bad breath and yellow teeth.

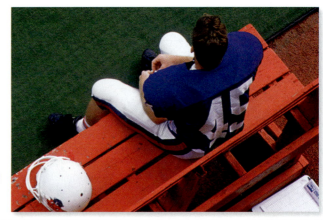
Figure 10 If you are caught smoking, you may not be allowed to participate in certain school activities and sporting events.

228

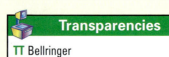 — GENERAL

Using Refusal Skills Read the following scenario to the students: "Philippe and Steve have been best friends for several years. Steve, who was on the school debate team, had been using chewing tobacco for a few months when his debate coach caught him. Philippe was with Steve at the time, and Steve told his coach that the can of tobacco belonged to Philippe. Philippe doesn't want Steve to get kicked off the debate team, but he doesn't feel right about lying to protect him." Ask the students what they think Philippe should do?
LS Auditory

Chapter Resource File
- Directed Reading BASIC
- Lesson Plan
- Lesson Quiz GENERAL

Transparencies
TT Bellringer

228   Chapter 11 • Teens and Tobacco

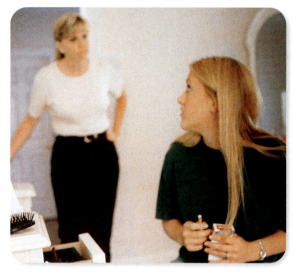

Figure 11 It is difficult to hide your smoking habit from other people.

Social Strain

Imagine being with someone who is underage when that person is trying to break the law and buy cigarettes. Even though you have done nothing wrong, you may be considered guilty because you are with that person. Or how about being around a group of people who insist on smoking even when it bothers other people? These people may not intend to hurt others but may simply find it too difficult to quit. These situations describe social strain. **Social strain** is when the use of tobacco causes awkward or risky situations and creates tension among family and friends. It is difficult for both parents and children to watch a loved one increase his or her chances of dying from a deadly disease. It is especially hard when that disease could have been prevented in the first place. Social strain also arises when pressure is placed on people to use tobacco even if they do not want to.

LIFE SKILLS ACTIVITY

ASSESSING YOUR HEALTH

As a class, find out what your school's policies are about tobacco use. If your school has no policies about tobacco use, find out the legal consequences of underage tobacco use through your local police department. Work in small groups to make posters to remind kids about these consequences.

Lesson Review

Using Vocabulary
1. What is social strain?

Understanding Concepts
2. What is the law regarding teen tobacco use?
3. Why does using tobacco lead to social strain?

Critical Thinking
4. **Making Inferences** Describe a specific example of how smoking may cause social strain.
5. **Making Predictions** How could the current law prohibiting smoking for people under 18 years of age be better enforced?

Lesson 4

Focus

Overview
Before beginning this lesson, review with your students the objectives listed under the What You'll Do head in the Student Edition. In this lesson, students will learn how physical addiction develops and how tolerance can lead to addiction. Students will also learn the symptoms of nicotine withdrawal.

Bellringer
Have students write three or four sentences describing what they think it might feel like to be addicted to something. **LS** Verbal

Answer to Start Off Write
Accept all reasonable answers. Sample answer: It is difficult to stop smoking because nicotine is a drug that people easily become addicted to.

Motivate

Discussion — GENERAL

Cravings Ask students to think about a time when they felt really thirsty or hungry. Ask them how easy it was to concentrate on other things and forget about their thirst or hunger. Ask students how they might feel if they could see other people eating and drinking but couldn't have any food or water themselves. Let students know that people can easily develop a craving for nicotine that feels similar to the need for food and water.
LS Auditory/Interpersonal

Lesson 4

What You'll Do
- Explain how an addiction develops.
- Explain how tolerance can lead to addiction.

Terms to Learn
- addiction
- tolerance
- withdrawal

Start Off Write
Why is it so difficult to stop smoking?

Forming a Tobacco Addiction

Among middle school students, about 15 percent currently smoke. Of these smokers, 55 percent said they want to stop smoking.

Nicotine: The Addictive Drug

Nicotine is a poisonous substance. After a person puffs on a cigarette, nicotine goes from the lungs into the bloodstream. It only takes seconds for the nicotine to reach the brain. Once in the brain, nicotine attaches to special structures on nerve cells. These structures are called *receptors*. When nicotine attaches to these receptors, chemical messages are sent throughout the body. These messages cause your heart to beat faster and your blood pressure to rise. The brain has to adapt to the nicotine by increasing the number of nicotine receptors in the brain. Therefore, tobacco users need more nicotine to fill these receptors.

The body gradually becomes used to the nicotine and cannot feel normal without it. This is because using nicotine causes an addiction. **Addiction** is a condition in which a person can no longer control his or her need or desire for a drug. The more a substance is used, the more it is needed. And people who try cigarettes are more likely to become addicted than people who try alcohol, cocaine, or heroin are.

Figure 12 The more nicotine that enters the body, the more nicotine that the body needs to satisfy the addiction.

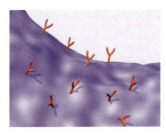

Nicotine receptors in the brain
When a person uses tobacco products for a long time, the brain develops more binding sites, or receptors, for nicotine.

Exposure to nicotine over a long time

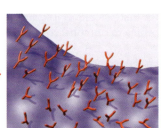

Increased number of nicotine receptors in the brain
When blood carries nicotine through the brain, these receptors catch the nicotine. With more receptors, the brain needs more nicotine to fill them.

Life SKILL BUILDER — BASIC

Practicing Wellness Ask students to take a deep breath and to hold it. Keep talking while the students are holding their breath. Tell the students they can breathe only when they really need to. Explain to students that to a person who is addicted to nicotine, the need for the drug is like the need to take a breath.
LS Kinesthetic

Chapter Resource File
- Directed Reading BASIC
- Lesson Plan
- Lesson Quiz GENERAL

 Transparencies
TT Bellringer
TT Nicotine Receptors

---

230 Chapter 11 • Teens and Tobacco

Figure 13 Facts About Smoking

Fact Studies have shown that once people are hooked on smoking their tolerance to nicotine never declines, even after years of not smoking.

Fact More than 90 percent of young people who use tobacco daily experience at least one symptom of nicotine withdrawal, such as difficulty concentrating and irritability.

Fact Three-fourths of young people who use tobacco daily report that they continue to use tobacco because they find it hard to stop using tobacco.

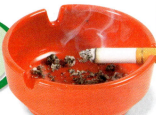

Tolerance, Dependence, and Withdrawal

Most long-time smokers smoke more cigarettes than beginning smokers do. This is because they have developed a tolerance to nicotine. **Tolerance** is a condition in which a user needs more of a drug to get the same effect. So, long-time smokers experience smaller and smaller effects, even with more cigarettes. As tolerance develops, smokers begin to feel more normal when using nicotine than when not using it. This leads to dependence. *Dependence* on a drug is when the user relies on the drug to feel normal. Dependence can be both physical and psychological. People who rely on tobacco products as an emotional crutch are psychologically dependent. If tobacco users have to go for a very long time without nicotine, they begin to feel sick, nervous, and irritable. These symptoms are examples of withdrawal. **Withdrawal** is the way in which the body responds when a dependent person stops using a drug. Tolerance and withdrawal are signs that a person has become physically dependent on tobacco products. Withdrawal usually includes uncomfortable physical and psychological symptoms. The main reason that it is difficult for long-time smokers to quit smoking is the discomfort of withdrawal.

Myth & Fact

Myth: I'm too young to get addicted. That only happens to adults.

Fact: Young people can get addicted to tobacco products just as easily as adults can.

Lesson Review

Using Vocabulary
1. What is addiction?
2. Define *tolerance*.

Understanding Concepts
3. What is the difference between physical and psychological dependence?
4. Explain how tolerance to nicotine leads to addiction.

Critical Thinking
5. **Making Inferences** What would be the best way to overcome psychological dependence on nicotine? Explain your answer.

internet connect
www.scilinks.org/health
Topic: Nicotine
HealthLinks code: HD4069
HEALTH LINKS. Maintained by the National Science Teachers Association

Lesson 5

Focus

Overview
Before beginning this lesson, review with your students the objectives listed under the What You'll Do head in the Student Edition. Students will learn how peer pressure can cause students to try tobacco. Students will also learn about how advertisements can influence someone's attitude toward tobacco.

Bellringer
Ask students to explain why it might be difficult to resist using tobacco if their friends are starting to use tobacco. (Students may say that they are afraid of losing their friends or that they don't want to be made fun of.) Verbal

Answer to Start Off Write
Sample answer: Most young people start using tobacco because of peer pressure.

Motivate

Discussion — GENERAL
Influence of Advertising Have students describe things they associate with cigarettes based on cigarette advertising and cigarette smoking in movies. You may want to bring in ads for brands of cigarettes to help generate discussion. Write the students' descriptions on the board. Then ask students to describe cigarettes based on what they have learned in this chapter. Write these descriptions on the board. Compare the two lists, and help students see how the media tries to make smoking appeal to an audience who is legally too young to even smoke. **LS Auditory/Visual**

Lesson 5 — Why People Use Tobacco

What You'll Do
- **Explain** how peer pressure can cause adolescents to try tobacco.
- **Explain** how advertisements can influence someone's attitude toward tobacco.

Terms to Learn
- peer pressure
- targeted marketing

Start Off Write
Why do most young people start using tobacco?

Bonnie was very hurt that Sue had laughed at her in front of a group of people just because she didn't want to try a cigarette. Bonnie couldn't believe that there could be so much pressure to use tobacco!

Pressure from friends is one of the main reasons teens begin to smoke. Having to say no to your friends is very difficult to do. In this lesson, you will learn about different influences on teens and why some teens eventually give in to smoking.

Influence from Others

Why would someone begin a habit that could cause serious health problems or death and is a very difficult habit to break? Experimenting with tobacco and risking addiction makes little sense—so why do people do it? There are many forces at work that influence people's decision to start using tobacco.

One of the most powerful forces comes from your peers. *Peers* are people of about the same age as you with whom you interact every day. **Peer pressure** is the feeling that you should do something because your friends want you to. Influence from peers is one of the main reasons that teens first try cigarettes. Most teens smoke because they want to be accepted by their peers. And they want to experiment with an "adult activity."

Sadly, most teens do not think they will become addicted. Nor do teenagers believe that they will have any serious tobacco-related health problems. Studies show that most teen smokers wish they could quit. And quitting is just as difficult for adolescent smokers as it is for adult smokers. Because adolescents are still growing and developing, they can seriously hurt their bodies by smoking.

TABLE 1 Reasons Why Kids Smoke	
Why kids smoke	Why that reason is bad
My friends smoke.	Just because your friends smoke doesn't make it a good idea!
It's cool to smoke.	Smoking doesn't make you cool—it makes you smell bad.
Smoking is fun.	Respiratory disease is not fun.

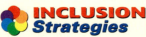 **INCLUSION Strategies** — BASIC

- Developmentally Delayed
- Attention Deficit Disorder

Make sure students understand the negative aspects of cigarette smoking by having them apply the effects of smoking to people in cigarette ads. Bring some cigarette ads to school. Provide brown, yellow, and black markers. Have students use the brown markers to apply wrinkles to smokers' faces, yellow markers to color their teeth, and black markers to create text balloons identifying odors, coughing, shortness of breath, and lung cancer. **LS Kinesthetic**

Chapter Resource File
- Directed Reading BASIC
- Lesson Plan
- Lesson Quiz GENERAL

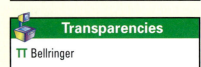 **Transparencies**

TT Bellringer

The Power of Advertising

Tobacco companies spend nearly $1 million *an hour* to advertise their products. Ads often use targeted marketing. Targeted marketing is advertising aimed at a particular group of people. Teenagers, sports fans, and outdoor enthusiasts are especially good targets. The ads make the companies' products and brands appealing to people in these groups. For example, most cigarette ads show very attractive people doing something very exciting while smoking their brand of cigarettes. Laws have been passed to ban tobacco advertising on TV, on billboards, and in certain magazines. But most people everywhere still recognize the name and packaging of popular cigarette brands.

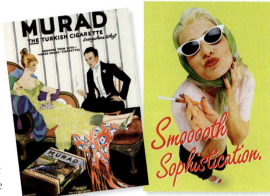

Figure 14 Tobacco companies create ads to make cigarette smoking look glamorous and accepted, but these ads are misleading.

Feeling Tempted

Peer pressure, family members who smoke, advertising, TV, and movies all influence your attitude about smoking. The movies and TV often make smoking look very glamorous. And, even though you know the dangers of tobacco use, it is difficult not to be curious about a product that is made to look so attractive. But people need to learn to see through these messages because once people begin to use tobacco, they will probably become addicted to nicotine.

Once people are addicted, the glamour of smoking quickly fades. Most smokers develop a nasty cough. And their clothes, hair, and breath smell of smoke. So, the next time you see ads that make smoking look cool, remember that this is what the advertisers want to emphasize, not the negative effects of smoking.

Health Journal
In your Health Journal, write about a time in which you saw an advertisement that made you want to buy something. Describe that ad, and explain why the advertisement appealed to you.

Lesson Review

Using Vocabulary
1. Define *peer pressure*.
2. Define *targeted marketing*.

Understanding Concepts
3. Describe three different influences that cause teens to try smoking.
4. Describe how advertisements influence your attitude about smoking.

Critical Thinking
5. **Applying Concepts** Using the power of peer pressure, write a convincing argument to another student about why he or she should quit smoking.

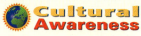
www.scilinks.org/health
Topic: Tobacco
HealthLinks code: HD4101
HEALTH LINKS. Maintained by the National Science Teachers Association

Lesson 6 Focus

Overview
Before beginning this lesson, review with your students the objectives listed under the What You'll Do head in the Student Edition. In this lesson, students will learn why it's difficult to quit using tobacco. Students will also learn strategies for quitting a tobacco habit. The lesson describes ways in which smoking can disrupt everyday life.

Bellringer
Have students write a description of two strategies to quit smoking. (Sample answer: chewing gum or eating candy, using nicotine gum or patches, or talking to a counselor.)

Answer to Start Off Write
Sample answer: A person can use nicotine gum or patches if he or she wants to quit smoking.

Motivate

Debate — GENERAL
Personal Rights Organize the class into two large groups. Have one group argue for the rights of smokers, and have the other group argue for the rights of nonsmokers. Have the students include the following issues in their arguments: ETS, laws regarding tobacco use, and health issues. **LS Auditory**

Lesson 6 — Quitting

What You'll Do
- **Explain** why it is difficult to quit using tobacco.
- **Describe** three strategies for quitting a tobacco habit.
- **Describe** how smoking causes disruptions in everyday life.

Terms to Learn
- nicotine replacement therapy (NRT)

Start Off Write
What can a person do if he or she wants to quit smoking?

Pawan hated smoking. He hated that he could not control his habit. Pawan had tried quitting before by gradually decreasing the number of cigarettes he smoked, but it hadn't worked.

It's Tough to Quit
Most people who use tobacco products wish they didn't. Every year, about 70 percent of adult smokers say they want to quit. Of the 50 percent of all adult smokers who try to quit, only about 7 percent of them are successful. By age 18, about two-thirds of teens who smoke say they regret having started smoking. And about half of these teens will try to quit but fail. Still, that means that many teens do successfully quit.

The younger a person is when they quit, the more that person's body can recover. Often, quitting takes several attempts. So, why is quitting so difficult? Once tobacco users quit using tobacco, withdrawal begins. They get headaches, become dizzy, have trouble sleeping, and get depressed. Withdrawal symptoms make it difficult to stay tobacco free. Even when withdrawal ends, many people still miss using tobacco. Some people crave tobacco products years after they've quit. But quitting has major health benefits even if the person is already sick with a smoking-related disease.

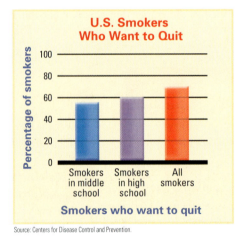

Figure 15 Quitting often requires several attempts, but it can be done.

INCLUSION Strategies — ADVANCED
- Gifted and Talented
- Behavior Control Issues

Have students research on the Internet or at the library additional methods that are used to stop smoking. Then, have students create posters that highlight ways to stop smoking. These posters should include the methods given in the textbook as well as the other methods they find in their research. On their posters, have students include an explanation of how each method helps a person quit smoking. **LS Kinesthetic**

Chapter Resource File
- Directed Reading **BASIC**
- Lesson Plan
- Lesson Quiz **GENERAL**

Transparencies
TT Bellringer

234 Chapter 11 • Teens and Tobacco

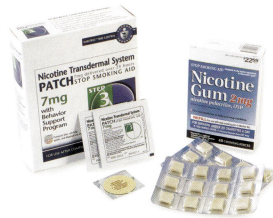

Figure 16 Many products on the market can help you quit smoking.

Tools That Can Help

For years, there was little help for people who wanted to quit using tobacco. Today, there are many tools to help smokers quit. Listed below are some of the tools that can help people who want to stop smoking.

- Support groups and counseling programs can provide encouragement for people who want to quit using tobacco.
- Nonprescription **nicotine replacement therapy**, or NRT, is a safe medicine that delivers a small amount of nicotine to the body. Many withdrawal symptoms are caused by a lack of nicotine in the body, so NRT was developed to help ease the symptoms. Nonprescription NRT is available as nicotine gum and nicotine patches.
- Prescription NRT can also help a person quit smoking. The latest prescription nicotine replacement therapies are nicotine inhalers and nicotine nasal sprays.
- A regular exercise program has helped many people quit smoking because it helps the person focus on his or her health. It also takes the person's mind off of the unpleasant side effects of quitting smoking.

Most of the prescription and nonprescription medicines available as aids to quit using tobacco have been tested only on adults. So, teens under 18 should talk to their doctor. It is important for smokers to know that a technique that works for one person may not always work for another person.

Sometimes, a combination of more than one method will work. For example, some people may use the nicotine patch while going to a support group. The nicotine patch can help with the physical addiction. The support group may help the person adjust mentally to not smoking. Anyone who really wants to quit will have to find the method that works best for him or her.

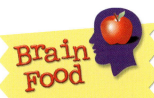

Brain Food

In one year, more than 800,000 cigarette butts were among the millions of pounds of debris collected along the U.S. coastline. These butts are responsible for the death of many birds and marine animals.

LIFE SCIENCE CONNECTION — ADVANCED

Patches Have interested students research how nicotine from a patch that is attached to a person's skin can enter the bloodstream. Have students answer the following questions in a written report: How long does it take for nicotine to reach the bloodstream after the patch is applied? Is this method faster or slower in delivering nicotine than smoking is? than chewing tobacco? Explain your answer. **LS Verbal**

Teach

Using the Figure — BASIC

Quitting Have students study the bar graph in the figure on the previous page. Use the following questions to guide a discussion:

- What does the bar graph tell us? (About 54 percent of smokers in middle school, about 59 percent of smokers in high school, and about 68 percent of all smokers want to quit smoking.)
- What are some reasons that smokers may want to quit? (Smokers begin to realize the toll that smoking is taking on their health as well as on their pocketbook. They also begin to see that it is no longer a socially acceptable thing to do.)
- Do you think that most people who start smoking think that they will someday have a difficult time quitting? Explain your answer. (Most people think they will be able to quit smoking whenever they want to. However, they soon find out that quitting is very difficult because nicotine is so addictive, and withdrawal from nicotine is very unpleasant.)
- What are some reasons people may find it difficult to quit smoking? (Nicotine withdrawal makes people sick and irritable.)

LS Visual/Auditory

Discussion — GENERAL

Comprehension Check Ask students to pair up and discuss how using a product that delivers nicotine in a form that is different than the one a person is used to could help someone break a tobacco addiction. (These products allow a person to slowly break the physical addiction, while the person also becomes psychologically used to the idea of not smoking.)

LS Interpersonal

Lesson 6 • Quitting

Teach, continued

Demonstration — GENERAL

Relaxation Exercise Tell students that one great way to relax in any situation is by focusing on deep breathing. Have students put their hands on their stomachs and take a deep breath through their nose, filling the lower part of their lungs first and then letting the air fill their chest. Let students know that they should feel their stomach expand under their hands. Have students pause with their lungs filled and then slowly release the air through their noses. Encourage students to try this focused breathing next time they need to relax, such as before a test or when they are having trouble falling asleep.
LS Kinesthetic

Discussion — GENERAL

Addiction Have students imagine that they have to use the bathroom every 45 minutes to an hour while they are awake. After about an hour of whatever they are doing (watching a movie, hanging out at the mall, sitting in class), they grow uncomfortable if they do not go to the bathroom (and the discomfort increases the longer they delay). Additionally, each time they use the bathroom, they have to pay 20 cents. Ask the students if they would see this situation as a problem or if this is something they would choose to do. Help students see the similarity between this situation and a cigarette addiction.
LS Auditory

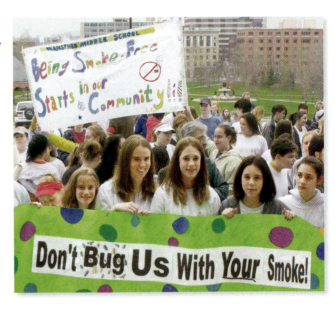

Figure 17 Teens across the country have joined organizations to show support for smoke-free youth.

LIFE SKILLS ACTIVITY

USING REFUSAL SKILLS

Work in a group of three or four people to write a skit about refusing tobacco. Think of multiple endings to the skit that show different ways to refuse tobacco.

Relaxing Without Tobacco

Hanging out with friends and enjoying life is much easier without tobacco. It's hard to relax and have fun when you know that you're breaking the law, becoming addicted to nicotine, and damaging your health as well as the health of others around you. Many everyday activities, such as playing sports, going to the movies, or shopping at the mall become a hassle when you're a tobacco user. Smokers often worry about what they will do in situations in which they can't smoke. It is difficult to travel on trains, buses, or planes now that smoking has been banned on them. Tobacco users face disruptions in their everyday lives because they have to find a place and time to smoke so that they won't have withdrawal symptoms.

Being addicted to nicotine means that if you don't get your nicotine fix you don't feel right. And that can be quite a problem. There are many times when you can't light up a cigarette or take a dip of snuff. Getting used to a tobacco-free life means making some changes in your lifestyle. You have to learn how to relax without tobacco. Some people need to stay away from places where other people will be using tobacco. It's hard to stay tobacco free when others around you are using tobacco. But over time, people find that they enjoy life more without tobacco. There is no more worrying about hiding your habit from parents or figuring out when and where you can smoke.

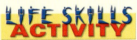

Answer
Student skits will vary, but they should all have at least two different endings to their scenario.

Extension: Ask students what they would do if the person offering the tobacco wouldn't take no for an answer.

Attention Grabber

Students may be surprised to know that tobacco use has been documented as far back as 600 to 1000 CE, but it wasn't until 1964 that the Surgeon General of the United States linked smoking and lung cancer.

236 Chapter 11 • Teens and Tobacco

Finding Healthy Habits

Many teens are first offered tobacco during middle and high school. Many of these teens will try it, get hooked, and ultimately die because of it. Understanding the dangers of tobacco and being prepared to refuse tobacco are the best ways to ensure a healthy life. The lifestyle choices that you make now will affect your future health and happiness. Make the right decisions about diet, exercise, and caring for your body—it's never too early to start practicing healthy habits. There are many fun, healthy things that you can do rather than use tobacco. A newfound feeling of physical health will come after the nicotine leaves your body. And you will also feel a well-deserved sense of accomplishment.

MATH ACTIVITY

Calculate how much it costs to smoke for one year if a pack of cigarettes cost $4.00, and a person smokes 1 pack a day.

How much would smoking cost over a lifetime if this same person started smoking at 16 years of age and lived to be 70? Assume that the price of cigarettes stays the same and this person keeps smoking 1 pack a day.

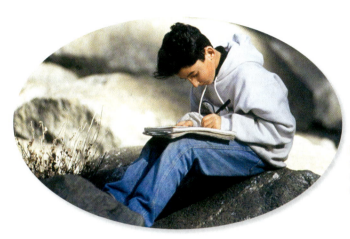

Figure 18 Plan ahead. Think of ways to say no when peers offer you tobacco, and write these ideas in your journal.

Lesson Review

Using Vocabulary
1. Define *NRT*. Explain how NRTs work.

Understanding Concepts
2. Describe withdrawal symptoms that make it difficult to stop smoking.
3. Identify three methods that can help a person quit smoking.
4. Identify three ways that smoking disrupts everyday life.

Critical Thinking
5. **Making Inferences** Do you think it is likely that a person could become addicted to nicotine gum or patches? Explain your answer.
6. **Making Predictions** Doug is a smoker and is flying across country. What problems may he face on the plane?

internet connect
www.scilinks.org/health
Topic: Smoking and Health
HealthLinks code: HD4090

HEALTH LINKS Maintained by the National Science Teachers Association

Lesson 7 Focus

Overview
Before beginning this lesson, review with your students the objectives listed under the What You'll Do head in the Student Edition. In this lesson, students will learn ways to refuse tobacco. The lesson will help students understand the difference between positive and negative peer pressure. Students will also identify ways to stay tobacco free.

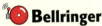

Have students write a description of a situation in which they have experienced peer pressure.
LS Verbal

Motivate

Group Activity
Peer Pressure Organize students into small groups. Have students discuss their perceptions and experiences of peer pressure. Ask students to describe how they think peer pressure works and why peer pressure is sometimes difficult to resist. Have each group brainstorm ways to handle pressure to try tobacco products. Ask for student volunteers from each group to role-play one of the ideas of how to handle pressure when tobacco is offered to them. **LS Interpersonal/Kinesthetic**

Lesson 7

What You'll Do
- **Demonstrate** three ways to refuse tobacco.
- **Explain** the difference between positive and negative peer pressure.
- **Identify** four reasons to stay tobacco free.

Start Off Write
How can positive peer pressure help you refuse tobacco?

Choosing Not to Use Tobacco

Lee knew that he didn't want to try chewing tobacco. When his friend Chris asked him if he wanted to try it, all Lee said was, "No, thanks," and Chris left him alone.

Refusing Tobacco

Most people will probably be offered tobacco at some time in their lives. Sometimes, it may be easy to refuse. However, other times it can be stressful, especially if peer pressure is used. Learning to say no can be a valuable tool. Your response could be a simple "No" or "No, thanks." Or you could reply, "Smoking is too dangerous—especially if my parents find out!" Whichever way you decide to handle the situation, don't feel that you have to explain why you refused or make excuses. And even if you've accepted tobacco in the past, you can still say no this time.

Peer pressure is not always a bad thing. If your friends do well in school, enjoy a particular sport, or choose not to use tobacco, you probably behave in a similar way. This is positive peer pressure. Positive peer pressure influences you to do something that benefits you. It is easier to stay tobacco free if none of your friends smoke. If your friends try to get you to smoke, they are using negative peer pressure. Negative peer pressure can harm you if you let it. You will want to avoid this kind of pressure.

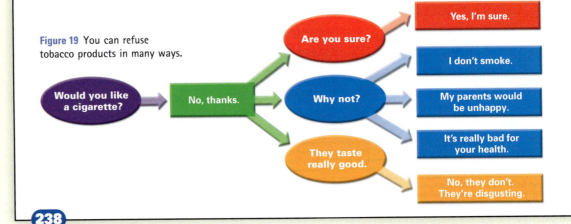

Figure 19 You can refuse tobacco products in many ways.

238

Answer to Start Off Write
Accept all reasonable answers. An example of how positive peer pressure can help you refuse tobacco is when your friends are with you when you are offered tobacco, and they refuse tobacco, too.

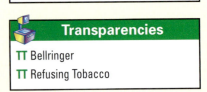

Chapter Resource File
- Directed Reading **BASIC**
- Lesson Plan
- Lesson Quiz **GENERAL**

Transparencies
TT Bellringer
TT Refusing Tobacco

238 Chapter 11 • Teens and Tobacco

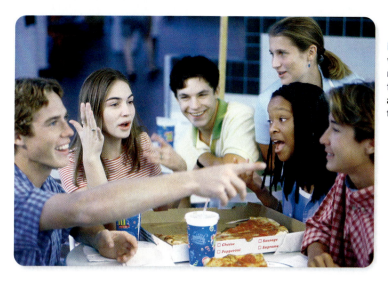

Figure 20 Having friends who don't use tobacco means you can have fun without worrying about being pressured to use tobacco.

A Tobacco-Free Life

If you have never used tobacco, don't start! The following is a list of reasons not to smoke.

- It is very easy to become addicted to nicotine. In fact, it is easier to become addicted to tobacco than to most other drugs.
- Using tobacco is deadly. Smoking is the leading preventable cause of death in the United States.
- Tobacco makes your skin, hair, breath, and clothing smell bad. It also makes your teeth yellow.
- Tobacco in any form is expensive, and it is getting more expensive every day.

Make a healthy choice to stay tobacco free. You won't regret it!

Health Journal
Write in your Health Journal five reasons why you will not start using tobacco products.

Lesson Review

Understanding Concepts
1. What are three ways to tell a friend that you don't want to try tobacco?
2. What is the difference between positive and negative peer pressure?
3. What are four reasons to never start using tobacco?

Critical Thinking
4. **Making Inferences** If tobacco has so many negative effects, explain why most people don't quit using it.
5. **Analyzing Ideas** Why do you think there are more people addicted to cigarettes and other forms of tobacco than are addicted to illegal drugs?

11 CHAPTER REVIEW

Assignment Guide

Lesson	Review Questions
1	1, 3, 6, 9, 13, 15, 16, 20, 22
2	4, 11, 17–18
3	10, 24
4	5, 8, 19
5	7, 14, 23
6	2, 12
7	21

ANSWERS

Using Vocabulary

1. additives
2. NRT
3. environmental tobacco smoke
4. cancer
5. dependent
6. nicotine
7. peer pressure

Understanding Concepts

8. Nicotine enters the body through the lungs. It then travels through the bloodstream to the rest of the body, including the brain.
9. If you are near someone who is smoking, you will likely inhale environmental tobacco smoke, which contains the same dangerous chemicals as the smoke a person inhales directly from a cigarette.
10. Answers may vary. Sample answer: Traveling by plane, going to the movies, and going shopping are difficult activities to do if you are a smoker.
11. Smoking damages the inside lining of the arteries. This damage can cause plaques to form inside the artery, which contributes to high blood pressure, heart disease, and stroke.
12. Nicotine replacement therapy supplies nicotine to a smoker's body. This helps tobacco users break their psychological addiction to tobacco products first, so they can work on their physical addiction.
13. The government has restricted tobacco advertising, made smoking illegal in many public places, and provided tobacco use prevention education.
14. Answers may vary. Sample answers: People might start smoking because their friends smoke, smoking is a rebellious act, and smoking looks like a grown-up thing.
15. People who smoke light cigarettes inhale smoke more deeply into the lungs and/or smoke more often.
16. Five types of tobacco products are cigarettes, pipe tobacco, chewing tobacco, snuff, and cigars. (Answers may vary; there are other tobacco products.)
17. Two common respiratory diseases are chronic bronchitis and emphysema.
18. The most common type of cancer caused by smokeless tobacco is mouth cancer.

11 CHAPTER REVIEW

Chapter Summary

- Tobacco products contain hundreds of chemicals. Additives make cigarettes more appealing to the user. ■ All tobacco products produce harmful health effects as soon as people start to use them. ■ ETS is harmful to people who are near someone who is smoking. ■ Respiratory diseases, cardiovascular diseases, and cancer are some of the major classes of illnesses caused by tobacco use. ■ Most smokers want to quit, but few can stop on the first try. ■ Using tobacco can create strain and tension between friends and family. Smoking is also against the law if you are under the age of 18.
- Peers often influence a person's decision to use tobacco.

Using Vocabulary

For each sentence, fill in the blank with the proper word from the word bank provided below.

additives, marketing, NRT, peer pressure, dependent, targeted, tolerance, cancer, nicotine, environmental tobacco smoke

1. Many ___ are put in cigarettes during processing to make them taste better.
2. ___ helps people quit smoking by providing nicotine.
3. ___ describes the smoke that is exhaled from the mouth of the smoker and comes from the tip of a burning cigarette.
4. Many of the chemicals in tobacco products are responsible for causing ___.
5. People can become physically and psychologically ___ on tobacco.
6. ___ is the substance in tobacco products to which people become addicted.
7. ___ is a feeling that you should do something because your friends want you to do it.

Understanding Concepts

8. How does nicotine enter the body when someone smokes a cigarette, and where does the nicotine go?
9. Why is it harmful to be near someone who is smoking even if you are not?
10. List three activities that are made more difficult by being a tobacco user.
11. Explain how smoking can damage the cardiovascular system.
12. Explain how nicotine replacement therapy helps people quit smoking.
13. What has the government done to try to control death and disease caused by tobacco?
14. List at least three reasons someone would choose to start using tobacco.
15. Explain why light cigarettes are just a dangerous as regular cigarettes.
16. Name five types of tobacco products.
17. List two common respiratory diseases.
18. What is the most common type of cancer caused by smokeless tobacco?

Critical Thinking

Analyzing Ideas

19. When Mary began smoking cigarettes, she promised she would limit herself to one a day, because she thought that would be less dangerous. She is now smoking a pack each day. Why wasn't she able to keep her original promise?

20. Yi-tee is a tobacco user and has just noticed some white sores on his gums and on the inside of his mouth. What product does Yi-tee likely use, and what has happened to his gums and mouth?

21. Antonio and his best friend, Dean, had been smoking for almost a year when they both decided to quit. Antonio quit without too much trouble. But Dean relapsed twice and is now smoking again. What may have caused Antonio and Dean to have different experiences with quitting?

22. Imagine that you find your younger sister smoking bidis with her friends. What can you tell her about bidis to help her decide not to use them?

Using Refusal Skills

23. Shari's family had just moved, and she was eager to make friends in her new school. One group of girls invited her to meet them after school so that they could get together, smoke some cigarettes, and chat. What should Shari do?

24. Some friends are thinking about going to a convenience store that they know sells cigarettes to teens without checking IDs. What should you say to your friends?

25. You and your best friend, Joe, play baseball for the same team. One night at a baseball game Joe tells you he has started using chewing tobacco, and he asks you if you want to try it. Joe also tells you that chewing tobacco won't cause lung cancer or any of the other diseases that smoking can cause. What should you tell your friend?

26. Use what you have learned in this chapter to set a personal goal. Write your goal, and make an action plan by using the Health Behavior Contract for ways to refuse tobacco. You can find the Health Behavior Contract at **go.hrw.com.** Just type in the keyword **HD4HBC09.**

Reading Checkup

Take a minute to review your answers to the Health IQ questions at the beginning of this chapter. How has reading this chapter improved your Health IQ?

Chapter Resource File

- Student Study Guide GENERAL
- Concept Mapping Worksheets GENERAL
- Performance Based Assessment GENERAL
- Chapter Test GENERAL

Critical Thinking

Analyzing Ideas

19. Mary became addicted to nicotine and developed a tolerance for nicotine. To satisfy her cravings for nicotine, she had to smoke more cigarettes.

20. Yi-tee probably uses a smokeless tobacco product, and the white sores can develop into cancer.

Using Refusal Skills

21. Antonio was determined to break his smoking habit, whereas Dean may not have really wanted to quit smoking. Dean may need to use an NRT or go to counseling to help him quit.

22. Answers may vary. Sample answer: I can tell my younger sister that bidis may be even more dangerous to her health because bidis are not filtered. I would explain that the health risks are the same for smoking regular cigarettes.

23. Answers may vary. Sample answer: Sarah could just say no, or she could say no and explain the dangers of smoking to her new friends.

24. Answers may vary. Sample answer: You should tell your friends that underage smoking is illegal and getting caught could result in a fine. You could also try to discourage them from smoking.

25. Sample answer: I should tell Joe that chewing tobacco is just as dangerous as smoking is because smokeless tobacco is the leading cause of mouth and lip cancer. Joe should also know that smokeless tobacco can cause cancer of the throat and neck.

Model

Introduce this activity by reminding students that using this Life Skill will help them take personal responsibility for their behavior. Then, review the scenario with the class.

Prepare students for this activity by modeling each of the steps of the skill. Make sure students understand each step before you move on to the next one.

Guided Practice: Practice with a Friend

Guided Practice is the stage in which you and the students analyze their approach to solving the problem given in the scenario and analyze their decision-making skills. Have students read Act 1. Discuss with the class the situation described and the way students are to act it out. Organize the class into groups of three. In each group, one person plays the role of Owen, another person plays Curtis, and the third person is the observer.

Proper pacing during the Guided Practice is important. The suggestions listed below will help you control the pace.

1. Stop after completing each step of making good decisions.
2. Discuss with each group the observer's comments.
3. Ask the other members of each group to listen to the observer's suggestions and to suggest ways to improve their decision-making skills.
4. Instruct students to repeat the steps that need improvement and to include their modifications.
5. Check to make sure that students understand each step before they move on to the next step.
6. If time permits, repeat the exercise three times, switching roles each time. Each student should have the opportunity to play each role. Co-op Learning

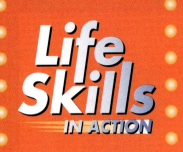

Life Skills IN ACTION

Making Good Decisions

You make decisions every day. But how do you know if you are making good decisions? Making good decisions is making choices that are healthy and responsible. Following the six steps of making good decisions will help you make the best possible choice whenever you make a decision. Complete the following activity to practice the six steps of making good decisions.

Tobacco Troubles

Setting the Scene

Owen and his friend Curtis are playing baseball in the park. During a break in the game, Curtis takes out a can of chewing tobacco and puts some in his mouth. Curtis offers some to Owen and says, "Try it, you will be like a real baseball player. Chewing tobacco isn't dangerous like smoking cigarettes." Owen is not sure what to do.

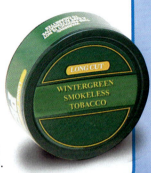

The 6 Steps of Making Good Decisions

1. Identify the problem.
2. Consider your values.
3. List the options.
4. Weigh the consequences.
5. Decide, and act.
6. Evaluate your choice.

Guided Practice

Practice with a Friend

Form a group of three. Have one person play the role of Owen and another person play the role of Curtis. Have the third person be an observer. Walking through each of the six steps of making good decisions, role-play Owen deciding whether or not to try the chewing tobacco. When Owen reaches step 5, he should tell Curtis his decision and explain his reasoning behind it. The observer will take notes, which will include observations about what the person playing Owen did well and suggestions of ways to improve. Stop after each step to evaluate the process.

242 Chapter 11 • Life Skills in Action

Independent Practice

Check Yourself

After you have completed the guided practice, go through Act 1 again without stopping at each step. Answer the questions below to review what you did.

1. What values should Owen consider before making his decision?
2. What options does Owen have in this situation?
3. What are the positive consequences and negative consequences of each of Owen's options?
4. How can Owen evaluate his choice?

On Your Own

Owen and Curtis are walking home after the game. Curtis tells Owen that he wants to get some more chewing tobacco. Curtis explains that he plans to shoplift the tobacco from a convenience store and he needs Owen to distract the cashier while he does it. Make a flowchart that illustrates how Owen could use the six steps of making good decisions to decide what to do in this situation.

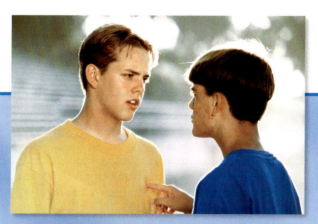

Independent Practice: Check Yourself

Instruct students to repeat Act 1 without stopping at each step. Remind students to apply what they learned in the Guided Practice to the Independent Practice.

Encourage students to use the Check Yourself questions as a starting point for reviewing and analyzing their Independent Practice. Remind students that as they change roles, the answers to these questions may change for each actor. Encourage students to create additional questions for checking their decision-making skills. When students have finished the Independent Practice, have them answer the Check Yourself questions in writing. Use their answers to assess their understanding of the steps of making good decisions and to assess their use of the steps to solve a problem.

Check Yourself Answers

1. Sample answer: Owen should consider if he values his health, staying out of trouble, and being a good friend.
2. Sample answer: Owen could refuse to use the chewing tobacco or he could agree to try some of it.
3. Sample answer: A positive consequence of refusing the tobacco is that Owen will not endanger his health. A negative consequence is that Curtis may call him a chicken. A positive consequence of agreeing to use the tobacco is that Owen will feel more like a real baseball player. A negative consequence is that Owen may get into trouble.
4. Sample answer: Owen could evaluate his choice by asking himself if he upheld his values and if he is happy with his decision.

Act 2: On Your Own

This additional scenario gives students an opportunity to apply what they have learned in both the Guided Practice and the Independent Practice to a new situation.

Suggest to students that they use the Check Yourself questions as a starting point for making good decisions in the new situation. Encourage students to be creative and to think of ways to improve their decision-making skills.

Assessment

Review the flowcharts that students have made as part of the On Your Own activity. The flowcharts should show that the students followed the steps of making good decisions in a realistic and effective manner. If time permits, ask student volunteers to draw one or more of their flowcharts on the blackboard. Discuss the flowcharts and the use of decision-making skills.

CHAPTER 12 — Teens and Alcohol
Chapter Planning Guide

PACING	CLASSROOM RESOURCES	ACTIVITIES AND DEMONSTRATIONS
BLOCK 1 • 45 min pp. 244–247 **Chapter Opener**	CRF Health Inventory * ■ GENERAL CRF Parent Letter * ■	SE Health IQ, p. 245 CRF At-Home Activity * ■
Lesson 1 Understanding Teens and Alcohol	CRF Lesson Plan * TT Bellringer *	CRF Life Skills Activity * ■ GENERAL CRF Enrichment Activity * ADVANCED
BLOCK 2 • 45 min pp. 248–251 **Lesson 2** Alcohol and Your Body	CRF Lesson Plan * TT Bellringer * TT Blood Alcohol Concentration and Its Effects * TT Factors Affecting Reactions to Alcohol *	TE Activities Slowed Reactions, p. 243F TE Activity Poor Coordination, p. 248 GENERAL TE Group Activity What's the Truth?, p. 250 BASIC CRF Enrichment Activity * ADVANCED
BLOCK 3 • 45 min pp. 252–257 **Lesson 3** Alcohol, You, and Other People	CRF Lesson Plan * TT Bellringer *	TE Activities What's the Message?, p. 243F TE Activity Practicing Wellness, p. 252 GENERAL TE Group Activity Skit, p. 253 GENERAL CRF Enrichment Activity * ADVANCED
Lesson 4 Drunk Driving	CRF Lesson Plan * TT Bellringer *	SE Math Activity, p. 257 CRF Enrichment Activity * ADVANCED
BLOCK 4 • 45 min pp. 258–263 **Lesson 5** Alcoholism	CRF Lesson Plan * TT Bellringer *	CRF Life Skills Activity * ■ GENERAL CRF Enrichment Activity * ADVANCED
Lesson 6 Resisting the Pressure to Drink	CRF Lesson Plan * TT Bellringer *	SE Life Skills in Action Refusal Skills, pp. 266–267 CRF Enrichment Activity * ADVANCED
Lesson 7 Alternatives to Alcohol	CRF Lesson Plan * TT Bellringer *	TE Group Activity Skit, p. 263 GENERAL TE Activity Guest Speaker, p. 263 BASIC CRF Enrichment Activity * ADVANCED

BLOCKS 5 & 6 • 90 min — Chapter Review and Assessment Resources

- SE Chapter Review, pp. 264–265
- CRF Concept Review * ■ GENERAL
- CRF Health Behavior Contract * ■ GENERAL
- CRF Chapter Test * GENERAL
- CRF Performance-Based Assessment * GENERAL
- OSP Test Generator
- CRF Test Item Listing *

Online Resources

Visit **go.hrw.com** for a variety of free resources related to this textbook. Enter the keyword **HD4AL7**.

Holt Online Learning
Students can access interactive problem solving help and active visual concept development with the *Decisions for Health* Online Edition available at **www.hrw.com**.

cnnstudentnews.com
Find the latest health news, lesson plans, and activities related to important scientific events.

Compression guide:
To shorten your instruction because of time limitations, omit Lesson 7.

KEY

TE Teacher Edition	CRF Chapter Resource File	* Also on One-Stop Planner
SE Student Edition	TT Teaching Transparency	■ Also Available in Spanish
OSP One-Stop Planner		♦ Requires Advance Prep

SKILLS DEVELOPMENT RESOURCES	LESSON REVIEW AND ASSESSMENT	STANDARDS CORRELATION
		National Health Education Standards
TE Life Skill Builder Making Good Decisions, p. 247 GENERAL CRF Directed Reading * BASIC	SE Lesson Review, p. 247 TE Reteaching, Quiz, p. 247 CRF Lesson Quiz * ■ GENERAL	1.1, 1.2, 1.4, 3.4, 4.2, 4.4, 6.2, 6.3
TE Inclusion Strategies, p. 248 BASIC SE Study Tip Word Origins, p. 250 TE Life Skill Builder Refusal Skills, p. 250 GENERAL CRF Cross-Disciplinary * GENERAL CRF Directed Reading * BASIC	SE Lesson Review, p. 251 TE Reteaching, Quiz, p. 251 TE Alternative Assessment, p. 251 GENERAL CRF Concept Mapping * GENERAL CRF Lesson Quiz * ■ GENERAL	1.1, 1.2, 3.4, 6.3
TE Life Skill Builder Making Good Decisions, p. 253 GENERAL TE Reading Skill Builder Paired Summarizing, p. 254 GENERAL TE Life Skill Builder Coping, p. 254 BASIC CRF Decision-Making * GENERAL CRF Directed Reading * BASIC	SE Lesson Review, p. 255 TE Reteaching, Quiz, p. 255 CRF Lesson Quiz * ■ GENERAL	1.1, 1.4, 3.4, 4.2, 4.4, 6.2, 6.3
TE Inclusion Strategies, p. 257 ♦ GENERAL CRF Cross-Disciplinary * GENERAL CRF Refusal Skills * GENERAL CRF Directed Reading * BASIC	SE Lesson Review, p. 257 TE Reteaching, Quiz, p. 257 CRF Lesson Quiz * ■ GENERAL	1.1, 3.4, 6.2, 6.3
CRF Directed Reading * BASIC	SE Lesson Review, p. 259 TE Reteaching, Quiz, p. 259 CRF Lesson Quiz * ■ GENERAL	1.1, 1.4, 3.4, 6.2, 6.3
TE Life Skill Builder Evaluating Media Messages, p. 261 GENERAL CRF Refusal Skills * GENERAL CRF Directed Reading * BASIC	SE Lesson Review, p. 261 TE Reteaching, Quiz, p. 261 CRF Concept Mapping * GENERAL CRF Lesson Quiz * ■ GENERAL	1.1, 1.4, 3.4, 4.2, 4.4, 6.2, 6.3
SE Life Skills Activity Making Good Decisions, p. 263 CRF Decision-Making * GENERAL CRF Directed Reading * BASIC	SE Lesson Review, p. 263 TE Reteaching, Quiz, p. 263 CRF Lesson Quiz * ■ GENERAL	1.1, 1.4, 3.4, 4.2, 4.4, 6.2, 6.3

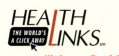

www.scilinks.org/health
Maintained by the **National Science Teachers Association**

Topic: Drug and Alcohol Abuse
HealthLinks code: HD4029
Topic: Drunk Driving
HealthLinks code: HD4032
Topic: Alcoholism
HealthLinks code: HD4007

Technology Resources

 One-Stop Planner
All of your printable resources and the Test Generator are on this convenient CD-ROM.

 Guided Reading Audio CDs

VIDEO SELECT
For information about videos related to this chapter, go to **go.hrw.com** and type in the keyword **HD4AL7V**.

Chapter 12 • Chapter Planning Guide

CHAPTER 12

Teens and Alcohol
Chapter Resources

Teacher Resources

TEACHING TRANSPARENCIES

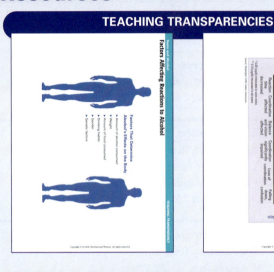
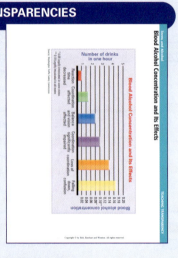

BELLRINGER TRANSPARENCIES

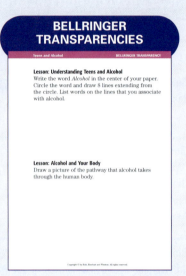

LESSON PLANS

PARENT LETTER

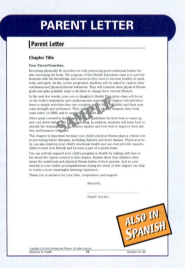

TEST ITEM LISTING

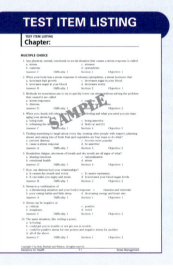

Meeting Individual Needs

DIRECTED READING

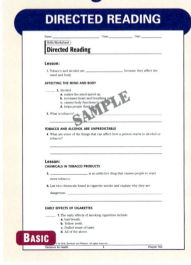

CONCEPT MAPPING

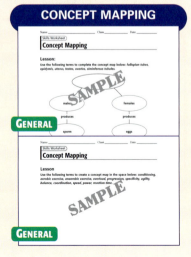

CONCEPT REVIEW

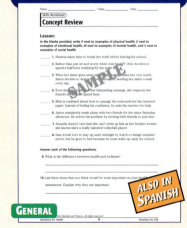

ENRICHMENT ACTIVITIES

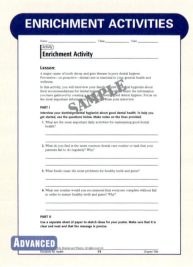

243C Chapter 12 • Teens and Alcohol

Resources

These worksheet pages can be found in the Chapter Resource File and the One-Stop Planner. The transparencies can be found in the Teaching Transparencies binder and on the One-Stop Planner.

Activities

LIFE SKILLS ACTIVITIES

AT-HOME ACTIVITY

DATASHEETS FOR IN-TEXT ACTIVITIES

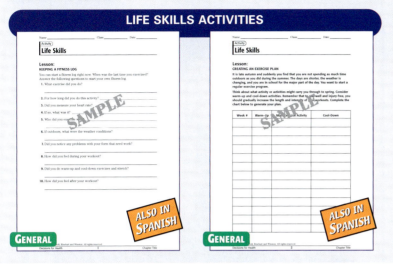
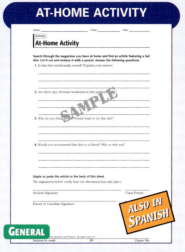
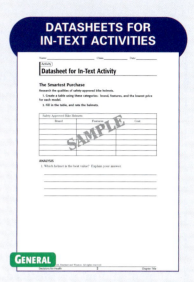

Applications

DECISION-MAKING

REFUSAL SKILLS

CROSS-DISCIPLINARY

HEALTH BEHAVIOR CONTRACT

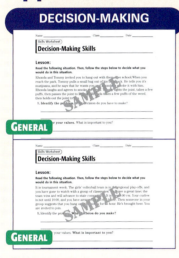
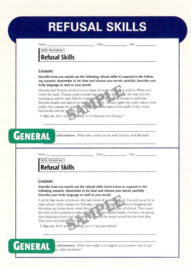
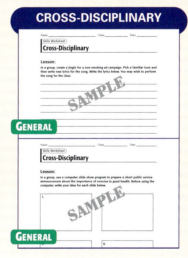
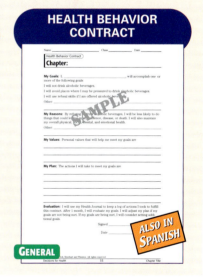

Assessments

HEALTH INVENTORY

LESSON QUIZZES

CHAPTER TEST

PERFORMANCE-BASED ASSESSMENT

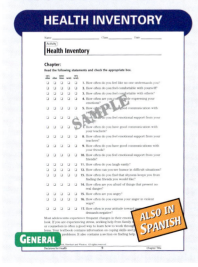
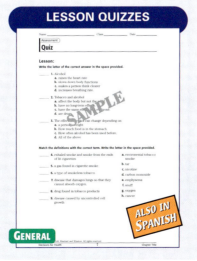
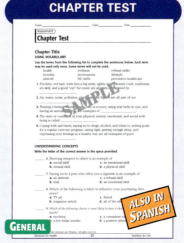
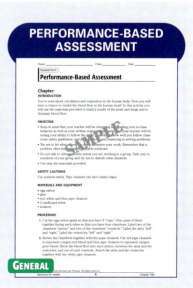

Chapter 12 • Chapter Resources and Worksheets   **243D**

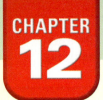

CHAPTER 12
Background Information

The following information focuses on alcohol and alcoholism. This material will help prepare you for teaching the concepts in this chapter.

Alcohol

- The term *alcohol* actually refers to a class of chemical compounds that contain atoms of carbon, hydrogen, and oxygen. In the mainstream, as well as this chapter, the term is synonymous with beverages containing a certain type of alcohol called *ethanol*. Ethanol, or ethyl alcohol, is a depressant drug contained in beer, wine, and liquor. It is also used as a solvent for chemical compounds and in the commercial preparation of detergents, flavorings, and fragrances.

- Alcoholic beverages are classified as either fermented drinks or distilled drinks. Ethyl alcohol makes up between 5 and 20% of fermented drinks such as beer and wine. Ethyl alcohol makes up between 10 and 50% of distilled drinks such as whiskey, gin, and vodka. *Proof* is the amount of ethyl alcohol contained in a distilled drink. In the United States, proof is double the percentage of ethyl alcohol in the beverage. A distilled drink that is classified as 100 proof contains 50% alcohol.

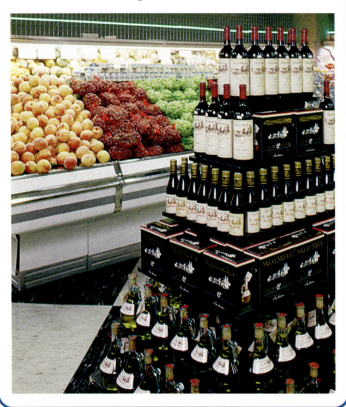

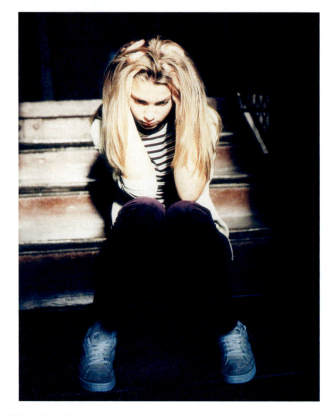

Alcoholism

- The National Council on Alcoholism and Drug Dependence reports that almost 14 million Americans 18 years and older have drinking problems. About 8 million of those are alcoholics, and males outnumber females 3 to 1.

- Research indicates that there may be a genetic disposition to alcoholism, especially in some males under age 25. Data show that children of alcoholics raised by non-alcoholic guardians are still more likely to become alcoholics than offspring of non-alcoholic parents.

- Nearly 11 million children under the age of 18 are offspring of alcoholics. In addition to an increased risk for alcoholism, these youngsters often deal with home environments filled with tension, fear, and stress. As a result, children of alcoholics often have high levels of anxiety, find it difficult to trust others, are uncomfortable demonstrating their feelings, and practice unhealthy living patterns.

> For background information about teaching strategies and issues, refer to the *Professional Reference for Teachers.*

ACTIVITIES

CHAPTER 12

Consider using the activities on this page as students explore the lessons of this chapter. Look for other activities throughout the Student Edition chapter.

What's the Message?

Procedure Organize the class into small groups. Ask each group to make a list of 10 movies in which a character or group of characters drink alcoholic beverages. After compiling the lists, groups should put a plus sign (+) next to the entries in which drinking somehow benefited the character or characters, a minus sign (−) next to the entries in which drinking had a harmful effect on the individuals, or a 0 next to the entries in which drinking had no effect one way or the other.

Analysis Have each group respond to the following questions:

- Why did some of the characters choose to drink alcohol? (Answers will vary based upon movies selected.)

- Did a majority of the movies listed show drinking alcohol as having a positive effect, negative effect, or no effect on the character or characters? (Answers will vary based upon movies selected.)

- Based on the movies you chose, do you think movies and the media in general accurately portray the causes and effects of teen drinking? (Answers will vary.)

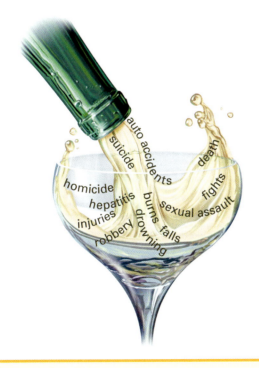

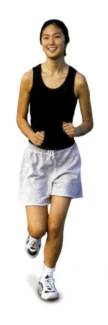

Slowed Reactions

Hands On

Procedure Pair up students so that at least one member of each pair is wearing shoes that tie. Have that student tie one shoe while his or her partner uses a stopwatch to time how long it takes to complete the task. (If both students are wearing shoes that tie, have students trade roles and repeat the activity.) Then have the student close his or her eyes and tie the shoe while the partner notes the time. You may even want the student to wear a blindfold when completing the task.

Analysis Have students respond to the following questions:

- How did closing your eyes affect the rate at which you were able to tie your shoe? (It took longer to complete the task.)

- How did tying your shoe with your eyes closed make you feel? (Answers will vary. Students may describe feeling uncomfortable and frustrated.)

Explain to students that drinking alcohol affects the drinker's coordination in a similar way that closing one's eyes affects his or her ability to complete a simple task. Tell them they will learn more about alcohol's effect on reaction time as they study this chapter.

Chapter 12 • Activities   243F

CHAPTER 12

Overview
Tell students that this chapter will help them understand the negative effect alcohol has on their bodies and on their relationships with other people. Students will explore reasons why some teens drink and examine ways to resist pressures to drink and alternatives to drinking.

Assessing Prior Knowledge
Students should be familiar with the following topics:
- refusal skills
- decision making
- communication skills
- mental and emotional health

Question Box

Students may feel more comfortable asking questions if you set up a Question Box to collect their questions. Have students write and anonymously submit their questions about alcohol, alcohol's effects, and alcoholism. Address these questions during class, or use these questions to introduce lessons that cover related topics.

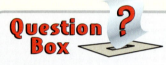

Check out *Current Health* articles and activities related to this chapter by visiting the HRW Web site at **go.hrw.com**. Just type in the keyword **HD4CH27T**.

Chapter Resource File
- Directed Reading BASIC
- Health Inventory GENERAL
- Parent Letter

CHAPTER 12 Teens and Alcohol

Check out **Current Health** articles related to this chapter by visiting **go.hrw.com**. Just type in the keyword **HD4CH27**.

Lessons

1	Understanding Teens and Alcohol	246
2	Alcohol and Your Body	248
3	Alcohol, You, and Other People	252
4	Drunk Driving	256
5	Alcoholism	258
6	Resisting the Pressure to Drink	260
7	Alternatives to Alcohol	262
	Chapter Review	264
	Life Skills in Action	266

Standards Correlations

National Health Education Standards

1.1 Explain the relationship between positive health behaviors and the prevention of injury, illness, disease, and premature death. (Lessons 1–7)

1.4 Analyze how the family, peers, and community influence the health of individuals. (Lessons 1, 3, and 5–7)

3.4 Develop strategies to improve or maintain personal, family, and community health. (Lessons 1–7)

4.2 Analyze how messages from media and other sources influence health behaviors. (Lessons 3 and 6–7)

4.4 Analyze how information from peers influences health. (Lessons 1 and 3)

6.2 Analyze how health-related decisions are influenced by individuals, family, and community values. (Lessons 3–7)

6.3 Predict how decisions regarding health behaviors have consequences for self and others. (Lessons 2–5)

> "My uncle is **addicted** to alcohol. When he drinks, he acts **stupid** and **crazy**. Sometimes he gets **violent**. In the last year, he has had to go to the hospital a couple of times, and he lost his job. I'm not going to drink."

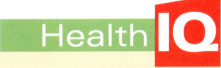

PRE-READING

Answer the following multiple-choice questions to find out what you already know about alcohol. When you've finished this chapter, you'll have the opportunity to change your answers based on what you've learned.

1. Reasons that teens drink alcohol include
   a. wanting to fit in.
   b. curiosity.
   c. wanting to look more adult.
   d. All of the above

2. Which is NOT an effect of drinking alcohol?
   a. relaxed, clear thinking
   b. reduced coordination
   c. poor concentration
   d. blurry vision

3. Your blood alcohol concentration measures
   a. the number of drinks you've had in an hour.
   b. the percentage of alcohol in your blood.
   c. the relationship between your weight and the number of drinks you have had.
   d. the amount of alcohol in the beverages you have drunk.

4. Alcoholism is an illness that
   a. can be completely cured with medicine.
   b. is treatable if the alcoholic wants treatment.
   c. only certain kinds of people get.
   d. lasts only a few weeks or months.

5. One way to avoid the pressure to drink is to
   a. have an interesting hobby.
   b. hang around with people who don't drink.
   c. recognize that alcohol can cause permanent damage to your brain.
   d. All of the above

ANSWERS: 1. d; 2. a; 3. b; 4. b; 5. d

Using the Health IQ

Misconception Alert
Answers to the Health IQ questions may help you identify students' misconceptions.

Question 3: Students may wonder how alcohol, which enters the body through the digestive system, winds up in the bloodstream. Explain that as most food and beverages pass through the digestive system, they are broken down into small molecules. The molecules pass from the digestive system and into the bloodstream through a process called absorption. The blood then moves the molecules throughout the body to supply body cells the materials they need to function. Alcohol, like some other substances, does not need to be broken down. It is absorbed directly into the bloodstream through the lining of the stomach and in the intestines.

Question 4: Students may have heard of alcoholism, but may not realize that alcoholism is a chronic illness that has no cure, that lasts a lifetime, and that can be treated only if the person with alcoholism wants treatment.

Answers
1. d
2. a
3. b
4. b
5. d

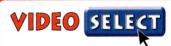

For information about videos related to this chapter, go to **go.hrw.com** and type in the keyword **HD4AL7V**.

Chapter 12 • Teens and Alcohol

Lesson 1

Focus

Overview
Before beginning this lesson, review with your students the objectives listed under the What You'll Do head in the Student Edition. In this lesson, students explore reasons why some teens drink and why some don't.

Bellringer
Have students write the term *Alcohol* in the middle of a sheet of paper. Then have them circle the term and draw 8 lines extending from the circle. Ask students to record words that they associate with *alcohol* on the lines. (Answers will vary, but may include reasons for drinking, alcoholism, and names of alcoholic beverages.)

Answer to Start Off Write
Accept all reasonable answers. Sample answer: curiosity, friends want them to, parents drink, want to be an adult, want to escape

Motivate

Discussion — GENERAL
Alcohol Advertising Discuss with students what they know about alcohol advertising. Ask students why companies pay large sums of money to advertise their products. Discuss with students how the advertisements may affect teens and adults. (by making alcohol seem exciting or fun, people may be convinced to try it and buy it) Finally, ask students which life skills might help them evaluate alcohol advertisements. (Evaluating a Media Message, Being a Wise Consumer, Making Good Decisions)
LS Verbal/Logical

Lesson 1

Understanding Teens and Alcohol

What You'll Do
- **List** three reasons why teens drink.
- **Identify** three reasons for not drinking.

Terms to Learn
- peer pressure

Start Off Write
Why do some teens drink alcohol?

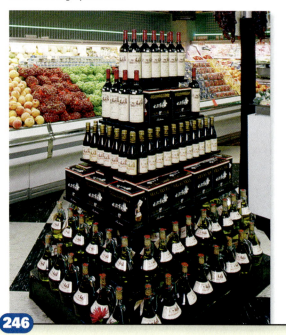

Figure 1 Beer and wine are often displayed in ways that encourage purchases.

Pascal loves to watch sports on TV. He thinks that some of the beer commercials are really cool. Pascal sees his dad drink beer, so Pascal decides to try it.

What things in Pascal's home encourage him to drink? What else in Pascal's life may tempt him to drink?

Why Teens Drink

There are many reasons why teens may drink. Many social settings encourage drinking. Beer ads showing images of people drinking and having a good time seem to be everywhere. Alcoholic beverages are often sold in grocery stores and convenience stores. And some adults may make alcohol easy to get or may even offer teens a drink.

Often, teens drink because they are curious about what other people are doing. They may see drinkers enjoying themselves, and want to try it. It is common for teens to see older family members, relatives, or family friends drinking alcoholic beverages after work, on the weekends, at parties, and on holidays. And it is perfectly normal for teens to be curious about drinking.

Some teens drink because of peer pressure. A *peer* is someone about your age with whom you interact every day. **Peer pressure** is a feeling that you should do something because your friends want you to. Teens do not want to feel left out. If friends are drinking and seem to be having a good time, it can be a challenge to resist the pressure to join in.

Some teens may think that drinking makes them look and feel like adults. They feel more mature with a drink in their hand. Some teens are unhappy and hope that alcohol will make them feel better. But there are no good reasons for teens to drink.

Cultural Awareness

Alcohol is a component of certain religious ceremonies. Stress to students that drinking wine during a traditional religious rite is vastly different from the types of alcohol consumption discussed in this chapter. In a religious rite, a small amount of alcohol is consumed to commemorate an event significant to the religious community. Often, a non-alcoholic substitute is available for those who do not drink. This chapter refers to drinking larger amounts of alcohol as a social activity.

Chapter Resource File
- Directed Reading BASIC
- Lesson Plan
- Lesson Quiz GENERAL

Transparencies
TT Bellringer

246 Chapter 12 • Teens and Alcohol

Teens and Alcohol

Why is alcohol bad for teens? One reason is because teens are still growing. Teens' bodies may continue to grow until they are in their early twenties. Teens' brains are still developing, and alcohol can have serious effects on a brain that is growing and changing.

Another reason is that teens' emotional responses are changing. Teens are making the change from being a child to being a young adult. Sometimes the emotional part of growing up is the hardest part of all. And alcohol may affect emotions in many ways. Alcohol may produce conflicting, unexpected, or even uncontrollable feelings. You can't predict what these feelings will be, or whether they will be pleasant or unpleasant.

But you do not have to drink. The truth is that most adults have less than one alcoholic drink a month or don't drink at all. People have a variety of reasons for not drinking. For some people, not drinking is a personal choice. Other people do not drink because they feel better able to meet their personal duties and responsibilities if they do not drink. Other people do not drink because of their religious beliefs, family values, or health problems. Any reason for not drinking is a good reason.

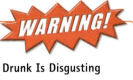

Drunk Is Disgusting

Being drunk can make you very unpopular with your friends and family. No one enjoys being around someone who is vomiting, violent, or out of control.

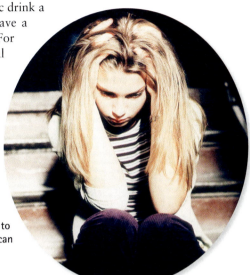

Figure 2 Some teens use alcohol to overcome sadness. But drinking can make sadness even worse.

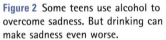

Lesson Review

Using Vocabulary
1. What is peer pressure?

Understanding Concepts
2. What are three reasons that teens may drink alcohol?
3. What are three reasons teens should not drink?

Critical Thinking
4. **Using Refusal Skills** What advice should you give to a friend who tells you he or she wants to start drinking?
5. **Analyzing Ideas** How may different social settings affect the feelings of a person who is drinking?

Teach

Life SKILL BUILDER — GENERAL

Making Good Decisions Have students apply their decision-making skills to the following scenario: You have just learned that your parent is changing jobs and that the family must move to another state. You don't want to leave your friends and are angry that no one seems to care about what you want. A friend invites you to a party where beer will be available. He promises that you will feel much better after a few drinks. What do you decide to do? Explain the steps you used to make your decision. **LS Logical**

Close

Reteaching — BASIC

Newspaper Article Have students write an article for your school newspaper titled "Teens and Alcohol." Encourage students to include the main ideas of this lesson in their articles.

Quiz — GENERAL

1. What effect may advertisements have on a teen's decision to drink alcohol? (Advertisements for alcohol make drinking look attractive and may influence a teen to try alcohol.)
2. Why is alcohol more harmful to teens than to adults? (A teen's body is still growing and changing, and alcohol can harm parts of the body, especially the brain, during this period of growth.)
3. How common is drinking alcoholic beverages among adults? (Most adults drink less than one drink a day, and as many as 1/3 of all adults do not drink at all.)

Answers to Lesson Review

1. Peer pressure is a feeling that you should do something because your friends want you to.
2. Some teens drink due to peer pressure, to appear mature, or to escape problems in their lives.
3. Teens should not drink because they are still growing and developing, and alcohol can cause lasting physical or mental damage. Alcohol is illegal and teens can get into trouble for drinking it. Finally, alcohol may produce strong or uncontrollable feelings that can harm relationships.
4. Answers will vary. Sample answer: I would ask my friend why he or she wants to drink, and I would try to explain the dangers of drinking to them. I would also tell my friend that I like him or her just the way he or she is, and not under the influence of alcohol.
5. In a social setting where few or no people are drinking, a person may decide not to have a drink because he or she doesn't want to stand out. At a party where everyone is drinking, a person may choose to have a drink, just to fit in.

Lesson 1 • Understanding Teens and Alcohol

Lesson 2

Focus

Overview
Before beginning this lesson, review with your students the objectives listed under the What You'll Do head in the Student Edition. In this lesson, students discover how the body processes alcohol. They explore both the short and long-term effects of alcohol on the body.

Bellringer
Have students draw a picture of alcohol's pathway through the human body.

Answer to Start Off Write
Accept all reasonable answers. Sample answer: Alcohol is a depressant and it slows brain and body functions.

Motivate

Activity — GENERAL
Poor Coordination Have right-handed students use their left hand and left-handed students use their right hand to write their names and addresses on a sheet of paper. When all students have completed the task, ask them to describe the experience. (Students will likely describe feeling strange, uncoordinated, and frustrated.) Guide students in recognizing that the activity models the effect drinking alcohol has on coordination.
LS Visual/Kinesthetic — English Language Learners

Lesson 2 — Alcohol and Your Body

What You'll Do
- **Describe** what happens to alcohol in the body.
- **Identify** three short-term effects of alcohol.
- **Describe** two effects of alcohol abuse.

Terms to Learn
- drug
- depressant
- blood alcohol concentration (BAC)
- intoxication
- reaction time
- alcohol abuse

Start Off Write
How does alcohol affect the body and the brain?

Trisha was confused—her aunt had gotten silly and sick from drinking alcohol at the family picnic. However, Trisha's uncle drank the same amount and he didn't seem to be affected by it at all.

How can people have such different reactions to the same amount of alcohol?

Alcohol in Your Body

Alcohol is a drug. A **drug** is any substance that changes how the mind or body works. And alcohol does have powerful effects on how your mind and body work.

As you drink alcohol, it goes from the mouth to the stomach and then to the small and large intestines. Most alcohol quickly enters the bloodstream through the intestines. Blood carries alcohol to every tissue and organ. Alcohol in the blood quickly reaches the brain, where its effects begin immediately. Blood also carries alcohol to the liver, where alcohol is converted into harmless waste products.

Even though alcohol is processed in your body as if it were food, alcohol has almost no nutritional value. In fact, when your body breaks down alcohol, your body stops making and storing glucose. Glucose is the sugar that your body uses as a source of energy. So, if you drink too much alcohol, your body cannot process your other food properly.

In addition to affecting your digestion, alcohol also is a depressant. A **depressant** is a drug that slows brain and body functions. Drinking too much alcohol is a drug overdose and may slow your bodily functions so much that they stop. This overdose and collapse is called *alcohol poisoning*.

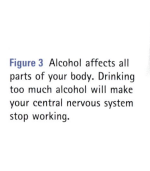
Figure 3 Alcohol affects all parts of your body. Drinking too much alcohol will make your central nervous system stop working.

248

 INCLUSION Strategies — BASIC

- Hearing Impaired   • Learning Disabled

Students with hearing impairments or learning disabilities can benefit from additional visual aids. Give each student a sheet of small circle stickers. Have them put stickers on the parts of their bodies (over their clothes) that are affected by alcohol. (All limbs and sense organs are fair game for receiving a sticker. Students may also place stickers on their clothes in the approximate location of internal organs, too.) Discuss that alcohol affects every part of the human body. **LS Kinesthetic**

Chapter Resource File
- Directed Reading BASIC
- Lesson Plan
- Lesson Quiz GENERAL

Transparencies
- TT Bellringer
- TT Alcohol's Effects on Different Bodies
- TT Effects of Blood Alcohol Concentration

248   Chapter 12 • Teens and Alcohol

Alcohol and the Brain

As a depressant, alcohol slows the activities of your body's central nervous system (CNS), which is made up of your brain and your spinal cord. Alcohol slows your thinking, your reactions, and your breathing. It slurs your speech, blurs your vision, and interferes with your muscle coordination. Alcohol also has negative effects on brain functions such as learning, motivation, and emotions. And the more alcohol in the blood, the more serious the effects on the CNS and all the things it controls. For example, alcohol slows the nerves that control your heart and your breathing. A fatal dose of alcohol will stop these functions.

How much alcohol is a fatal dose? That depends on the person and how much alcohol is in his or her blood. Generally, a blood alcohol concentration of 0.40 or above will be fatal to most people. **Blood alcohol concentration (BAC),** also called *blood alcohol level,* is the percentage of alcohol in a person's blood. For example, a BAC of 0.10 percent means that you have 10 parts of alcohol per 10,000 parts of blood in your body. A drinker's BAC is affected by a number of factors, such as his or her weight, how many drinks he or she has had, and whether he or she has eaten recently. But even one drink in an hour produces effects on the brain in many drinkers. The figure below shows how BAC, the number of drinks in one hour, and the effects of those drinks are related. For example, the BAC of a person who has three drinks in an hour will be about 0.10 to 0.12. At that level, the person's muscle coordination, reaction time, vision, and balance are all significantly impaired. A person with a BAC of 0.10 is legally drunk in all states.

WARNING!

Brain Changes

Even with as few as two drinks in an hour, recognizable changes in the brain occur. A person may feel lightheaded and giddy. Their coordination may be slightly altered, and driving becomes significantly more dangerous.

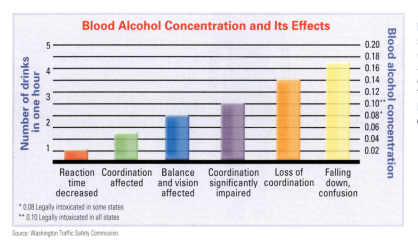

Figure 4 This graph shows alcohol's effects on a body after a number of drinks in one hour. The approximate BAC caused by those drinks is also shown.

REAL-LIFE CONNECTION — GENERAL

Alcohol and Death Research shows that the average age at which teens begin experimenting with alcohol is between 11 and 13 and that some students continue drinking throughout high school. A survey of high school seniors showed that 80% of the respondents had used alcohol and 62% had been drunk. Have students research how alcohol is related to causes of death among young people ages 10–19. (Students should find that alcohol-related accidents, automobile crashes, and violence are among the most frequent causes of death in this age group.) **LS** Verbal

LIFE SCIENCE CONNECTION — ADVANCED

Depressants Invite interested students to research other types of depressant drugs such as barbiturates, tranquilizers, and narcotics. Have students determine the short and long term effects of each type of drug, how it is taken, and whether there are legalized uses of the drug. Students can present their findings to the class in a poster or pamphlet. **LS** Visual/Logical

Teach

Discussion — BASIC

Comprehension Check
Reinforce understanding of these two pages by asking the following questions: Why is alcohol classified as a drug? (Like all other drugs, alcohol changes the functioning of one's mind and body.) What category of drug is alcohol? (depressant) What effect do depressants such as alcohol have on the body? (Depressants slow down the actions of the central nervous system.) Is it possible to die from drinking too much alcohol? (Yes, drinking a great deal of alcohol may cause an individual's body systems to stop working completely.) **LS** Verbal/Auditory

Using the Figure — BASIC

BAC Have students study the graph on this page. Ask students the following questions about the graph: What does BAC stand for? (blood alcohol concentration) What does BAC measure? (the percentage of alcohol in a person's blood) At what BAC level does driving becoming dangerous? (0.05) What is the average number of drinks a person would have to drink in an hour to yield a BAC of 0.05? (2 drinks) What BAC level would be fatal to half of the population? (0.40) What does a BAC of 0.50 indicate? (The person's blood contains 50 parts of alcohol to every 10,000 parts of blood.) What does the statement "lethal dose for 75% of the population mean"? (75% of the average population, or 3 out of 4 people, would not be able to survive a BAC of 0.50) **LS** Logical/Visual English Language Learners

Lesson 2 • Alcohol and Your Body

Teach, continued

Group Activity —— BASIC

What's the Truth? Read the following statements about the short-term effects of alcohol and have students respond by holding up one hand if the statement is true or both hands if the statement is false: Alcohol affects every male differently. (t); One drink makes some people feel less anxious. (t); Females usually drink less alcohol than males before becoming intoxicated. (t); A person's physical and mental abilities get worse as his or her BAC increases. (t); A drinker's weight has no relationship to his or her BAC. (f) **LS Verbal**

Life SKILL BUILDER —— GENERAL

Refusal Skills Share the following scenario with students: While visiting her relatives, Angela attends a party with her married cousin, Tina, and her husband. Tina's husband drove them to the party. During the party, Angela watched Tina's husband drink two beers. When he opened his third can, Angela asked Tina if it was wise for her husband to be drinking since he was their only driver. Tina laughed and told Angela, "Don't worry about him. He can hold his beer." But Tina is still concerned about getting into a car with him. What should she do? **LS Logical**

STUDY TIP for better reading

Word Origins Look up the definition of the word *intoxicate*. What is the root word in *intoxicate*? What does that root word mean? How does that root word relate to the meaning of *intoxicate*?

Short-Term Reactions to Alcohol

Each body reacts differently to alcohol. As BAC rises, intoxication occurs. **Intoxication** is the physical and mental changes produced by drinking alcohol. At lower BAC levels—after one or two drinks—some people experience increased energy, positive feelings, and less anxiety. Other people feel less shy or cautious. But other people are more quiet and calm. They may feel sad or negative. And some people, after one or two drinks, feel few effects at all.

Several factors affect the way a body reacts to alcohol. For example, a person who has several drinks in a short time is likely to be affected more than a person who has a single drink in the same time. Food in a drinker's stomach can also slow alcohol absorption into the blood. Finally, women absorb and process alcohol differently from men. Women achieve a higher BAC than do men who drink the same amount.

As BAC increases, mental and physical abilities decline. Moods are affected first, then physical abilities, then memory. Muscle coordination, especially important for walking and driving, decreases. Vision becomes blurred. Speech and memory are impaired. Reaction time slows. **Reaction time** is the amount of time that passes from the instant when your brain detects an external stimulus until the moment you respond.

At higher BAC levels, your central nervous system slows down so much that you might pass out or even die. And nothing speeds the process to sober you up—not coffee, cold showers, or exercise.

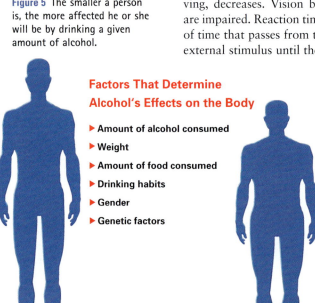

Figure 5 The smaller a person is, the more affected he or she will be by drinking a given amount of alcohol.

Factors That Determine Alcohol's Effects on the Body
▶ Amount of alcohol consumed
▶ Weight
▶ Amount of food consumed
▶ Drinking habits
▶ Gender
▶ Genetic factors

Attention Grabber

Binge Drinking It is estimated that 20% of underage drinkers engage in *binge drinking*. Binge drinking is defined as drinking 5 or more drinks at one sitting (for males; for females, it is 4 or more drinks at one sitting). About 16% of those heavy drinkers have experienced "black outs," after which they could not remember what had occurred the previous evening.

Alcohol Abuse

Young people who start drinking alcohol at an early age or who drink regularly are more likely to abuse alcohol later in life. **Alcohol abuse** is the inability to drink in moderation or at appropriate times. And regular, heavy alcohol use causes many drinkers to develop some tolerance to alcohol's effects. *Tolerance* for alcohol means that a person needs more alcohol to produce the same effects. Tolerance is a sign of a drinking problem.

Young people who drink alcohol may damage their brain and nervous system. Young drinkers are likely to show impaired memory and to perform poorly in school. Their verbal skills may be reduced and never catch up. And long-term alcohol abuse increases the risk of illnesses such as stroke, heart disease, cancer, and liver diseases such as hepatitis and cirrhosis.

Alcohol abuse doesn't only mean drinking too much. It also means drinking at the wrong time. Even one drink at the wrong time or wrong place may be alcohol abuse. Alcohol abuse can lead to car crashes, or to death through drowning or overdose. Your risk of injury or permanent disability grows with every drink. As your mental and physical abilities are impaired, you are less able to protect yourself and others. You are more likely to become a victim of physical or sexual assault. The consequence of an assault may be pregnancy or sexually transmitted diseases, including HIV infection. Alcohol abuse also makes depression, family problems, and violence more likely.

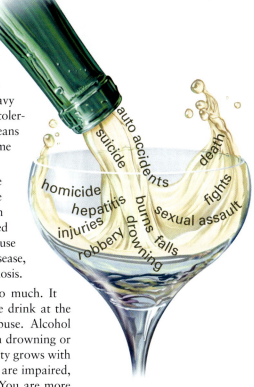

Figure 6 Alcohol abuse contributes to a wide range of social and personal problems.

Lesson Review

Using Vocabulary
1. What is a depressant?
2. What does BAC measure?

Understanding Concepts
3. What happens to alcohol in the body?
4. Describe three short-term effects of alcohol.

Critical Thinking
5. **Making Good Decisions** After drinking several beers at the picnic, Tricia's aunt said she wanted to go swimming. She wanted Tricia to walk down to the lake and swim with her. What should Tricia do? Why?
6. **Analyzing Ideas** Describe two results of alcohol abuse that might affect a young person differently from an adult.

internet connect
www.scilinks.org/health
Topic: Drug and Alcohol Abuse
HealthLinks code: HD4029
HEALTH LINKS. Maintained by the National Science Teachers Association

Lesson 3 Focus

Overview
Before beginning this lesson, review with your students the objectives listed under the What You'll Do head in the Student Edition. In this lesson, students will discover that drinking alcohol is linked to making bad decisions and to violence. Students will also learn about fetal alcohol syndrome and its causes.

Bellringer
Have students reflect on a time when they made a decision that ultimately proved to be unwise. Ask them to recall and write down the other options available at the time and what factors influenced their final decision.

Answer to Start Off Write
Accept all reasonable answers. Sample answer: If you drink, you may say something that either hurts someone's feelings or that makes them angry. If the person gets angry, he or she may get violent and hurt you.

Motivate

Activity — GENERAL
Practicing Wellness Have students work in pairs and scan newspapers and magazines for stories describing situations in which an individual made a decision that proved costly. Have each pair summarize the story for the class by identifying the problem, the decision, and the result. After each presentation, have students brainstorm more suitable ways that the individual might have handled the situation. **LS Verbal/Logical** — English Language Learners

---

Lesson 3 — Alcohol, You, and Other People

What You'll Do
- **Explain** how alcohol can lead to bad decisions and violence.
- **Explain** how a person's decision to drink alcohol may affect other people.
- **Identify** three effects of fetal alcohol syndrome.

Terms to Learn
- binge drinking
- fetal alcohol syndrome (FAS)

Start Off Write
Why does alcohol make violence more likely?

Sarah has noticed that when her college-age brother is with his friends, they are usually friendly and fun. But, when they have been drinking, they argue more, have more fights, and sometimes get violent.

Does everyone behave the way that Sarah's brother and his friends do when they drink? Why would they behave this way?

Alcohol and Decision Making
Alcohol makes it more difficult to think clearly about your choices. It makes remembering all your options less likely. For example, if you have had a couple of drinks, you may get into a car with a drunk driver. You may not even think about all the safer ways you could get home.

Alcohol affects your memory. You may forget what you said or did. Alcohol also affects your ability to process information. As a result, you may ignore, misunderstand, or not recognize a dangerous situation. You may not notice that the driver of the car is drunk, or you may not care. Either way, alcohol has affected your ability to make a good decision.

Alcohol harms your coordination, slows your reactions, and changes the way you see situations. As a result, low risk situations may become high risk ones. For example, activities such as swimming or cycling become more difficult and dangerous. You may take risks you usually do not take and increase your chances of having a serious, or even deadly, accident.

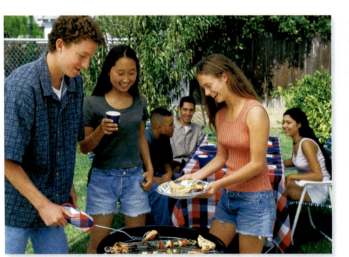

Figure 7 If alcohol harms a person's ability to make a good decision, even a small amount of alcohol may indirectly cause harm to others.

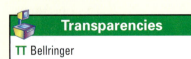

Chapter Resource File
- Directed Reading **BASIC**
- Lesson Plan
- Lesson Quiz **GENERAL**

Transparencies
TT Bellringer

252   Chapter 12 • Teens and Alcohol

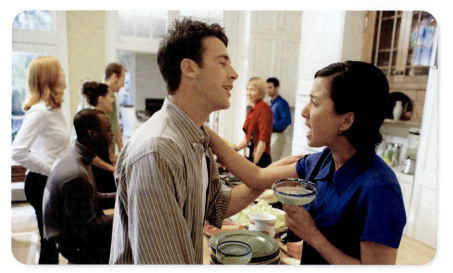

Figure 8 Alcohol affects your emotions and your relationships with other people.

Alcohol and Social Decisions

Alcohol also affects the decisions you make in social situations. What's fun for a drinker may be seen as obnoxious to those nearby. Intoxicated people are less likely to think about how their decisions will influence their lives. Intoxication can easily lead to dangerous decisions and dangerous behaviors. For example, drinking makes you less careful about your sexual behaviors. The chances increase for unplanned, unprotected, and unwanted sex. And with the increased chances of sexual activity, the chances for getting sexually transmitted diseases (STDs) or for becoming pregnant also increase. Such consequences can be life changing.

Alcohol may change your feelings. You may become very happy and silly. Or you may become very sad, very angry, or even violent. Alcohol may make you forget your values. As a result, you may say or do things that you regret later on. For example, drinking is often associated with fights, arguments, and injuries. You may start a fight with a friend, someone you would usually never fight with. Or you may start a fight with someone you do not even know.

Alcohol's social effects are even stronger in people who binge drink. **Binge drinking** for men is drinking five or more drinks in one sitting, and for women is drinking four or more drinks in one sitting. Binge drinking increases the chances that the drinkers will be involved in violence or other harmful behavior. But even one drink can lead to unpleasant and unhappy results.

Myth & Fact

Myth: It is safer to drink beer than it is to drink whiskey or wine.

Fact: Any kind of alcohol can make you drunk, sick, and at risk for serious problems. A beer may affect you just as much as a glass of wine or a drink that contains whiskey does.

SOCIAL STUDIES CONNECTION — GENERAL

Recent studies have shown that the average age for first trying alcohol is 11 for boys and 13 for girls. Ask students to research reasons why some young people try alcohol at such an early age and how drinking at an early age affects their chances of developing alcohol dependence. **LS Interpersonal/Intrapersonal**

Teach

Life SKILL BUILDER — GENERAL

Making Good Decisions Have students work in pairs and apply their decision-making skills to the following scenario: You have made plans to go fishing with a friend. When you get to the lake, you find your friend waiting by his family's boat. He immediately tells you that you will have to do the rowing because he has "a buzz on" from drinking. One problem: You've never been in a rowboat before! What do you do? **LS Logical** — English Language Learners

Group Activity — GENERAL

Skit Have small groups of students work cooperatively to write and perform a skit in which a teen tries to act cool by drinking and then behaves in a manner that causes peers to reject him or her. **LS Interpersonal/Kinesthetic** — English Language Learners

Discussion — BASIC

Friends Ask students to identify traits of a good friend. (possible responses include honesty, loyalty, trustworthiness, and dependability) Then ask students to describe what a "good friend" would do in the following scenario: Jill goes to a party with a friend. She spends most of the evening drinking beer with a guy from another school. Late in the evening, Jill tells her friend to go home without her because she is leaving with the guy. **LS Interpersonal/Logical**

Lesson 3 • Alcohol, You, and Other People

Teach, continued

READING SKILL BUILDER — GENERAL

Paired Summarizing Have students work in pairs to read these two pages about alcohol and violence and alcohol and pregnancy. One student should read a paragraph aloud, then the other student should summarize its key points. Have students trade roles and repeat this procedure for each paragraph. **English Language Learners**
LS **Verbal/Auditory**

REAL-LIFE CONNECTION — ADVANCED

Support Groups If appropriate for your class, tell students that a number of organizations provide support for individuals victimized by a family member's drinking. Encourage students to survey your local community for the names and phone numbers of such support groups. Have students compile their findings in a poster that can be displayed in your classroom or the school's guidance office. **English Language Learners**
LS **Verbal/Visual**

Life SKILL BUILDER — BASIC

Coping Share the following scenario with students and discuss possible actions that Mica could take: Mica and Leah have been best friends for years. Recently, Leah confided that her father was out of work and spent most of his time drinking. She also told Mica that after a few beers, her father became angry and violent. Leah said the situation was so bad that she was considering running away from home. LS **Intrapersonal/Interpersonal**

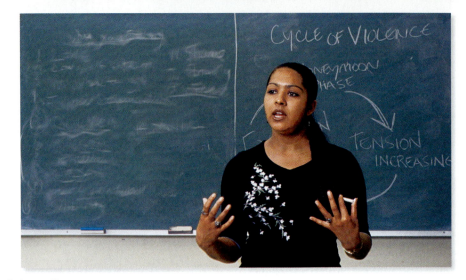

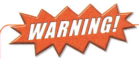

Figure 9 Alcohol can affect family life. When violence occurs in the home, the family may need counseling or other help.

Alcohol Harms Everyone

Drinkers are not the only ones who may be harmed by alcohol use. Those around them, such as family and friends, are at increased risk for alcohol-related harm.

Alcohol and Violence

Alcohol and violence often go together because alcohol can reduce a drinker's self-control. In fact, some people think drinking causes their behaviors. And some people use alcohol as an excuse for their actions. For example, some people drink so that they can lose control and act in ways that they normally wouldn't. But silliness, rude behavior, fighting, and sexual aggression are not caused by drinking. The way that you behave when you are drunk is heavily influenced by your personal values, your expectations of what will happen, and the social setting where you are drinking. Drinking is never an excuse for violence.

Alcohol does not cause violence, but it does make violence more likely. Alcohol makes conflict more difficult to control by making emotions and behaviors seem stronger. Some people who drink become upset or angry easily. They become rude or want to argue. Insults, careless threats, arguments, and fights become more likely. Someone who is drinking may have trouble understanding what other people are trying to say. He or she may imagine an insult or feel threatened. He or she may want to start a fight without worrying about who gets hurt. And in some cases, an intoxicated person who is depressed or unhappy may even try to harm himself or herself.

Someone who is drinking is also more likely to become a victim of violence. That's because intoxication reduces your ability to defend yourself. Drinking also reduces your alertness to danger signs or risky situations. When you are intoxicated, you become an easier target for assault, battering, robbery, or rape.

Background

Alcohol and Date Rape A report by the U.S. Department of Health and Human Services showed that alcohol use is implicated in one to two-thirds of sexual assault and acquaintance or "date" rape cases among teens and college students.

Alcohol and Pregnancy

Alcohol poses special risks for a fetus. A fetus has its own blood supply. But when a pregnant woman drinks alcohol, all of the alcohol in the mother's blood passes into the fetus's blood. **Fetal alcohol syndrome (FAS)** is a group of birth defects that can happen when a pregnant woman drinks alcohol. The child's birth defects range from mild, such as small size at birth, to severe. The more-severe effects may include brain damage, mental retardation, and severe emotional problems as the child grows up. Individuals with FAS often have difficulties with learning, memory, attention, problem solving, and interacting with other people in social situations. There is no known safe level of drinking during pregnancy. Not drinking totally prevents FAS.

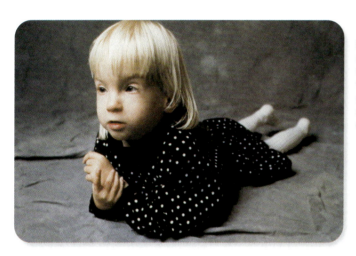

Figure 10 The little girl has fetal alcohol syndrome. Her condition causes her small size and distinct facial characteristics. But the condition's greatest effects are on behavior and mental development.

Lesson Review

Using Vocabulary
1. What is binge drinking?

Understanding Concepts
2. What are three effects of fetal alcohol syndrome?
3. Explain how alcohol can lead to bad decisions and violence.
4. How can a person's decision to drink alcohol affect other people?
5. How does drinking alcohol make a person more likely to become a victim of violence?

Critical Thinking
6. **Analyzing Ideas** Why is drinking alcohol never an excuse for rude, dangerous, or violent behavior?

Lesson 4

Focus

Overview
Before beginning this lesson, review with your students the objectives listed under the What You'll Do head in the Student Edition. In this lesson, students examine how drinking alcohol affects one's ability to drive safely. They also identify ways to prevent drinking and driving.

Bellringer
Ask students to list five behaviors they associate with driving safely. Next to each entry, have students note how drinking alcohol affects the behavior.

Answer to Start Off Write
Accept all reasonable answers. Sample answer: Drinking slows a driver's reaction time, affects vision, and impairs muscle coordination.

Motivate

Discussion — GENERAL

SADD Guest Speaker Invite a representative of SADD (Students Against Destructive Decisions) to speak to your students about the organization and its history, goals, and activities. Encourage the speaker to include descriptions of actions your students can take to prevent drivers from getting behind the wheel while intoxicated. **LS Auditory**

Lesson 4

What You'll Do
- Explain how alcohol affects a person's ability to drive.
- Identify two ways that you can prevent drinking and driving.

Terms to Learn
- driving under the influence (DUI)

Write
How does drinking impair a person's ability to drive?

Figure 11 The combination of alcohol and motor vehicles can be deadly. A drunk driver is not the only one who may be hurt.

Drunk Driving

In a recent year, 14 percent—about 1 out of 7—of 16- to 20-year-old drivers involved in fatal crashes were legally drunk.

And 26 percent—more than 1 out of every 4—of 21- to 24-year-old drivers were legally drunk. *Legally drunk* means that the driver's BAC is higher than the limit set by the state.

Drinking and Driving Is Dangerous!
Alcohol makes driving and other activities, such as skateboarding and riding a bike, so dangerous because alcohol affects every part of the body and mind that a person needs for safe driving or riding. Alcohol makes driving mistakes and crashes more likely. These often lead to injuries and death.

After a single drink, a driver may not feel or look drunk, but he or she already can't drive as safely as before having the drink. His or her vision and muscle coordination may be impaired. Even one drink slows a driver's reaction time. For example, one drink increases the time between when a driver sees the light turn red and when the driver moves to put on the brakes.

Every state has laws that make driving under the influence of alcohol illegal. **Driving under the influence (DUI)** happens when a person who is legally intoxicated or who is using illegal drugs drives a motor vehicle. In most states, a person is legally intoxicated when his or her BAC is greater than 0.08. A few states set the limit at 0.10. In all states, a person under age 21 is legally intoxicated if his or her BAC is above 0.00. People convicted of DUI, whatever their age, may lose their driver's license or permit. A DUI conviction may mean no more driving for months or years.

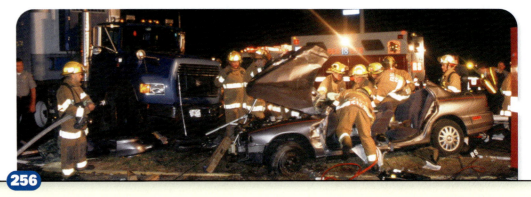

REAL-LIFE CONNECTION — GENERAL

DUI Have students work in pairs to research the DUI laws in your state. Ask each pair to determine the BAC level that determines if a person is legally drunk and is driving under the influence. Students should include the penalties imposed for DUI violations. Have each pair share its findings with the class in an oral report, a poster, or a pamphlet. **LS Logical/Verbal**

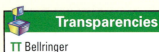

Chapter Resource File
- Directed Reading BASIC
- Lesson Plan
- Lesson Quiz GENERAL

Transparencies
TT Bellringer

256 Chapter 12 • Teens and Alcohol

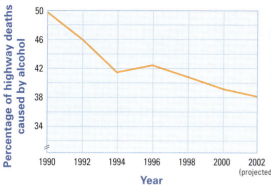

Figure 12 Efforts by many people in the last few years have helped reduce the number of deaths due to DUI.

Source: Washington Traffic Safety Administration FARS data

What Can You Do About Drunk Driving?

Would you walk in front of a car steered by a drunk driver? Probably not. You can't always control what other people do, but you can control and protect yourself. Don't ride with a drunk driver. Get home some other way, or try to arrange a ride beforehand. Avoid situations in which there might be drinking. You can help protect others, too. If a friend is about to drive after drinking, try to stop him or her. Do not ride along. And if someone is drinking, don't let him or her skateboard or bike ride. No matter what you hear, there is no way for anyone to sober up quickly. So be safe, not sorry.

What else can you do to prevent drunk driving? You can join others in a group to prevent DUI, such as SADD (Students Against Destructive Decisions) or MADD (Mothers Against Drunk Driving). Stay away from people who drink and drive. Take control of your life and stay safe.

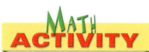

Have students research the latest statistics on alcohol-related highway deaths. Then have them copy the graph in the figure above and revise it to incorporate the latest information. Ask students to make a second graph that shows their state's information on alcohol-related deaths.

Lesson Review

Using Vocabulary
1. What is DUI?

Understanding Concepts
2. Why is driving after drinking so dangerous?
3. How can a reaction time that is slowed by alcohol cause problems?
4. What are two ways that you can prevent drinking and driving?

Critical Thinking
5. **Making Inferences** What do you think are the reasons that some state DUI laws make 0.00 the BAC limit for people under 21?

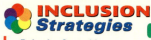

www.scilinks.org/health
Topic: Drunk Driving
HealthLinks code: HD4032

HEALTH LINKS. Maintained by the National Science Teachers Association

---

Answers to Lesson Review

1. DUI means "driving under the influence" of alcohol or illegal drugs.
2. Drinking alcohol slows the functioning of a driver's body and mind. Drinking may also make a driver feel like taking chances that he or she would not take if he or she was sober.
3. If a driver's reaction time is slowed, his or her ability to respond to and avoid hazards is impaired or reduced and the chances of injury and death are increased.
4. Ways of preventing drinking and driving include not allowing drinking to occur in or on a motorized vehicle, including snowmobiles or personal water craft, that you operate or ride in, never getting into a car with a person who has been drinking, and stopping friends from driving after drinking.
5. Because alcohol affects teens more than it does adults, because teens lack experience driving, and because it is illegal for people under the age of 21 to drink, all state DUI laws make 0.00 the BAC limit for people under 21.

Teach

INCLUSION Strategies — GENERAL

- Behavior Control Issues
- Learning Disabled

Manipulatives Use flashcards that simulate a yield sign and a stop sign to clarify the concept of *delayed reaction time*. Make one card with a large yellow circle and one with a large red circle. Have students slap their desk after the yield sign but before the stop sign. Using both hands, show the yield sign and then immediately show the stop sign. Practice a couple of times to make sure students can get "stopped" in time. Then, tell students to simulate delayed reaction time by counting *1001, 1002* before slapping the desk. Discuss the driving problems created by delayed reaction times.

LS Verbal/Kinesthetic — English Language Learners

Close

Reteaching — BASIC

Concept Map Have students create a concept map or other graphic organizer of the important concepts in this lesson.

LS Verbal/Visual — English Language Learners

Quiz — GENERAL

1. What is the BAC level used by most states to classify a driver as DUI? (a BAC level 0.08 or above)
2. What happens to a driver who is convicted of DUI? (The driver's driving privileges are revoked for a period of time.)
3. Is it possible to ride a bicycle or skateboard safely after drinking alcohol? Explain why or why not. (No; Alcohol impairs a drinker's vision, reaction time, muscle coordination, and judgment.)

Lesson 4 • Drunk Driving

Lesson 5

Focus

Overview
Before beginning this lesson, review with your students the objectives listed under the What You'll Do head in the Student Edition. In this lesson, students examine factors that can contribute to a person becoming an alcoholic. They also explore how alcoholism may affect an alcoholic's family.

Bellringer
Ask students to list some times when they benefited from the help or support of a family member, such as a parent or older sibling.

Answer to Start Off Write
Accept all reasonable answers. Sample answer: Alcoholism may make parents angry or violent.

Motivate

Discussion — GENERAL

Families Ask students to name teams to which they belong. (Responses will likely include sports teams, such as baseball or football, and academic teams, such as debate.) Then ask students to define the term *team*. (Possible response: a group of individuals who work together for a common goal) Discuss the idea that the effectiveness of a team depends on each member doing his or her part. Ask students if a family is a type of team. (yes) Discuss the concept that as with all types of teams, the actions of each family member affects all the other family members. **Intrapersonal/Interpersonal**

Lesson 5 — Alcoholism

Bobby is happy that his Uncle Frank has recovered from years of alcoholism. But Bobby is concerned because his uncle still has a lot of problems to deal with.

Why is Bobby still concerned about his uncle if Uncle Frank has recovered? Is alcoholism different from an illness such as the flu?

What Is Alcoholism?

Alcoholism is an illness. **Alcoholism** is a physical and emotional addiction to alcohol. Like other illnesses, alcoholism has certain symptoms. Alcoholism's main symptoms are a strong need for a drink, an inability to stop or limit drinking, an increasing tolerance for alcohol, and a physical dependence on alcohol. *Physical dependence* means that your body needs alcohol to function normally. Like other illnesses, alcoholism may get worse if it is not treated. Alcoholism may eventually lead to death.

Alcoholism has different causes. Frequent heavy drinking can change your body's reactions to alcohol and result in dependence. Alcoholism may be hereditary, because certain genes seem to make alcoholism more likely. But family environment, especially in childhood, and your choice of friends may be stronger influences. For example, friends and relatives may offer you alcohol and encourage drinking.

But alcoholism is not automatic. It occurs in families with and without a history of alcoholism. And not all children whose parents have alcoholism become alcoholics. People who start drinking as adults are less likely to develop alcoholism than people who start drinking in their teens are.

Alcoholism is an illness that affects individuals. But alcoholism also affects everyone in an alcoholic's life. A person with alcoholism may become violent and hurt other family members, or may be moody and unpredictable. Family members don't know what to expect from their loved one. Parents with alcoholism cannot meet their duties or provide emotional support to their children. They may lose their job and create serious financial problems for the family.

What You'll Do
- Identify three factors that can contribute to a person developing alcoholism.
- Explain how alcoholism may affect an alcoholic's family.

Terms to Learn
- alcoholism
- recovery

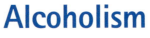
How can alcoholism affect a family?

Figure 13 Alcoholism is a lifelong illness. But many people with alcoholism can recover and live productive, happy lives.

Sensitivity ALERT

Families and Alcoholism Some of your students may come from families where alcoholism is present. These students may be sensitive about some of the material in this chapter. If it is appropriate for your class, as you teach this lesson, you may want to post local contact numbers for support groups such as Al-Anon and Alateen in the classroom.

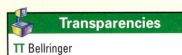

Chapter Resource File
- Directed Reading BASIC
- Lesson Plan
- Lesson Quiz GENERAL

Transparencies
TT Bellringer

258 Chapter 12 • Teens and Alcohol

Overcoming Alcoholism

There is no cure for alcoholism, but alcoholism is treatable. Not drinking at all, or *abstinence from alcohol,* is the best treatment. When a person with alcoholism stops drinking, he or she may experience withdrawal. *Withdrawal* is the reaction the body goes through when it does not get a drug that it is addicted to. A person with alcoholism going through withdrawal may experience severe headaches, extreme nervousness, shaking, or seizures (SEE zuhrz). Medical help may be needed to get through withdrawal.

A person with alcoholism will always be addicted to alcohol. But many people with alcoholism do recover and stay sober by seeking treatment and help. **Recovery** is learning to live without alcohol. Recovery means that the drinker—not alcohol—is in control. But recovery from alcoholism requires that the person wants to stop drinking. Recovery is possible with medication, and with the support and help of other people. Treatment consists of medical help and counseling. Groups, such as Alcoholics Anonymous, may provide help and support for the person with alcoholism.

Counseling also helps families affected by alcoholism. Alanon and Alateen help families cope with alcoholism's effects. Teenage children whose parent has alcoholism can ask a trusted adult for help. Together, they can find a program that provides assistance for teens.

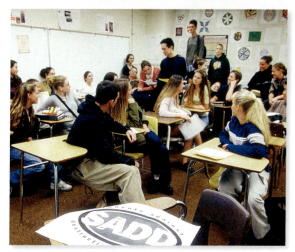

Figure 14 Every member of the family is affected by the disease of alcoholism. But help is available for every family member.

teen talk

Teen: I've heard that once you start drinking, nothing you do will stop you from becoming a person with alcoholism.

Expert: One drink does not cause alcoholism. But alcoholism is a lot less likely if you don't drink until you are an adult. If you think you are at risk for alcoholism, avoid it by not drinking.

Lesson Review

Using Vocabulary
1. Define *alcoholism*.

Understanding Concepts
2. What are three factors that can contribute to a person developing alcoholism?
3. Can alcoholism be cured? Explain.

Critical Thinking
4. **Making Inferences** Explain how alcoholism may affect many people other than the alcoholic.
5. **Identifying Relationships** How might the recovery of a person who has alcoholism benefit his or her family?

internet connect
www.scilinks.org/health
Topic: Alcoholism
HealthLinks code: HD4007
HEALTH LINKS. Maintained by the National Science Teachers Association

Answers to Lesson Review
1. Alcoholism is an illness characterized by a physical and emotional addiction to alcohol.
2. Factors that contribute to alcoholism include inherited traits, childhood environment, and frequent, heavy drinking.
3. No, but a person with alcoholism can recover from the illness. A person with alcoholism must learn to live without alcohol, and may need medicine and support groups to help.
4. Alcoholism affects friends and family members because they must deal with the erratic behavior of the person who has alcoholism and the person's inability to meet his or her social and financial responsibilities.
5. Sample answer: Through recovery, a person with alcoholism breaks free of his or her dependence on alcohol. This reduces the physical, emotional, and financial stress on his or her family members.

Teach

Discussion — GENERAL
Dependence Assess students' understanding of the lesson by asking the following questions: What is physical dependence on a drug? (when a person's body requires the drug in order to work function) What happens when a person with alcoholism stops drinking? (the body goes through withdrawal that may include severe headaches, nervousness, shaking, and seizures) How is physical dependence related to withdrawal? (A person who is physically dependent on a substance needs the substance in order to function. During withdrawal, when the body does not have the substance, it becomes sick and cannot function.)
LS Verbal/Logical

Close

Reteaching — BASIC
Friend Needs Help Have students write a letter to a friend who believes that a family member's alcoholism is his or her fault. Encourage students to support their friend by explaining the causes of alcoholism and suggesting ways the friend can get help for himself and his family member.

Quiz — GENERAL
1. What is one reason that alcoholism may run in families? (Studies indicate that certain genes may increase a person's chances of becoming an alcoholic if he or she chooses to drink.)
2. What are some symptoms of withdrawal from alcohol? (During withdrawal, an alcoholic may experience severe headaches, nervousness, shaking, or even seizures.)
3. What are some factors that increase the likelihood of recovery from alcoholism? (Support groups, such as Alcoholics Anonymous, and medication increase the likelihood of successful recovery from alcoholism.)

Lesson 6 Focus

Overview
Before beginning this lesson, review with your students the objectives listed under the What You'll Do head in the Student Edition. In this lesson, students examine how pressure from different sources, such as peers or the media, is exerted on teens to drink. Students also explore ways of avoiding alcohol.

Bellringer
Have students think about advertisements for alcoholic beverages they are familiar with. Ask students to list things these ads may have in common.

Answer to Start Off Write
Accept all reasonable answers. Sample answer: Beer commercials make drinking look like fun or they make you laugh so you will buy the beer and laugh and have fun, too.

Motivate

Discussion — GENERAL
Debate: Beer Commercials
Discuss with students that some companies spend a lot of money to advertise beer on television, even though these companies know that beer may cause health risks. Have students debate whether a law should be passed banning beer advertising from television.
LS Logical/Verbal

Lesson 6 — Resisting the Pressure to Drink

What You'll Do
- **Identify** three pressures to drink that teens face.
- **Explain** how people can be influenced by advertisements for alcohol.
- **Identify** three questions that can help you resist the pressures to drink.

Start Off Write
How do beer commercials try to convince you to drink?

Rudy was angry with his friend Shanna. Rudy knew that Shanna didn't drink alcohol, but then he saw Shanna drinking beer at a party.

What should Rudy do? He doesn't know why Shanna decided to drink. What may have made Shanna change her mind?

Pressures to Drink
Society provides all kinds of pressures to drink. For teens, peer pressure may be the strongest pressure of all. Peers may make you feel that if you don't drink, you'll be left out and alone. You want to be accepted by groups that have the same interests you do. So, if some of the people you are with start drinking, you may feel pressure to drink, too. That peer pressure is what Shanna felt at the party. Resisting peer pressure is one of the hardest things for teens to do. That is why choosing friends who do not drink is so important.

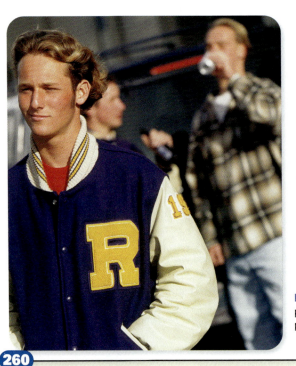

Another source of pressure to drink is advertisements for alcohol. Alcohol advertising is in magazines and on TV and radio. There are ads at sports arenas and on buses and trucks. Drinking is shown in movies and on TV. The message in the ads is that alcohol is a normal part of life. The ads want to convince you that drinking is fun. That's why they never show sick, unhappy, injured, or lonely drinkers. People in the ads are good-looking, smart, happy, athletic, and popular. Sometimes, teens hope that drinking will make them look like the adults in the ad. Some teens may actually think that drinking is the only way to have a good time.

Figure 15 Social and peer pressures influence many people to take a drink.

LIFE SCIENCE CONNECTION — ADVANCED
 Have students research alcohol's effects on a person's physical and emotional growth and development between the ages of 10 and 19. Have students prepare a poster, a brochure, or a pamphlet describing how alcohol can harm this growth and development, and giving suggestions to teens about ways to resist the pressure to drink and avoid the damage caused by alcohol. **LS Verbal/Visual**

Chapter Resource File
- Directed Reading **BASIC**
- Lesson Plan
- Lesson Quiz **GENERAL**

Transparencies
TT Bellringer

Knowing What You Want

Sometimes, messages in ads for alcohol may make knowing what you really want more difficult. After all, alcohol advertising targets parts of you that you may not feel good about, such as appearance or popularity. The ads aim for your fears or your hopes. Or, if you're bored, the ads make drinking seem exciting and fun. How can you make it through all the messages about drinking that you get? You can start by knowing what is right for you.

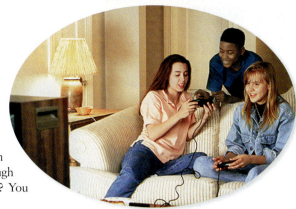

Figure 16 Friends can support your decision not to drink by joining you in healthy alternatives.

Knowing what you want is a lot easier if you take some time to think about it. Try to sort it out with the help of someone you trust. Remember, no matter what the ads tell you, most adults and teens either don't drink at all or drink very rarely.

To drink or not to drink is only one of thousands of choices that teens have to make. Knowing what's best for you helps you make smart choices. Ask yourself the following questions, and write down your answers.

- What makes you happy?
- What do you do to feel good or to feel adult and in charge?
- How can drinking hurt you or get you in trouble?
- What pressures to drink do you feel?
- How can you avoid or stop those pressures?

If you've already decided not to drink, or not to drink again, good for you. But answer the questions anyway. The answers will help you focus on the important things in your life and will help you make good decisions about many different things.

Health Journal

In your Health Journal, write why your decision about whether or not to use alcohol should be based only on your own ideas rather than on what someone else thinks.

Lesson Review

Understanding Concepts

1. What are three questions that might help you resist pressures to drink?
2. Identify three kinds of pressure to drink that teens face.
3. Identify two steps that you would take in making the decision about whether to drink or not.

Critical Thinking

4. **Analyzing Viewpoints** Explain why you should be very careful about believing advertisements for alcohol.
5. **Making Good Decisions** Brandi was eating dinner at her best friend's house. Brandi's friend offered her a glass of wine with dinner. Brandi doesn't drink. What should Brandi do?

Lesson 7 Focus

Overview
Before beginning this lesson, review with your students the objectives listed under the What You'll Do head in the Student Edition. In this lesson, students discover sources of help for people with drinking problems. They also explore ways of having fun and avoiding alcohol use.

🔔 Bellringer
Have students make a list of 5 hobbies or activities they would like to try and the reasons they would like to try it. (Answers will vary.)

Answer to Start Off Write
Accept all reasonable answers. Sample answer: A hobby or other interest will let you be with friends who do not drink and do things that challenge or interest you.

Motivate

Discussion — GENERAL
Exploring Hobbies Invite volunteers to speak to the class about a particular hobby, such as rock climbing or skateboarding, they enjoy. Encourage the speakers to describe the activity, the necessary equipment, how they became interested in the activity, and how people who want to try the activity can get started. Extend students' exposure to hobbies by inviting members of your community to speak to the class about unique leisure-time activities such as origami, fossil hunting, and cooking.
LS Intrapersonal/Auditory

Lesson 7

What You'll Do
- **Describe** two ways to have fun without using alcohol.
- **Identify** three sources of help for drinking problems.

Terms to Learn
- hobby

Start Off Write
How might a hobby or other interest help you avoid using alcohol?

Alternatives to Alcohol

```
SuLinda left her first rock-climbing lesson
with a huge smile on her face. She was
thrilled by the chance to try something new
and exciting outdoors.
```

What do you think SuLinda liked about rock climbing? What other kinds of activities would be exciting for SuLinda or other teens?

Friends and Fun
If you are struggling with a decision about drinking alcohol, one of your best sources of help may be your friends. Friends are usually people you like, trust, talk to, and have a good time with. Your real friends will not pressure you to drink. And you will want to go with your friends to places where you can do things you enjoy. Being with friends who do not drink will keep the pressure to drink off of you. So, pick your friends carefully.

Many activities, such as sports teams, school and religious groups, and community volunteering, provide fun ways to avoid alcohol. Join a group that does things you enjoy, and you may not have time to worry about drinking. Every community has fun things to do, so look around.

Another way to prevent the pressure to drink from getting to you is to find a hobby. A **hobby** is something you like to do or to study in your spare time. Only you can say what interests you and what bores you. If physical challenges, such as rock climbing, excite you, look for places to learn these skills and do them safely. Or maybe you like astronomy or painting. Look for clubs or groups focused on an activity that you enjoy. These are good places to meet new friends.

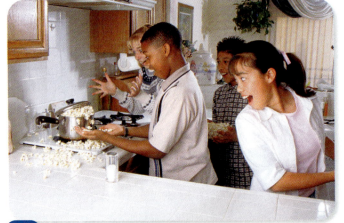

Figure 17 Having fun with friends who share your values is a way to avoid alcohol.

REAL-LIFE CONNECTION — GENERAL
Volunteers Teens can often explore careers they might be interested in by volunteering. For example, a teen that thinks she wants to be a veterinarian may help out at an animal shelter or in a vet's clinic. Have students research opportunities for volunteers in their community, and have them make a poster showing the careers that these opportunities may relate to. **LS** Verbal/Logical

Chapter Resource File
- Directed Reading BASIC
- Lesson Plan
- Lesson Quiz GENERAL

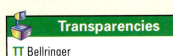

Transparencies
TT Bellringer

262 Chapter 12 • Teens and Alcohol

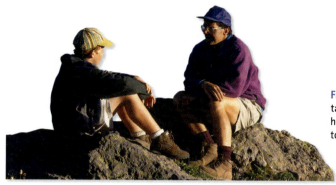

Figure 18 Sometimes, just talking to someone can help you find alternatives to alcohol.

Resources for Emotional Problems

If you have a problem with alcohol, talking to someone you trust may help. Major problems may require more help than your friends can provide. But there is help around you. Adults may have some experience and suggestions about help for drinking problems that they can offer you. A trusted teacher, coach, or guidance counselor can help. You can also talk to your parents, a relative, or another adult you trust. For many teens, talking with a religious or spiritual leader about the mental and emotional problems related to alcohol is best. And for any physical problems related to alcohol, seek help from a parent, school nurse, or family doctor. Don't wait. If you need help, ask someone you trust.

Sometimes, it is a friend who needs help. Be a good listener. Don't judge him or her. And if the alcohol problems are too difficult for you or your friends to handle, help your friend find someone who can help. Seeking professional help is especially important for problems involving alcohol. If you don't know where to start, ask a trusted adult for suggestions.

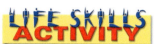

MAKING GOOD DECISIONS

Make a list of the top ten fun things you like to do that don't involve alcohol. With your classmates, make a class list of fun activities on the board. Put a star by any new ideas that appeal to you. Try new activities when you are bored or tempted to drink alcohol.

Lesson Review

Using Vocabulary
1. What is a hobby? Name a few examples.

Understanding Concepts
2. What are two ways to have fun without drinking?
3. List three sources of help for drinking problems.

Critical Thinking
4. **Identifying Relationships** Why is it important to have friends who have the same interests and values that you have?
5. **Using Refusal Skills** Describe two realistic ways to avoid alcohol in the next week.

Answers to Lesson Review
1. A hobby is something you like to do in your spare time such as painting, rock climbing, or collecting stamps.
2. join a sports team or do volunteer work, and take up a hobby
3. Sample answer: teachers, family members, coaches, counselors, religious advisors, and friends
4. Having friends who share your interests and values reduces the chances of peer pressure to try risky activities and increases the chances you will have someone to support you if you need help.
5. Sample answer: Stay away from people and places where you know alcohol will be present, and do things to keep busy so you will not feel pressured to try alcohol.

Teach

Group Activity — GENERAL
Skit Have small groups of students work together to write and perform a skit in which a teen tells a good friend that he thinks he has a drinking problem. Encourage the groups to incorporate the main ideas of this lesson in their skits.
LS **Interpersonal/Kinesthetic**   *English Language Learners*

Activity — BASIC
Guest Speaker Invite the guidance counselor to speak about school and community support services available to students whose lives are touched by alcohol. Ask the speaker to explain how a student in need can obtain assistance in a confidential manner.
LS **Auditory/Interpersonal**

Close

Reteaching — BASIC
Resisting Peer Pressure Have students write a letter to a younger student explaining how he or she can resist peer pressure and can make healthy decisions. LS **Verbal/Logical**

Quiz — GENERAL
1. What are some benefits of joining a hobby club? (Sample answer: A hobby club helps a person develop new skills, meet new people, and avoid peer pressure to drink.)
2. What are some enjoyable leisure-time activities available to teens in your community? (Answers will vary but may include sports teams and hobby clubs.)
3. What are some benefits of being a volunteer? (Sample answer: helping others, meeting new people, developing new skills, exploring possible career paths, and avoiding peer pressure to drink.)

Lesson 7 • Alternatives to Alcohol

CHAPTER 12 REVIEW

Assignment Guide

Lesson	Review Questions
1	12
2	1, 3, 4, 9, 18
3	7, 8, 14, 15
4	10, 13
5	2, 5, 11
6	19
7	6
1–2 and 5	16
2–3	17
3–4	20

ANSWERS

Using Vocabulary

1. Sample answer: Mr. Potter's BAC was only 0.02, so he was not arrested for DUI. Alcohol's depressant effect made Ali clumsy and sleepy.
2. Sample answer: Alcoholism is a disease in which a person needs alcohol in order to function.
3. intoxication
4. alcohol abuse
5. Recovery
6. hobby
7. fetal alcohol syndrome (FAS)
8. binge drinking

Understanding Concepts

9. Alcohol slows down the action of the central nervous system.
10. Because alcohol slows down a drinker's central nervous system, it impairs the person's coordination, concentration, vision, and reaction time. Impaired functioning in these areas increases the likelihood of automobile crashes.
11. While there is no cure for alcoholism, the disease can be treated if a person abstains from alcohol and enters recovery from alcoholism.
12. Sample answer: to seem more adult, to experience something the media portrays as enjoyable, and to be accepted by peers; Alcohol is illegal, alcohol can cause physical and emotional damage, and alcohol may make you a victim of violence.
13. Sample answer: never getting into a car with a drunk driver, calling someone to come and drive everyone home, and stopping friends or passengers in your car from drinking
14. Drinking increases the likelihood of violence because alcohol can trigger powerful emotions, affect one's ability to process information and make wise decisions, and cause a person to say or do things he or she would not do when sober.
15. When a pregnant woman drinks alcohol, some of the alcohol gets to the developing fetus, where it may cause the birth defects known as fetal alcohol syndrome.

Chapter Summary

- Teens drink alcohol for a variety of reasons, including to fit in and to feel more adult.
- Alcohol is a depressant drug that affects the central nervous system.
- Blood alcohol concentration (BAC) is a measure of the amount of alcohol in the blood.
- Alcohol's effects on the brain may make a person more likely to be involved in violence.
- Alcohol's long-term effects include alcohol abuse and liver diseases, such as hepatitis and cirrhosis.
- Alcohol's effects on the body and brain make it extremely dangerous to drink and drive or do any other complex activity.
- Alcoholism is an illness in which a person is physically and psychologically dependent on alcohol.
- You can resist the pressure to drink by considering your options and by understanding the dangers of drinking alcohol.

Using Vocabulary

1. Use each of the following terms in a separate sentence: *blood alcohol concentration (BAC)* and *depressant*.
2. In your own words, write a definition for the term *alcoholism*.

For each sentence, fill in the blank with the proper word from the word bank provided below.

binge drinking
alcohol abuse
blood alcohol concentration
fetal alcohol syndrome (FAS)
hobby
intoxication
recovery
reaction time

3. The physical and mental changes produced by drinking alcohol are ___.
4. The inability to drink in moderation is ___.
5. ___ is learning to live without alcohol.
6. Something you like to do in your spare time is a(n) ___.
7. The possible physical and mental effects on a fetus that has been exposed to alcohol are called ___.
8. Drinking several drinks in one sitting is ___.

Understanding Concepts

9. Describe how alcohol acts as a depressant.
10. How does alcohol affect a person's ability to drive?
11. Explain the statement, "There is no cure for alcoholism, but alcoholism is treatable."
12. Give three reasons that teens drink alcohol, and three reasons for not drinking.
13. How can you prevent someone from drinking and driving?
14. Why might drinkers become involved with violence more easily than nondrinkers?
15. Why is it dangerous for a pregnant woman to drink alcohol?

Critical Thinking

Inferring Conclusions

16. Marie's uncle is an alcoholic, and Marie's father drinks a lot. Marie's college-age brother also seems to drink quite a bit, but usually only on the weekends. Would you predict that Marie will become an alcoholic? Why or why not?

17. Brian's older brother, David, is a binge drinker. David drinks heavily on Friday nights on his way home from work, and on Saturday nights at home with his family. The rest of the time, David doesn't drink. Brian thinks that David abuses alcohol. Explain why you agree or disagree with Brian.

18. Imagine that you are at a family reunion and see your cousin have a couple of drinks in a very short time. About half an hour later, your cousin seems a bit clumsy and a little sleepy. Is it possible the alcohol has anything to do with your cousin's condition? Explain.

Making Good Decisions

19. Imagine that you see a very funny beer commercial on TV. Using the steps for making good decisions, describe how you would react to the ad.

20. At the family reunion, you run into some cousins and their spouses, all in their twenties and thirties. Some of them have been drinking. They have decided to go shopping at a nearby mall, then stop and get some ice cream. They invite you to go with them. Discuss in detail how you would decide whether to go or not.

Interpreting Graphics

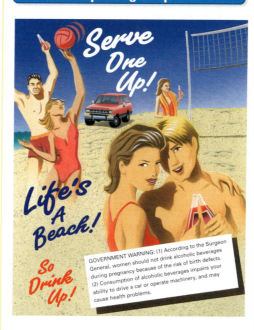

Use the figure above to answer questions 21–24.

21. Who is this ad trying to reach?
22. Why do you think a company would make an ad like this to advertise an alcoholic beverage?
23. Is this ad misleading? Why or why not?
24. What information should an ad for an alcoholic beverage contain?

Reading Checkup

Take a minute to review your answers to the Health IQ questions at the beginning of this chapter. How has reading this chapter improved your Health IQ?

Critical Thinking

Inferring Conclusions

16. Marie is in an environment where alcohol is abused and where there is alcoholism. Her family may have a genetic disposition to alcoholism. These factors increase the chances that Marie will also turn to alcohol. However, Marie can overcome these pressures by making a conscious decision to abstain from alcohol.

17. Accept all reasonable answers. Sample answer: I agree with Brian's assessment of his brother. By drinking heavily and then driving, and by drinking heavily around his family, David is abusing alcohol.

18. The cousin's behavior may definitely be the result of drinking a couple of drinks in a short amount of time. Clumsy actions and sleepiness occur as alcohol slows down the actions of the central nervous system.

Making Good Decisions

19. Students should describe reasons for and against drinking, examine their goals and values, determine whether drinking alcohol supports those goals and values, consider additional consequences of their actions, and then make a final decision.

20. Answers will vary, but students should be concerned about getting into a car with a driver who has been drinking. They should describe refusing to accompany the group to the mall and also attempting to persuade the group not to make the trip, or at least urge the group to find someone who had not been drinking to be the driver.

Interpreting Graphics

21. The ad is trying to appeal to young, active, athletic people, or to people who want to be young, active, and athletic.

22. Companies make ads like this because they want people to buy their products. If people think the product will make them like the beautiful people in the ad, people may buy the product.

23. Yes, the ad is misleading because drinking alcohol will not make you younger, more athletic, or more active.

24. Ads for alcoholic beverages should describe the risks of physical, mental, emotional, and social harm that come with drinking alcohol. They should also state that it is illegal to use alcohol before the age of 21.

Chapter Resource File

- Concept Review GENERAL
- Concept Mapping GENERAL
- Performance-Based Assessment GENERAL
- Chapter Test GENERAL

Model

Introduce this activity by reminding students that using this Life Skill will help them take personal responsibility for their behavior. Then, review the scenario with the class.

Prepare students for this activity by modeling each of the steps of the skill. Make sure students understand each step before you move on to the next one.

Guided Practice: Practice with a Friend

Guided Practice is the stage in which you and the students analyze their approach to solving the problem given in the scenario and analyze their use of refusal skills. Have students read Act 1. Discuss with the class the situation described and the way students are to act it out. Organize the class into groups of three. In each group, one person plays the role of Sophie, another person plays Faith, and the third person is the observer.

Proper pacing during the Guided Practice is important. The suggestions listed below will help you control the pace.

1. Stop after completing each step of using refusal skills.
2. Discuss with each group the observer's comments.
3. Ask the other members of each group to listen to the observer's suggestions and to suggest ways to improve their refusal skills.
4. Instruct students to repeat the steps that need improvement and to include their modifications.

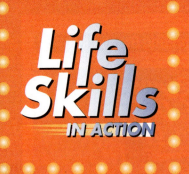

Life Skills IN ACTION

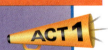 ACT 1

Using Refusal Skills

Using refusal skills is saying no to things you don't want to do. You can also use refusal skills to avoid dangerous situations. Complete the following activity to develop your refusal skills.

Sophie and the Secret Alcohol

Setting the Scene

Sophie is at a high school football game with her friend Faith and Faith's older brother. During the game, Faith and her brother go to buy snacks and drinks. When they return, Faith tells Sophie that her brother managed to sneak in some alcohol. He poured some alcohol into each of the soda cups so that no one would know. Faith hands Sophie a cup and laughs as she tells Sophie to enjoy her soda.

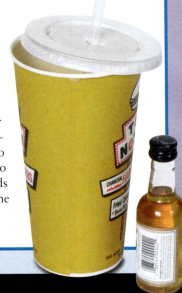

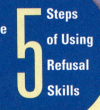

The 5 Steps of Using Refusal Skills

1. Avoid dangerous situations.
2. Say "No."
3. Stand your ground.
4. Stay focused on the issue.
5. Walk away.

Guided Practice

Practice with a Friend

Form a group of three. Have one person play the role of Sophie and another person play the role of Faith. Have the third person be an observer. Walking through each of the five steps of using refusal skills, role-play Sophie telling Faith that she does not want to drink alcohol. Faith should try to convince Sophie that drinking alcohol is okay. The observer will take notes, which will include observations about what the person playing Sophie did well and suggestions of ways to improve. Stop after each step to evaluate the process.

5. Check to make sure that students understand each step before they move on to the next step.
6. If time permits, repeat the exercise three times, switching roles each time. Each student should have the opportunity to play each role. Co-op Learning

Independent Practice

Check Yourself

After you have completed the guided practice, go through Act 1 again without stopping at each step. Answer the questions below to review what you did.

1. Which refusal skill will not work in this situation? Explain.
2. What could Sophie say to Faith when she is standing her ground?
3. What plan could Sophie have to get out of this situation?
4. How would you say no to your friends if they offered you alcohol?

ACT 2

On Your Own

The next weekend, Faith calls Sophie to invite her over to her house. Faith says that her parents went out for the evening and her brother is having a few of his friends over to hang out. Sophie doesn't want to go to Faith's house because she thinks Faith's brother and his friends will be drinking. Write a skit about the conversation between Sophie and Faith. Sophie should use the five steps of using refusal skills during the conversation.

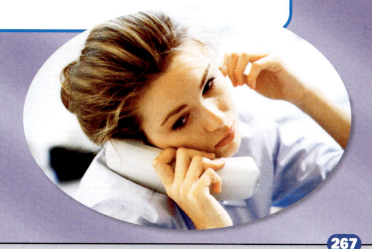

Independent Practice: Check Yourself

Instruct students to repeat Act 1 without stopping at each step. Remind students to apply what they learned in the Guided Practice to the Independent Practice. Students do not have to use every step to refuse successfully.

Encourage students to use the Check Yourself questions as a starting point for reviewing and analyzing their Independent Practice. Remind students that as they change roles, the answers to these questions may change for each actor. Encourage students to create additional questions for checking their use of refusal skills. When students have finished the Independent Practice, have them answer the Check Yourself questions in writing. Use their answers to assess their understanding of the steps of using refusal skills and to assess their use of the steps to solve a problem.

Check Yourself Answers

1. Sample answer: Avoiding dangerous situations will not work in this situation because Sophie is already at the game with Faith.
2. Sample answer: Sophie could say, "No, I don't want to drink alcohol. It is illegal and we could get in trouble."
3. Sample answer: Sophie could call her parents or a trusted adult and ask to be picked up from the game.
4. Sample answer: I would tell my friends that I'm not interested in drinking alcohol and then suggest doing something else.

Act 2: On Your Own

This additional scenario gives students an opportunity to apply what they have learned in both the Guided Practice and the Independent Practice to a new situation.

Suggest to students that they use the Check Yourself questions as a starting point for using refusal skills in the new situation. Encourage students to be creative and to think of ways to improve their use of refusal skills.

Assessment

Review the skits that students have written as part of the On Your Own activity. The skits should include a realistic conversation and should show that the students applied one or more refusal skills in a realistic and effective manner. If time permits, ask student volunteers to act out one or more of the skits. Discuss the conversation and the use of refusal skills.

Chapter 13: Teens and Drugs
Chapter Planning Guide

PACING	CLASSROOM RESOURCES	ACTIVITIES AND DEMONSTRATIONS
BLOCK 1 • 45 min pp. 268–273 **Chapter Opener**	CRF Health Inventory * ■ GENERAL CRF Parent Letter * ■	SE Health IQ, p. 269 CRF At-Home Activity * ■
Lesson 1 Using Drugs	CRF Lesson Plan * TT Bellringer *	TE Activities Truth Vs. Fiction, p. 267F ◆ TE Activity, pp. 270, 272 GENERAL TE Demonstration, pp. 271, 272 ◆ CRF Life Skills Activity * ■ GENERAL CRF Enrichment Activity * ADVANCED
BLOCK 2 • 45 min pp. 274–279 **Lesson 2** The Use of Drugs as Medicine	CRF Lesson Plan * TT Bellringer * TT Reading a Prescription Medicine Label *	TE Activity Reading Labels, p. 275 ◆ BASIC CRF Enrichment Activity * ADVANCED
Lesson 3 Drug Misuse and Abuse	CRF Lesson Plan * TT Bellringer *	TE Activity Skit, p. 276 GENERAL CRF Enrichment Activity * ADVANCED
Lesson 4 Drug Addiction	CRF Lesson Plan * TT Bellringer *	TE Group Activity Poster Project, p. 278 GENERAL CRF Enrichment Activity * ADVANCED
BLOCK 3 • 45 min pp. 280–285 **Lesson 5** The Consequences of Drug Abuse	CRF Lesson Plan * TT Bellringer * TT The Effects of Drug Abuse on the Body *	SE Science Activity, p. 282 TE Group Activity Drugs and Death, p. 282 ADVANCED SE Life Skills in Action Coping, pp. 296–297 CRF Enrichment Activity * ADVANCED
Lesson 6 Stimulants and Depressants	CRF Lesson Plan * TT Bellringer *	CRF Enrichment Activity * ADVANCED
BLOCK 4 • 45 min pp. 286–289 **Lesson 7** Marijuana	CRF Lesson Plan * TT Bellringer *	TE Activity Skit, p. 286 GENERAL CRF Enrichment Activity * ADVANCED
Lesson 8 Hallucinogens and Inhalants	CRF Lesson Plan * TT Bellringer *	TE Group Activity Optical Illusions, p. 288 ◆ GENERAL CRF Life Skills Activity * ■ GENERAL CRF Enrichment Activity * ADVANCED
BLOCK 5 • 45 min pp. 290–293 **Lesson 9** Staying Drug Free	CRF Lesson Plan * TT Bellringer *	TE Activities Working Together to Stay Drug Free, p. 267F ◆ SE Hands-on Activity, p. 291 CRF Datasheets for In-Text Activities * GENERAL TE Activity Poster Project, p. 291 BASIC CRF Enrichment Activity * ADVANCED

BLOCKS 6 & 7 • 90 min Chapter Review and Assessment Resources

- SE Chapter Review, pp. 294–295
- CRF Concept Review * ■ GENERAL
- CRF Health Behavior Contract * ■ GENERAL
- CRF Chapter Test * ■ GENERAL
- CRF Performance-Based Assessment * GENERAL
- OSP Test Generator
- CRF Test Item Listing *

Online Resources

Visit go.hrw.com for a variety of free resources related to this textbook. Enter the keyword **HD4DR7**.

Students can access interactive problem solving help and active visual concept development with the *Decisions for Health* Online Edition available at **www.hrw.com**.

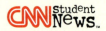

cnnstudentnews.com

Find the latest health news, lesson plans, and activities related to important scientific events.

Chapter 13 • Teens and Drugs

Compression guide:
To shorten your instruction because of time limitations, omit Lessons 1 and 6–8.

KEY

TE Teacher Edition	**CRF** Chapter Resource File	***** Also on One-Stop Planner
SE Student Edition	**TT** Teaching Transparency	■ Also Available in Spanish
OSP One-Stop Planner		◆ Requires Advance Prep

SKILLS DEVELOPMENT RESOURCES	LESSON REVIEW AND ASSESSMENT	STANDARDS CORRELATION
		National Health Education Standards
TE Life Skill Builder Practicing Wellness, p. 270 ADVANCED TE Reading Skill Builder Anticipation Guide, p. 271 BASIC TE Life Skill Builder Evaluating Media Messages, p. 271 ◆ ADVANCED CRF Directed Reading * BASIC	SE Lesson Review, p. 273 TE Reteaching ◆, Quiz, p. 273 TE Alternative Assessment, p. 273 GENERAL CRF Lesson Quiz * ■ GENERAL	
TE Life Skill Builder Being a Wise Consumer, p. 274 GENERAL TE Inclusion Strategies, p. 274 GENERAL CRF Cross-Disciplinary * GENERAL CRF Directed Reading * BASIC	SE Lesson Review, p. 275 TE Reteaching, Quiz, p. 275 CRF Lesson Quiz * ■ GENERAL	
TE Inclusion Strategies, p. 276 ◆ SE Life Skills Activity Practicing Wellness, p. 277 CRF Refusal Skills * GENERAL CRF Directed Reading * BASIC	SE Lesson Review, p. 277 TE Reteaching, Quiz, p. 277 CRF Lesson Quiz * ■ GENERAL	
TE Life Skill Builder Evaluating Media Messages, p. 279 ◆ GENERAL CRF Directed Reading * BASIC	SE Lesson Review, p. 279 TE Reteaching, Quiz, p. 279 CRF Concept Mapping * GENERAL CRF Lesson Quiz * ■ GENERAL	
SE Life Skills Activity Making Good Decisions, p. 281 TE Life Skill Builder, pp. 281, 281 GENERAL TE Reading Skill Builder Paired Reading, p. 281 BASIC CRF Decision-Making * GENERAL CRF Directed Reading * BASIC	SE Lesson Review, p. 283 TE Reteaching, Quiz, p. 283 TE Alternative Assessment, p. 283 GENERAL CRF Concept Mapping * GENERAL CRF Lesson Quiz * ■ GENERAL	6.3
CRF Cross-Disciplinary * GENERAL CRF Directed Reading * BASIC	SE Lesson Review, p. 285 TE Reteaching, Quiz, p. 285 CRF Lesson Quiz * ■ GENERAL	
CRF Directed Reading * BASIC	SE Lesson Review, p. 287 TE Reteaching, Quiz, p. 287 CRF Lesson Quiz * ■ GENERAL	
TE Life Skill Builder Making Good Decisions, p. 289 GENERAL CRF Directed Reading * BASIC	SE Lesson Review, p. 289 TE Reteaching, Quiz, p. 289 CRF Lesson Quiz * ■ GENERAL	
TE Life Skill Builder, pp. 291, 291, 292 GENERAL SE Study Tip Reviewing Information, p. 292 CRF Decision-Making * GENERAL CRF Refusal Skills * GENERAL CRF Directed Reading * BASIC	SE Lesson Review, p. 293 TE Reteaching ◆, Quiz, p. 293 TE Alternative Assessment, p. 293 GENERAL CRF Lesson Quiz * ■ GENERAL	3.6

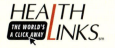
www.scilinks.org/health

Maintained by the **National Science Teachers Association**

Topic: Drugs
HealthLinks code: HD4030
Topic: Medicine Safety
HealthLinks code: HD4066
Topic: Drug Addiction
HealthLinks code: HD4028
Topic: Drugs and Drug Abuse
HealthLinks code: HD4031

Technology Resources

One-Stop Planner
All of your printable resources and the Test Generator are on this convenient CD-ROM.

 Guided Reading Audio CDs

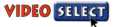
For information about videos related to this chapter, go to **go.hrw.com** and type in the keyword **HD4DR7V**.

Chapter 13 • Chapter Planning Guide **267B**

Chapter 13: Teens and Drugs
Chapter Resources

Teacher Resources

TEACHING TRANSPARENCIES

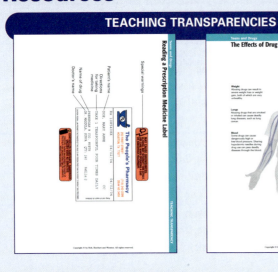
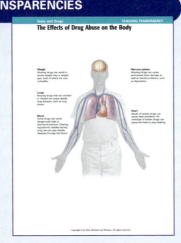

BELLRINGER TRANSPARENCIES

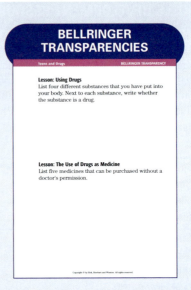

LESSON PLANS
PARENT LETTER
TEST ITEM LISTING

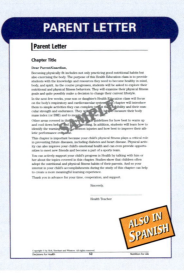
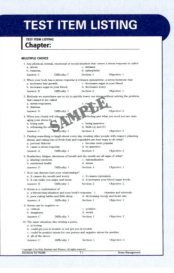

Meeting Individual Needs

DIRECTED READING
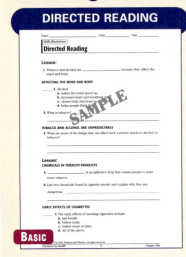
BASIC

CONCEPT MAPPING
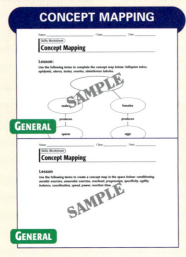
GENERAL

CONCEPT REVIEW
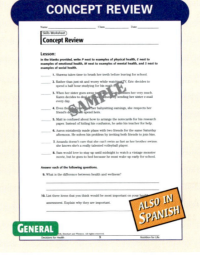
GENERAL

ENRICHMENT ACTIVITIES
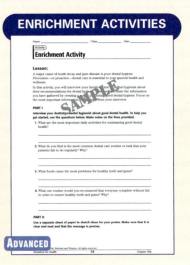
ADVANCED

267C Chapter 13 • Teens and Drugs

Resources

These worksheet pages can be found in the Chapter Resource File and the One-Stop Planner. The transparencies can be found in the Teaching Transparencies binder and on the One-Stop Planner.

Activities

LIFE SKILLS ACTIVITIES

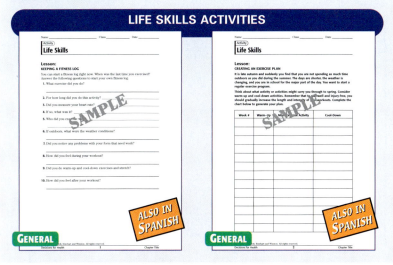

AT-HOME ACTIVITY

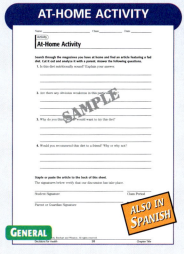

DATASHEETS FOR IN-TEXT ACTIVITIES

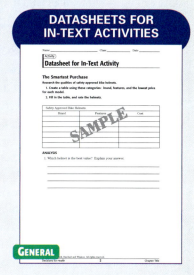

Applications

DECISION-MAKING

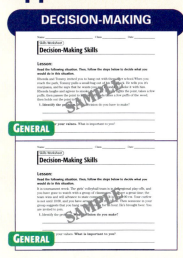

REFUSAL SKILLS

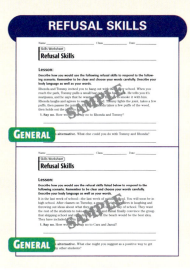

CROSS-DISCIPLINARY

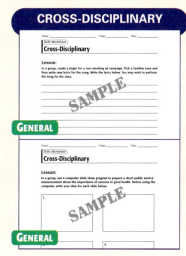

HEALTH BEHAVIOR CONTRACT

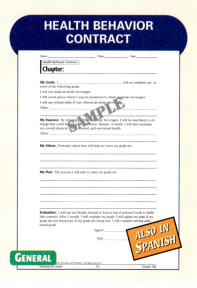

Assessments

HEALTH INVENTORY

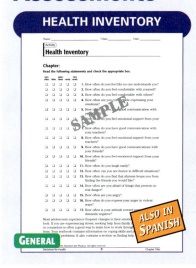

LESSON QUIZZES

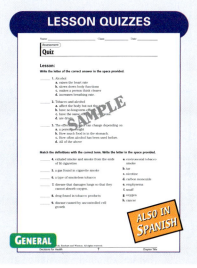

CHAPTER TEST

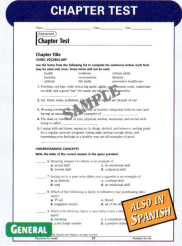

PERFORMANCE-BASED ASSESSMENT

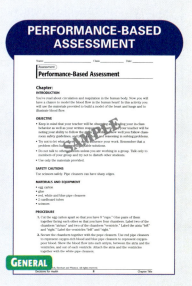

Chapter 13 • Chapter Resources and Worksheets 267D

Chapter 13 — Background Information

The following information focuses on over-the-counter medicines and designer drugs. This material will help prepare you for teaching the concepts in this chapter.

Over-the-Counter Medicines

- One group of common over-the-counter medicines is analgesics. Analgesics are mainly used to treat pain or reduce fevers. The three most commonly used analgesics are aspirin, acetaminophen, and ibuprofen. Aspirin is also used to treat arthritis and as a preventive medicine for people with heart disease. Aspirin's side effects include nausea, heartburn, and bleeding ulcers. Aspirin can cause Reye's syndrome in children with flu or chicken pox. In addition to treating other types of pain, acetaminophen is used to relieve pain from menstrual cramps. Acetaminophen has few side effects when taken in normal doses. Large doses of acetaminophen can cause rashes, fever, or changes in the blood. Ibuprofen can be used to treat pain as well as muscle strain, arthritis, and menstrual cramping. Side effects of ibuprofen include dizziness, drowsiness, headache, upset stomach, and ringing in the ears.

- Over-the-counter cold medicines are designed to treat specific cold symptoms and to temporarily relieve discomfort. They do not cure colds. Types of medicines that treat cold symptoms include antihistamines, decongestants, antitussives, and expectorants. Over-the-counter cold medicines may contain one or more of these types of medicines. Antihistamines and decongestants are used to relieve itchy, watery eyes or to reduce congestion caused by allergies, colds, and flu. Side effects of antihistamines are drowsiness and excitability. Antitussives and expectorants are used to treat coughs. Antitussives suppress coughs. Expectorants clear out mucus from the respiratory system. Some cold medicines contain alcohol or narcotics to reduce pain and help the person sleep. Because of the narcotics and alcohol, some cold medicines are addictive.

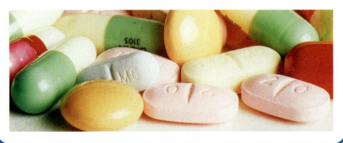

Designer Drugs or Club Drugs

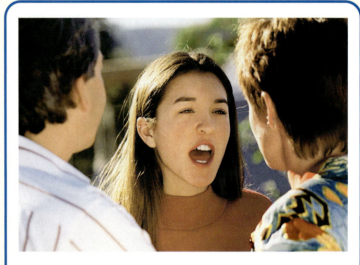

- A group of drugs that your students may be familiar with are designer drugs. Designer drugs are drugs that are produced by making a small chemical change to a drug that already exists. A designer drug has many of the same effects as its parent drug, but also may have other effects. Because some designer drugs are so new, they are not illegal. However, this does not mean that those drugs are safe to use.

- Designer drugs are often called *club drugs* because they are commonly found in nightclubs or at all night parties called *raves*. Three popular club drugs are Ecstasy, Ketamine, and GHB. Rohypnol, LSD, nitrous oxide, and methamphetamine are also considered to be club drugs although they fit under other categories of drugs as well. Sometimes club drugs are used in combination to produce varied effects. Many teens and young adults are attracted to club drugs because they believe the drugs to be safe. However, club drugs can cause memory loss, paranoia, amnesia, coma, heart problems, and death.

- Some club drugs are used as date-rape drugs because they cause people to become unconscious, to enter dreamlike states, or to forget events that happened while under the influence of the drugs. GHB, Ketamine, and Rohypnol are examples of date-rape drugs. They are colorless, odorless, and tasteless and therefore can be added to a person's drink without his or her knowledge.

For background information about teaching strategies and issues, refer to the *Professional Reference for Teachers*.

ACTIVITIES

CHAPTER 13

Consider using the activities on this page as students explore the lessons of this chapter. Look for other activities throughout the Student Edition chapter.

Truth Vs. Fiction

Hands on

Procedure To introduce this activity, ask students to think about something they once thought was true and later discovered was not true. For example, students may think about the tooth fairy. Ask them how they learned the truth, what it was like to discover the truth, and how knowing the truth changed them. Next, organize the students into groups. Give each group a newspaper, tabloid, or magazine article that is either very factual and informative or very misleading and filled with inaccuracies. Instruct each group to read the article together, research the information in the article, and write a paragraph explaining why they believe the article is accurate or inaccurate. Have each group share the group's findings.

Analysis Ask students the following questions:

- What methods did you use to determine if the article was accurate or inaccurate? (Sample answer: We checked on the Internet and with other sources.)

- How does it feel to know that an article may be inaccurate? (Sample answer: I was disappointed that people would print something that is inaccurate.)

- Some information you hear about drugs and alcohol is inaccurate. What methods can you use to determine if information you hear about drugs is accurate or inaccurate? (Sample answers: I could do research on drugs and alcohol, or I could ask a doctor for more information.)

- What should you do if you hear some information about drugs from a friend? (Sample answer: I would try to determine if it was true before believing it.)

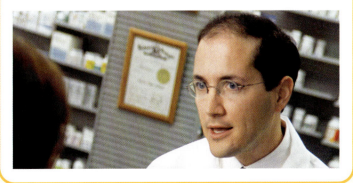

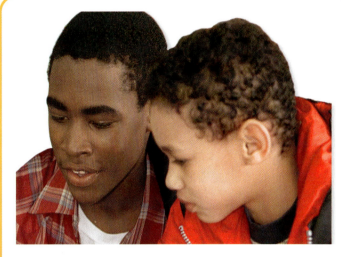

Working Together to Stay Drug Free

Hands on

Procedure Organize the class into teams of four. Provide a large open space for the students to work in. Blindfold all students. Then, give each team a rope that is at least 20 feet long. Tell students that each team has to make a square using a rope, with each team member holding one corner of the square. Tell students that they need to discuss their strategy and plan how to proceed. Explain that they can talk to each other and help each other until they have succeeded but that they cannot remove the blindfolds until instructed to do so.

Analysis Ask students the following questions:

- What positive things took place in your group? (Answers may vary. Sample answer: We worked together to accomplish a group goal.)

- Did you succeed in creating a square? What strategies helped or hindered making the square? (Answers may vary. Sample answer: We were able to make the square because one person walked along the rope to make sure it was in the right shape.)

- What does this activity teach you about solving problems versus turning to drugs or alcohol? (Answers may vary. Sample answer: If you become stressed or frustrated when trying to reach a goal, you can ask other people for help or support. As a result, you won't be tempted to use drugs or alcohol to relieve your stress.)

Chapter 13 • Activities 267F

CHAPTER 13

Overview
Tell students that this chapter will help them learn about drugs and how drugs are used, misused, and abused. Students will learn about the use of drugs as prescription and over-the-counter medicines. Students will also learn about specific types of drugs, including stimulants, depressants, marijuana, inhalants, and hallucinogens. Finally, students learn ways to stay drug free.

Assessing Prior Knowledge
Students should be familiar with the following topics:
- refusal skills
- decision-making skills
- communication skills
- health effects of tobacco smoke

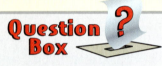

Students may feel more comfortable asking questions if you set up a Question Box to collect their questions. Have students write and anonymously submit their questions about drugs, medicine, and drug abuse. Address these questions during class, or use these questions to introduce lessons that cover related topics.

Current Health
Check out *Current Health* articles and activities related to this chapter by visiting the HRW Web site at **go.hrw.com.** Just type in the keyword **HD4CH28T.**

Chapter Resource File
- Directed Reading **BASIC**
- Health Inventory **GENERAL**
- Parent Letter

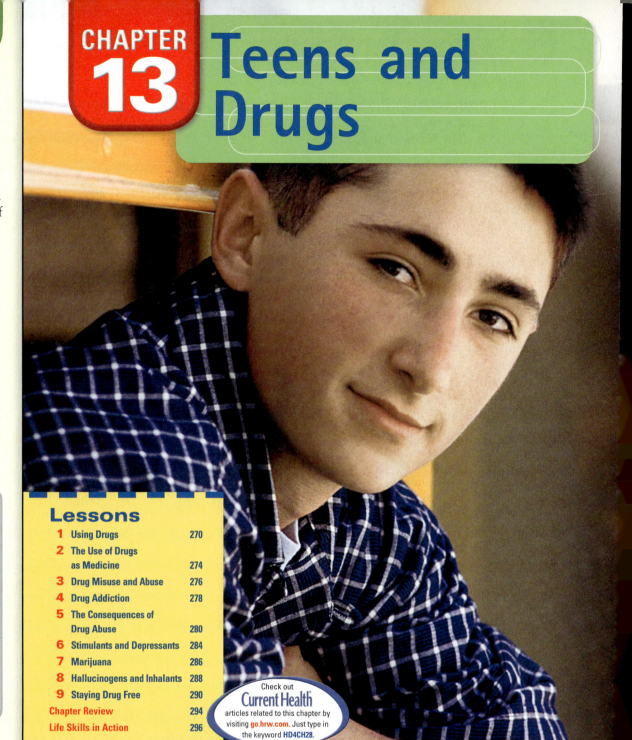

CHAPTER 13 Teens and Drugs

Lessons
1	Using Drugs	270
2	The Use of Drugs as Medicine	274
3	Drug Misuse and Abuse	276
4	Drug Addiction	278
5	The Consequences of Drug Abuse	280
6	Stimulants and Depressants	284
7	Marijuana	286
8	Hallucinogens and Inhalants	288
9	Staying Drug Free	290
Chapter Review		294
Life Skills in Action		296

Check out **Current Health** articles related to this chapter by visiting **go.hrw.com.** Just type in the keyword **HD4CH28.**

Standards Correlations

National Health Education Standards

3.6 Demonstrate ways to avoid and reduce threatening situations (Lesson 9)

6.3 Predict how decisions regarding health behaviors have consequences for self and others. (Lesson 5)

" I used to be the **best player** on my school's **basketball** team. Then, I started **smoking marijuana.** Before long, I got out of breath whenever I played. I also started skipping practice to go smoke marijuana with my friends. Last week, the coach told me that I was off the team. I wish I had never started using drugs. "

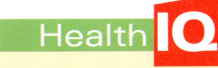

PRE-READING
Answer the following multiple-choice questions to find out what you already know about drugs. When you've finished this chapter, you'll have the opportunity to change your answers based on what you've learned.

1. Which of the following statements about drugs is true?
   a. Food is a drug.
   b. A medicine is not a drug.
   c. Drugs do not provide your body with any nutrients that you need to live.
   d. All drugs can be purchased legally with a prescription.

2. Which statement about prescription drugs is NOT true?
   a. You need a doctor's approval to use prescription drugs.
   b. Prescription drugs should never be shared with another person.
   c. People can get addicted to prescription drugs.
   d. Prescription drugs are always legal, even if they are used improperly.

3. When a person's body has a chemical need for a drug, the person has
   a. a physical dependence.
   b. a psychological dependence.
   c. a drug prescription.
   d. used a stimulant.

4. Marijuana is
   a. made in a laboratory.
   b. a plant.
   c. harmless if it is used properly.
   d. a relatively new drug.

5. Which of the following statements is a good reason to avoid drugs?
   a. Drugs are illegal.
   b. Using drugs can damage your relationships.
   c. Drugs can damage your health.
   d. all of the above

6. Ways to refuse drugs include
   a. saying, "No, thank you."
   b. giving a reason.
   c. suggesting another activity.
   d. All of the above

ANSWERS: 1. c; 2. d; 3. a; 4. b; 5. d; 6. d

Using the Health IQ

Misconception Alert
Answers to the Health IQ questions may help you identify students' misconceptions.

Question 2: Students may not think that prescription drugs can be addictive. Tell students that many prescription drugs—especially opiate painkillers—can be addictive. Because of this, patients must always follow their doctors' instructions when taking prescription medicine.

Question 4: Some students may believe that marijuana is harmless because it is a natural drug. Tell students that marijuana causes physical and psychological problems. For example, marijuana use can decrease a person's coordination, motivation, and ability to concentrate. Furthermore, people who use marijuana for a long time can become dependent on it.

Answers
1. c
2. d
3. a
4. b
5. d
6. d

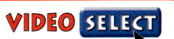

For information about videos related to this chapter, go to **go.hrw.com** and type in the keyword **HD4DR7V**.

Chapter 13 • Teens and Drugs

Lesson 1

Focus

Overview
Before beginning this lesson, review with your students the objectives listed under the What You'll Do head in the Student Edition. In this lesson, students will learn the definition of the term *drug*. Students will also learn different ways that drugs are taken into the body.

Bellringer
Ask students to list four different substances that they have taken into their body. Next to each substance, have students write whether or not the substance is a drug. (Accept all reasonable answers. Sample answer: food—not a drug, drinks—not a drug, medicines—drug, and air—not a drug. Students may note that certain foods and drinks contain drugs.) **LS Logical**

Answer to Start Off Write
Accept all reasonable answers. Sample answer: Drugs can be taken orally, by injection, by smoking, or by inhaling.

Motivate

Activity — GENERAL
Poster Project Have groups of students brainstorm a list of common drugs and a list of substances that are taken into the body that are not drugs. Then, have students create a poster that illustrates how to distinguish between substances that are drugs and those that are not drugs. **LS Visual**

Lesson 1: Using Drugs

What You'll Do
- **Explain** what a drug is.
- **Describe** five different ways in which drugs can enter the body.

Terms to Learn
- drug

Write
What are some ways that drugs can be taken?

Jamal's head was pounding. Jamal had a math test and a big soccer game that day. He was afraid that with the headache, he wouldn't be able to pass the test or run well. Jamal's mother gave him a painkiller, and his headache went away. Did Jamal use a drug?

When he took the painkiller, Jamal used a drug. A **drug** is any substance other than food that changes a person's physical or psychological state. When many people think of drugs, they think of harmful, illegal drugs that can cause serious problems. But there are many different kinds of drugs. Some, such as aspirin and other painkillers, are legal. Others, such as marijuana and cocaine, are illegal. It can also be easy to forget that many drugs, such as the painkiller that cured Jamal's headache, are used to treat diseases and pain. So, what exactly is a drug?

Is It a Drug or Not?

Not everything you take into your body is considered a drug. Food and water provide your body with chemicals, vitamins, and nutrients that your body needs to live. Without food and water, you cannot survive. Unlike food, drugs do not provide your body with any nutrients that are necessary for life. But many foods do contain drugs, although food itself is not a drug. For example, chocolate and cola both contain the drug caffeine.

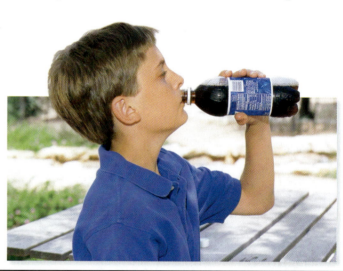
Figure 1 Drugs are contained in many products, including the soft drink that this teen is drinking.

Practicing Wellness The body needs six basic nutrients for survival: proteins, carbohydrates, fats, vitamins, minerals, and water. All six of these nutrients can be found in foods. Encourage interested students to research the essential nutrients and to determine how the body uses them. Have students summarize their findings in a report. **LS Logical**

Chapter Resource File
- Directed Reading BASIC
- Lesson Plan
- Lesson Quiz GENERAL

Transparencies
TT Bellringer

Taking Drugs Orally

The painkiller that Jamal took was taken *orally*, which means that it was taken through the mouth. Swallowing, chewing, and drinking are all ways of taking drugs orally. These are the simplest ways to take drugs. Drugs taken orally may be pills, capsules, or liquid. Pills, sometimes called *tablets*, are medicine in a solid form. Capsules are tiny containers that hold a drug in powdered or liquid form.

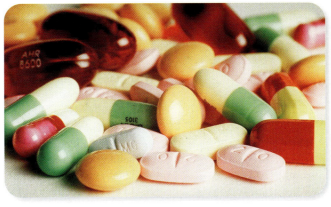

Figure 2 Many drugs can be taken orally.

After a pill or a capsule is swallowed, it is dissolved by the chemicals in the stomach. The medicine is absorbed from the stomach into the bloodstream. The blood carries the drug to the body's cells, where it begins to take effect.

Some capsules have a coating that makes them dissolve more slowly. These capsules are called *controlled-release capsules*. A controlled-release capsule allows the body's cells to take in the medicine over a long period of time, rather than all at once. These capsules enter the small intestine. There, as the container dissolves, the medicine is absorbed slowly into the bloodsteam.

Taking Drugs by Injection

At some point in your life, you have probably gotten a shot—and you probably didn't like it. A shot is an injection of a drug into the body through a special needle called a *hypodermic needle* (HIE poh DUHR mik NEED'l). A doctor often gives an injection when he or she wants a drug to act quickly or when a drug won't work properly if it is taken orally. Drugs are usually injected into a muscle in the thigh, upper arm, or buttocks. On rare occasions, drugs are injected directly into a vein.

Some illegal drugs are taken by injection. Injection is the fastest and most powerful way for the drug to reach the brain. People who abuse injected drugs usually inject the drugs directly into a vein to get a greater effect from the drug. They also often share hypodermic needles. If one person has an infectious disease, he or she can pass the disease to others who use the same needle.

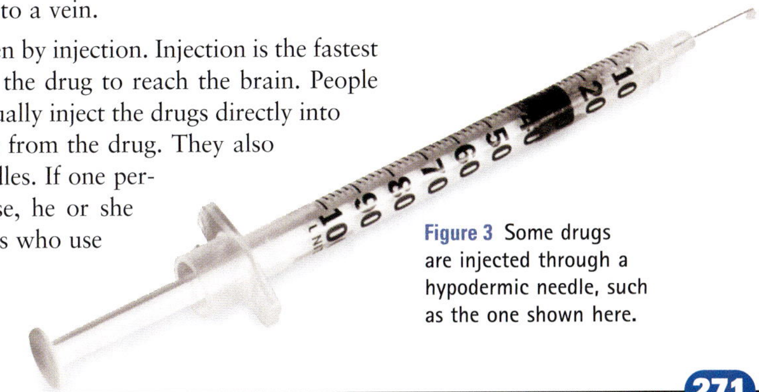

Figure 3 Some drugs are injected through a hypodermic needle, such as the one shown here.

Teach

READING SKILL BUILDER — BASIC

Anticipation Guide Before students read this lesson, ask them to predict the answers to the following true/false questions:

- Some drugs are necessary nutrients for life. (false)
- Drugs given with a needle are usually injected directly into a vein. (false)
- Some illegal drugs are taken by injection. (true)
- Smoking drugs is different from inhaling drugs. (true)
- All drugs enter the bloodstream. (false)

Give students a chance to review the questions and their answers after they finish reading the lesson. **LS Verbal**

Demonstration — GENERAL

Drugs Taken Orally Display a variety of oral medicines in the front of the room. Be sure to have pills, capsules, gel tablets, chewable pills, liquids, and medicine for children in the form of a lollypop. Tell students that the medicines they see are examples of the many ways a person can take drugs through the mouth. Explain that some oral medicines can be found in different forms because some people have difficulties swallowing pills and other people dislike the taste of liquids. Show students the lollypop, and ask them why medicine in this form is both good and bad. (Sample answer: It is good because it makes it easy for a child to take medicine. It is bad because the child may think it is candy and eat it when he or she is not sick.) If you wish, you can open a capsule or cut open a gel tablet so that students can see what is inside. When doing this, be sure to wear protective gloves and safety goggles. **LS Visual**

Life SKILL BUILDER — ADVANCED

Evaluating Media Messages Have students cut out two media messages about drugs from magazines or newspapers. Tell them to find one positive message and one negative message. Ask students the following questions:

- What are the differences between the positive message and the negative message?
- What ideas are conveyed by each media message?
- What are the sources of each message?
- Do you believe what each message is telling you? Explain your reasoning. **LS Logical**

LIFE SCIENCE CONNECTION — GENERAL

Into the Bloodstream After a drug is taken into the body, the drug enters the bloodstream. The blood carries the drug to body cells in different parts of the body. Most drugs pass through cell membranes into cells, where the drugs affect the cells in some way. Display a diagram of the human body that shows the internal organs. Have volunteers trace the path that drugs follow to get to certain body cells. Repeat this process for the five ways that drugs are taken into the body. **Note:** Topical drugs, such as ointments and eyedrops, do not enter the bloodstream. **LS Visual**

Lesson 1 • Using Drugs

Teach, continued

Debate — ADVANCED
Tobacco and Television Tell students that TV commercials for cigarettes and other tobacco products used to be very common until they were banned in 1969. However, people can still see actors of all ages smoking cigarettes on TV shows. Encourage interested students to research the effects of media messages about smoking on teens. Then, have students debate the benefits and drawbacks of having characters smoking on TV shows. **LS Verbal**

Demonstration — BASIC
Inhalers Have a student with asthma demonstrate how his or her inhaler works. Explain to the class what asthma is and why inhalers are the fastest way to deliver medicine to the lungs. Tell the class that asthma is a very common condition in people of all ages. Also tell students that people with asthma usually carry their inhalers with them at all times and that the inhalers allow them to live normal lives. Finally, warn students never to borrow their friend's inhaler. If a student thinks he or she might have asthma, he or she should see a doctor. **LS Visual**

Activity — GENERAL
Role-Play Have students role-play the following scenario: "Mario has a part-time job in a convenience store. Peter comes in and wants to buy cigarettes. Mario thinks that Peter is too young to buy cigarettes, but Peter insists that he is old enough. What should Mario do?" **LS Kinesthetic**

Myth & Fact
Myth: Using tobacco in the form of chewing tobacco or snuff is much safer than smoking.

Fact: Although chewing tobacco doesn't cause lung diseases like smoking does, it does cause other serious diseases, such as mouth cancer.

Taking Drugs by Smoking
Nicotine, which is found in tobacco, is the most common drug that is smoked. Some illegal drugs, such as marijuana and crack cocaine, are also smoked. When a person smokes, the chemicals in the drug enter the lungs and pass through tiny blood vessels into the bloodstream. From there, they are carried throughout the body.

All smoke contains poisonous substances. Tobacco smoke contains nicotine, carbon monoxide, and tar. Tar increases the smoker's chance of getting lung diseases, such as cancer and emphysema (EM fuh SEE muh). Carbon monoxide increases the likelihood of heart disease and blood vessel disease. Regular use of marijuana has effects on the lungs that are similar to those caused by tobacco.

Inhaling Drugs
If you or a friend has asthma, you are probably familiar with taking a drug by inhaling, which means breathing in the drug. Some drugs, such as those used to treat asthma, are stored in air or gas and are then breathed in through a device called an *inhaler*. Each time the inhaler is pumped, a certain amount of the drug is released. After the drug is inhaled into the lungs, it is absorbed into the bloodstream and taken to the body cells. Other drugs, such as those used to relieve nasal congestion, are dissolved in water and inhaled through the nose. In an operating room or a dentist's office, anesthetics (AN es THEHT iks)—drugs used to numb patients during medical procedures—are sometimes given by having the patient inhale the drugs.

Inhaling drugs is different from taking in drugs by smoking. When a drug is inhaled, the user breathes the drug directly into the lungs. In smoking, the drug is burned, and the resulting smoke is then inhaled.

Many harmful drugs, such as nitrous oxide, are abused by inhaling. Inhaling substances to get "high" is extremely dangerous. In fact, it can cause heart failure, brain damage, suffocation, and instant death.

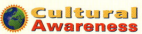

Figure 4 This teen is treating her asthma by using an inhaled drug.

Background
Needle-Free Vaccines Because most people hate receiving shots, scientists are currently working on developing new ways to administer medicines and vaccines through the skin. One method is a skin patch that has hundreds of short, tiny needles that pierce the top layer of skin and deliver medicine to the bloodstream without any pain. Another painless method uses a helium gas jet to force powdered medicines through the skin.

Cultural Awareness — ADVANCED
Folk Remedies Some of the medicines used today were developed from folk remedies known to different cultures from around the world. For example, scientists are developing a weight loss drug from a cactus plant found in southwest Africa. The plant is called *hoodia* and was identified by a nomadic tribe called the San. The San use hoodia to stave off hunger and thirst during long journeys. Have students research folk remedies that led to the development of drugs. Students can summarize their findings in a report. **LS Verbal**

Other Ways That Drugs Are Taken

There are many other ways to take drugs. One way is called a *transdermal patch* (tranz DUHR muhl PACH). A transdermal patch sticks to the skin like a bandage. The medicine contained in the patch is slowly released into the skin and absorbed into the bloodstream.

Some drugs do not need to enter the bloodstream to be effective. For example, ointments are applied directly to the skin and do not enter the bloodstream. Drops of medicine used for infections in the ears or eyes also do not enter the bloodstream.

Same Drug, Different Forms

Some drugs can be taken in more than one form. The way in which a drug is taken can change the effects it has. For example, the antibiotic drug penicillin may be taken orally in either pill or liquid form, or it may be injected. When penicillin is injected, it has a much stronger and faster effect than when it is taken orally. Another example is nicotine, which is generally taken by smoking cigarettes or is taken orally in the form of chewing tobacco. People who are trying to stop smoking may take nicotine orally by chewing nicotine gum. Or they may use a transdermal patch, which releases nicotine slowly through the skin. Nicotine gum and transdermal patches do not hurt the body as much as tobacco does because they do not contain many of the poisons that tobacco contains.

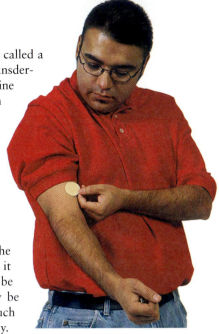

Figure 5 This patch is delivering medicine to the body through the skin.

Lesson Review

Using Vocabulary

1. What is a drug?

Understanding Concepts

2. What are five different ways that drugs can be taken?
3. How do medicines and other drugs get to the body's cells?
4. Do all drugs enter the bloodstream? Explain.

Critical Thinking

5. **Analyzing Ideas** Chocolate contains caffeine, but chocolate is also food. If you eat chocolate, are you taking a drug? Explain your answer.
6. **Making Good Decisions** Imagine that you have a bad headache. Your father offers you a choice between medicine in a liquid form and medicine in a controlled-release capsule. Which would you choose? Explain your answer.

internet connect
www.scilinks.org/health
Topic: Drugs
HealthLinks code: HD4030
HEALTH LINKS. Maintained by the National Science Teachers Association

Lesson 2 Focus

Overview

Before beginning this lesson, review with your students the objectives listed under the What You'll Do head in the Student Edition. In this lesson, students will learn how drugs are used as medicines and how to distinguish between prescription and over-the-counter medicines.

Bellringer

Have students list five medicines that can be purchased without a doctor's permission. **(Sample answer: aspirin, cough drops, antibiotic ointments, nasal sprays, and rubbing alcohol)** LS Logical

Answer to Start Off Write

Accept all reasonable answers. Sample answer: Some medicines require a doctor's permission and supervision. Other medicines don't require a doctor's permission because they are safer and are taken in smaller doses than prescription medicines are.

Motivate

Life SKILL BUILDER — GENERAL

Being a Wise Consumer Tell students that there are many different over-the-counter medicines available in drugs stores and grocery stores. Ask students to describe how they could determine which medicine to buy to treat a cold. **(Sample answer: Different cold medicines often relieve different symptoms. I would read the labels of the medicines to find medicines that treat only the symptoms that I have. I could also ask a pharmacist to help me find the right medicine.)** LS Logical

Lesson 2 — The Use of Drugs as Medicine

What You'll Do

- **Explain** the difference between prescription medicines and over-the-counter medicines.

Terms to Learn

- medicine
- prescription medicine
- over-the-counter medicine

Start Off Write

Why must you have a prescription to buy certain medicines, but not to buy others?

Brain Food

The Rx symbol that often appears on prescription medicine labels stands for the word *recipe*, which means "to take" in Latin. Pharmacists now use the symbol to indicate that a medicine can be bought only with a prescription.

Melissa had a bad cough. She took cough medicine from the drugstore, but it didn't help. When Melissa went to the doctor, he gave her a different cough medicine. Melissa soon started to feel better.

Many drugs are used as medicine. A **medicine** is any substance used to treat disease, injury, or pain. Different kinds of medicine are used to treat different problems. As Melissa discovered, treating an illness or a disease requires finding the right medicine.

Prescription Medicine

Medicine that can be bought only if a doctor orders its use is called **prescription medicine.** To get prescription medicine, you must have written instructions from your doctor, known as a *prescription* (pree SKRIP shuhn). A prescription contains the patient's name, the medicine's name, and the doctor's signature. It also contains information on the proper dosage (DOHS ij), or how much of the medicine to take and when to take it. As with any medicine, taking prescription medicine exactly as instructed is important. Taking too much of the drug can be harmful. Taking too little of the drug or taking it incorrectly can keep it from working.

Figure 6 Reading a Prescription Medicine Label

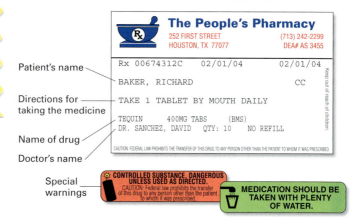

INCLUSION Strategies — GENERAL

- Developmentally Delayed
- Learning Disabled

Some students may be unsure of which medicines are over-the-counter medicines and which are prescription medicines. Help clarify this difference by reading drug names or types of drugs to the class and by having students identify whether each is available as a prescription medicine, an over-the-counter (OTC) medicine, or both. Some possible medicines include aspirin **(OTC)**, cough syrup **(both)**, penicillin **(prescription)**, calamine lotion **(OTC)**, allergy medicine **(both)**, and asthma medicine **(prescription)**. LS Logical

Chapter Resource File

- Directed Reading BASIC
- Lesson Plan
- Lesson Quiz GENERAL

Transparencies

- TT Bellringer
- TT Reading a Prescription Medicine Label

274 Chapter 13 • Teens and Drugs

Figure 7 Reading an Over-the-Counter Medicine Label

List of ingredients

Directions for taking the medicine

Special warnings

COUGH SUPPRESSANT/EXPECTORANT
ACTIVE INGREDIENTS (in each 5 mL tsp): Dextromethorphan HBr, USP 10 mg; Guaifenesin, USP 100 mg. See carton for complete list of inactive ingredients.
USES: Temporarily relieves cough due to minor throat and bronchial irritation as may occur with a cold; helps loosen phlegm (mucus) and thin bronchial secretions to make coughs more productive.
DIRECTIONS: Do not take more than 6 doses in any 24 hour period. Adults and children 12 years and over — 2 teaspoonfuls every 4 hours as needed. Children 6–12 years of age —1 teaspoonful every 4 hours as needed.
WARNINGS: Do not take if you are now taking a prescription monoamine oxidase inhibitor (MAOI) (certain drugs for depression, psychiatric, or emotional conditions, or Parkinson's disease), or for 2 weeks after stopping the MAOI drug. If you do not know if your prescription drug contains MAOI, ask a doctor or pharmacist before taking this product.
Keep this and all drugs out of reach of children. In case of accidental overdose, get medical help or contact a poison control center immediately.
Store at 20-25°C (68-77°F), alcohol free, dosage cup provided.
Made in U.S.A. 8685-22/21A
LOT 011954 Exp 5 2004

Over-the-Counter Medicine

Any medicine that can be purchased without a prescription is called **over-the-counter medicine.** These drugs are sold without a prescription because they are safer and are in smaller doses than prescription medicines are. Thousands of over-the-counter medicines exist, including pain relievers and cold and cough medicines.

If used improperly, over-the-counter medicines can be harmful. You should take over-the-counter medicines just as carefully as you take prescription medicines. Following the medicine's instructions is important. Make sure you take the right dosage at the right time. Taking too much of any medicine, even an over-the-counter medicine, can be very dangerous.

Health Journal
Write about a time when you used an over-the-counter medicine to treat pain or an illness. How did you feel after taking the medicine?

Lesson Review

Using Vocabulary
1. What is a medicine?
2. What is the difference between prescription medicines and over-the-counter medicines?

Understanding Concepts
3. What information is included in a prescription?

Critical Thinking
4. **Making Inferences** Some medicines are sold in both prescription and over-the-counter forms. What might be the difference between these forms?
5. **Analyzing Ideas** Why is it important for a prescription to contain a doctor's signature?

Answers to Lesson Review
1. A medicine is any substance used to treat disease, injury, or pain.
2. Prescription medicines can be bought only with a doctor's permission, but over-the-counter medicines can be purchased at any time.
3. A prescription contains the patient's name, the medicine's name, the doctor's signature, the proper dosage, and information about when to take the medicine.
4. Accept all reasonable answers. Sample answer: The prescription form may have more of the amount of medicine in it.
5. Accept all reasonable answers. Sample answer: The doctor's signature shows the person who is selling the medicine that a patient is allowed to take the medicine and is under a doctor's supervision.

Teach

Activity — BASIC
Reading Labels Provide students with empty containers from a variety of over-the-counter medicines, including eardrops and ointments. Have students group each medicine by how it is taken. Have students read the labels and record the name of each medicine, the recommended dose, and the possible side effects of each medicine.
LS Verbal

Answer to Health Journal
Answers may vary. This Health Journal may be a good way to close the lesson.

Close

Reteaching — BASIC
Dosage Schedule Write the following dosage for a medicine on the board: "This medicine must be taken five times a day and must be taken at least one hour before eating or two hours after eating." Have students create a schedule of meal times and times that the medicine should be taken. (Sample answer: 7 A.M., medicine; 8 A.M., breakfast; 11 A.M., medicine; 12 noon, lunch; 2 P.M., medicine; 5 P.M. medicine; 6 P.M., dinner; 9 P.M. medicine) Ask students to explain why it is important to stick to the schedule. (Sample answer: It is important to follow directions when taking any medicine.) **LS** Logical

Quiz — GENERAL
1. What is a prescription medicine? (medicine that can only be bought and taken if a doctor orders its use)
2. What can happen if the wrong amount of a drug is taken? (Too much of a drug can be harmful, and not enough may keep it from working properly.)
3. What should you do if you are taking an over-the-counter medicine? (You should read and follow the medicine's instructions.)

Lesson 2 • The Use of Drugs as Medicine

Lesson 3

Focus

Overview
Before beginning this lesson, review with your students the objectives listed under the What You'll Do head in the Student Edition. In this lesson, students will learn how to distinguish between drug misuse and drug abuse. Students will also learn four rules for taking medicines properly.

Bellringer
Have students list three things they should do when taking a medicine to treat an illness. (Accept all reasonable answers. Sample answer: I should take the correct dosage, take it at the correct time, and use it only for its proper purpose.) **LS** Logical

Answer to Start Off Write
Accept all reasonable answers. Sample answer: The first thing you should do is read the instructions and make sure that you understand them.

Motivate

Activity — GENERAL
Skit Have students work in small groups to write and perform a skit about a teen who starts using a medicine properly and then begins to misuse it. After students present their skits to the class, lead a discussion on how to avoid misusing medicines.
LS Kinesthetic

Lesson 3 — Drug Misuse and Abuse

What You'll Do
- Explain what drug misuse is.
- List four rules for using medicines properly.
- Explain how drug misuse can turn into drug abuse.

Terms to Learn
- drug misuse
- drug abuse

Start Off Write
What should you do before you take any medicine? Explain.

Tyla had allergies and she took an allergy medicine to stop her symptoms. But she also liked the way the medicine made her feel. Pretty soon, she was ignoring the instructions and taking the medicine whenever she felt like it. Before long, she was taking it all the time.

When Tyla started ignoring the instructions that came with her medicine, she began misusing the medicine. Pretty soon, this misuse turned into abuse.

Using Medicines Improperly

Any use of a medicine that is different from the intended use is **drug misuse.** This includes not following the directions. Whenever you take any kind of medicine, take it exactly as instructed. Misuse can sometimes lead to overdose, drug abuse, or addiction. If you're not sure how to take a medicine, talk to your doctor or pharmacist. When taking medicine, follow these rules:

- Follow all instructions, not just the ones that are convenient.
- Never increase the amount of the medicine that you take without your doctor's permission.
- Don't stop taking a prescription medication without your doctor's permission, even if your symptoms are gone.
- Never take someone else's prescription medicine.

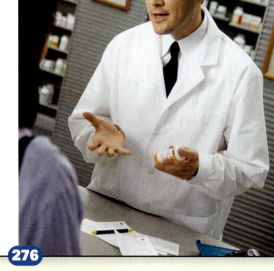

Figure 8 If you have questions about how to take a medicine properly, you may talk to a pharmacist.

INCLUSION Strategies — GENERAL
- Learning Disabled   • Developmentally Delayed

Students with learning disabilities or developmental delays may have difficulties reading and comprehending complicated information, such as the directions for taking medicines. Review specific directions from a selection of common over-the-counter medications, and explain what each direction means. Then, ask students to work in pairs to discuss when a person would use each medicine.

Chapter Resource File
- Directed Reading BASIC
- Lesson Plan
- Lesson Quiz GENERAL

Transparencies
TT Bellringer

---

276   Chapter 13 • Teens and Drugs

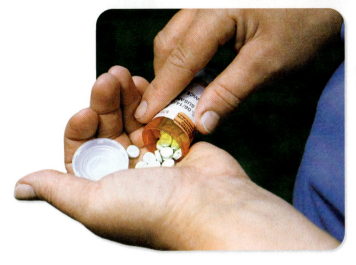

Figure 9 Misusing a drug can sometimes lead to drug abuse.

When Does Misuse Become Abuse?

When Tyla started taking her cough medicine to feel good rather than to stop coughing, she started abusing the drug. **Drug abuse** is misusing a legal drug on purpose or using any illegal drug. Misuse of a drug often involves taking too much of the drug. The person becomes used to the higher dosage and craves more of the drug when he or she takes the correct dosage. The person begins to take more of the drug more often. This is how drug abuse often starts.

People abuse drugs for many reasons. Often, like Tyla, they like how the drug makes them feel. Sometimes, people abuse a drug because they feel that the drug helps them perform better. All drugs are dangerous if misused or abused. If you think you have been misusing or abusing a drug, talk to a doctor or a trusted adult right away.

LIFE SKILLS ACTIVITY

PRACTICING WELLNESS

Find an over-the-counter medicine at your home. Read the instructions for taking this medicine. How much should be taken? How often? Are there any special warnings?

Lesson Review

Using Vocabulary
1. What is drug misuse?
2. In your own words, explain the difference between drug misuse and drug abuse.

Understanding Concepts
3. What kinds of medicines can be misused or abused?
4. Describe how drug misuse can lead to drug abuse.

Critical Thinking
5. **Making Inferences** Steven lost the label from his bottle of prescription medicine. How could this lead to drug misuse?

internet connect
www.scilinks.org/health
Topic: Medicine Safety
HealthLinks code: HD4066
HEALTH LINKS. Maintained by the National Science Teachers Association

Lesson 3 • Drug Misuse and Abuse 277

Lesson 4 Focus

Overview
Before beginning this lesson, review with your students the objectives listed under the What You'll Do head in the Student Edition. In this lesson, students learn what drug addiction is and how it happens. Students also learn the difference between physical and psychological addiction.

Bellringer
Ask students to explain the difference between the adjectives *psychological* and *physical*. (Sample answer: *Psychological* refers to emotions or a person's mental state, and *physical* refers to the body.)

Motivate

Group Activity — GENERAL
Poster Project Ask students to research how a drug addiction affected the life of someone famous, such as a sports star or an actor. Have students answer the following questions: How did the addiction affect the person's career and relationships? How did the person start getting involved with drugs? Was the person able to overcome his or her addiction? How? Have students present the information they gathered in a poster. They can include pictures of their chosen celebrity, timelines of the person's career and drug usage, and—in the case of sports stars—statistics of the athlete's performance on the playing field. Display these posters in the hallway to share with all the students in the school. **LS Visual**

Lesson 4

What You'll Do
- **Describe** what drug addiction is, and explain how it happens.
- **Describe** the difference between physical dependence and psychological dependence.

Terms to Learn
- drug addiction
- withdrawal
- physical dependence
- psychological dependence

Start Off Write
Why is it difficult for some people to stop abusing drugs?

Drug Addiction

Tom had knee surgery and was given a prescription painkiller. At first, he liked the way the medicine relieved his pain. But soon, he found that he had to take more of the medicine to feel better and would become anxious if he didn't take it.

Tom couldn't stop taking his medicine because he was addicted to it. Tom's addiction happened very quickly, and it made him do things he would not have done before, such as misusing the medicine. But how did Tom's addiction happen?

What Is Addiction?
The effects that some drugs produce can cause people to want to use the drug over and over. When a person cannot control his or her use of a drug, that person has a drug addiction. **Drug addiction** is the uncontrollable use of a drug. Someone who is addicted to a drug continues to take it even if the drug is harming his or her health and relationships.

A person with an addiction cannot control his or her use of a drug because he or she has become dependent on the drug. *Dependence* on a drug means needing the drug in order to function properly. If the person stops taking the drug, he or she will experience withdrawal. **Withdrawal** is the negative symptoms that result when a drug-dependent person stops taking a drug. There are two types of dependence: physical dependence and psychological dependence.

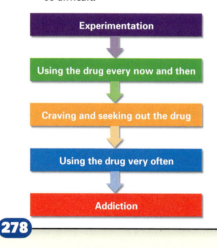

Figure 10 The path to drug addiction may be easy, but recovery can be difficult.

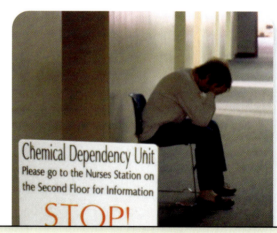

Answer to Start Off Write
Accept all reasonable answers. Sample answer: It is difficult for some people to stop abusing drugs because they are dependent on the drugs.

Chapter Resource File
- Directed Reading BASIC
- Lesson Plan
- Lesson Quiz GENERAL

Transparencies
TT Bellringer

Physical Dependence

When a person abuses a drug long enough, his or her body gets used to the drug. In fact, chemical changes take place in the body. These changes make the body need a regular supply of the drug to keep functioning normally. This type of dependence is called physical dependence. **Physical dependence** is the body's chemical need for a drug. If a person with a physical dependence suddenly stops taking the drug, he or she will quickly go into withdrawal. A person in physical withdrawal may experience vomiting, muscle and joint pain, fever, chills, anxiety, and many other symptoms.

Psychological Dependence

Some people are addicted to drugs without being physically dependent on the drug. This type of addiction is called psychological dependence. **Psychological** (SIE kuh LAHJ i kuhl) **dependence** is a person's emotional or mental need for a drug. A person with psychological dependence craves the drug and feels that he or she can't get along without the drug. Psychological dependence is sometimes even harder to overcome than physical dependence.

Psychological dependence can also cause withdrawal symptoms. These symptoms may include sleeplessness, nervousness, irritability, and depression.

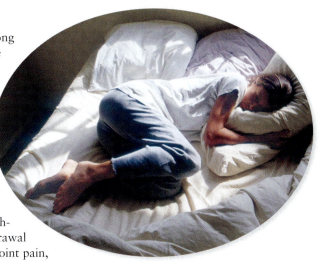

Figure 11 Even psychological dependence can lead to withdrawal symptoms, such as being unable to sleep.

Lesson Review

Using Vocabulary
1. What is drug addiction?
2. Describe the difference between physical and psychological dependence.
3. What is withdrawal? When does it happen?

Understanding Concepts
4. How does physical dependence happen?

Critical Thinking
5. **Analyzing Ideas** Is it possible to be addicted to a legal drug? Explain your answer.

internet connect
www.scilinks.org/health
Topic: Drug Addiction
HealthLinks code: HD4028
HEALTH LINKS. Maintained by the National Science Teachers Association

Answers to Lesson Review
1. Drug addiction is the uncontrollable use of a drug.
2. Physical dependence is the body's chemical need for a drug. Psychological dependence is a person's emotional or mental need for a drug.
3. Withdrawal is the negative symptoms that result when a drug-dependent person stops taking a drug.
4. Physical dependence happens when a person abuses a drug for a long time and his or her body gets used to it.
5. yes; People can become addicted to legal drugs such as nicotine. People who are addicted to nicotine suffer from withdrawal if they try to stop smoking.

Teach

Life SKILL BUILDER — GENERAL
Evaluating Media Messages
Show an episode of a TV show in which a main character (preferably a teen) becomes addicted to drugs. As students watch the show, have them take notes on the effect of the drug addiction and the character's recovery from the addiction. Ask students the following questions:
- How quickly did the character become addicted to drugs? Was it realistic?
- How did the character behave once he or she was addicted?
- How quickly did the character recover from the addiction? Was the recovery easy for the character?

Tell students that characters on TV shows usually recover from addictions much more rapidly and easily than a real person would. **LS Visual**

Close

Reteaching — BASIC
Dependence Have students write each of the various symptoms of physical dependence and psychological dependence on a separate index card. Have students place the cards face down and mix them up. As students turn each card over, have them put it into a pile marked "physical dependence" or "psychological dependence." **LS Logical**

Quiz — GENERAL
1. What does it mean to be dependent on a drug? (Dependence on a drug means that you need the drug in order to function properly.)
2. List four symptoms of physical withdrawal. (Symptoms of physical withdrawal include vomiting, muscle and joint pain, fever, chills, and anxiety.)
3. List four symptoms of psychological withdrawal. (Symptoms of psychological withdrawal include sleeplessness, nervousness, irritability, and depression.)

Lesson 4 • Drug Addiction

Lesson 5

Focus

Overview
Before beginning this lesson, review with your students the objectives listed under the What You'll Do head in the Student Edition. In this lesson, students will learn about the consequences that can result from drug abuse.

🔔 Bellringer
Have students write the term *DRUG ABUSE* vertically down the left side of a paper. Next to each letter, have them write a word or phrase that they associate with the term. For example, next to the letter *S*, they may write "stealing from others." **LS** Verbal

Answer to Start Off Write
Accept all reasonable answers. Sample answer: If you abuse drugs, you may have difficulties concentrating and your grades may drop.

Motivate

Discussion ——— GENERAL
A Family Affair Have students imagine a family in which one of the three teens in the family abuses drugs. Ask students to describe problems that may arise in the family. (Sample answer: The teen may steal from family members, may become violent, or may be difficult to get along with.) Ask students how the other people in the family may feel about the situation. (Sample answer: The parents may be worried about the teen, and the other teens may be angry with their sibling.) **LS** Interpersonal

---

Lesson 5 — The Consequences of Drug Abuse

What You'll Do
- **Describe** five types of problems that can arise because of drug abuse or addiction.

Start Off Write
How can drug abuse affect your performance in school?

Trish and her brother Doug used to talk about everything, but lately Doug has been acting strangely. Then, after Trish's last baby-sitting job, all the money was gone from her purse. Trish suspects that Doug stole the money to buy drugs, and she isn't sure she can trust him anymore.

When a person abuses or becomes addicted to drugs, his or her relationships usually suffer. But damaged relationships, such as the one between Trish and Doug, are just one of the consequences of abusing drugs.

Problems with Family and Friends

Drug abuse does not affect just the people using drugs. It also affects the people in their lives. Drug abuse causes changes in a person's behavior, which can lead to problems at home. Teens who use drugs are likely to show anger toward family members. People who abuse drugs often have serious mood swings, which can make them difficult to talk to. They may have violent outbursts and become verbally or even physically abusive. Because they need money for drugs, people who abuse drugs often steal from family members. All of these behaviors can permanently damage family relationships.

Problems with other people aren't limited to the family. Teenagers who abuse or become addicted to drugs lose interest in activities that were once important to them. They also may begin to care less about the friends with whom they shared these activities. Friendships fall apart. At first, people who abuse drugs will spend time with new friends who share their interest in drugs. Eventually, they may find that they do not have any friends at all.

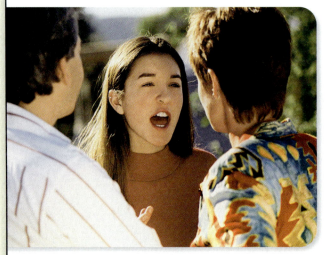

Figure 12 This teen's moods are affected by drug abuse. Her behavior is seriously damaging her family relationships.

REAL-LIFE CONNECTION ADVANCED

Many people have stereotypes of who they believe is a typical drug abuser. To help students understand that drug abuse affects all types of people, have interested students read stories about people who abused drugs. Such stories can be found in newspapers, magazines, and antidrug literature. Have students select a person from one of the stories and create a poster about that person. The posters should include information about the background of the person and about how he or she started using drugs. Display the posters around the room. **LS** Visual

Chapter Resource File
- Directed Reading **BASIC**
- Lesson Plan
- Lesson Quiz **GENERAL**

Transparencies
TT Bellringer
TT The Effects of Drug Abuse on the Body

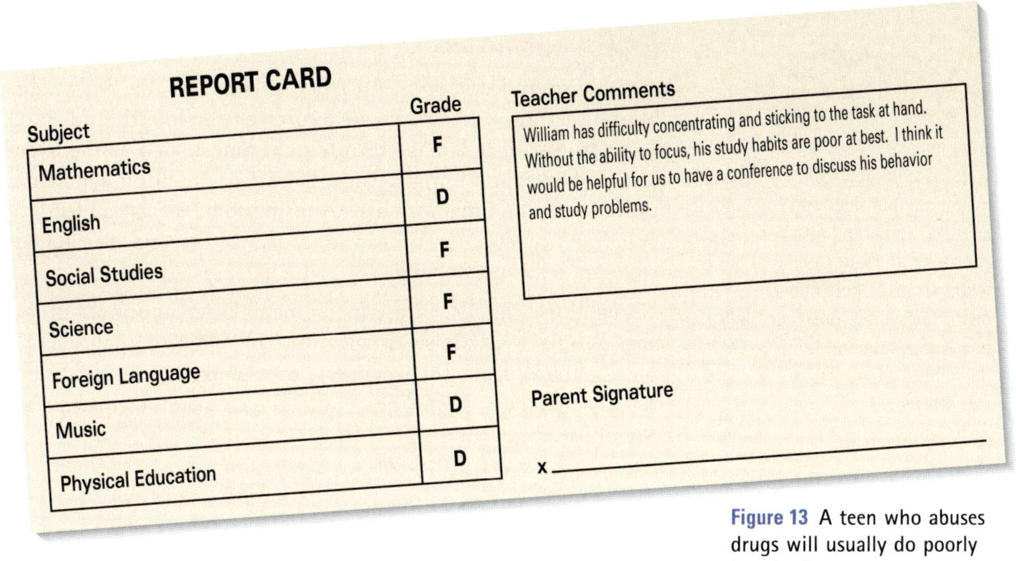

REPORT CARD

Subject	Grade
Mathematics	F
English	D
Social Studies	F
Science	F
Foreign Language	F
Music	D
Physical Education	D

Teacher Comments

William has difficulty concentrating and sticking to the task at hand. Without the ability to focus, his study habits are poor at best. I think it would be helpful for us to have a conference to discuss his behavior and study problems.

Parent Signature

x ______________________

Figure 13 A teen who abuses drugs will usually do poorly in school.

Problems at School

Most teens who abuse drugs begin to have serious problems at school. Most people who abuse drugs do not think or care about the future, and they lose their interest in education. In addition, learning becomes difficult for a person who abuses drugs. A person who abuses drugs will have difficulty concentrating, and he or she may forget from one day to the next what happened in class. Teens who abuse drugs usually stop doing homework, and their grades drop. They often skip school and school-related activities. When they are in school, they may interfere with the learning of others by disrupting classes. Teens who abuse drugs often get in trouble with school authorities. Many teens who abuse or become addicted to drugs eventually drop out of school.

Money Problems

Abusing drugs is expensive. Drugs cost a lot of money. As a person's drug problem gets worse, he or she will need more and more money. People who abuse or are addicted to drugs will often do anything to get money. Sometimes, the things they do are harmful to other people. They will lie or cheat. They will borrow or steal money or property from family members, friends, strangers, and even stores. A person who abuses drugs doesn't think about the possible consequences of these acts. To a person with a drug problem, respecting others' property is less important than getting drugs.

LIFE SKILLS ACTIVITY

MAKING GOOD DECISIONS

Research on the Internet or in the library how much money a person with a drug addiction spends on drugs each month. Then write a paper about how the money could be better spent. Give examples of other things that the money could be spent on.

281

MATH CONNECTION — GENERAL

The Cost of Drugs Have students do research to find out how much a person with a drug addiction may spend each day on drugs. Students may find information about the use of more than one kind of drug. Then, have students calculate how much addiction to a particular drug costs per week, per month, and per year. LS Logical

Life SKILL BUILDER — GENERAL

Practicing Wellness Lead a class discussion about how the consequences of drug abuse may provide clues to others that a person may be abusing drugs. Then, have students use these clues to create a poster illustrating the warning signs of drug abuse. Tell students that it is important for them to be able to recognize the signs of drug abuse. Tell students that if students suspect that someone they know is abusing drugs, they should tell a trusted adult. LS Interpersonal

Teach

Life SKILL BUILDER — GENERAL

Making Good Decisions Have students apply their decision-making skills to the following scenario: "You spend the night at your best friend's house. Your friend tells you that his or her older sister might be abusing drugs. Your friend also tells you that he or she isn't sure and wants you to keep it a secret. When you are home the next day, you discover that you are missing some money from your wallet. What should you do?" LS Intrapersonal

LIFE SKILLS ACTIVITY

Answer

Answers may vary.

Extension: Ask students how problems with money may affect an addicted person's relationships with others. (Sample answer: Money problems can hurt an addicted person's relationships with others because he or she may steal money or property from his or her friends and family.)

READING SKILL BUILDER — BASIC

Paired Reading Pair each student with a partner. Have the pairs read this lesson silently and use sticky notes to mark passages that they do not understand. After they finish reading, students should help each other understand passages that one or both marked with a sticky note. Have one student in each pair summarize the main ideas of the lesson aloud to his or her partner. Have the partner listen to the retelling and point out any mistakes and omissions in it. LS Verbal

Teach, continued

Using the Figure — GENERAL
The Effects of Drug Abuse on the Body Have students study the figure on this page of the Student Edition. Tell students that the figure shows only some of the physical effects of drug abuse. Tell students that drug abuse can also cause permanent damage to the liver and kidneys, and can cause mental and emotional problems. Finally, remind students that some permanently damaged organs can be replaced with transplanted organs, but tell them that finding healthy organs to use is difficult and many people die every year waiting for transplants. **LS Visual**

Group Activity — ADVANCED
Drugs and Death Ask interested students to investigate the connection between drugs and the leading causes of death and injury among teens. One student may contact the local police station for information, another may contact a local chapter of SADD or MADD, and a third may do research on the Internet. Have students pool their information and write a report to present to the class. Have them include a pie chart or other visual of the data they collected. **LS Verbal** Co-op Learning

MISCONCEPTION ALERT
Some students may think that drugs that come from natural sources are safe. Explain to students that many drugs that come from natural sources are not safe. Marijuana and opiates are examples of dangerous drugs that come from natural sources.

SCIENCE ACTIVITY
Drug abuse can damage your internal organs, including your liver and kidneys. Research how your liver and kidneys work. Write a short paper describing what your liver and kidneys do and how damage to these organs could affect the way your body works.

Answer to Science Activity
Accept all reasonable answers. Sample answer: The liver aids in digestion and stores glucose, vitamins, and minerals. The liver also removes drugs and alcohol from the blood. The kidneys have several functions including maintaining fluid levels in the body and filtering blood to remove poisons and waste materials. Damage to either the liver or kidneys can cause drugs and poisons to build up in the body.

Health Problems

Drug abuse and addiction are very harmful to the body. The abuse of certain drugs may cause sores on the mouth and skin. Many drugs cause damage to internal organs, such as the liver, kidneys, heart, and brain. Drugs that affect the brain can cause brain damage and memory loss. Abusing some drugs can lead to dangerous infections. For example, using dirty needles to do drugs can lead to HIV infection, which causes AIDS.

Drug abuse can also cause many mental and emotional problems. People who abuse drugs run a high risk of depression. Emotional problems, such as nervousness and fear, are also common. The chances of suicide or attempted suicide increase with drug abuse.

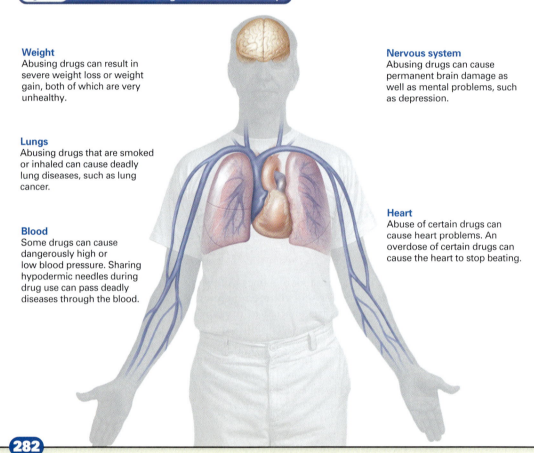

Figure 14 The Effects of Drug Abuse on the Body

Weight Abusing drugs can result in severe weight loss or weight gain, both of which are very unhealthy.

Lungs Abusing drugs that are smoked or inhaled can cause deadly lung diseases, such as lung cancer.

Blood Some drugs can cause dangerously high or low blood pressure. Sharing hypodermic needles during drug use can pass deadly diseases through the blood.

Nervous system Abusing drugs can cause permanent brain damage as well as mental problems, such as depression.

Heart Abuse of certain drugs can cause heart problems. An overdose of certain drugs can cause the heart to stop beating.

MUSIC CONNECTION — BASIC
Music for a Drug-Free Life Tell students that some popular musicians celebrate drugs and drug use in their music. Invite students to share their opinions about this. Then, have teams of students choose a song and work together to write new lyrics about the consequences of drug addiction and the benefits of staying drug free. **LS Auditory**

Problems with the Law

Some drugs are illegal. Even legal prescription drugs can be illegal if they are used improperly. Developing a problem with drug abuse or addiction can quickly lead to problems with the law. Getting arrested and going to court can affect a person's entire life. For example, if you have been convicted of a crime, it may be harder to find a job because many employers do not want to hire someone with a criminal record. A conviction for illegal drug use or a drug-related crime can also result in a jail sentence. Sentences for having or using illegal drugs are becoming more and more serious. And when it comes to illegal drugs, you have to get caught only once to go to jail. Time spent in jail not only means a loss of freedom. It can also mean the loss of dreams for the future.

Drug abuse can lead to other crimes as well. People with drug problems often steal to get drug money. They may begin by stealing from family members, but later they may steal from others. Theft and burglary are very serious crimes, and they carry very harsh punishments.

Another type of crime associated with drug abuse is driving under the influence, or DUI. When a person under the influence of drugs operates a car, he or she puts everyone on the road in danger. The law takes this action very seriously, especially if anyone is hurt or killed in a car accident.

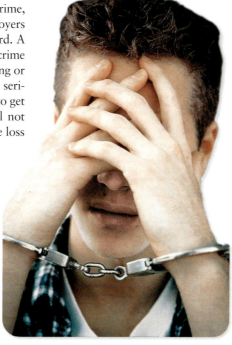

Figure 15 This teen has been arrested for having illegal drugs.

Lesson Review

Understanding Concepts
1. What types of problems can arise as a consequence of drug abuse?
2. How can drug abuse damage family relationships?
3. Why do people who abuse drugs have problems with money?
4. What are three ways that a person who uses drugs can get into trouble with the law?

Critical Thinking
5. **Making Inferences** Imagine that your dream is to become a professional athlete. Describe how drug abuse could affect these plans.
6. **Making Inferences** Driving under the influence puts others in danger. Describe another situation in which one person's drug use could put other people in danger.

internet connect
www.scilinks.org/health
Topic: Drugs and Drug Abuse
HealthLinks code: HD4031
HEALTH LINKS. Maintained by the National Science Teachers Association

---

Close

Reteaching — BASIC
Drugs and Relationships On the board, draw a stick figure of a person and write around it the words *family, school, money, health,* and *police,* or draw simple pictures to symbolize them. Write the word *DRUGS* above the diagram. Then, ask students to tell how drug addiction affects the relationships between the person in the middle and each of the things surrounding him or her. (Students should describe ways that the relationships change and worsen.) **LS Visual**

Quiz — GENERAL
1. Why is a person who abuses drugs willing to steal? (A person who abuses drugs needs money for drugs and doesn't think about the consequences of stealing.)
2. Why do drug abusers have trouble in school? (Sample answer: Drug abusers have trouble in school because they may have trouble concentrating or remembering things and may stop doing their homework.)
3. What are six health problems that can arise from using drugs? (Sample answer: Six health problems that can arise from using drugs are severe weight loss or weight gain, sores, damage to internal organs, memory loss, infections such as HIV, and mental and emotional problems.)

Alternative Assessment — GENERAL
Short Story Have students write a short story about a family with a teen who abuses drugs. The story should describe how the teen's drug addiction affects each person in the family. **LS Verbal**

Answers to Lesson Review
1. Problems can arise with friends and family, school, money, health, and the law.
2. Family relationships can be damaged when a drug abuser steals from family members, becomes verbally or physically violent, and is difficult to get along with.
3. Drugs are expensive, and people who abuse drugs need a lot of money to buy drugs. Sometimes people who abuse drugs steal from others to get money.
4. A drug abuser can be arrested for having illegal drugs, for committing other crimes such as theft or burglary, or for driving while under the influence of drugs.
5. Accept all reasonable answers. Sample answer: Drug abuse can lead to many serious health problems. Some of these problems can affect your performance in sports.
6. Accept all reasonable answers. Sample answer: Operating heavy machinery while under the influence of drugs can put other people in danger.

Lesson 5 • The Consequences of Drug Abuse

Lesson 6 Focus

Overview
Before beginning this lesson, review with your students the objectives listed under the What You'll Do head in the Student Edition. In this lesson, students will learn how stimulants and depressants affect the body and will learn the dangers of using stimulants and depressants.

🔔 Bellringer
Ask students to write definitions for the following pairs of words: *stimulus/stimulate* and *depress/depression*. (Sample answers: A stimulus is something that causes a reaction. *Stimulate* means "to cause a reaction." *Depress* means "to press down." A depression is a sunken area or an emotional state in which a person is sad.)

Motivate

Discussion — GENERAL
Tell students that caffeine is a type of drug called a *stimulant*. Lead a discussion about caffeine by asking the following questions:

- What foods and drinks have you consumed that contain caffeine? (Sample answers: chocolate, some soft drinks, and iced tea)
- How does caffeine affect you? (Sample answer: Caffeine makes me more alert and keeps me awake at night.)
- What happened when someone you knew tried to stop consuming caffeine? (Sample answer: He was in a bad mood all the time.)

LS Verbal

Lesson 6 — Stimulants and Depressants

What You'll Do
- **Describe** the effects of stimulants.
- **Identify** dangers associated with the use of stimulants.
- **Describe** the effects of depressants.
- **Identify** dangers associated with the use of depressants.

Terms to Learn
- stimulant
- depressant

Start Off Write
Why do people drink coffee in the morning? How does this relate to stimulants?

Dorie drank a can of cola at dinner. After dinner, she found that it was easier to pay attention to her homework. But when it was time to go to bed, Dorie couldn't sleep.

Dorie was experiencing the effects of caffeine, a drug found in the cola she drank. Caffeine is one drug in a group of drugs called *stimulants*. Stimulants (STIM yoo luhnts) and another group of drugs called *depressants* (dee PREHS uhnts) include some of the most commonly used and abused drugs.

Stimulants
Any drug that speeds up the activity of the body and the brain is a **stimulant.** Stimulants increase blood pressure and heart rate and tighten blood vessels. Stimulants also raise the level of sugar in the blood. All of these changes make a user feel more awake and alert. Dangers of using stimulants include heart failure, brain damage, and stroke. Stimulants include legal drugs, such as caffeine and nicotine, and illegal drugs, such as cocaine and methamphetamine.

TABLE 1 Common Stimulants

Name	How it is taken	Effects	Dangers
Caffeine	found in many foods, such as chocolate and cola, and in some over-the-counter medicines; taken orally	alertness, energy, and ability to think more clearly	causes users to experience a "crash," or a feeling of illness or lack of energy after the drug has worn off
Nicotine	found in all tobacco products; can be smoked or taken orally	alertness, feeling of calm, mild *euphoria* (yoo FOR ee uh), or a sense of well-being	is very addictive; people addicted to nicotine abuse tobacco products, which can cause cancer and heart disease
Cocaine	taken by *snorting*, (inhaling through the nose), by injection, or by smoking	euphoria, alertness, or feeling of increased strength; causes users to crash and to crave more of the drug	is very addictive; can cause heart disease or sudden heart failure; can also cause brain damage or strokes
Methamphetamine (crystal meth)	can be snorted, smoked, or injected	euphoria, alertness, or feeling of increased strength; effects last several hours	is very addictive; can cause heart disease, sudden heart failure, brain damage, or stroke

Answer to Start Off Write
Accept all reasonable answers. Sample answer: People drink coffee in the morning because coffee contains caffeine. Caffeine is a stimulant that helps people stay alert and awake.

Chapter Resource File
- Directed Reading BASIC
- Lesson Plan
- Lesson Quiz GENERAL

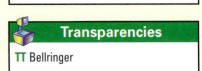
Transparencies
TT Bellringer

Depressants

Any drug that causes activity in the body and brain to slow is called a **depressant.** The effects of depressants are opposite of the effects of stimulants. Depressants reduce heart rate, blood pressure, and breathing. People who take depressants become relaxed or sleepy and react slowly.

Many depressants are prescription drugs, such as Valium™ (VAL ee uhm) and Xanax™ (ZAN aks), that doctors use to treat problems with nervousness and sleeplessness. These drugs are all extremely addictive. Taking too much of a depressant can cause brain damage, heart failure, or death.

The most commonly used depressant is alcohol. Alcohol can cause health problems such as heart disease and liver damage. When taken with another depressant, alcohol is very dangerous. Misuse or abuse of any depressant can lead to both physical and psychological dependence.

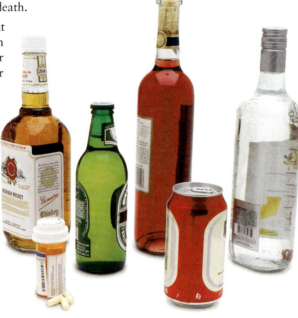

Figure 16 Depressants include different drugs, including alcohol, which is the most commonly used depressant.

Lesson Review

Using Vocabulary
1. What is a stimulant?
2. What is a depressant?

Understanding Concepts
3. Compare the effects of stimulants and depressants.
4. Describe three dangers of using stimulants and three dangers of using depressants.

Critical Thinking
5. **Making Inferences** How could you tell the difference between somebody who was using stimulants and somebody who was using depressants?
6. **Applying Concepts** Why is it dangerous to drive a car or operate heavy machinery while under the influence of alcohol?

Teach

Using the Figure — BASIC

Common Stimulants The table on the previous page of the Student Edition shows some common stimulants, their effects, and their dangers. Have students identify which of these drugs are legal and which are illegal. (Caffeine and nicotine are legal; cocaine and methamphetamine are illegal.) Ask students what the appeal of these drugs is for people. Ask them what the dangers are. Use the table to help them focus on the addictive nature of these drugs, as well as the ways that the drugs can harm the body. **LS** Visual

Close

Reteaching — BASIC

Study Chart Have students create a chart to review the material in this lesson. The chart should have two columns, one labeled "Stimulants" and the other labeled "Depressants." In the columns, students should write how each type of drug affects the body, the dangers of each type of drug, and names of drugs that belong to each category. Tell students they can use their charts to study for the lesson quiz and chapter test.
LS Visual

Quiz — GENERAL

1. Why would a person want to take a stimulant such as caffeine? (Sample answer: The person may take the stimulant to stay awake or alert.)
2. What are some legal uses of depressants? (Depressants are used to treat problems with nervousness and sleeplessness.)
3. What is the most commonly used depressant? (Alcohol is the most commonly used depressant.)

Answers to Lesson Review

1. A stimulant is any drug that speeds up the activity of the body and the brain.
2. A depressant is any drug that causes activity in the body and brain to slow down.
3. The effects of stimulants and depressants are opposite. Stimulants increase blood pressure and heart rate, tighten blood vessels, and raise the blood sugar level. Depressants reduce heart rate, blood pressure, and breathing.
4. Sample answer: Three dangers of using stimulants are stroke, heart failure, and brain damage. Three dangers of depressants are brain damage, heart failure, and death.
5. Someone using stimulants would be very active and alert. Someone using depressants would react slowly and be sleepy.
6. Alcohol is a depressant and can cause you to react slowly. If you drive a car or operate heavy machinery when under the influence of alcohol, you may not be able to react quickly enough to avoid accidents.

Lesson 6 • Stimulants and Depressants

Lesson 7 Focus

Overview
Before beginning this lesson, review with your students the objectives listed under the What You'll Do head in the Student Edition. In this lesson, students will learn what marijuana is and how it affects the body. Students will also learn the dangers of marijuana use.

Bellringer
Ask students to write a brief paragraph about what they know about marijuana. (Answers may vary. Students may mention nicknames for marijuana, ways people take in marijuana, and misconceptions they have about marijuana.)

Answer to Start Off Write
Accept all reasonable answers. Sample answer: no; Marijuana can cause both physical and psychological problems including decreased coordination and the inability to concentrate.

Motivate

Activity — GENERAL
Skit Have students work in small groups to write a skit about a teen who starts using marijuana. The skit should focus on how marijuana affects the teen both physically and psychologically and on how these effects interfere with the teen's daily life. **LS** Verbal

---

Lesson 7

What You'll Do
- **Describe** the effects of marijuana.
- **Identify** the dangers of using marijuana.

Terms to Learn
- marijuana
- THC

Start Off Write
Is marijuana harmless? Explain your answer.

Marijuana

Ben wanted Samuel to smoke marijuana with him. Ben said he'd done it dozens of times and it was great. He told Samuel not to worry, nothing bad would happen. Samuel didn't know what to do.

Samuel needed more information about marijuana. Many people, such as Ben, will tell you that marijuana is totally harmless. But anyone who tells you that isn't telling you the whole truth.

What Is Marijuana?
Of all illegal drugs, marijuana may be the most widely used. But what is marijuana? **Marijuana** (mar uh WAH nuh) is the dried flowers and leaves of the *Cannabis* plant. Marijuana has a long history of use and now grows almost everywhere in the world. Marijuana has more than 200 slang names, including pot, grass, weed, green, and Mary Jane. Marijuana is usually smoked, although it can also be eaten.

The active chemical in marijuana is called **THC.** The way marijuana affects a person depends on how much THC the marijuana contains, how the marijuana is taken, and what the user's expectations are. Some people feel nothing. Others feel relaxed or happy. Still others have severe panic attacks or feel unable to move. Drinking alcohol or using other drugs at the same time increases the effects of marijuana.

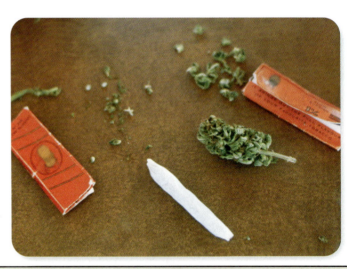

Figure 17 Marijuana is often wrapped in paper and smoked.

Attention Grabber
Although THC is known to be the main active chemical in marijuana, marijuana leaves and flowers also contain more than 400 other chemicals. The effects of these chemicals on the body are not well known.

Chapter Resource File
- Directed Reading BASIC
- Lesson Plan
- Lesson Quiz GENERAL

Transparencies
TT Bellringer

286   Chapter 13 • Teens and Drugs

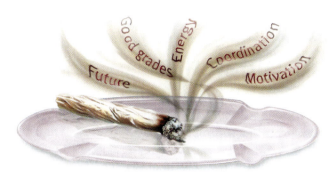

Figure 18 Smoking marijuana makes your health and dreams go up in smoke.

Is Marijuana Harmful?

Marijuana can cause many problems, both physical and psychological. The most common problems are the inability to concentrate and lack of motivation. For this reason, many people who use marijuana perform poorly in school or at work. Marijuana also affects coordination and the ability to react quickly. This effect makes many activities, such as driving and sports, difficult.

People who use marijuana for a long time become psychologically dependent on the drug. People who are psychologically dependent on marijuana are often irritable or unable to sleep if they do not use the drug. Long-term users also need to take more of the drug in order to get the same effect.

Long-term use of marijuana also causes physical damage. Smoking the drug can cause lung problems, including coughing, frequent colds, and lung cancer.

Lesson Review

Using Vocabulary
1. Describe the relationship between marijuana and THC.

Understanding Concepts
2. What are some of marijuana's effects? What can affect a person's reaction to this drug?
3. What physical and psychological problems can happen because of long-term marijuana use?

Critical Thinking
4. **Making Inferences** Some of the harmful effects of marijuana come from smoking the drug. Does that mean eating marijuana is safe? Explain your answer.
5. **Analyzing Ideas** If you could remove all of the THC from marijuana, would it be completely safe? Explain your answer.

Teach

LIFE SCIENCE CONNECTION — ADVANCED

Marijuana as Medicine
Recently, several states passed laws that allow marijuana to be used for medical purposes. Marijuana has been used for many years to treat the symptoms of illnesses such as cancer, AIDS, and glaucoma. Have students research why most health professionals oppose the use of marijuana as medicine. Students should present their research to the class as an oral report. **LS Logical**

Close

Reteaching — BASIC

Graphic Organizer Have students write the words "marijuana" in one circle and "THC" in a second circle. Have them draw a third circle that touches both of these circles. In the third circle, have them write all the ways that the two words are connected. **LS Logical**

Quiz — GENERAL

1. What types of activities are difficult when a person is using marijuana? (Driving, sports, and other activities that require coordination and the ability to react quickly are difficult when a person uses marijuana.)
2. What can increase the effects of marijuana? (Drinking alcohol or using other drugs at the same time increases the effects of marijuana.)
3. What is marijuana? (Marijuana is the dried flowers and leaves of the *Cannabis* plant.)

Answers to Lesson Review
1. THC is the active chemical in marijuana. The amount of THC in a sample of marijuana is one factor that determines how the drug affects a person.
2. Marijuana can cause people to feel relaxed or happy, to have severe panic attacks, or to feel unable to move. A person's reaction is affected by the amount of THC in the marijuana, how the drug is taken, and the person's expectations.
3. Long-term use can lead to psychological dependence, irritability, sleeplessness, and lung problems including coughing, colds, and lung cancer.
4. no; Eating marijuana will still cause you to suffer from many of the physical and psychological effects of marijuana.
5. Sample answer: no; You will still suffer from lung problems associated with smoking.

Lesson 8

Focus

Overview
Before beginning this lesson, review with your students the objectives listed under the What You'll Do head in the Student Edition. In this lesson, students will learn what hallucinogens and inhalants are and how they affect the body.

Bellringer
Ask students to define the term *hallucinate*. (Sample answer: *Hallucinate* means "to see or hear things that are not actually present.") Invite volunteers to share their definitions with the class.

Answer to Start Off Write
Accept all reasonable answers. Sample answer: Household products contain chemicals that can damage your brain.

Motivate

Group Activity —— GENERAL
Optical Illusions Tell students that looking at optical illusions is similar to hallucinating because a person sees something that does not really exist. Show students a few optical illusions to illustrate this idea. You can find examples in books and on the Internet. Have students work in small groups to find more optical illusions. Students should draw copies of the optical illusions on a poster board and write a brief description of what a person can see in each illusion. Display the posters around the room. **LS Visual**

Lesson 8 — Hallucinogens and Inhalants

What You'll Do
- Identify the dangers of using hallucinogens.
- Identify the dangers of using inhalants.

Terms to Learn
- hallucinogen
- inhalant

Start Off Write
Why is it dangerous to inhale household products?

Cameron's friend talked him into taking a drug called LSD at a party. Before long, Cameron was seeing and hearing things that didn't exist. He became very frightened and had to be taken to the hospital.

LSD, the drug Cameron took, is also called *acid* and belongs to a group of drugs called *hallucinogens*. Hallucinogens (huh LOO si nuh juhns) and another group of drugs called *inhalants* (in HAY luhntz) can produce very strong effects. These effects come with some serious dangers.

Hallucinogens

Drugs that cause a person to sense things that don't actually exist are called **hallucinogens**. Examples of hallucinogens include LSD and magic mushrooms, also called *psilocybin*. Hallucinogens cause the user to experience events in a distorted way or to sense things that don't exist. Hallucinogens also affect the emotions. A person may feel several emotions at once or may swing rapidly from one emotion to another. Being on hallucinogens is often frightening and can cause panic or dangerous actions. Physical reactions to hallucinogens may include nausea, increased heart rate and blood pressure, and sweating.

One long-term effect of hallucinogens is called a flashback. A *flashback* is a sudden reliving of the hallucinogen experience. Flashbacks can happen any time—even months or years after a hallucinogen was last used.

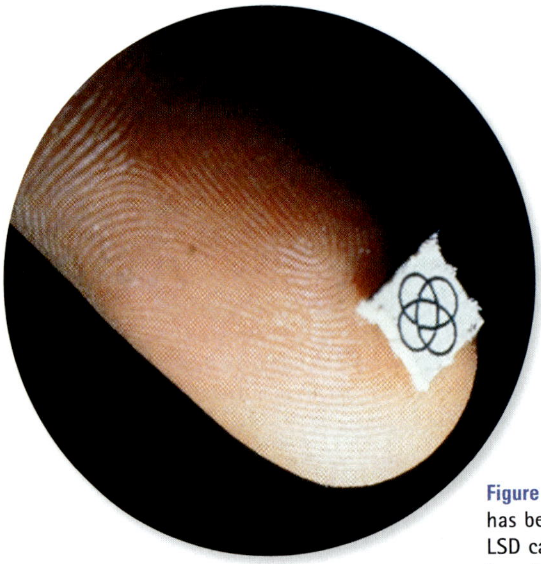

Figure 19 This piece of paper has been soaked in LSD. LSD can make you see or hear things that don't exist.

MISCONCEPTION ALERT

Huffing Some students may believe that inhaling, or huffing, household chemicals is not dangerous. In fact, some of your students may have experimented with huffing cleaning supplies or sniffing glue. Tell your students that inhaling household chemicals can be as dangerous as inhaling illegal drugs.

Chapter Resource File
- Directed Reading **BASIC**
- Lesson Plan
- Lesson Quiz **GENERAL**

Transparencies
TT Bellringer

288 Chapter 13 • Teens and Drugs

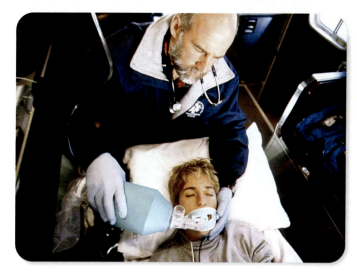

Figure 20 This teen tried inhalants only once, but that was all it took to damage her brain and almost kill her.

Inhalants

A very dangerous group of drugs that is increasing in popularity is called inhalants. **Inhalants** are drugs that are inhaled directly and that enter the bloodstream through the lungs. Inhalants do not include drugs that are smoked. Many products, including common household cleaning supplies, contain chemicals that can be used as inhalants.

When breathed in, inhalants replace the oxygen that goes to the brain. Because they prevent oxygen from reaching your brain, inhalants damage your brain with each use. Some inhalants can cause breathing to stop. Immediate death, coma, or serious brain damage can result from using inhalants just once.

The effects of inhalants are very intense but very short-lived. These effects can include hallucinations, numbness, and the inability to move.

Myth & Fact

Myth: Inhalants stay in your body for only a minute or two, which isn't long enough to do any real damage.

Fact: While the effects of inhalants last only a short while, these chemicals can remain in your body for weeks. Even if they were to remain in your body for only a minute or two, that length of time is more than enough time to kill brain cells, damage your lungs, or even stop your heart.

Lesson Review

Using Vocabulary
1. Define *hallucinogen*.
2. What is an inhalant?

Understanding Concepts
3. What are the main short-term and long-term dangers of using hallucinogens?
4. How do inhalants work on the body?
5. List five dangers of using inhalants.

Critical Thinking
6. **Analyzing Ideas** What kind of dangers could a hallucinogen flashback produce, even if it happened years after the drug was used?

Answers to Lesson Review
1. A hallucinogen is a drug that causes a person to sense things that don't actually exist.
2. An inhalant is a drug that is inhaled directly and that enters the bloodstream through the lungs.
3. The short-term effects of hallucinogens include nausea, increased heart rate and blood pressure, and sweating. One long-term effect of hallucinogens is a flashback.
4. Inhalants affect the body by replacing the oxygen that goes to the brain.
5. Five dangers of using inhalants are brain damage, immediate death, coma, hallucinations, and the inability to breathe.
6. Accept all reasonable answers. Sample answer: If a person experiences a flashback while driving a car, he or she may panic and may get into a car accident.

Teach

Life SKILL BUILDER — GENERAL

Making Good Decisions Have students role-play the following scenario: "You are at the birthday party of your best friend. During the party, your friend opens a helium balloon, inhales some of the gas from the balloon, and starts to sing. His voice is very squeaky, and everyone laughs. Several other people start opening balloons. Your friend hands you his balloon and urges you to try it. What should you do?"
LS **Kinesthetic**

Close

Reteaching — BASIC

Where the Air Goes Have students hold their hand on their chest and breathe deeply. Ask students what they felt. (My chest went out when I breathed in and went back in when I breathed out.) Tell students that although it feels like all the air that they breathe in comes back out, some of the air stays in the body. Explain that the chemicals that make up the air they breathe are absorbed into the bloodstream through blood vessels in the lungs. Once in the bloodstream, the chemicals travel to all parts of the body. LS **Kinesthetic**

Quiz — GENERAL

1. What are some of the effects of using inhalants? (Inhalants can cause hallucinations, numbness, and the inability to move.)
2. What is a flashback? (A flashback is a sudden reliving of a hallucinogen experience, which may occur months or years after using the hallucinogen.)
3. What are some examples of hallucinogens? (LSD and magic mushrooms are two examples of hallucinogens.)

Lesson 8 • **Hallucinogens and Inhalants**

Lesson 9 Focus

Overview
Before beginning this lesson, review with your students the objectives listed under the What You'll Do head in the Student Edition. In this lesson, students will learn five reasons to stay drug free. Students will also learn ways to refuse drugs, and activities and skills that can help them avoid drugs.

Bellringer
Have students write down three reasons why they should remain drug free. (Accept all reasonable answers. Sample answer: I will be healthier, I will do better in school, and my parents will be happy with me.)

Answer to Start Off Write
Accept all reasonable answers. Sample answer: Using drugs could damage my health, could destroy my relationships with others, or could cause me to end up in jail.

Motivate

Discussion — GENERAL
Hopes and Dreams Invite student volunteers to share their goals and dreams for the future. (Sample answer: I want to succeed in sports, school, and work.) Ask students how becoming addicted to drugs would affect each of these dreams. (Sample answer: Becoming addicted to drugs will make it difficult to achieve my goals.) Ask students to suggest some ways they can stay drug free. (Sample answer: I can stay involved in activities, and I can stay away from situations where people might be using drugs.)
LS Intrapersonal

Lesson 9

What You'll Do
- **List** four reasons to remain drug free.
- **Identify** five ways to refuse drugs.
- **Describe** activities and skills that can help one avoid drugs.

Start Off Write
How could using drugs negatively affect your plans for the future?

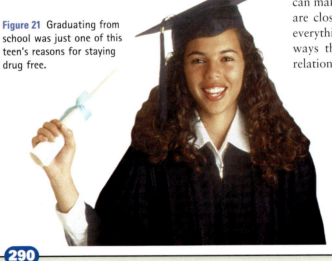

Figure 21 Graduating from school was just one of this teen's reasons for staying drug free.

Staying Drug Free

Raoul is a very fast runner. One day, he hopes to make it to the Olympics. Raoul turns down drugs when they are offered to him because he knows that using drugs could make his dream impossible.

Raoul has a reason to stay drug free. He also knows how to resist the pressure to do drugs. By staying drug free, Raoul has a much better chance of making his dream come true.

Reasons to Be Drug Free
No one else is quite like you. Because you are unique, you will have your own reasons for wanting to stay drug free. Here are some of the best reasons to stay drug free. Perhaps one of these reasons works for you. Or maybe they all do!

- Drugs can damage your health. They can cause permanent effects, such as heart disease, brain damage, or emotional problems. Some drugs can even kill you.
- Drugs can mess up your body and your mind. They can interfere with your ability to succeed in sports and other activities. Drugs can also damage your memory and destroy your desire to accomplish things. As your ability to learn decreases, so will your success in school. A poor school record can limit your choices both now and later in life.
- Drugs can destroy your relationships. They can make you forget about the people who are close to you. You can lose interest in everything except drugs and can behave in ways that are harmful to you and your relationships with your family and friends.
- Drugs are illegal. Even legal drugs, such as nicotine and alcohol, are illegal for someone your age. If you use illegal drugs, you could be arrested. Using drugs can also lead to other illegal behaviors. Going to jail can ruin your future.

Chapter Resource File
- Directed Reading **BASIC**
- Lesson Plan
- Lesson Quiz **GENERAL**

Transparencies
TT Bellringer

290 Chapter 13 • Teens and Drugs

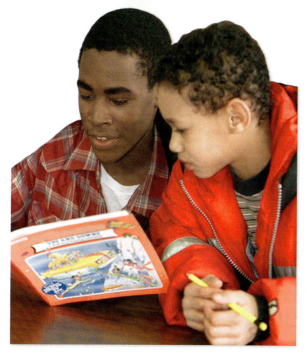

Figure 22 This teen is staying away from drugs by volunteering in his community.

Ways to Stay Drug Free

One of the best ways to protect yourself from drugs is to be involved in activities with others who want to stay drug free. Another way to stay drug free is to stay away from situations where there may be pressure to use drugs. Here are some ways to stay drug free.

- Participate in sports or get involved in school clubs or activities, such as drama or music.
- Develop a hobby, such as doing magic tricks, gardening, or making video movies.
- Get involved in community service by volunteering at a local daycare center or animal shelter.
- Play games with friends, read a book, or write a story.
- Identify students who you think are using drugs, and stay away from them. They may pressure you to do drugs.
- Identify places and situations where drugs are likely to be used, and stay away from these situations.
- Learn ways to handle stress in your life so you won't feel tempted to try to feel better by using drugs.
- Stay connected to a trusted adult, such as a parent, a coach, a relative, or a teacher.

Hands-on ACTIVITY

WHY STAY DRUG FREE?

1. Work in groups of two. Interview 10 people, which consist of both adults and students.
2. Ask each person why he or she wants to stay drug free. Record their answers.

Analysis
1. Categorize your results into four or five areas, such as health, family, education, and other responsibilities.
2. Illustrate your results by making a pie graph. What was the most popular reason for staying drug free?

Teach

Life SKILL BUILDER — GENERAL

Assessing Your Health Have students count the number of times they see advertisements for alcohol or tobacco in one week. During the same week, have students count the number of times they face peer pressure to use drugs, tobacco, or alcohol. Student can make tally marks in a journal to count these incidents. At the end of the week, have students discuss how exposure to advertisements and peer pressure affects them physically and emotionally. **LS Intrapersonal**

Activity — BASIC

Poster Project Have students brainstorm a list of activities they can do to help themselves stay drug free. Ask each student to pick five activities from the list and make a poster illustrating the activities. Encourage students to draw themselves participating in the activities they chose. Have students write a sentence explaining how the activity helps them stay drug free under each illustration. **LS Visual**

REAL-LIFE CONNECTION — ADVANCED

Drug Myths There are many myths about drugs. For example, many people think that marijuana is not addictive. Invite teams of students to interview other students to learn what the other students think are true statements about drugs. Have the teams do research to determine which statements are true and which are not true. Then, have the teams create a brochure about drug myths and facts. Students can make copies of their brochure and distribute it in school or in other public places. **LS Logical**

Life SKILL BUILDER — GENERAL

Communicating Effectively Ask students to brainstorm a list of people with whom they would talk if they thought that a friend may be using drugs. (Sample answers: parents, teachers, counselors, coaches, and other adults) Ask students what they would want to hear from the person in whom they confided. (Sample answer: I would want the person to help me find a way to help my friend.) Ask students what they should do if the person they confided in cannot help them. (Sample answer: I would talk to someone else.) **LS Interpersonal**

Hands-on ACTIVITY

Answer
Answers may vary.

Extension: Ask students to compare the responses given by adults to the students' responses. (Answers may vary. Sample answer: Adults gave more responses related to health and family, and students gave more responses related to education.)

Lesson 9 • Staying Drug Free   291

Teach, continued

Using the Figure — BASIC
Different Ways to Refuse Drugs
The table on the next page of the Student Edition lists some refusal skills and describes how they work. Ask students which of the refusal skills would be the most effective and most comfortable for them to use. Ask students to give an example of a situation in which each of these refusal skills may work. Finally, have students suggest other refusal skills and explain how they would work. **LS Verbal**

Group Activity — GENERAL
Brochure Tell students that teaching young children about the dangers of drugs and teaching them how to refuse drugs is very important. Have students work in groups of three to design brochures for children in elementary school about drugs and refusal skills. Tell students to make their brochures easy to read and eye-catching. One student can write the text of the brochure, one student can draw the illustrations, and one student can create the layout of the brochure. Students fluent in another language can write the text in both English and their other language.
LS Interpersonal
Co-op Learning | English Language Learners

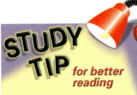

STUDY TIP *for better reading*

Reviewing Information
As you read the different ways to refuse drugs in the table on the next page, make a chart of your own. Draw a line down the middle of a sheet of paper. On one side, write down the ways to refuse drugs. On the other side, write a personal example of each way.

Refusing Drugs
At some point, people you know may pressure you to use drugs. If so, you are not alone. Even adults have this problem. Often, the people who pressure you are your friends, which can make it even more difficult to say no. When this type of situation arises, it is important to remember the reasons that you have decided to stay drug free. Think about all of the things that you could be giving up if you use drugs. Remember that it is up to you to protect your dreams and your future.

Knowing how to refuse drugs and get out of a pressure situation is also very important. You never know when you might be offered drugs, so it is best to be prepared. The table on the next page shows several different ways to refuse drugs.

Saying No Is OK
Once you've decided to refuse drugs, you can take pride in your decision. By refusing to take drugs, you are saying that you refuse to damage your mind, your relationships, and your future. You will discover that you are not alone in your decision.

Not everyone is using drugs. In fact, most young people are NOT using drugs.

If someone stops being your friend just because you refuse to take drugs, that person was not a true friend to begin with. Remember that friendship is based on respect. Anyone who would force you to do something that could hurt you doesn't respect you.

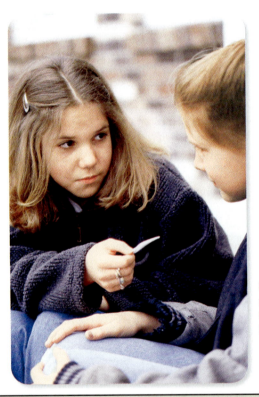

Figure 23 Knowing how to refuse drugs is important, especially when your friends pressure you to use drugs.

292

Life SKILL BUILDER — GENERAL
Practicing Wellness Have students brainstorm a list of the different ways they could say no to someone who wants them to take drugs. Encourage them to use their imagination and their sense of humor. Then have each student choose one way of saying no and create a cartoon drawing showing someone using it. Display the cartoons in the classroom.
LS Visual

Career
Drug Enforcement Agent The U.S. Drug Enforcement Administration (DEA) is the federal organization that locates and arrests illegal drug users and dealers. DEA agents enforce federal drug laws in the United States and also lead drug investigations abroad. Agents work on criminal investigations, carry out surveillance of suspected drug dealers, and use undercover techniques to infiltrate illegal drug organizations. Drug enforcement agents also work with state and local governments.

292 Chapter 13 • Teens and Drugs

TABLE 2 Different Ways to Refuse Drugs

Refusal skill	How it works
Say, "No, thank you."	Very clearly explain to the person who is offering you drugs that you don't want to take them. This is the clearest and easiest way to refuse drugs.
Give a reason.	Explain to the person why you can't take the drugs or why you don't want to take them. Say something like, "I have a big test tomorrow," or "I'm on the track team, and that stuff will just slow me down."
State the consequences.	Describe some of the consequences that may occur if you used the drug offered to you. Say something like, "I would be grounded for a month if I did drugs," or "That stuff could mess up my mind or even kill me!" This might make the person offering the drugs think twice about using the drugs.
Suggest another activity.	Come up with an idea for something that you could do that doesn't involve taking drugs. You could suggest going to a movie, playing a game, going shopping, going to get something to eat, or going for a walk in the park. Try to suggest something fun so that the temptation to use drugs will be less.
Walk away.	If all of your other strategies fail, just walk away from the situation. Nobody can pressure you to do drugs if you aren't there.

Health Journal
Describe a time when you had to say no to a friend. What did you say to convince your friend that you meant no?

Lesson Review

Understanding Concepts
1. How can using drugs affect a person's future?
2. What are four different actions you can take to help keep yourself drug free?
3. List five ways to refuse drugs.
4. What is one reason that you want to stay drug free? Use a reason that is not listed in the text.

Critical Thinking
5. **Analyzing Ideas** Describe an out-of-school activity that you might be interested in. Describe how this activity could make you less likely to use drugs.
6. **Using Refusal Skills** Suppose a friend of yours is trying to get you to smoke marijuana, and he won't take no for an answer. Describe how you would handle this situation.

Answer to Health Journal
Answers may vary. This Health Journal can be used to begin a class discussion on refusal skills. Remember that some students may be uncomfortable sharing personal information.

Close

Reteaching — BASIC
Drug-Free Collage Provide students with old magazines. Have students cut out pictures that show reasons to stay drug free and ways to stay drug free. Have students glue the pictures on a poster board to create a collage. **LS Visual**

Quiz — GENERAL
1. What is the clearest and easiest way to refuse drugs? (The clearest and easiest way to refuse drugs is to say "No, thank you.")
2. Why is learning to handle stress a way to stay drug free? (If you know how to handle stress, you won't be tempted to use drugs to feel better.)
3. How can drugs affect your grades in school? (Drugs can damage your memory and destroy your desire to accomplish things. As your ability to learn decreases, your success in school will decrease.)
4. What should you do if you face pressure to use drugs? (Accept all reasonable answers. Sample answer: You should remember your reasons for staying drug free and use refusal skills to say no.)

Alternative Assessment — GENERAL
Skit Have students work in small groups to write and perform a skit about a teen who faces pressure to use drugs. In the skit, the teen should discuss his or her reasons to stay drug free and should use refusal skills to say no to the people who are pressuring him or her. **LS Kinesthetic**

Answers to Lesson Review
1. Using drugs can affect a person's future by damaging his or her health or mind or by causing him or her to go to jail.
2. Accept all reasonable answers. Sample answer: Four actions that will help you stay drug free are participating in sports, developing a hobby, learning how to handle stress, and staying connected with a trusted adult.
3. Five ways to refuse drugs are saying "No, thank you," giving a reason, stating the consequences, suggesting another activity, and walking away.
4. Accept all reasonable answers. Sample answer: I want to stay drug free to set a good example for my little brother.
5. Accept all reasonable answers. Sample answer: I would like to go hiking in state parks. The hikes would help me relieve stress so that I won't be tempted to use drugs to feel better.
6. Accept all reasonable answers. Sample answer: I would explain why I don't want to smoke marijuana, and then I would walk away.

Lesson 9 • Staying Drug Free

13 CHAPTER REVIEW

Chapter Summary

- A drug is any substance other than food that changes a person's physical or psychological state. ■ Drugs can enter your body in several different ways. ■ Some medicines require a prescription from a doctor, while others do not. ■ Carefully follow all instructions when taking any medicine. ■ Drug abuse is misusing a legal drug on purpose or using any illegal drug. ■ Drug abuse can lead to drug addiction. ■ Drug addiction can cause problems with relationships, money, health, and the law. ■ There are many good reasons to stay drug free, and everyone's reasons will be different. ■ Knowing how to avoid drugs and how to refuse drugs will help you stay drug free.

Using Vocabulary

For each pair of terms, describe how the meanings of the terms differ.

1. drug/medicine
2. prescription medicine/over-the-counter medicine
3. drug misuse/drug abuse
4. physical dependence/psychological dependence

For each sentence, fill in the blank with the proper word from the word bank provided below.

hallucinogen   stimulant
medicine   marijuana
drug addiction withdrawal

5. A drug that is used to treat disease, injury, or pain is a(n) ___.
6. A drug that speeds up the activity in your body is a(n) ___.
7. A(n) ___ is a drug that can make a person sense things that don't exist.
8. The dried leaves and flowers of the *Cannabis* plant are better known as ___.

Understanding Concepts

9. List the five ways that drugs enter the body, and briefly describe each way.
10. What four rules should you follow when taking medicine?
11. What is drug addiction, and how is it related to dependence?
12. What is withdrawal?
13. What dangers are involved in using marijuana?
14. In your own words, compare the effects of stimulants with the effects of depressants.
15. Explain how inhalants work and how this process presents dangers.
16. What are four reasons to stay drug free?
17. How can certain activities help keep you drug free?
18. Describe five ways to refuse drugs, and give an example of each.
19. What are the most common problems experienced by marijuana users?

---

13 CHAPTER REVIEW

Assignment Guide

Lesson	Review Questions
1	9
2	2, 5, 20
3	3, 10, 21, 24–25
4	4, 11–12
5	
6	6, 14
7	8, 13, 19, 23
8	7, 15, 22
9	16–18
1 and 2	1
2 and 9	26

ANSWERS

Using Vocabulary

1. A drug is any substance other than food that changes a person's physical or psychological state. A medicine is a drug that is used to treat disease, injury, or pain.

2. A prescription medicine can be bought only if a doctor orders its use. An over-the-counter medicine can be purchased at any time.

3. Drug misuse is any use of a medicine other than its intended use, while drug abuse is the intentional misuse of a legal drug or any use of an illegal drug.

4. Physical dependence is the body's chemical need for a drug, and psychological dependence is a person's emotional or mental need for a drug.

5. medicine
6. stimulant
7. Hallucinogens
8. marijuana

Understanding Concepts

9. Five ways that drugs enter the body are orally, by injection, by smoking, by inhaling, and with a transdermal patch. Students should include a description of each.

10. follow all instructions, never increase the amount of medicine that you take, don't stop taking a prescription without your doctor's permission, and never take someone else's prescription medicine

11. Drug addiction is the uncontrollable use of a drug. A person with a drug addiction cannot control his or her use of a drug because he or she has a dependence on the drug.

12. Withdrawal is the negative symptoms that result when a drug-dependent person stops taking a drug.

13. Sample answer: Marijuana affects coordination and the ability to react quickly.

14. Stimulants increase the activity of the body and the brain. Depressants decrease the activity of the body and brain.

15. Inhalants replace the oxygen that goes to the brain. Because of this, brain damage can occur.

294 Chapter 13 • Teens and Drugs

Critical Thinking

Analyzing Ideas

20. Some medicines are sold in over-the-counter and prescription forms. What differences would you expect between these two forms of a medicine?

21. Pilar has been taking a prescription asthma medicine for a few days. She knows that she is supposed to use the medicine only twice a day, but she uses it four times a day because it really helps her asthma. Is Pilar misusing or abusing this drug? What should she do?

22. People who have used hallucinogens in the past may have a flashback at any time. What kind of dangers could an unexpected flashback cause?

23. Tyler is the captain of his school's academic team. Recently, Tyler's friends have started asking him to smoke marijuana with them. How could smoking marijuana affect Tyler's position on the team? Explain your answer.

Making Good Decisions

24. Imagine that a friend of yours has a prescription for a headache medicine. One day, you are having a bad headache, and you complain about it to your friend. He says that you should take some of his medicine because it works very well. He also says that it's safe for you to take the medicine because he has a prescription for it from a doctor. Is your friend right? Should you take his medicine? Explain your answer.

25. Alice has a prescription for a certain medicine. When she took the medicine to school, the label on the medicine fell off and she lost it. Alice is pretty sure that she remembers all of the instructions, but she isn't positive. Should she keep taking the medicine anyway? Explain.

26. Use what you have learned in this chapter to set a personal goal. Write your goal, and make an action plan by using the Health Behavior Contract for drugs. You can find the Health Behavior Contract at go.hrw.com. Just type in the keyword HD4HBC15.

Reading Checkup

Take a minute to review your answers to the Health IQ questions at the beginning of this chapter. How has reading this chapter improved your Health IQ?

Chapter Resource File

- Concept Review GENERAL
- Concept Mapping GENERAL
- Performance-Based Assessment GENERAL
- Chapter Test GENERAL

---

16. Drugs can damage your health, can mess up your mind, can destroy relationships, are illegal, and can interfere with your ability to succeed in activities.

17. Certain activities help you stay drug free by keeping you away from people who use drugs and situations where drugs may be available.

18. say "No, thank you," give a reason, state the consequences, suggest another activity, and walk away; Student answers should also include examples of each refusal skill.

19. The most common problems experienced by marijuana users are the inability to concentrate and a lack of motivation.

Critical Thinking

Analyzing Ideas

20. The prescription medicine probably has a higher dosage than the over-the-counter medicine does.

21. Pilar is abusing the drug. She should stop taking the medicine four times a day.

22. Sample answer: If a person becomes frightened by a flashback, he or she may accidentally hurt himself or herself or others while reacting to what he or she sees or hears.

23. Sample answer: Using marijuana could negatively affect Tyler's ability to concentrate, which would make it hard for him to study and to take the tests.

Making Good Decisions

24. no; You should never take someone else's prescription medicine.

25. no; Alice may accidentally take the wrong amount of the medicine. She should contact her doctor before taking the medicine again.

26. Accept all reasonable responses. **Note:** A Health Behavior Contract for each chapter can be found in the Chapter Resource File and at the HRW Web site, go.hrw.com.

Model

Introduce this activity by reminding students that using this Life Skill will help them take personal responsibility for their behavior. Then, review the scenario with the class.

Prepare students for this activity by modeling each of the steps of the skill. Make sure students understand each step before you move on to the next one.

Guided Practice: Practice with a Friend

Guided Practice is the stage in which you and the students analyze their approach to solving the problem given in the scenario and analyze their coping skills. Have students read Act 1. Discuss with the class the situation described and the way students are to act it out. Organize the class into groups of three. In each group, one person plays the role of Sasha, another person plays one of Sasha's parents, and the third person is the observer.

Proper pacing during the Guided Practice is important. The suggestions listed below will help you control the pace.

1. Stop after completing each step of coping.
2. Discuss with each group the observer's comments.
3. Ask the other members of each group to listen to the observer's suggestions and to suggest ways to improve their coping skills.
4. Instruct students to repeat the steps that need improvement and to include their modifications.

5. Check to make sure that students understand each step before they move on to the next step.
6. If time permits, repeat the exercise three times, switching roles each time. Each student should have the opportunity to play each role. `Co-op Learning`

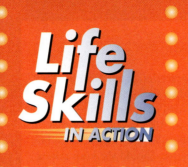

Life Skills IN ACTION

ACT 1

The 5 Steps of Coping

1. Identify the problem.
2. Identify your emotions.
3. Use positive self-talk.
4. Find ways to resolve the problem.
5. Talk to others to receive support.

296

Coping

At times, everyone faces setbacks, disappointments, or other troubles. To deal with these problems, you have to learn how to cope. Coping is dealing with problems and emotions in an effective way. Complete the following activity to develop your coping skills.

The Drug Problem

Setting the Scene

Sasha's older sister Michelle is addicted to drugs. Their parents know about the problem and have been working with Michelle to break her habit. Michelle is having a hard time quitting, and she is often very moody. Michelle yells at Sasha a lot and sometimes refuses to talk to her. Sasha is unhappy about the situation with Michelle. She used to look up to Michelle, and they used to be good friends.

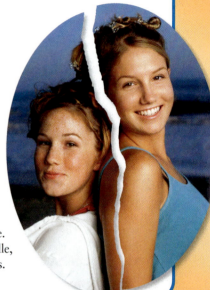

Guided Practice

Practice with a Friend

Form a group of three. Have one person play the role of Sasha and another person play the role of one of Sasha's parents. Have the third person be an observer. Walking through each of the five steps of coping, role-play Sasha dealing with Michelle's drug addiction. When you reach step 5, Sasha should talk to one of her parents. The observer will take notes, which will include observations about what the person playing Sasha did well and suggestions of ways to improve. Stop after each step to evaluate the process.

Independent Practice

Check Yourself

After you have completed the guided practice, go through Act 1 again without stopping at each step. Answer the questions below to review what you did.

1. What are some emotions that Sasha may have?
2. What could Sasha say to herself when using positive self-talk?
3. What are some ways that Sasha could solve her problem?
4. Why is it important for Sasha to talk to someone to receive support for her problem?

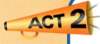

On Your Own

Sasha's family has been planning to take a long vacation at the beach. A week before they are scheduled to leave, Sasha's father tells her that they will not be going after all. Michelle is still receiving treatment for her drug problem, and her counselor thinks it would be best for Michelle if the entire family stays home. Sasha is very disappointed and wishes that Michelle wasn't her sister anymore. Write a short story that describes how Sasha uses the five steps of coping to deal with the cancelled vacation plans.

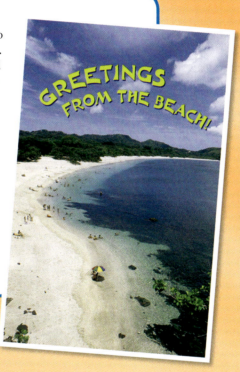

Independent Practice: Check Yourself

Instruct students to repeat Act 1 without stopping at each step. Remind students to apply what they learned in the Guided Practice to the Independent Practice. Students do not have to use every step to cope successfully, nor do they have to follow steps 2–5 in order.

Encourage students to use the Check Yourself questions as a starting point for reviewing and analyzing their Independent Practice. Remind students that as they change roles, the answers to these questions may change for each actor. Encourage students to create additional questions for checking their coping skills. When students have finished the Independent Practice, have them answer the Check Yourself questions in writing. Use their answers to assess their understanding of the steps of coping and to assess their use of the steps to solve a problem.

Check Yourself Answers

1. Sample answer: Some emotions that Sasha may feel include sadness, anger, and disappointment.
2. Sample answer: Sasha could tell herself that Michelle's behavior is a result of Michelle's drug addiction and that Michelle is not really angry with her. Sasha could also tell herself that things will be normal again after Michelle recovers from the addiction.
3. Sample answer: Sasha should not become upset when Michelle yells at her and should try to understand what Michelle is going through.
4. Sample answer: It is important for Sasha to talk to someone so she can express her emotions in a healthy way. Talking with someone may also help her find ways to cope with her problem.

Act 2: On Your Own

This additional scenario gives students an opportunity to apply what they have learned in both the Guided Practice and the Independent Practice to a new situation.

Suggest to students that they use the Check Yourself questions as a starting point for coping in the new situation. Encourage students to be creative and to think of ways to improve their coping skills.

Assessment

Review the short stories that students have written as part of the On Your Own activity. The stories should show that the students applied their coping skills in a realistic and effective manner. If time permits, ask student volunteers to read aloud one or more of the stories. Discuss the stories and the use of coping skills.

CHAPTER 14
Infectious Diseases
Chapter Planning Guide

PACING	CLASSROOM RESOURCES	ACTIVITIES AND DEMONSTRATIONS
BLOCK 1 • 45 min pp. 298–301 **Chapter Opener**	**CRF** Health Inventory * ■ GENERAL **CRF** Parent Letter * ■	**SE** Health IQ, p. 299 **CRF** At-Home Activity * ■
Lesson 1 What Is an Infectious Disease?	**CRF** Lesson Plan * **TT** Bellringer *	**TE** Activities Modeling Antibiotic Resistance, p. 297F **SE** Hands-on Activity, p. 301 **CRF** Datasheets for In-Text Activities * GENERAL **CRF** Enrichment Activity * ADVANCED
BLOCK 2 • 45 min pp. 302–305 **Lesson 2** Bacterial Infections	**CRF** Lesson Plan * **TT** Bellringer * **TT** Exponential Growth Pattern of Bacteria *	**TE** Group Activity Debate, p. 302 GENERAL **TE** Activity Research Project, p. 303 ADVANCED **TE** Group Activity Group Report, p. 304 GENERAL **CRF** Enrichment Activity * ADVANCED
BLOCK 3 • 45 min pp. 306–309 **Lesson 3** Viral Infections	**CRF** Lesson Plan * **TT** Bellringer * **TT** Sizes of a Bacterium and Several Viruses *	**TE** Activity Virus ID, p. 306 GENERAL **TE** Activity Poster Project, p. 307 ◆ ADVANCED **SE** Science Activity, p. 308 **CRF** Life Skills Activity * ■ GENERAL **CRF** Enrichment Activity * ADVANCED
BLOCK 4 • 45 min pp. 310–315 **Lesson 4** Sexually Transmitted Diseases	**CRF** Lesson Plan * **TT** Bellringer * **TT** Estimated Number of People Living with HIV/AIDS Worldwide *	**TE** Activity Matching Information, p. 310 ◆ GENERAL **TE** Activity Poster Project, p. 312 GENERAL **TE** Activity Discussion, p. 313 GENERAL **CRF** Enrichment Activity * ADVANCED
Lesson 5 Preventing the Spread of Infectious Diseases	**CRF** Lesson Plan * **TT** Bellringer *	**TE** Activities Making a Public Service Advertisement, p. 297F **TE** Demonstration Hand Washing, p. 314 ◆ BASIC **SE** Life Skills in Action Making Good Decisions, pp. 318–319 **CRF** Life Skills Activity * ■ GENERAL **CRF** Enrichment Activity * ADVANCED

BLOCKS 5 & 6 • 90 min Chapter Review and Assessment Resources

- **SE** Chapter Review, pp. 316–317
- **CRF** Concept Review * ■ GENERAL
- **CRF** Health Behavior Contract * ■ GENERAL
- **CRF** Chapter Test * ■ GENERAL
- **CRF** Performance-Based Assessment * GENERAL
- **OSP** Test Generator
- **CRF** Test Item Listing *

Online Resources

Visit **go.hrw.com** for a variety of free resources related to this textbook. Enter the keyword **HD4ID7**.

Students can access interactive problem solving help and active visual concept development with the *Decisions for Health* Online Edition available at **www.hrw.com**.

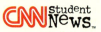

cnnstudentnews.com

Find the latest health news, lesson plans, and activities related to important scientific events.

Chapter 14 • Infectious Diseases

Compression guide:
To shorten your instruction because of time limitations, omit Lessons 2–3.

KEY
- **TE** Teacher Edition
- **SE** Student Edition
- **OSP** One-Stop Planner
- **CRF** Chapter Resource File
- **TT** Teaching Transparency
- * Also on One-Stop Planner
- ■ Also Available in Spanish
- ◆ Requires Advance Prep

SKILLS DEVELOPMENT RESOURCES	LESSON REVIEW AND ASSESSMENT	STANDARDS CORRELATION
		National Health Education Standards
TE Inclusion Strategies, p. 301 `BASIC` **CRF** Cross-Disciplinary * `GENERAL` **CRF** Directed Reading * `BASIC`	**SE** Lesson Review, p. 301 **TE** Reteaching, Quiz, p. 301 **CRF** Lesson Quiz * ■ `GENERAL`	1.8
TE Reading Skill Builder Reading Hint, p. 303 **TE** Life Skill Builder Being a Wise Consumer, p. 304 `ADVANCED` **SE** Study Tip Word Origins, p. 305 **TE** Inclusion Strategies, p. 305 `BASIC` **CRF** Decision-Making * `GENERAL` **CRF** Directed Reading * `BASIC`	**SE** Lesson Review, p. 305 **TE** Reteaching, Quiz, p. 305 **CRF** Concept Mapping * `GENERAL` **CRF** Lesson Quiz * ■ `GENERAL`	
SE Life Skills Activity Practicing Wellness, p. 309 **CRF** Decision-Making * `GENERAL` **CRF** Directed Reading * `BASIC`	**SE** Lesson Review, p. 309 **TE** Reteaching, Quiz, p. 309 **CRF** Lesson Quiz * ■ `GENERAL`	
TE Life Skill Builder Coping, p. 311 `GENERAL` **TE** Reading Skill Builder Anticipation Guide, p. 312 `BASIC` **CRF** Cross-Disciplinary * `GENERAL` **CRF** Refusal Skills * `GENERAL` **CRF** Directed Reading * `BASIC`	**SE** Lesson Review, p. 313 **TE** Reteaching, Quiz, p. 313 **CRF** Concept Mapping * `GENERAL` **CRF** Lesson Quiz * ■ `GENERAL`	1.4, 3.3, 6.3
TE Life Skill Builder Practicing Wellness, p. 315 `GENERAL` **CRF** Refusal Skills * `GENERAL` **CRF** Directed Reading * `BASIC`	**SE** Lesson Review, p. 315 **TE** Reteaching, Quiz, p. 315 **CRF** Lesson Quiz * ■ `GENERAL`	1.4, 1.8, 2.5, 3.4

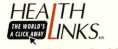

www.scilinks.org/health

Maintained by the **National Science Teachers Association**

Topic: Bacteria — HealthLinks code: HD4012
Topic: Viruses — HealthLinks code: HD4104
Topic: AIDS — HealthLinks code: HD4005
Topic: HIV — HealthLinks code: HD4055

Technology Resources

One-Stop Planner
All of your printable resources and the Test Generator are on this convenient CD-ROM.

Guided Reading Audio CDs

VIDEO SELECT
For information about videos related to this chapter, go to **go.hrw.com** and type in the keyword **HD4ID7V**.

Chapter 14 • Chapter Planning Guide

Chapter 14

Infectious Diseases
Chapter Resources

Teacher Resources

TEACHING TRANSPARENCIES

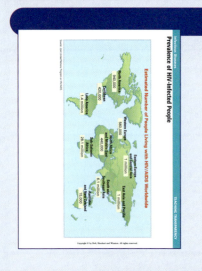
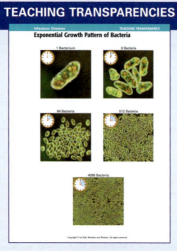
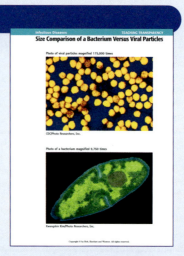

BELLRINGER TRANSPARENCIES

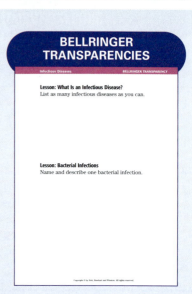

LESSON PLANS

PARENT LETTER

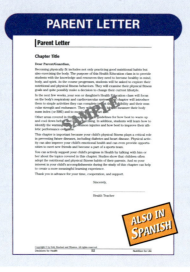

TEST ITEM LISTING

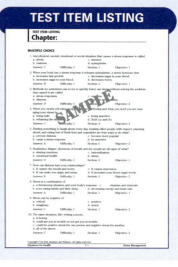

Meeting Individual Needs

DIRECTED READING

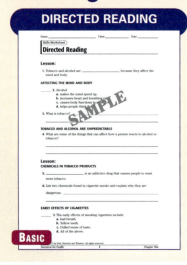

CONCEPT MAPPING

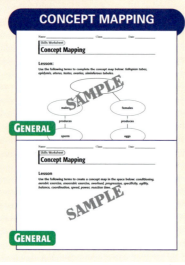

CONCEPT REVIEW

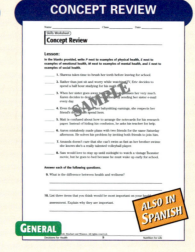

ENRICHMENT ACTIVITIES

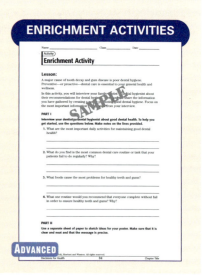

Resources

These worksheet pages can be found in the Chapter Resource File and the One-Stop Planner. The transparencies can be found in the Teaching Transparencies binder and on the One-Stop Planner.

Activities

LIFE SKILLS ACTIVITIES
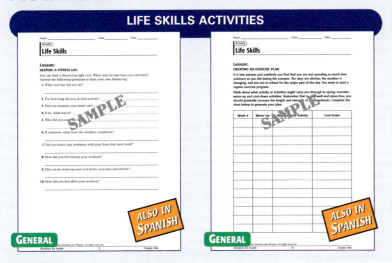

AT-HOME ACTIVITY
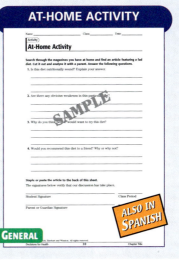

DATASHEETS FOR IN-TEXT ACTIVITIES
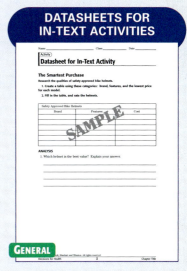

Applications

DECISION-MAKING
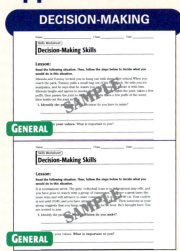

REFUSAL SKILLS
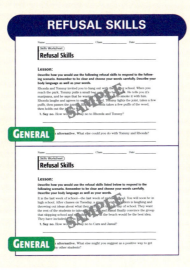

CROSS-DISCIPLINARY
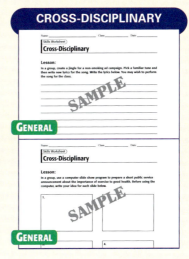

HEALTH BEHAVIOR CONTRACT
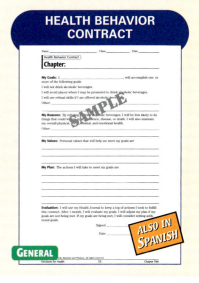

Assessments

HEALTH INVENTORY
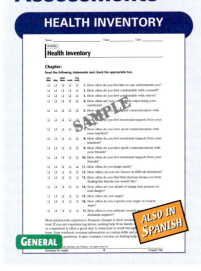

LESSON QUIZZES
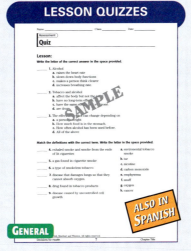

CHAPTER TEST
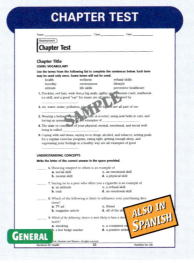

PERFORMANCE-BASED ASSESSMENT
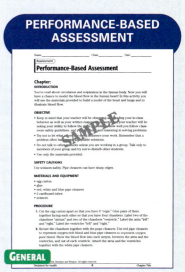

Chapter 14 • Chapter Resources and Worksheets 297D

Chapter 14: Background Information

The following information focuses on the reproductive cycle of a virus. Also included is a list of viral diseases and their symptoms. This material will help prepare you for teaching the concepts in this chapter.

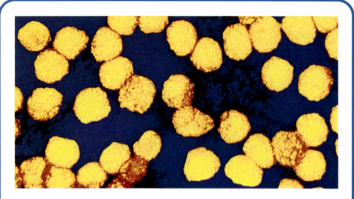

How a Virus Reproduces

- Most scientists agree that viruses are not living things. All living things are made of cells, are guided by information stored in their DNA, and are able to grow and reproduce on their own. Because viruses are acellular and do not grow and reproduce on their own, they are not classified as living things. Viruses are only able to reproduce inside a host.

- Viruses depend on a host cell's enzymes and organelles to reproduce. A virus has no control over its movements; it is spread by wind, water, and food. Once a virus comes in direct contact with a host, the virus can begin its life cycle. One method by which an animal virus enters its host is by endocytosis. Endocytosis occurs when vesicles, which are small membrane-bound sacs, pull materials in and release materials from cells.

- Once inside a cell, a virus may use one of several mechanisms to complete its life cycle. Some viruses may enter a lytic cycle in which the virus enters a host cell, replicates itself inside the cell, and then destroys the cell and releases new viruses. This cycle causes tissue and organ damage to the organism.

- Other viruses enter into a cycle in which the virus may incorporate its own DNA into the host's DNA. Every time the host cell divides, the viral DNA divides as well, resulting in more infected cells. The viral DNA can be activated by many things, such as carcinogens and UV sunlight. When the viral DNA becomes activated, it will then detach from the host DNA. The virus then enters a lytic cycle and new viral particles are produced.

- There are other less common mechanisms that viruses use when infecting cells. Some viruses have RNA instead of DNA and do not go through a DNA stage when reproducing. Other viruses enter a cell but do not reproduce or incorporate their DNA into the host genome. Although this would appear to cause no harm, the immune system recognizes these infected cells and soon destroys them.

Some Viral Diseases and Their Symptoms

The following infectious diseases are not covered in this chapter. However, students may ask questions about these diseases, many of which can be fatal.

- Chickenpox produces symptoms that include blisters, rash, muscle soreness, and fever.

- Rubella produces symptoms that include a rash, swollen glands, and fever.

- Mumps produce a painful swelling in the salivary glands.

- Smallpox produces symptoms including blisters, lesions, fever, malaise, blindness, and scars.

- Hepatitis produces symptoms that include fever, chills, nausea, swollen liver, yellow skin color, and painful joints. Liver cancer may result from some forms of hepatitis.

- Polio produces symptoms including fever, headache, stiff neck, and possible paralysis.

- Rabies produces symptoms including depression, fever, restlessness, difficulty swallowing, paralysis, and convulsions.

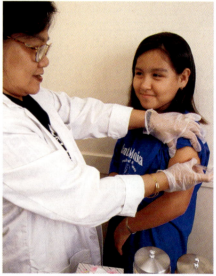

For background information about teaching strategies and issues, refer to the *Professional Reference for Teachers.*

ACTIVITIES

CHAPTER 14

Consider using the activities on this page as students explore the lessons of this chapter. Look for other activities throughout the Student Edition chapter.

Modeling Antibiotic Resistance

Hands on

Procedure Organize students into two large groups of equal numbers. Designate one group as the bacteria and the other group as the antibiotics. Put the groups on opposite sides of the room. One by one, send an antibiotic over to remove one bacterium from the group. After half of the antibiotics have taken their turn, tell the class that the symptoms of the disease have disappeared, and have the antibiotics stop removing the bacteria. Then, have other students replace the bacteria that were removed. Tell the class the symptoms have returned, and send the remaining antibiotics over. After all of the antibiotics have removed a bacterium, there will be several bacteria left. This demonstration shows the importance of taking a full course of antibiotics, even when the symptoms disappear.

Analysis Ask students the following questions:

- How does the first part of this demonstration resemble the way antibiotics work? (Antibiotics destroy disease-causing bacteria.)

- What happens when a person doesn't take all the antibiotics prescribed? (Not all bacteria are killed. Basteria that are resistant to the antibiotics survive and reproduce.)

- Why is it dangerous to not take all the prescribed antibiotics? (Some of the remaining bacteria may be resistant to the antibiotic. Because they were not killed, they have the opportunity to produce a large number of resistant bacteria. When these antibiotic-resistant bacteria reproduce, the new cells will also be resistant to the antibiotics. Thus, a new and different antibiotic must be used. Eventually, there may be no more effective antibiotics, so people will be defenseless against some bacterial infections.)

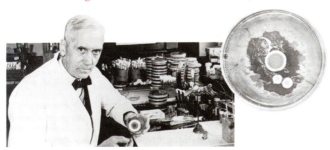

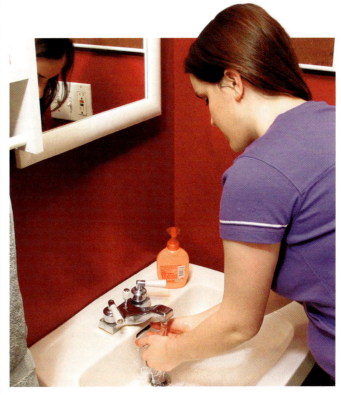

Making a Public Service Advertisement

Procedure Organize students into groups. Have students research common bacterial or viral diseases and their effects on the human body. Each group should explore a different disease. Students should research how the disease is transmitted, its symptoms, and how the disease is treated. Have each group present their findings to the class. The presentation should include a visual aid that can later serve as a poster. The poster should be a public service advertisement that raises awareness of a particular disease.

Analysis Ask students the following questions:

- What is the most common method of transmission? (Direct contact with an infected person is the most common method.)

- How can these kinds of advertisements be effective? (Images or statistics of the effects of a disease can teach people how easy it is to contract the disease, perhaps changing their behavior to avoid contracting the disease.)

Chapter 14 • Activities   **297F**

CHAPTER 14

Overview
Students will learn what an infectious disease is. They will learn about bacterial infections, viral infections, and sexually transmitted diseases. Students will also learn how antibiotics are used to treat bacterial infections. After reading this chapter, students will know how to protect themselves against infectious diseases.

Assessing Prior Knowledge
Students should be familiar with the following topics:
- decision making
- refusal skills
- body systems

Question Box
Students may feel more comfortable asking questions if you set up a Question Box to collect their questions. Have students write and anonymously submit their questions about infectious diseases, and ways to prevent the spread of these diseases. Address these questions during class, or use these questions to introduce lessons that cover related topics.

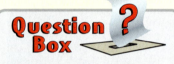

Check out *Current Health* articles and activities related to this chapter by visiting the HRW Web site at go.hrw.com. Just type in the keyword HD4CH29T.

Chapter Resource File
- Directed Reading BASIC
- Health Inventory GENERAL
- Parent Letter

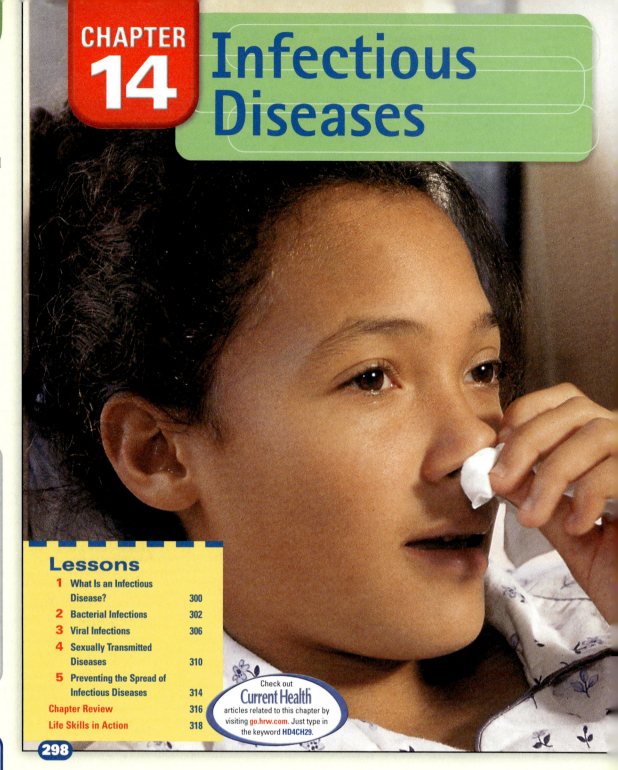

CHAPTER 14 Infectious Diseases

Lessons
1. What Is an Infectious Disease? 300
2. Bacterial Infections 302
3. Viral Infections 306
4. Sexually Transmitted Diseases 310
5. Preventing the Spread of Infectious Diseases 314

Chapter Review 316
Life Skills in Action 318

Check out **Current Health** articles related to this chapter by visiting go.hrw.com. Just type in the keyword HD4CH29.

Standards Correlations

National Health Education Standards

1.4 Explain how appropriate health care can prevent premature death and disability. (Lessons 4–5)

1.8 (partial) Describe how lifestyle, pathogens, family history, and other risk factors are related to the cause or prevention of disease and other health problems. (Lessons 1 and 5)

2.5 Describe situations requiring professional health services. (Lesson 5)

3.3 Distinguish between safe and risky or harmful behaviors in relationships. (Lesson 4)

3.4 Demonstrate strategies to improve or maintain personal and family health. (Lesson 5)

6.3 Predict how decisions regarding health behaviors have consequences for self and others. (Lesson 4)

" Last year, I got a **flu shot** and was one of the only kids in my class who didn't get **sick** and miss several days of **school**. This year, I wasn't so **lucky**. "

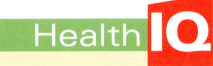

PRE-READING

Answer the following true/false questions to find out what you already know about infectious diseases. When you've finished this chapter, you'll have the opportunity to change your answers based on what you've learned.

1. The term *infectious diseases* refers to diseases that can be passed from person to person.

2. All infectious diseases are caused by tiny organisms called *bacteria*.

3. Antibiotics are drugs that are used to kill bacteria.

4. A common cold is actually an illness that is caused by many different viruses.

5. There is no way to prevent catching viral diseases.

6. *Abstinence* means "being very careful about who you have sex with."

7. HIV infection from blood transfusions is rare now, thanks to testing of donor blood.

8. HIV and AIDS exist only in America and Africa.

9. Frequent hand washing is a very useful tool against catching an infectious disease.

10. If you have a contagious disease, you should avoid public places, such as school.

11. Strep throat is caused by a virus.

12. There is no cure for AIDS at this time.

13. Tuberculosis is a disease of the past and is rarely seen today.

ANSWERS: 1. false; 2. false; 3. true; 4. true; 5. false; 6. false; 7. true; 8. false; 9. true; 10. true; 11. false; 12. true; 13. false

Using the Health IQ

Misconception Alert
Answers to the Health IQ questions may help you identify students' misconceptions.

Question 1: Students may confuse an infectious disease, which is any disease caused by a microorganism, with a contagious disease, which is a disease that can be spread directly from one person to another.

Question 3: Many people are under the impression that antibiotics can be used to treat any type of infectious disease. However, they are only effective against diseases caused by bacteria. Even then, any antibiotic is effective only against certain bacteria.

Question 7: Some students may think that blood transfusions, and even donating blood, can put them at risk for HIV in this country. Blood that is donated is carefully screened for HIV, and the equipment used for donating blood is carefully sterilized to be made free of any infection. The blood supply in the United States is very safe.

Answers

1. false
2. false
3. true
4. true
5. false
6. false
7. true
8. false
9. true
10. true
11. false
12. true
13. false

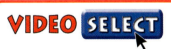

For information about videos related to this chapter, go to **go.hrw.com** and type in the keyword: **HD4ID7V**.

Lesson 1 Focus

Overview
Before beginning this lesson, review with your students the objectives listed under the What You'll Do head in the Student Edition. In this lesson, students will define an infectious disease and explain the difference between infectious diseases and contagious diseases. This lesson also explains different ways that infections can be spread.

Bellringer
Ask students to write down the names of two contagious diseases. (Sample answers: Strep throat, a cold, and the flu are contagious diseases.)

Answer to Start Off Write
Sample answer: A cold or flu is spread through direct or indirect contact with a sick person.

Motivate

Discussion — GENERAL
Infectious Talk Have students describe the last time that they had an infection. They should describe the type of disease they had, how they think they became infected, and the symptoms they experienced. Students should also include what they did to become well, as well as how they can prevent getting the infection again.
LS Auditory

Lesson 1 — What Is an Infectious Disease?

What You'll Do
- **Describe** the difference between infectious diseases and contagious diseases.
- **List** four common ways that contagious diseases spread.

Terms to Learn
- infectious disease

Start Off Write
How does a cold or flu spread from one person to another?

Daryl went to visit his friend Hector, who had been sick for several days. Daryl stayed and talked to Hector for only a few minutes. A few days later, Daryl had the same illness that Hector had. Why did Daryl get sick?

Daryl became ill because the tiny organisms that were making his friend sick infected Daryl's body, too.

Infectious Diseases
Daryl caught an infectious disease. An **infectious disease** (in FEK shuhs dih ZEEZ) is an illness that is caused by microorganisms. *Microorganisms* (MY kroh AWR guhn iz uhmz) are very small things that are found everywhere. Most microorganisms do not cause disease. In fact, there are millions of microorganisms in your body all of the time. Many of these microorganisms help your body function normally.

However, certain microorganisms do cause infectious diseases. Infectious diseases that can spread directly or indirectly from one person to another are called *contagious* diseases. Contagious diseases include sexually transmitted diseases (STDs) and many common infections, such as colds and influenza. However, not all infectious diseases are contagious.

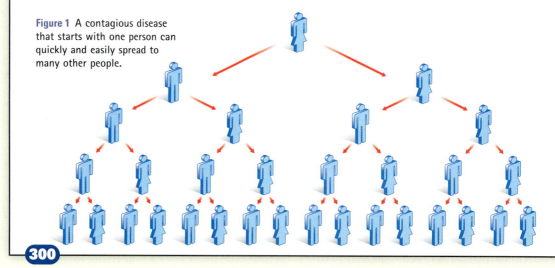

Figure 1 A contagious disease that starts with one person can quickly and easily spread to many other people.

Sensitivity ALERT
Be aware that some students may not want to discuss certain diseases or infections. Reassure the students that this discussion is voluntary.

Chapter Resource File
- Directed Reading **BASIC**
- Lesson Plan
- Datasheet for In-Text Activities
- Lesson Quiz **GENERAL**

Transparencies
TT Bellringer

---

300 Chapter 14 • Infectious Diseases

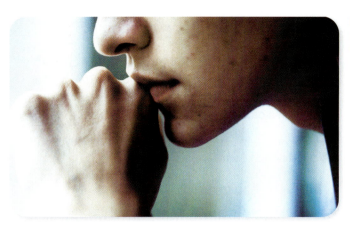

Figure 2 Touching your face passes germs from your hands to your mouth, nose, or eyes.

How Diseases Spread

Infections can come from another person, an animal, or an object. Once you have an infection, you can spread it in many ways. Here are a few of the most common ways that infections are spread.

- **Touching** Your hands are often covered in germs. Germs can be easily passed to people or objects by touching.
- **Coughing or Sneezing** Coughing or sneezing releases many germs into the air. Nearby people can inhale these germs.
- **Sharing** Sharing is usually a good thing, but sharing an infection is not. You can easily catch or spread an infection by sharing objects or food and drink with another person.
- **Sexual Contact** Certain infections are spread through sexual contact.

Hands-on ACTIVITY

INFECTIOUS HANDSHAKE

1. Your teacher will secretly select a member of your class to be a "disease carrier." This person will give a special handshake.
2. Everybody will shake hands. If you receive the secret handshake, you must give this handshake to anyone else whose hand you shake.
3. After everyone has shaken hands with five people, the people who received the secret handshake will raise their hands.

Analysis

1. Figure out the percentage of students who caught the "disease."

Lesson Review

Using Vocabulary

1. List three infectious diseases that can be passed from person to person.
2. What is a *contagious* disease?

Understanding Concepts

3. List four ways that contagious diseases can be spread. Give three examples of contagious diseases.

Critical Thinking

4. **Identifying Relationships** Not all infectious diseases are contagious. Are all contagious diseases infectious? Explain your answer.
5. **Making Inferences** Steven caught an infectious disease from eating a piece of meat that had gone bad. Is this type of disease contagious? Explain your answer.

Answers to Lesson Review

1. Examples are a cold, the flu, and strep throat.
2. A contagious disease is a disease that can spread from one person to another by direct contact.
3. Touch, coughing or sneezing, sharing food and drink, and sexual contact are ways to spread diseases.
4. All contagious diseases are infectious, as they are caused by microorganisms being spread directly from person to person.
5. No, this disease is not contagious. A person could only get the disease from eating the bad meat. This disease doesn't spread directly from person to person.

Hands-on ACTIVITY

Note: Tell students not to shake hands with the same person twice.

Answer

The percentage of students who caught the "disease" will depend on the size of the class.

Teach

INCLUSION Strategies — BASIC

- Attention Deficit Disorder
- Behavior Control Issues

Students with attention deficit disorders and behavior control issues are more comfortable when they are allowed to spend time out of their seats. Have students choose a partner. Ask each pair to act out a scenario demonstrating how a person can show a sick friend that he or she cares without exposing himself or herself to an infectious disease. (Examples of scenarios are talking on the phone, sending flowers or gifts, dropping off food, or bringing homework to the student.) **LS Kinesthetic**

Close

Reteaching — BASIC

Spreading Disease Ask for a student volunteer. Draw a stick figure on the board to represent the student. Ask the student how many family members he or she lives with. Draw that number of stick figures under the original stick figure, and connect the new stick figures to the original stick figure. Now, draw another stick figure next to the original to represent another student in the class. Draw a line between the two figures. Explain that if the original student had a contagious disease, he or she could spread it to family members and classmates. Continue the exercise by adding classmates and each classmate's family and friends to show how a disease can spread. **LS Visual**

Quiz — GENERAL

1. Are all microorganisms bad for your health? Explain. (No, many microorganisms play important roles in the health of people.)
2. How can sneezing spread an infection? (Sneezing releases many germs into the air, which can be inhaled by other people.)

Lesson 1 • What Is an Infectious Disease?

Lesson 2

Focus

Overview
Before beginning this lesson, review with your students the objectives listed under the What You'll Do head in the Student Edition. This lesson explains what bacteria are and describes some common bacterial infections. Students will also learn how antibiotics are used to treat bacterial infection.

🔔 Bellringer
Ask students to describe one bacterial infection. (Answers may vary. Sample answers are strep throat, tetanus, and food poisoning.)

Answer to Start Off Write
Sample answer: Antibiotics are usually used to treat bacterial infections.

Motivate

Group Activity —— GENERAL
Debate Organize the students into two large groups. Have students research safety issues and risks involved with ear piercing. Have students debate the issue on ear piercing. Tell students to include in their debate information on safety procedures, the risks of ear piercing, and ways that the risks could be reduced. **LS Kinesthetic**

Lesson 2 — Bacterial Infections

What You'll Do
- **Identify** three common bacterial infections and their symptoms.
- **List** five ways to avoid bacterial infections.
- **Describe** one way to treat bacterial infections.

Terms to Learn
- bacteria
- antibiotic

Start Off Write
How are bacterial infections treated?

Tina's throat started hurting so badly that Tina could barely swallow. She also had a fever. Her doctor told her that she had an illness called strep throat.

Strep throat is a bacterial infection. But what are bacteria, and how do they make a person ill?

What Are Bacteria?
Some of the most common infectious diseases are caused by bacteria. **Bacteria** (bak TIR ee uh) are very simple single-celled microorganisms that are found everywhere. Bacteria reproduce very quickly by dividing in half. One bacterium can divide into two identical bacteria in as little as 20 minutes. Because they can reproduce so rapidly, a few bacteria can often cause a serious infection very quickly. Bacteria invade a host, such as a human, animal, or plant. Once inside the host, the bacteria get nutrients from the host's cells. In the process, the bacteria may cause damage to the host. If left untreated, bacterial infections can be very serious or deadly.

1 Bacterium
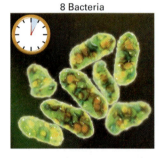

8 Bacteria
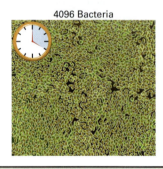

Figure 3 A single bacterium can double once every 20 minutes. At this rate, a single bacterium may become 4,096 bacteria in only 4 hours.

64 Bacteria
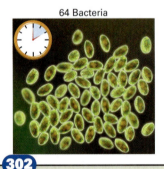

512 Bacteria
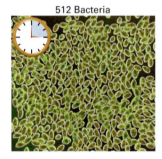

4096 Bacteria

302

Background
Ancient Bacteria Students may be interested to know that bacteria are probably the oldest known life-forms on Earth. While the bacteria may seem too small to form a fossil of any kind, one kind of bacteria, called *Cyanobacteria* or *"blue-green algae,"* have left a fossil record. This type of bacteria dates back to the Precambrian era, which was as long ago as 3.5 billion years and which makes them the oldest known fossils.

Chapter Resource File
- Directed Reading **BASIC**
- Lesson Plan
- Lesson Quiz **GENERAL**

Transparencies
- TT Bellringer
- TT Exponential Growth Pattern of Bacteria

302 Chapter 14 • Infectious Diseases

Strep Throat

Strep throat is caused by a type of bacterium called *streptococcus* (STREP tuh CAHK uhs). Although strep throat infections most commonly cause pain in the throat, these infections can also cause body aches elsewhere. The main symptom of strep throat is pain when you try to swallow. Most people also have a fever with strep throat.

If your doctor thinks you might have strep throat, he or she may take a throat culture. A *throat culture* is a test in which a doctor uses a cotton swab to wipe the back of the throat. The material on the swab is then tested for strep throat bacteria. If the throat culture shows that you have strep throat, the doctor will give you a medicine to fight the bacteria. You should take all of the medicine even if you feel better in a few days. You must take all of the medicine to make sure that all infectious bacteria have been killed. If strep throat infections are not treated properly, they can cause a condition called *rheumatic fever*. This disease can affect your heart valves and can make you very sick long after the sore throat is gone.

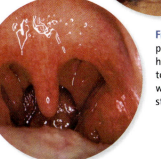

Figure 4 The throat in the picture on the bottom is healthy. The throat in the top picture is infected with bacteria that cause strep throat.

Sinus Infections

The *sinuses* (SIEN uhs uhz) are spaces located within the front of the skull. There are several pairs of sinuses located in the front of the head, above the mouth. Most, but not all, of the sinuses have a small tube that drains fluid down into the nose or throat. If this tube gets blocked by something, the sinus can become clogged. Clogging of the sinuses can cause the sinuses to become inflamed, which means that they swell and begin to hurt. This inflammation of a sinus is called *sinusitis* (SIEN uhs IET is).

Sinusitis is often caused by bacterial infections. These infections can be caused by many different types of bacteria. Bacterial sinus infections are rarely transmitted from person to person. In other words, bacterial sinus infections are usually not contagious. Often, sinusitis may be confused with colds or flu. The symptoms of sinusitis include congestion, a runny nose, a fever, or a headache. If you have bacterial sinusitis, your doctor will give you medicine to kill the bacteria.

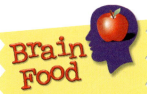

Brain Food

Most bacteria are completely harmless. In fact, there are millions of bacteria in your body right now. Some of these bacteria are necessary for your body to work correctly. For example, bacteria in your intestines play an important role in providing nutrients during digestion of your food.

Teach, continued

Discussion —— GENERAL

Carriers Tuberculosis, which usually affects the lungs, can spread to other parts of the body, such as the kidneys and brain. Only about 10 percent of people infected with *Mycobacterium* get "active" TB, which means they exhibit symptoms of the disease. Bacteria may remain dormant in the lungs of some people. These people are called *carriers* because they do not exhibit any symptoms of the disease. Often, carriers can get rid of the bacteria by taking medicine, but sometimes the bacteria survive. Then, the best defense against getting the active disease is to live a healthy lifestyle. Ask the students what they consider to be a healthy lifestyle and what extra steps carriers could take to prevent an active infection.
LS Auditory

Group Activity —— GENERAL

Group Report Organize students into groups, and have them research information on both a harmful and a helpful type of bacteria. Each group should write a report about a harmful bacterium and a helpful bacterium, including the name of each type of bacterium, where the bacterium can be found, and why the bacterium is either helpful or harmful. Have the groups present their reports to the class. (Sample answer: *Clostridium tetani* is a bacterium found in the soil and if the bacterium enters through a cut in the skin, it can cause tetanus. *Escherichia coli* is found in the intestinal tract and helps the body digest food.)
LS Interpersonal

Myth & Fact

Myth: Tuberculosis used to be a dangerous disease, but people rarely get it anymore.

Fact: Tuberculosis is on the rise. In the United States in the year 2000, more than 16,000 cases of tuberculosis were reported.

Tuberculosis

Tuberculosis is a serious disease caused by a slow-growing bacterium. This bacterium is in the family of long, thin bacteria called *mycobacteria*. People who have tuberculosis may feel very tired and may have a fever, night sweats, and a cough. Tuberculosis is usually spread through a very contagious cough. However some people with tuberculosis have few or no symptoms. These people are called *carriers*. Even though a carrier does not have symptoms of the disease, he or she can pass the disease to others. Your doctor can find out if you have been exposed to tuberculosis by doing a simple test. During this test, your doctor injects a small amount of a special fluid under your skin. If you have been exposed to tuberculosis, your skin will have a reaction to this fluid. Tuberculosis kills about 3 million people a year worldwide. Because tuberculosis is so contagious, all cases must be reported to the health department.

Avoiding Bacterial Infections

There are many ways to reduce your chances of getting a bacterial infection. The best ways are listed below.

- Limit your contact with people who have a bacterial infection.
- Avoid sharing food or drink with others, especially if they have an infection.
- Wash your hands frequently and carefully with soap and warm water.
- Take warm showers frequently.
- Be sure to eat properly and get enough sleep. Then your body will be stronger and more able to fight infections.

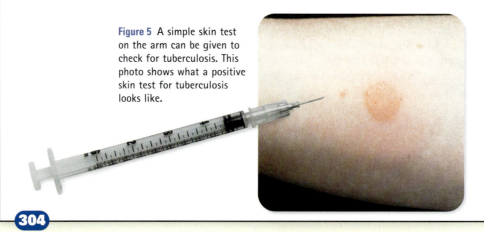

Figure 5 A simple skin test on the arm can be given to check for tuberculosis. This photo shows what a positive skin test for tuberculosis looks like.

Life SKILL BUILDER —— ADVANCED

Being a Wise Consumer Most grocery stores have sections devoted to liquid hand-soaps that contain antibacterial products. But these soaps can be harmful, scientists believe. Have students research the effects of overuse of antibacterial soaps and present their findings to the class. (The harsh detergent action can leave you vulnerable to hand eczema, which can cause the spread of harmful bacteria. The soaps can also contribute to the increase of bacteria that are resistant to antibacterial treatments.) **LS Verbal**

Attention Grabber

Most students doubt the existence of extraterrestrial life on Earth, so the following information may surprise them. Many scientists think that over millions of years, bacteria have traveled to Earth from Mars in meteorites. Recent experiments support the theory that bacteria, which used to inhabit Mars, could survive the long journey between the two planets.

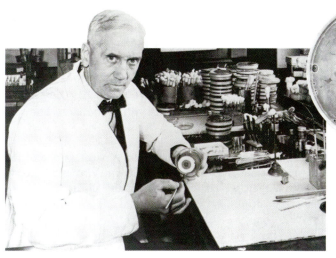

Figure 6 Alexander Fleming discovered penicillin when he noticed that bacteria in a dish were dying around a spot where a mold was growing.

Antibiotics

Fortunately for the millions of people who develop bacterial infections each year, doctors can treat these infections with antibiotics. An **antibiotic** is a drug that can kill bacteria or slow the growth of bacteria. Antibiotics are made naturally by many different organisms, such as other bacteria and molds. Humans have used these substances to fight dangerous bacteria. Penicillin, the first antibiotic, was discovered by accident in 1928. This discovery happened when a scientist named Alexander Fleming noticed that bacteria in a Petri dish were dying where a mold was growing. But it wasn't until the 1940's that antibiotics became available to many people. If you take an antibiotic, you should follow the doctor's instructions carefully. Complete all of the antibiotics. This will ensure that you get rid of all of the bacteria that are making you sick.

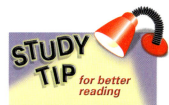

STUDY TIP for better reading

Word Origins The word *antibiotic* comes from two root words: *anti-*, meaning "against," and *biotic*, meaning "life." So *antibiotic* means "against life." This name refers to the ability of antibiotics to kill small living organisms, particularly bacteria.

Lesson Review

Using Vocabulary
1. What are bacteria?
2. What is an antibiotic?

Understanding Concepts
3. Identify three common bacterial infections, and describe their symptoms.
4. What are five things you can do to keep from catching or spreading a bacterial infection?

Critical Thinking
5. **Making Inferences** Look at the figure on the first page of this lesson. Why were so many more bacteria produced in the fourth hour than were produced in the first hour?

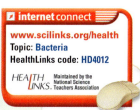

internet connect
www.scilinks.org/health
Topic: Bacteria
HealthLinks code: HD4012

Answers to Lesson Review
1. Bacteria are a group of very simple single-celled organisms that are found everywhere.
2. An antibiotic is a drug that can kill or slow the growth of bacteria.
3. Strep throat causes pain when you swallow as well as fever and body aches. Sinus infections cause inflamed sinuses, congestion, runny nose, fever, and headache. Tuberculosis causes a fever, tiredness, night sweats, and a cough.
4. You can limit contact with people who are infected and avoid sharing food or drink with others, especially if they have an infection. You can also wash your hands frequently and carefully. And you can eat properly and get enough sleep.
5. The first hour started with only one bacterium dividing. The fourth hour started with 512 bacteria dividing.

INCLUSION Strategies — BASIC
- Developmentally Delayed
- Learning Disabled

Give all students a chance to successfully take part in a data-collection activity so that they can understand the relative regularity of the common cold, the flu, and mononucleosis (mono). Organize the class into teams of four or five students. Place students of different abilities on each team. Ask students to create a chart to show how often teachers have had the cold, flu, and mono in the last 2 years. Have teams survey at least 25 teachers of varying ages and then report their findings to the class. Require that all team members actively participate.
LS Kinesthetic

Close

Reteaching — BASIC
Bacterial Infections Have students work together in pairs and write a description of the three types of bacterial infections in this lesson. Students should include the symptoms and the treatment for each disease. Students should also explain how to prevent the spread of bacterial infections. Have the students quiz each other over the information they wrote.
LS Verbal

Quiz — GENERAL
1. Where do bacteria that have invaded a host get their nutrients? (from the host's cells)
2. What can result if strep throat goes untreated? (An untreated strep throat infection can cause a condition called *rheumatic fever*, which can affect the heart valves.)
3. What was the first antibiotic known to man? (penicillin)
4. What is a carrier of a disease? (It is a person who is infected with the bacteria that cause the disease, but who shows no symptoms of that disease.)

Lesson 2 • Bacterial Infections

Lesson 3 Focus

Overview
Before beginning this lesson, review with your students the objectives listed under the What You'll Do head in the Student Edition. This lesson explains what a virus is and how it infects the human body. Students will learn about common viral infections. This lesson also describes how vaccines can help prevent viral infections.

🔔 Bellringer
Ask students about the last time they had a cold. Ask them how long their cold lasted, and what they used to treat their symptoms.
LS *Verbal*

Answer to Start Off Write
Accept all reasonable answers. Sample answer: A cold, flu, AIDS, or herpes are examples of viral infections.

Motivate

Activity — GENERAL
Virus ID Have students work in groups to create a list of diseases that they think are caused by viruses. Ask students to write how they think that disease is contracted next to each disease listed. Students should also give a written description of the symptoms of each disease. (Diseases may include the common cold, influenza, AIDS, chickenpox, the mumps, mononucleosis, and rabies. Symptoms vary.) Discuss the lists with the class.
LS *Verbal*

Lesson 3 — Viral Infections

What You'll Do
- **Explain** how viruses infect the body.
- **Identify** three common viral infections and their symptoms.
- **Describe** how vaccines protect against disease.

Terms to Learn
- virus
- vaccine

Start Off Write
What is an example of a viral infection?

One of the most common infections in the world is the cold. You have probably had a cold several times. But what causes the common cold?

The common cold is caused by a virus. A **virus** is one of the smallest and simplest disease-causing agent. Viruses are everywhere, and they are responsible for many diseases, some of which can be deadly.

Are Viruses Alive?
Most scientists do not consider viruses to be living things. Like living things, viruses contain proteins and genetic material. *Genetic material* is chemical information that is passed on during reproduction. However, unlike living things, a virus cannot reproduce on its own. A virus must reproduce by invading a living thing, such as an animal or person. The virus then uses the organism's cells to produce more viruses. When viruses invade your cells and use them to produce more viruses, a viral infection occurs. Viral infections can be transmitted in many ways. Viruses can be passed by touching living or nonliving objects, coughing, sneezing, insect bites, blood, or sexual contact.

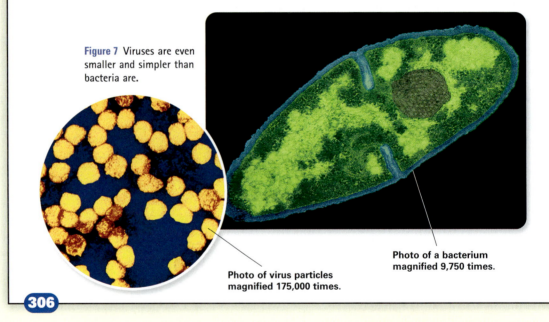

Figure 7 Viruses are even smaller and simpler than bacteria are.

Photo of virus particles magnified 175,000 times.

Photo of a bacterium magnified 9,750 times.

Background
Beginning Virology Though scientists had been studying bacteria for some time, it wasn't until the end of the 19th century that scientists discovered the existence of viruses. At the time, scientists lacked the technology to thoroughly study something as small as a virus. Viruses were thought to be tiny ancestors of bacteria until 1935 when Wendell Stanley isolated the tobacco mosaic virus (TMV), which causes stunted growth in tobacco plants. Stanley's work suggested that viruses were chemicals rather than a life form. Although some of Stanley's assumptions were false, his work led to the modern understanding of viruses.

Chapter Resource File
- Directed Reading **BASIC**
- Lesson Plan
- Lesson Quiz **GENERAL**

Transparencies
- TT Bellringer
- TT Sizes of a Bacterium and Several Viruses

---

306 Chapter 14 • Infectious Diseases

TABLE 1 The Symptoms of Common Infections

Infections	Symptoms
A common cold	congestion, runny nose, sore throat, sneezing, and coughing
Influenza	body aches, headaches, high fever, chills, congestion, cough, and sore throat
Viral sinus infection	congestion, runny nose with thick mucus, high fever, and headache

The Common Cold

The most common viral infection is the cold. The common cold is actually caused by two or three different kinds of viruses. On average, each person gets about two colds a year. Colds are spread from person to person by coughing, sneezing, or touching. The symptoms of a cold include congestion, a runny nose, a sore throat, sneezing, and coughing. There are many medicines that can treat the symptoms of a cold, and just recently, a medicine that can cure the common cold is available. If you have a cold, you should drink a lot of fluid and get plenty of rest. Because colds are very contagious, you should also stay away from school or other public places if you have a cold.

Influenza

Influenza, or the "flu," is a viral infection that is very common in the winter months. There are three types of influenza, each of which has many different *strains*, or variations. Like the common cold, the flu is spread by touching, coughing, or sneezing. The symptoms of the flu include body aches, headaches, a high fever, chills, congestion, cough, and a sore throat. When you have the flu, you may have any or all of these symptoms. Many of these symptoms are similar to cold symptoms. A high fever is the main difference between the two viral infections. If you think that you might have the flu, you should talk to your doctor right away.

It is hard to predict when an influenza outbreak will happen. The number of flu cases varies from year to year. One way to avoid the flu is to be given a vaccine. A **vaccine** is a substance that helps the body build a resistance to a certain disease. Vaccines cannot completely stop the spread of a virus. In fact, a new flu vaccine must be developed every year because new strains of the flu develop every year. Receiving the flu shot one year does not guarantee that you will be protected against the flu the next year.

Myth & Fact

Myth: You catch a cold when you are out in cold or wet weather.

Fact: Colds are caused by viruses, not by the weather.

Health Journal

Have you ever received a flu vaccine? How did you feel after you received the shot? Did you get the flu that season? Write about the experience in your Health Journal.

REAL-LIFE CONNECTION — ADVANCED

Chickenpox and Shingles Chickenpox is a highly contagious viral disease that results in a fever and a skin rash. After the symptoms have disappeared, the chickenpox viruses continue to live in the nerve cells of the body, but the viruses are kept inactive by the body's immune system. As people age, their immune system weakens, and the virus can be activated. This results in a disease called *shingles*. Shingles is very painful. Symptoms associated with shingles include a fever and a severe localized rash. Pneumonia can result from the weakened immune system. Although shingles is not contagious, contact with a person who has shingles can cause chickenpox in someone who has never had it. **LS Auditory**

Teach, continued

Discussion — ADVANCED

Electronic Viruses As the use of computers spreads to all parts of our society, the risk of and damage caused by electronic viruses becomes more severe. Ask students to debate the similarities and the differences between electronic viruses and biological viruses. Ask students, "What makes each of them so destructive?" (Examples of similarities are as follows: Both types of viruses depend on a host—a body or a computer—for reproduction and for being spread from one body or computer to another. A biological virus can cause harm to a person's body or to a society during an epidemic. And an electronic virus can damage a person's computer or cause damage to a business whose systems are infected. A biological virus can damage organ systems, and a computer virus can damage important data systems.) **LS Auditory**

Using the Figure — GENERAL

Ask students how the remedies pictured in the figure on this page can help a person recover from the flu. Ask students whether these remedies destroy the virus. (Tell students that these remedies do nothing to destroy the virus itself, they merely treat the symptoms. Flu remedies can help relieve body aches, fever, congestion, cough, and sore throat, but a person's immune system must fight the infection itself. Recently, antiviral medications have become available to specifically treat the flu.) **LS Visual**

Answer to Science Activity
The Epstein-Barr Virus has been associated with Burkitt's lymphoma and Chronic Fatigue Syndrome.

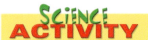

The Epstein-Barr virus has been linked to diseases other than mono. Research this virus, and describe two other diseases (or syndromes) associated with EBV.

Mononucleosis

Mononucleosis (MAHN oh NOO klee OH sis), also known as *mono* or the *kissing disease*, is caused by a virus called the *Epstein-Barr virus,* or EBV. In the United States, mono is most common in older teens and young adults. EBV is spread from person to person by coughing, sneezing, kissing, or sharing food and drink. Mononucleosis can make you tired for weeks. It can also give you a bad sore throat, a fever, a swollen spleen, and swollen lymph nodes. *Lymph nodes* are small organs located throughout the body that help remove harmful substances from your body. About three-fourths of the people who get infected with mononucleosis have no symptoms at all. People who have mononucleosis but have no symptoms can still pass the disease to others.

Fighting Viral Infections

Most viral infections will make you uncomfortable but will do little harm. However, some viral infections can cause more serious problems, especially for babies, older people, and people who get sick easily. Your body has many defenses and natural chemicals that successfully fight off viral infections. For example, your saliva contains chemicals that help kill some viruses. The mucus in your nose also traps viruses and keeps them from getting into your body. Antiviral drugs are now available to treat a few viral infections. Most viral infections run their course while you take care of your body with extra rest.

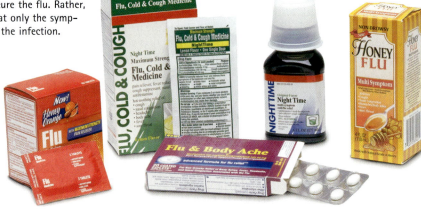

Figure 8 Most flu "remedies" do not cure the flu. Rather, they treat only the symptoms of the infection.

Background

Emerging Viruses A virus that is dangerous to humans and that forms and evolves in an isolated area of the world is called an *emerging virus.* Emerging viruses are one of the world's major health issues. While many of these viruses, such as the Ebola virus and the Lassa virus, originated in Africa, a virus called the Hanta virus has emerged in the southwestern United States. This virus spreads through the droppings or urine of rodents. The virus, which is often fatal to humans, is contracted by inhaling viral particles. **LS Auditory**

Attention Grabber

Students probably know that the flu can be dangerous, but they may be surprised to know how many deaths that it has caused. In 1918, more than 21 million deaths were attributed to the flu worldwide. Each year, 20,000 deaths are associated with the flu in the United States.

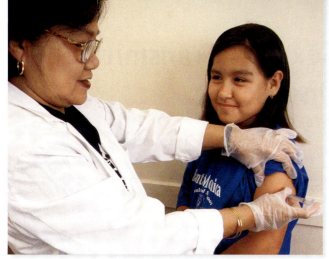

Figure 9 Getting a vaccination is less painful than getting a viral infection.

Getting Your Shots

The best tools available to prevent viral diseases are vaccines. Today, vaccines are used all over the world to prevent many serious diseases. A vaccine contains viruses or parts of viruses that have been specially treated so that they don't make you sick. Instead of infecting you with a virus, vaccines fool your body into thinking it has been infected. This causes your body to produce chemicals to fight the infection. These chemicals then give you protection from the real virus. Although common vaccines can sometimes—though very rarely—cause harm, their benefits far outweigh their risks. Students are often legally required to get vaccines before they are allowed to go to school. Some vaccines require only one or two doses, but others, like the flu vaccine, should be received every year. Your doctor can tell you if you have had all of the shots that you need.

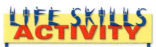

PRACTICING WELLNESS

Talk to your parents or guardians about which vaccinations you have had recently. Find out when you were vaccinated and when you are supposed to receive additional vaccinations. Make a chart for yourself that contains all of this information.

Lesson Review

Using Vocabulary
1. What is a virus?
2. What is a vaccine?

Understanding Concepts
3. How do viruses reproduce?
4. Identify three common viral infections, and describe the symptoms of each one.
5. How do the symptoms of influenza differ from the symptoms of a common cold?

Critical Thinking
6. **Making Good Decisions** Your mom has made an appointment for you to get a flu shot at the clinic. But you just had one last year. Will last year's shot prevent the flu this year? Explain your answer.

internet connect
www.scilinks.org/health
Topic: Viruses
HealthLinks code: HD4104
HEALTH LINKS. Maintained by the National Science Teachers Association

---

Answers to Lesson Review
1. A virus is a small, simple disease-causing agent.
2. A vaccine is a substance that helps the body build resistance to a disease.
3. A virus enters a cell and uses the host's cell to produce more viruses.
4. The symptoms of a common cold are runny nose, congestion, sore throat, and cough. Flu symptoms are the same as cold symptoms, but include body aches and high fever. Symptoms of mononucleosis are sore throat, fever, and swollen lymph nodes.
5. Additional symptoms of the flu are headaches, high fever, body aches, and chills.
6. This year's flu may not be caused by the same strain of virus, so last year's shot will not protect you.

Cultural Awareness — GENERAL

Vaccines Abroad Have students work in groups. Students should choose an underdeveloped country and research the following questions: What kinds of viral diseases are most prevalent in this country? Do children receive vaccinations for these diseases? How many children die because of these diseases? Have students present their findings to the class. Students should include a visual aid, such as a poster, in their oral report.
LS Verbal

Close

Reteaching — BASIC

Viral Infections Have students write a short story about a viral infection. They can tell the story from their own perspective by explaining how they contracted and fought off the disease, or they can tell the story from the perspective of their body's defenses. They can also tell the story from the perspective of the virus by describing how the virus enters and infects the body. Students fluent in another language may be interested in writing a story in their other language. **English Language Learners**
LS Verbal

Quiz — GENERAL

1. Why do scientists believe that viruses are not living things? (A virus cannot reproduce on its own and is not composed of cells.)
2. Why can't the common cold be treated with antibiotics? (Antibiotics only work on bacterial infections, and the common cold is a viral infection an antiviral drug is needed for a cold.)
3. What are two of your body's natural defenses against viral infections? (Saliva contains chemicals that kill some viruses; mucus in your nose traps viruses.)

Lesson 4

Focus

Overview
Before beginning this lesson, review with your students the objectives listed under the What You'll Do head in the Student Edition. This lesson defines a sexually transmitted disease and describes the symptoms and consequences of common STDs. Students will learn about the difference between HIV and AIDS and how HIV can be transmitted. Students will also learn that abstinence is the most effective way to avoid contracting STDs.

🔔 Bellringer
Ask students where they would go to get reliable information about STDs and why they think these sources are reliable. **LS** Verbal

Answer to Start Off Write
Sample answers: STDs that I have heard of are AIDS, gonorrhea, syphilis, and genital warts.

Motivate

Activity — GENERAL
Matching Information Have students work in pairs. Ask one student in each pair to write the names of all of the STDs in the table on this page on separate 3 in. × 5 in. cards. Have the other student write the long-term consequences of each disease on separate 3 in. × 5 in. cards. The students should then try to match each STD with its corresponding long-term consequence. **LS** Verbal

---

Lesson 4 — Sexually Transmitted Diseases

What You'll Do
- **Explain** what a sexually transmitted disease is.
- **Identify** seven common sexually transmitted diseases.
- **Explain** the difference between HIV and AIDS.
- **Identify** four ways that HIV can be passed from person to person.

Terms to Learn
- sexually transmitted disease (STD)
- sexual abstinence
- AIDS
- HIV

Write
How many STDs have you heard of? List them.

One in every four people newly infected with a sexually transmitted disease is a teenager!

Every year there are millions of new cases of diseases that are spread through sexual contact. Many of these diseases not only are painful, but several of them also have no cure.

What Are STDs?

Herpes is just one of the incurable diseases that can be sexually transmitted. A **sexually transmitted disease** (STD) is any disease that can be passed from person to person by any form of sexual contact. STDs can be caused by bacteria, viruses, fungi, or parasites.

The symptoms of STDs vary. Some STDs cause very serious and painful symptoms. Other STDs cause no symptoms at all in some people. This means that a person with an STD can sometimes not know that he or she has the infection. This person can then unknowingly spread the disease to others. If untreated, some STDs can cause lasting pain and *infertility*, or the inability to produce children. Other STDs can cause brain damage, paralysis, and death. The only sure way to protect yourself from these diseases is to practice sexual abstinence. **Sexual abstinence** is the refusal to take part in sexual activity.

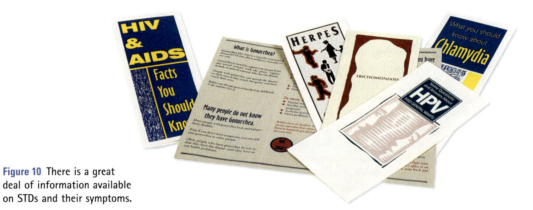

Figure 10 There is a great deal of information available on STDs and their symptoms.

Sensitivity ALERT
Some students may know someone who is suffering from AIDS or who has died from AIDS. Be sensitive to their feelings, and remember that it may upset them to talk about this topic with the class.

Chapter Resource File
- Directed Reading **BASIC**
- Lesson Plan
- Lesson Quiz **GENERAL**

Transparencies
- TT Bellringer
- TT Estimated Number of People Living with HIV/AIDS Worldwide

310 Chapter 14 • Infectious Diseases

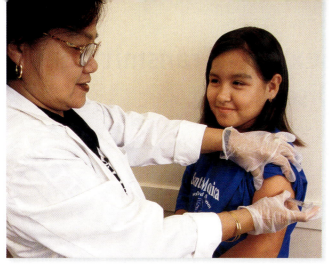

Figure 9 Getting a vaccination is less painful than getting a viral infection.

Getting Your Shots

The best tools available to prevent viral diseases are vaccines. Today, vaccines are used all over the world to prevent many serious diseases. A vaccine contains viruses or parts of viruses that have been specially treated so that they don't make you sick. Instead of infecting you with a virus, vaccines fool your body into thinking it has been infected. This causes your body to produce chemicals to fight the infection. These chemicals then give you protection from the real virus. Although common vaccines can sometimes—though very rarely—cause harm, their benefits far outweigh their risks. Students are often legally required to get vaccines before they are allowed to go to school. Some vaccines require only one or two doses, but others, like the flu vaccine, should be received every year. Your doctor can tell you if you have had all of the shots that you need.

LIFE SKILLS ACTIVITY

PRACTICING WELLNESS

Talk to your parents or guardians about which vaccinations you have had recently. Find out when you were vaccinated and when you are supposed to receive additional vaccinations. Make a chart for yourself that contains all of this information.

Lesson Review

Using Vocabulary
1. What is a virus?
2. What is a vaccine?

Understanding Concepts
3. How do viruses reproduce?
4. Identify three common viral infections, and describe the symptoms of each one.
5. How do the symptoms of influenza differ from the symptoms of a common cold?

Critical Thinking
6. **Making Good Decisions** Your mom has made an appointment for you to get a flu shot at the clinic. But you just had one last year. Will last year's shot prevent the flu this year? Explain your answer.

internet connect
www.scilinks.org/health
Topic: Viruses
HealthLinks code: HD4104
HEALTH LINKS. Maintained by the National Science Teachers Association

---

Answers to Lesson Review

1. A virus is a small, simple disease-causing agent.
2. A vaccine is a substance that helps the body build resistance to a disease.
3. A virus enters a cell and uses the host's cell to produce more viruses.
4. The symptoms of a common cold are runny nose, congestion, sore throat, and cough. Flu symptoms are the same as cold symptoms, but include body aches and high fever. Symptoms of mononucleosis are sore throat, fever, and swollen lymph nodes.
5. Additional symptoms of the flu are headaches, high fever, body aches, and chills.
6. This year's flu may not be caused by the same strain of virus, so last year's shot will not protect you.

Cultural Awareness — GENERAL

Vaccines Abroad Have students work in groups. Students should choose an underdeveloped country and research the following questions: What kinds of viral diseases are most prevalent in this country? Do children receive vaccinations for these diseases? How many children die because of these diseases? Have students present their findings to the class. Students should include a visual aid, such as a poster, in their oral report.
LS Verbal

Close

Reteaching — BASIC

Viral Infections Have students write a short story about a viral infection. They can tell the story from their own perspective by explaining how they contracted and fought off the disease, or they can tell the story from the perspective of their body's defenses. They can also tell the story from the perspective of the virus by describing how the virus enters and infects the body. Students fluent in another language may be interested in writing a story in their other language. **English Language Learners**
LS Verbal

Quiz — GENERAL

1. Why do scientists believe that viruses are not living things? (A virus cannot reproduce on its own and is not composed of cells.)
2. Why can't the common cold be treated with antibiotics? (Antibiotics only work on bacterial infections, and the common cold is a viral infection an antiviral drug is needed for a cold.)
3. What are two of your body's natural defenses against viral infections? (Saliva contains chemicals that kill some viruses; mucus in your nose traps viruses.)

Lesson 3 • Viral Infections

Lesson 4 Focus

Overview
Before beginning this lesson, review with your students the objectives listed under the What You'll Do head in the Student Edition. This lesson defines a sexually transmitted disease and describes the symptoms and consequences of common STDs. Students will learn about the difference between HIV and AIDS and how HIV can be transmitted. Students will also learn that abstinence is the most effective way to avoid contracting STDs.

🔔 Bellringer
Ask students where they would go to get reliable information about STDs and why they think these sources are reliable. **LS** Verbal

Answer to Start Off Write
Sample answers: STDs that I have heard of are AIDS, gonorrhea, syphilis, and genital warts.

Motivate

Activity — GENERAL
Matching Information Have students work in pairs. Ask one student in each pair to write the names of all of the STDs in the table on this page on separate 3 in. × 5 in. cards. Have the other student write the long-term consequences of each disease on separate 3 in. × 5 in. cards. The students should then try to match each STD with its corresponding long-term consequence. **LS** Verbal

---

Lesson 4 — Sexually Transmitted Diseases

What You'll Do
- **Explain** what a sexually transmitted disease is.
- **Identify** seven common sexually transmitted diseases.
- **Explain** the difference between HIV and AIDS.
- **Identify** four ways that HIV can be passed from person to person.

Terms to Learn
- sexually transmitted disease (STD)
- sexual abstinence
- AIDS
- HIV

Start Off Write
How many STDs have you heard of? List them.

One in every four people newly infected with a sexually transmitted disease is a teenager!

Every year there are millions of new cases of diseases that are spread through sexual contact. Many of these diseases not only are painful, but several of them also have no cure.

What Are STDs?
Herpes is just one of the incurable diseases that can be sexually transmitted. A **sexually transmitted disease** (STD) is any disease that can be passed from person to person by any form of sexual contact. STDs can be caused by bacteria, viruses, fungi, or parasites.

The symptoms of STDs vary. Some STDs cause very serious and painful symptoms. Other STDs cause no symptoms at all in some people. This means that a person with an STD can sometimes not know that he or she has the infection. This person can then unknowingly spread the disease to others. If untreated, some STDs can cause lasting pain and *infertility*, or the inability to produce children. Other STDs can cause brain damage, paralysis, and death. The only sure way to protect yourself from these diseases is to practice sexual abstinence. **Sexual abstinence** is the refusal to take part in sexual activity.

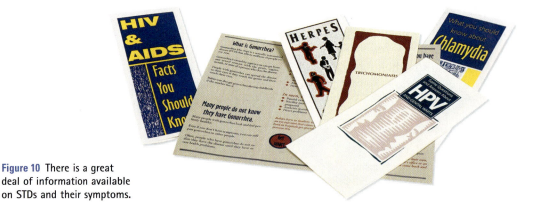
Figure 10 There is a great deal of information available on STDs and their symptoms.

Sensitivity ALERT
Some students may know someone who is suffering from AIDS or who has died from AIDS. Be sensitive to their feelings, and remember that it may upset them to talk about this topic with the class.

Chapter Resource File
- Directed Reading **BASIC**
- Lesson Plan
- Lesson Quiz **GENERAL**

Transparencies
- TT Bellringer
- TT Estimated Number of People Living with HIV/AIDS Worldwide

Common STDs

You might think that STDs are dangerous but rare. Nothing could be farther from the truth. STDs are very common. In fact, statistics show that one out of every five people in the United States has an STD. Because STDs are so common, practicing sexual abstinence is very important. Sexual abstinence is the only way to stay completely safe from STDs. Table 2 gives information on the most common STDs and what they do to your body.

TABLE 2 Common Sexually Transmitted Diseases

Disease	Symptoms	Treatment or cure	Long-term consequences
Chlamydia (kluh MID ee uh)	Some people show no symptoms, especially women; others have a discharge from the genitals, painful urination and severe abdominal pain.	Chlamydia can be cured with antibiotics taken by mouth.	If left untreated, chlamydia can cause sterility, inflammation of the testicles, and complications during pregnancy.
Human papillomavirus (HPV) (HYOO muhn PAP i LOH muh vie ruhs)	Some people show no symptoms, others have warts on the genital area, and women have an abnormal Pap-smear test.	HPV can be treated, but not cured; sometimes, warts can be removed; Pap-smear tests help to identify precancerous conditions.	If left untreated, HPV can cause cervical cancer in women.
Genital herpes (JEN i tuhl HUHR PEEZ)	Symptoms include outbreaks of painful blisters or sores around the genital area that recur, swelling in the genital area, and burning during urination.	Genital herpes cannot be cured. Treatment with antiviral medicines can decrease the length and frequency of outbreaks, and can decrease the spread of herpes.	Herpes may cause cervical cancer in women; can cause deformities in unborn babies.
Gonorrhea (GAHN uh REE uh)	Some people show no symptoms; others have a discharge from the genitals, painful urination, and severe abdominal pain.	Gonorrhea can be cured with antibiotics, although a new strain of this bacteria has shown resistance to antibiotics.	If left untreated, gonorrhea can cause sterility, can cause liver disease, and can spread to the blood and joints.
Syphilis (SIF uh lis)	Symptoms, if present, may include sores, fever, body rash, and swollen lymph nodes.	Syphilis can be cured with antibiotics.	If left untreated, syphilis can cause mental illness, heart and kidney damage, and death.
Trichomoniasis (TRIK oh moh NIE uh sis)	Symptoms include itching, discharge from the genitals, and painful urination.	Trichomoniasis can be cured with medication.	Trichomoniasis has been linked to an increased risk of infection by HIV.

Career

Epidemiologist A scientist who figures out what causes a certain disease and why some people get the disease and other people don't is called an epidemiologist. This person often works in a lab and looks for viruses or bacteria in blood samples. Other epidemiologists work in a city where an outbreak of some disease has occurred. They talk to the people who are ill and try to find out how and why they became ill.

Life SKILL BUILDER — GENERAL

Coping Have students write a letter to an imaginary friend who has told them that he or she has an STD but is afraid to tell his or her parents and doesn't know where to go for treatment. The letter should try to convince the friend to tell his or her parents so that he or she can begin treatment for the disease.
LS Verbal

Teach

Using the Figure — GENERAL
Ask students to identify some of the common treatments for the various STDs described in the table on this page. Ask students why they think some of these diseases can be cured with antibiotics while others cannot be. (The treatments will depend on the STD. Some diseases can be cured with antibiotics if they are caused by bacteria. Viral diseases cannot be cured with antibiotics.)
LS Visual

Discussion — GENERAL
Hidden Danger Point out to students that some people can be infected with an STD without experiencing any physical symptoms associated with that disease. Ask students to explain why they think it can be more dangerous for a person infected with an STD to show no symptoms than it is for an infected person to show some symptoms. (An infected person who has no symptoms might not know he or she is infected and could spread the disease without meaning to, whereas a person showing symptoms would know he or she is infected and could take steps to cure the disease or at least keep from spreading it.)
LS Auditory

Debate — ADVANCED
STDs and Crime Have students debate whether it should be a crime if a person engages in sexual activity while knowing that he or she has an STD. (Half of the states in the United States have passed a law making it a crime to engage in unprotected sex if you know you are infected with HIV and your partner is unaware of your infection.)
LS Auditory

Lesson 4 • Sexually Transmitted Diseases

Teach, continued

Activity —— GENERAL

Poster Project Have students read the Myth and Fact on this page. Then, ask students if they have heard any other information about HIV or AIDS that they think might be false. Have interested students create a poster that defines some other myths about HIV and AIDS. Posters should have two columns, one titled "Myth" and the other titled "Fact." Have students present their findings to the class. (Some other myths report that HIV can be spread by casual contact, such as a handshake or the sharing of food or drinks. In fact, HIV can only be spread through sexual intercourse or by exchanging blood with an infected person. Another myth is that HIV can be spread by mosquito bites. No case of HIV has ever been traced to bug bites. There may not be enough infected blood in the bite of a mosquito to be able to spread the disease or HIV may be inactivated in the mosquito.)
LS Kinesthetic

READING SKILL BUILDER —— BASIC

Anticipation Guide Before students read this page, ask them to predict the major differences between AIDS and other STDs. (The major differences are that presently there is no cure for AIDS, and AIDS is usually a fatal disease.)

HIV and AIDS

Even though many STDs are painful and often incurable, they are not usually fatal diseases. However, unlike most STDs, AIDS is a deadly disease. **AIDS,** or acquired immune deficiency syndrome (uh KWIERD im MYOON dee FISH uhn see SIN DROHM), is a disease that is caused by HIV (human immunodeficiency virus), an infectious virus. **HIV** is a virus that attacks the immune system, which is the group of cells and tissues that defends your body against disease. As HIV infects a person, it slowly destroys the person's ability to fight disease. Once a person is infected with HIV, the infection does not go away. Eventually, the patient starts to develop the symptoms of AIDS. The symptoms of AIDS vary widely and can include such things as fever, weight loss, and sores covering the body. Once a person develops AIDS, he or she becomes gradually more and more ill. Eventually, he or she dies. People who die from AIDS actually die from secondary infections, such as pneumonia, that AIDS has left their body unable to fight. There are now combinations of drugs to treat HIV and AIDS as well as the related infections. Although very unpleasant and expensive, these treatments have extended the lives of many patients. However, as of the writing of this book, there is no cure for HIV or AIDS.

How HIV Is Spread

You can protect yourself from AIDS by avoiding exposure to HIV. HIV is spread in several of the following ways:

- **Sexual Contact** HIV is most often spread through exchange of bodily fluids during sexual intercourse.
- **Mother to Child** A mother can spread HIV to her unborn child while she is pregnant or to her child while she is breast-feeding.
- **Drug Use** Many people are infected by sharing hypodermic needles while using illegal drugs.
- **Blood Transfusion** Some people are infected through blood transfusions at hospitals. This type of infection is now extremely rare, because all blood in this country is tested for diseases before it is used.

Myth & Fact

Myth: You can get HIV by using a toilet after somebody who has HIV.

Fact: HIV can only be passed in certain ways. You cannot get HIV by using a toilet after anybody.

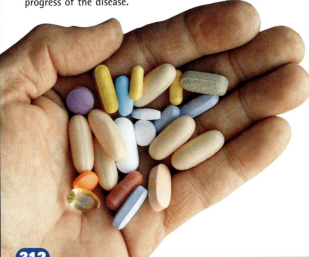

Figure 11 People who have HIV or AIDS often take dozens of pills every day to slow the progress of the disease.

SOCIAL STUDIES CONNECTION —— ADVANCED

AIDS in Africa AIDS has had serious consequences in most parts of the world, but it has been the most devastating in Africa. In 1999, there were 5.4 million new HIV infections worldwide, and 4 million of them were in Africa. Of the 2.8 million people who died from AIDS in 1999, 85 percent were in Africa. Millions of African children have been orphaned by the disease. And the spread of the disease has reduced life expectancy in the part of Africa below the Sahara desert to 45 years of age. Government programs and international aid are providing medicine and education, but the African continent is far from recovering from this epidemic. Have interested students research new programs that have been implemented by the African government to halt the epidemic. Students should also find out what the Worldwide Health Organization (WHO) and other countries, such as the United States, are doing to help Africa. **LS** Verbal

312   Chapter 14 • Infectious Diseases

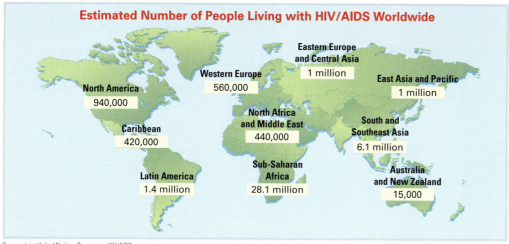

Figure 12 Since the HIV/AIDS epidemic started, the disease has spread to every continent and has claimed tens of millions of victims.

The HIV/AIDS Problem

Since the first AIDS cases were reported in 1981, the disease has spread worldwide. Cases are now reported from virtually every country in the world. Africa has been hit very hard, but the number of cases is rising everywhere. HIV infection is increasing most quickly in poorer countries, where education and healthcare are lacking.

If you think you might have been exposed to HIV, you should be tested for the virus. There are several very simple tests to detect HIV infection. HIV is not transmitted by casual contact. So do not be afraid to show your love to people who are infected with this deadly disease.

Lesson Review

Using Vocabulary
1. What is a sexually transmitted disease?
2. Define *sexual abstinence* in your own words.

Understanding Concepts
3. What are some symptoms common among the STDs listed in the table on the second page of this lesson?
4. What is the difference between HIV and AIDS?
5. Describe four ways that HIV can spread from person to person.

Critical Thinking
6. **Making Inferences** HIV is spreading more quickly now than it was in the early 1980s. Why might HIV spread to more people per year now than it did in the 1980s?

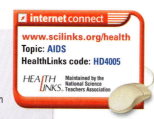

www.scilinks.org/health
Topic: AIDS
HealthLinks code: HD4005

Lesson 5

Focus

Overview
Before beginning this lesson, review with your students the objectives listed under the What You'll Do head in the Student Edition. Students will learn the importance of staying clean to avoid infectious disease. Students will also learn ways to avoid infection and ways to prevent infectious diseases from spreading to others.

 Bellringer
Perfect attendance is very important to some students. Ask students if they think it's more important to attend school every day or to stay at home when they become ill. Tell students to explain their answer. **LS Verbal**

Answer to Start Off Write
Accept all reasonable answers. Sample answer: Ways to prevent the spread of infection are to cover your mouth when you sneeze and to wash your hands after going to the bathroom.

Motivate

Demonstration — **BASIC**
Hand Washing Show students that there is a big difference between just washing your hands and washing them properly. Hands should be washed front and back up to the wrist, not just the palms. Hands should be washed with soap in warm water for at least 20 seconds. Also, care should be taken to wash between all the fingers and on the backsides of fingers, not just the inside. Thorough rinsing and drying completes the process.
LS Visual

Lesson 5 — Preventing the Spread of Infectious Diseases

What You'll Do
- **Discuss** the role of hygiene in avoiding infectious diseases.
- **Identify** ways to avoid infection.
- **Describe** ways to prevent infectious diseases from spreading to others.

Start Off Write
What can you do to prevent the spread of a disease?

Angelo remembers last winter, when almost half of his classmates caught the flu around the same time. Is there anything that Angelo's classmates could have done to keep from catching this disease?

There are several things that Angelo's classmates could have done to slow the spread of this disease. No matter what you do, you will get sick sometimes. However, if you follow certain rules, you can seriously lower your chances of catching an infection.

Keeping Clean

The first step you can take to prevent the spread of a disease is to practice good hygiene. Remember that contagious infections are spread more often by touch than by any other method. Wash your hands before you eat. Germs that collect on your hands can infect you when you touch your mouth, eyes, or nose or when you eat. Every time you use the bathroom, wash your hands with soap and warm water. If your hands get dirty, wash them as soon as you can. Also be sure to take warm showers regularly. Showering with soap washes off many of the germs that are on your body, lowering your risk of infection.

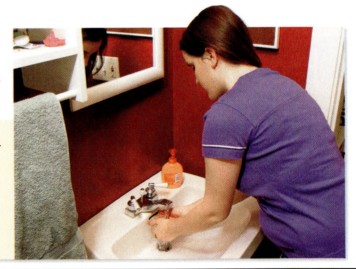

Figure 13 Washing your hands regularly with soap and warm water lowers your risk of infection.

▶ Always use soap because washing your hands with water alone does not kill germs.
▶ Use warm water.
▶ Scrub your hands with soap for at least 20 seconds. Pay attention to your fingernails, where germs may be trapped.

Attention Grabber

Most students don't realize the importance of hand washing. A recent study in Detroit showed that school children who washed their hands four times each day had 24 percent fewer sick days from respiratory infections and 51 percent fewer sick days from upset stomachs than children who did not wash their hands. The common cold and flu are not the only diseases that can be kept from spreading by hand washing. The spread of more serious diseases such as hepatitis A, meningitis, and infectious diarrhea can be prevented by simply washing your hands.

Chapter Resource File
- Directed Reading **BASIC**
- Lesson Plan
- Lesson Quiz **GENERAL**

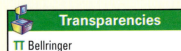 **Transparencies**
TT Bellringer

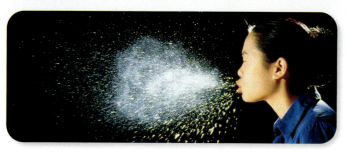

Figure 14 When a person sneezes, he or she can release millions of germs into the air.

Avoiding Infection

The only sure way to avoid an infectious disease is to stay away from the source of the infection. However, this is not always possible. If you must be around somebody who has a contagious infection, do the following things to protect yourself:

- Keep distance so that you don't get infected by a cough or sneeze.
- Avoid sharing food or drink with the infected person.
- If you touch the infected person or objects that he or she has touched, wash your hands with soap and warm water.

Protecting Others

When you have a contagious illness, you should do certain things to keep from infecting others. First, if you feel ill, you should stay away from school or other public places until you start to feel better. By going to school, you could spread the infection to many of your classmates. If you do have to be around other people, remember not to touch others or share food and drink with them. Also, remember to cover your mouth when you cough or sneeze.

Myth & Fact

Myth: You should cover your mouth and nose with your hand when coughing or sneezing.

Fact: You should cover your mouth or nose with the inner part of your elbow or with a tissue. This keeps the germs from getting on your hands, where they could be easily passed to others.

Lesson Review

Understanding Concepts

1. How does washing your hands lower your risk of catching an infectious disease?
2. How should you protect yourself if somebody around you has a contagious infection?
3. What are three things you can do to protect others from infection?

Critical Thinking

4. **Making Good Decisions** Imagine that you are on the soccer team. You have a big game coming up. You need to go to practice, but you are sick. You don't feel that bad, though. And you don't have a fever. Should you go to practice anyway? Explain.

internet connect
www.scilinks.org/health
Topic: HIV
HealthLinks code: HD4055

Lesson 5 • Preventing the Spread of Infectious Diseases

CHAPTER 14 REVIEW

Assignment Guide

Lesson	Review Questions
1	1, 9
2	5, 7, 11–12, 25
3	4, 13–14, 18, 21, 23
4	3, 6, 8, 15–17, 19, 22, 24, 26
5	10, 19
2 and 3	2, 20

ANSWERS

Using Vocabulary

1. An infectious disease is an illness caused by microorganisms. A contagious disease is an infectious disease that can be spread directly from one person to another.
2. Bacteria are a group of single-celled microorganisms. Viruses are disease-causing agents that cannot reproduce on their own.
3. AIDS is a disease in humans that is caused by the virus, HIV.
4. EBV
5. antibiotic
6. abstinence
7. throat culture
8. infertility

Understanding Concepts

9. Microorganisms cause infectious diseases.
10. A cough or a sneeze can release millions of germs into the air.
11. Symptoms of strep throat are pain when swallowing, fever, and body aches.
12. Sinuses are spaces located in the front of the skull, many of which have small tubes that drain fluids down into the nose or throat. If these tubes get blocked, the sinuses can become infected.
13. A virus must use a host cell in which to reproduce, and a virus is not composed of cells.
14. Both cause congestion, sore throat, and coughing. A cold causes sneezing, a runny nose, and congestion while influenza causes headaches, chills, body aches, and a high fever.
15. Some people can have an STD and not show any symptoms. They are still infected and can pass the disease to others.
16. HIV is the virus that causes the disease AIDS.
17. Sexual intercourse is the most common way that HIV is spread.
18. A vaccine fools the body into thinking it is being attacked by a disease-causing microorganism. The body produces chemicals to fight the disease, which then builds resistance to the disease.
19. These practices help to cleanse your body of germs and prevent the spread of germs, which cause infectious disease.
20. Antibiotics can be prescribed to treat bacterial infections but not viral infections. There are medications that can treat the symptoms of an infection caused by a virus. Certain antiviral drugs are now available, but they are specific for only certain viral infections, such as herpes.

CHAPTER REVIEW 14

Chapter Summary

- Infectious diseases are caused by microorganisms and viruses.
- Some infectious diseases are contagious, which means that they can be passed from person to person.
- Many common infections are caused by bacteria, which are single-celled organisms that can reproduce quickly.
- Antibiotics are drugs that kill bacteria or slow the growth of bacteria.
- Many common infections are caused by viruses, which are extremely small disease-causing agents.
- Some infections are passed from person to person through sexual contact.
- AIDS is a deadly disease that is caused by HIV, a virus.
- You cannot avoid all infections, but certain behaviors can lower your risk of infection.
- If you have a contagious infection, you should try to avoid passing it to others.

Using Vocabulary

For each pair of terms, describe how the meanings of the terms differ.

1. infectious disease/contagious disease
2. bacteria/virus
3. AIDS/HIV

For each sentence, fill in the blank with the proper term from the word bank provided below.

HIV	antibiotic
infertility	EBV
throat culture	chlamydia
influenza	sexual abstinence

4. ___ is the virus that causes mononucleosis.
5. A drug that kills bacteria or slows the growth of bacteria is called a(n) ___.
6. Avoiding all sexual contact is called ___.
7. If a doctor thinks that you might have strep throat, he or she will give you a test called a(n) ___.
8. If untreated, some STDs can cause ___, or the inability to have children.

Understanding Concepts

9. What causes infectious diseases?
10. How can coughing or sneezing pass contagious infections?
11. Describe the symptoms of strep throat.
12. What are the sinuses, and how can they become infected?
13. Why are viruses not considered living things?
14. How do the symptoms of influenza differ from the symptoms of the common cold?
15. Do all people who have an STD get sick? Explain.
16. Describe the relationship between HIV and AIDS.
17. What is the most common way that HIV is passed from person to person?
18. How does a vaccine work?
19. How does washing your hands and taking warm showers lower your risk of catching an infectious disease?
20. Compare and contrast bacterial infections and viral infections.

Critical Thinking

Applying Concepts

21. If you vaccinated every living thing that a certain virus could infect, could you be sure that the virus would be eliminated? Explain your answer.
22. Does everybody that has HIV also have AIDS? Explain your answer.
23. Imagine that one morning in January, you wake up feeling sick. Your head hurts, you have a sore throat, your muscles ache, and you have a very high fever. What disease do you most likely have? Explain your answer.

Making Good Decisions

24. A man speaks to your school about HIV. During his speech, he tells everybody that he is HIV positive, meaning that he is infected with HIV. After the speech, you want to shake the man's hand, but you are afraid of catching HIV. Should you shake the man's hand or not? Explain your answer.
25. Your doctor prescribes an antibiotic for your strep throat. You take the medicine for a few days, and you start feeling better. The instructions for the medicine say that you should keep taking it until it is gone. During the last few days, the medicine has been giving you stomachaches. What should you do in this situation? Explain your answer.
26. If you were in charge of lowering the rate of HIV infection in your city, what three things would you do? Explain your answer.

Interpreting Graphics

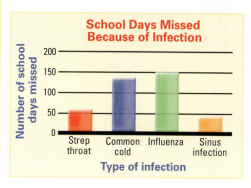

School Days Missed Because of Infection

The graph above shows the number of missed days that were caused by each different infection. Use this graph to answer questions 27–31.

27. How many days of school were missed because of bacterial infections?
28. How many days of school were missed because of viral infections?
29. Which infection caused the most missed school days?
30. Fewer students at the school caught influenza than common colds, yet the cold caused less total missed days. What would explain this?
31. About how many more days of school were missed because of strep throat infections than were missed because of sinus infections?

Reading Checkup

Take a minute to review your answers to the Health IQ questions at the beginning of this chapter. How has reading this chapter improved your Health IQ?

Critical Thinking

Applying Concepts

21. No, vaccines are not always 100 percent effective. Also, many viruses continually change, which means that new vaccines may have to be made.
22. No. AIDS is a group of symptoms that come from infection with HIV. All people infected with HIV do not show symptoms of AIDS.
23. The symptoms described are probably caused by influenza, a disease that is common in that time of year.

Making Good Decisions

24. You should shake his hand. HIV cannot be spread by casual contact such as a handshake.
25. Consult your doctor immediately. He may change the type of antibiotic you are taking.
26. Answers will vary, but should include testing for HIV infections, education, and promotion of safe sexual practices.

Interpreting Graphics

27. 102 (about 57 from strep and 45 from sinus infections)
28. 280 (about 130 from the cold and 150 from the flu)
29. Influenza caused the most missed days of school.
30. The symptoms of influenza are more severe, and many people don't stay home because of a cold.
31. About 15 more days of school were missed because of strep throat infections.

Chapter Resource File

- Concept Review GENERAL
- Concept Mapping GENERAL
- Performance-Based Assessment GENERAL
- Chapter Test GENERAL

Model

Introduce this activity by reminding students that using this Life Skill will help them take personal responsibility for their behavior. Then, review the scenario with the class.

Prepare students for this activity by modeling each of the steps of the skill. Make sure students understand each step before you move on to the next one.

Guided Practice: Practice with a Friend

Guided Practice is the stage in which you and the students analyze their approach to solving the problem given in the scenario and analyze their decision-making skills. Have students read Act 1. Discuss with the class the situation described and the way students are to act it out. Organize the class into groups of three. In each group, one person plays the role of Juan, another person plays Juan's mother, and the third person is the observer.

Proper pacing during the Guided Practice is important. The suggestions listed below will help you control the pace.

1. Stop after completing each step of making good decisions.
2. Discuss with each group the observer's comments.
3. Ask the other members of each group to listen to the observer's suggestions and to suggest ways to improve their decision-making skills.
4. Instruct students to repeat the steps that need improvement and to include their modifications.
5. Check to make sure that students understand each step before they move on to the next step.
6. If time permits, repeat the exercise three times, switching roles each time. Each student should have the opportunity to play each role. Co-op Learning

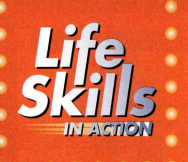

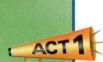

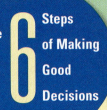

The 6 Steps of Making Good Decisions

1. Identify the problem.
2. Consider your values.
3. List the options.
4. Weigh the consequences.
5. Decide, and act.
6. Evaluate your choice.

Making Good Decisions

You make decisions every day. But how do you know if you are making good decisions? Making good decisions is making choices that are healthy and responsible. Following the six steps of making good decisions will help you make the best possible choice whenever you make a decision. Complete the following activity to practice the six steps of making good decisions.

Juan's Illness

Setting the Scene

Juan does not feel very well this morning. His body aches, and he thinks he has a fever. Juan's mother suggests that he stay home from school because he might have the flu. But Juan tells her that he wants to go to school because the school band is having solo tryouts. He has been practicing on his trumpet for weeks, and he doesn't want to miss his chance to audition.

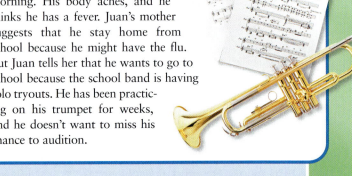

Guided Practice

Practice with a Friend

Form a group of three. Have one person play the role of Juan and another person play the role of Juan's mother. Have the third person be an observer. Walking through each of the six steps of making good decisions, role-play Juan deciding whether or not to go to school. Juan's mother can help him brainstorm options and weigh the consequences of each option. The observer will take notes, which will include observations about what the person playing Juan did well and suggestions of ways to improve. Stop after each step to evaluate the process.

Independent Practice

Check Yourself

After you have completed the guided practice, go through Act 1 again without stopping at each step. Answer the questions below to review what you did.

1. What values should Juan consider while making his decision?
2. What options does Juan have?
3. What are the possible consequences of Juan's options?
4. Think about a time when you went to school while you were ill. What were the consequences of your decision? Would you make the same decision again?

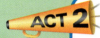

On Your Own

One day during band practice, Juan drops his trumpet. When he picks it up, he discovers that it is badly dented. Juan starts to worry about what will happen when he tells his parents. Then, his friend Mark tells Juan that he thinks he can fix the trumpet in the school's metal shop. Make an outline that shows how Juan could use the six steps of making good decisions to decide what to do about his trumpet.

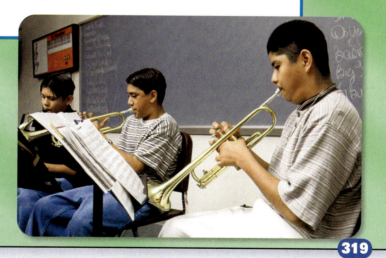

Act 2: On Your Own

This additional scenario gives students an opportunity to apply what they have learned in both the Guided Practice and the Independent Practice to a new situation.

Suggest to students that they use the Check Yourself questions as a starting point for making good decisions in the new situation. Encourage students to be creative and to think of ways to improve their decision-making skills.

Assessment

Review the outlines that students have written as part of the On Your Own activity. The outlines should show that the students followed the steps of making good decisions in a realistic and effective manner. If time permits, ask student volunteers to write one or more of their outlines on the blackboard. Discuss the outlines and the use of decision-making skills.

Independent Practice: Check Yourself

Instruct students to repeat Act 1 without stopping at each step. Remind students to apply what they learned in the Guided Practice to the Independent Practice.

Encourage students to use the Check Yourself questions as a starting point for reviewing and analyzing their Independent Practice. Remind students that as they change roles, the answers to these questions may change for each actor. Encourage students to create additional questions for checking their decision-making skills. When students have finished the Independent Practice, have them answer the Check Yourself questions in writing. Use their answers to assess their understanding of the steps of making good decisions and to assess their use of the steps to solve a problem.

Check Yourself Answers

1. Sample answer: Juan should consider if he values his health and the health of other people. He should also consider how important playing a solo is to him.
2. Sample answer: Juan can stay home or he can go to school.
3. Sample answer: Consequences of staying home from school include getting rest that will help Juan recover from his illness, not being able to audition for a solo, and falling behind in school. Consequences of going to school include being able to audition for a solo, causing other people to become sick, and slowing Juan's recovery from his illness.
4. Sample answer: I took a test when I was ill and did very poorly on the test. I would not make the same decision again. I would rather make up the work I missed than get a bad grade on it.

Chapter 14 • Making Good Decisions

Chapter 15: Noninfectious Diseases and Disorders
Chapter Planning Guide

PACING	CLASSROOM RESOURCES	ACTIVITIES AND DEMONSTRATIONS
BLOCK 1 • 45 min pp. 320–323 **Chapter Opener**	**CRF** Health Inventory * ■ GENERAL **CRF** Parent Letter * ■	**SE** Health IQ, p. 321 **CRF** At-Home Activity * ■
Lesson 1 Noninfectious Diseases and Body Systems	**CRF** Lesson Plan * **TT** Bellringer * **TT** Body Organs and Systems *	**TE** Activities Introduction to Body Systems, p. 319F **TE** Activity Analyzing Lifestyle, p. 322 GENERAL **SE** Life Skills in Action Coping, p. 344–355 **CRF** Enrichment Activity * ADVANCED
BLOCK 2 • 45 min pp. 324–329 **Lesson 2** Circulatory System	**CRF** Lesson Plan * **TT** Bellringer * **TT** A Healthy Artery and a Blocked Artery *	**TE** Activity Heart Rate, p. 324 ◆ GENERAL **SE** Hands-on Activity, p. 326 **CRF** Datasheets for In-Text Activities * GENERAL **TE** Activity Analyzing Lifestyle, p. 327 GENERAL **CRF** Life Skills Activity * ■ GENERAL **CRF** Enrichment Activity * ADVANCED
Lesson 3 Respiratory System	**CRF** Lesson Plan * **TT** Bellringer *	**TE** Activity Lung Cancer Poster Project, p. 328 GENERAL **CRF** Enrichment Activity * ADVANCED
BLOCK 3 • 45 min pp. 330–335 **Lesson 4** Nervous System	**CRF** Lesson Plan * **TT** Bellringer *	**TE** Activity Using the Figure, p. 330 GENERAL **CRF** Enrichment Activity * ADVANCED
Lesson 5 Endocrine System	**CRF** Lesson Plan * **TT** Bellringer *	**TE** Activity Insulin and Diabetes, p. 333 GENERAL **CRF** Enrichment Activity * ADVANCED
Lesson 6 Digestive System	**CRF** Lesson Plan * **TT** Bellringer *	**TE** Activities Food for Health, p. 319F **TE** Group Activity Digestive Health, p. 334 GENERAL **CRF** Enrichment Activity * ADVANCED
BLOCK 4 • 45 min pp. 336–341 **Lesson 7** Urinary System	**CRF** Lesson Plan * **TT** Bellringer *	**TE** Demonstration How Kidneys Work, p. 336 ◆ GENERAL **CRF** Enrichment Activity * ADVANCED
Lesson 8 Skin, Bones, and Muscles	**CRF** Lesson Plan * **TT** Bellringer *	**TE** Activity Prime Movers, p. 338 GENERAL **SE** Hands-on Activity, p. 339 ◆ **CRF** Datasheets for In-Text Activities * GENERAL **CRF** Life Skills Activity * ■ GENERAL **CRF** Enrichment Activity * ADVANCED
Lesson 9 Eyes and Ears	**CRF** Lesson Plan * **TT** Bellringer *	**TE** Activity Binocular Vision, p. 340 GENERAL **TE** Activity Sound and Hearing Damage, p. 341 GENERAL **CRF** Enrichment Activity * ADVANCED

BLOCKS 5 & 6 • 90 min Chapter Review and Assessment Resources

- **SE** Chapter Review, pp. 342–343
- **CRF** Concept Review * ■ GENERAL
- **CRF** Health Behavior Contract * ■ GENERAL
- **CRF** Chapter Test * ■ GENERAL
- **CRF** Performance-Based Assessment * GENERAL
- **OSP** Test Generator
- **CRF** Test Item Listing *

Online Resources

Visit **go.hrw.com** for a variety of free resources related to this textbook. Enter the keyword **HD4ND7**.

Students can access interactive problem solving help and active visual concept development with the *Decisions for Health* Online Edition available at **www.hrw.com**.

CNN Student News
cnnstudentnews.com
Find the latest health news, lesson plans, and activities related to important scientific events.

Compression guide:
To shorten your instruction because of time limitations, omit Lesson 9.

KEY

TE Teacher Edition	**CRF** Chapter Resource File	* Also on One-Stop Planner
SE Student Edition	**TT** Teaching Transparency	■ Also Available in Spanish
OSP One-Stop Planner		♦ Requires Advance Prep

SKILLS DEVELOPMENT RESOURCES	LESSON REVIEW AND ASSESSMENT	STANDARDS CORRELATION
		National Health Education Standards
CRF Cross-Disciplinary * GENERAL **CRF** Directed Reading * BASIC	**SE** Lesson Review, p. 323 **TE** Reteaching, Quiz, p. 323 **CRF** Concept Mapping * GENERAL **CRF** Lesson Quiz * ■ GENERAL	1.1, 1.3, 1.8, 6.3
TE Life Skill Builder Assessing Your Health, p. 325 GENERAL **CRF** Directed Reading * BASIC	**SE** Lesson Review, p. 327 **TE** Reteaching, Quiz, p. 327 **CRF** Lesson Quiz * ■ GENERAL	1.1, 1.2, 1.3, 1.6, 1.8, 3.1, 6.3
SE Life Skills Activity Making Good Decisions, p. 329 **CRF** Refusal Skills * GENERAL **CRF** Directed Reading * BASIC	**SE** Lesson Review, p. 329 **TE** Reteaching, Quiz, p. 329 **CRF** Lesson Quiz * ■ GENERAL	1.1, 1.3, 1.5, 1.6, 1.8, 3.1, 6.3
TE Inclusion Strategies, p. 331 GENERAL **CRF** Refusal Skills * GENERAL **CRF** Directed Reading * BASIC	**SE** Lesson Review, p. 331 **TE** Reteaching, Quiz, p. 331 **CRF** Lesson Quiz * ■ GENERAL	1.1, 1.3, 1.5, 1.6, 1.8, 3.1, 6.3
SE Life Skills Activity Being a Wise Consumer, p. 333 **CRF** Cross-Disciplinary * GENERAL **CRF** Directed Reading * BASIC	**SE** Lesson Review, p. 333 **TE** Reteaching, Quiz, p. 333 **CRF** Lesson Quiz * ■ GENERAL	1.1, 1.3, 1.5, 1.8, 3.1, 6.3
CRF Decision-Making * GENERAL **CRF** Directed Reading * BASIC	**SE** Lesson Review, p. 335 **TE** Reteaching, Quiz, p. 335 **CRF** Lesson Quiz * ■ GENERAL	1.1, 1.3, 1.5, 1.6, 1.8, 3.1, 6.3
CRF Directed Reading * BASIC	**SE** Lesson Review, p. 337 **TE** Reteaching, Quiz, p. 337 **TE** Alternative Assessment, p. 337 GENERAL **CRF** Concept Mapping * GENERAL **CRF** Lesson Quiz * ■ GENERAL	1.1, 1.3, 1.5, 1.6, 1.8, 3.1, 6.3
TE Life Skill Builder Assessing Your Health, p. 339 GENERAL **CRF** Directed Reading * BASIC	**SE** Lesson Review, p. 339 **TE** Reteaching, Quiz, p. 339 **CRF** Lesson Quiz * ■ GENERAL	1.1, 1.3, 1.8, 6.3
TE Inclusion Strategies, p. 340 ADVANCED **CRF** Decision-Making * GENERAL **CRF** Directed Reading * BASIC	**SE** Lesson Review, p. 341 **TE** Reteaching, Quiz, p. 341 **CRF** Lesson Quiz * ■ GENERAL	1.1, 1.3, 1.8, 6.3

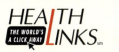

www.scilinks.org/health

Maintained by the **National Science Teachers Association**

Topic: Inherited Diseases
HealthLinks code: HD4062
Topic: Noninfectious Diseases
HealthLinks code: HD4070
Topic: Asthma
HealthLinks code: HD4011

Technology Resources

 One-Stop Planner
All of your printable resources and the Test Generator are on this convenient CD-ROM.

 Guided Reading Audio CDs

VIDEO SELECT
For information about videos related to this chapter, go to **go.hrw.com** and type in the keyword **HD4ND7V**.

Chapter 15 • Chapter Planning Guide **319B**

Chapter 15

Noninfectious Diseases and Disorders
Chapter Resources

Teacher Resources

TEACHING TRANSPARENCIES

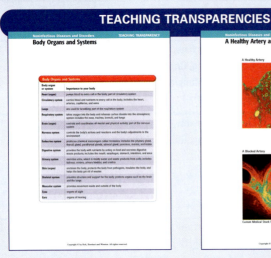
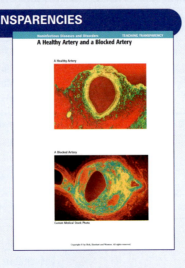

BELLRINGER TRANSPARENCIES

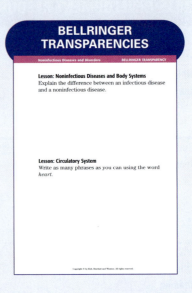

LESSON PLANS

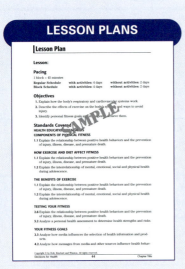

PARENT LETTER (ALSO IN SPANISH)

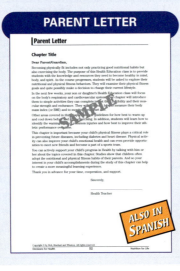

TEST ITEM LISTING

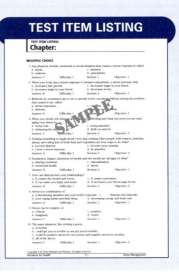

Meeting Individual Needs

DIRECTED READING (BASIC)

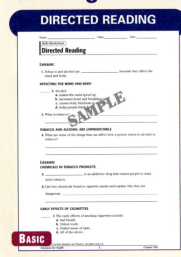

CONCEPT MAPPING (GENERAL)

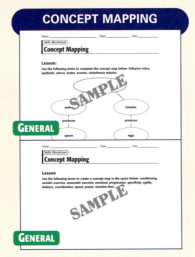

CONCEPT REVIEW (GENERAL) (ALSO IN SPANISH)

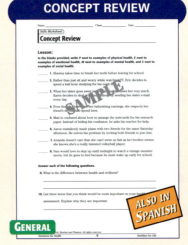

ENRICHMENT ACTIVITIES (ADVANCED)

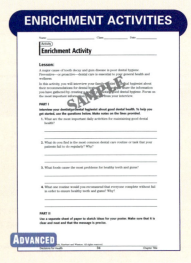

Chapter 15 • Noninfectious Diseases and Disorders

Resources

These worksheet pages can be found in the Chapter Resource File and the One-Stop Planner. The transparencies can be found in the Teaching Transparencies binder and on the One-Stop Planner.

Activities

LIFE SKILLS ACTIVITIES
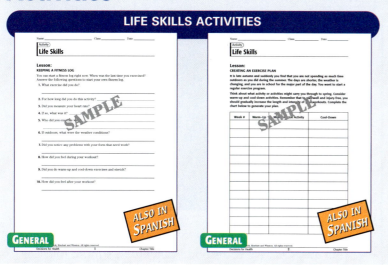

AT-HOME ACTIVITY
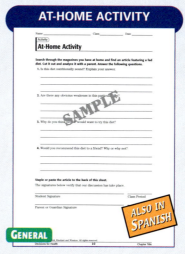

DATASHEETS FOR IN-TEXT ACTIVITIES
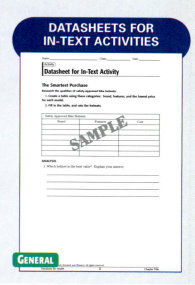

Applications

DECISION-MAKING
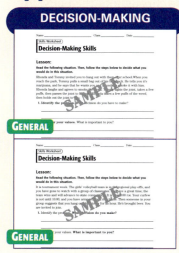

REFUSAL SKILLS
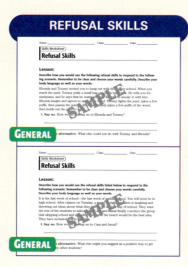

CROSS-DISCIPLINARY
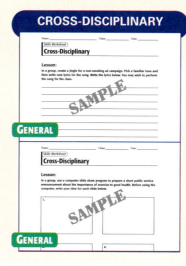

HEALTH BEHAVIOR CONTRACT
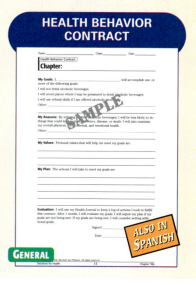

Assessments

HEALTH INVENTORY
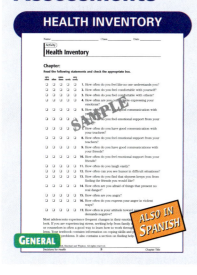

LESSON QUIZZES
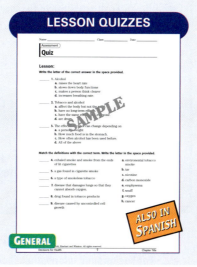

CHAPTER TEST
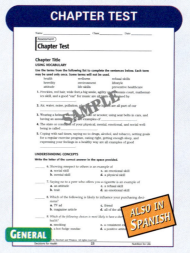

PERFORMANCE-BASED ASSESSMENT
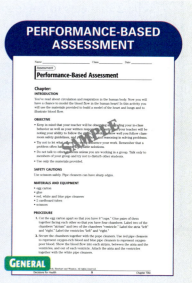

Chapter 15 • Chapter Resources and Worksheets   **319D**

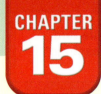

Chapter 15: Background Information

The following information focuses on type 2 diabetes and how nerves work. This material will help prepare you for teaching the concepts in this chapter.

Type 2 Diabetes

- Type 2 diabetes, also called non-insulin dependent diabetes (NIDD) or adult onset diabetes, is a major health problem facing Americans today. Type 2 diabetes is linked to hereditary factors and is directly related to obesity.

- Specialized cells in the pancreas release *insulin*, a hormone that helps your body store and use sugar from food you eat. When the pancreas doesn't produce enough insulin, or when the body doesn't properly use the insulin produced, diabetes results.

- Symptoms of type 2 diabetes include increased thirst and hunger, dry mouth, fatigue, frequent urination, blurred vision, numbness of hands and feet, and even loss of consciousness. People with type 2 diabetes may also exhibit slow-healing cuts or sores, itchy skin, and recent weight gain.

- Sometimes people with type 2 diabetes show no symptoms at all, which can be dangerous. The disease may go undetected until it damages the kidneys, causes failure of the nervous or circulatory systems, or results in diabetic coma or death.

- Diabetes may cause or aggravate vision problems, such as glaucoma and *retinopathy*, a disease that damages the retina and may lead to blindness.

- Type 2 diabetes is usually found in people over 40 years old and who are overweight. But the increase in the number of American children who are overweight or obese has been accompanied by a rise in type 2 diabetes in some groups of younger people. Type 2 diabetes now occasionally occurs in elementary and middle school children.

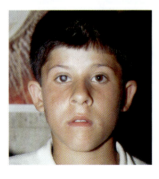

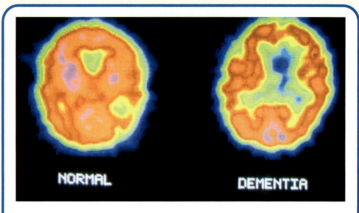

How Neurons Work

- Your body is able to respond quickly to stimuli that come from the environment because of your nervous system. A complex system of nerve cells, known as *neurons*, transmits information throughout the body. Neurons are the basic cell of the nervous system. *Sensory neurons* carry messages toward the spinal cord and brain. *Motor neurons* carry messages to the muscles and other tissue.

- Neurons have structures called *dendrites* that act as antennae. They enable the neurons to receive information from other body cells. Neurons carry information in the form of electrical impulses along structures called *axons*.

- The junction of a neuron with another neuron is a small gap known as a *synapse*. At these junctions, information in the form of electrical energy is transformed into chemical energy, carried across the synapse by a chemical neurotransmitter, and then converted back into electrical energy.

- The peripheral nervous system (PNS) carries information to the central nervous system (CNS), which includes the spinal cord and the brain. The information in the PNS is carried by *nerves*, which are bundles of axons.

- The brain processes all of the information and commands other body parts, through information passed by neurons, to respond accordingly. Movement, thought, perception, emotion, learning, communicating—all of these things are possible because of neurons.

For background information about teaching strategies and issues, refer to the *Professional Reference for Teachers*.

ACTIVITIES

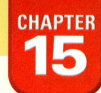

CHAPTER 15

Consider using the activities on this page as students explore the lessons of this chapter. Look for other activities throughout the Student Edition chapter.

Food for Health

Procedure Organize students into groups. Have one group research the recommended daily nutritional intake for their age group. This group should explain how good nutrition helps prevent noninfectious diseases. Have them present their findings in a chart or a poster to the class. Direct each of the other groups to choose a fast-food restaurant or a type of commonly eaten fast food, such as hamburgers, tacos, or french fries. Have each group then research the nutritional value of foods offered by the restaurant or the nutritional value of various brands of the same type of fast food. Information about the food choices should include the serving size of each food item, calories per serving, grams of carbohydrates, protein, and fat per serving, milligrams of cholesterol per serving, and milligrams of sodium per serving. Students should organize the results of their research into a chart or poster that can be presented to the class. Discuss with students how they wish to display their results and establish a format for everyone to follow. This will make it easier for the groups to compare their information.

Analysis How healthy is fast food? (Answers will vary.)

- Have students compare the results of the restaurant and fast food research to the results of the recommended nutritional intake of the first group. How do fast-food restaurants and fast food measure up to a recommended healthy diet?

- Ask students how eating frequently at fast-food restaurants, or eating a lot of fast food, can cause one or more noninfectious diseases.

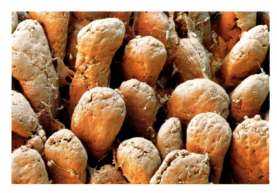

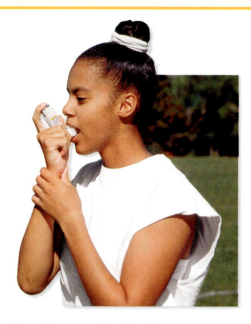

Introduction to Body Systems

Procedure Have each student choose a different body system. They can choose from the circulatory system; the respiratory system; the nervous system; the endocrine system; the digestive system; the urinary system; the skeletal system; the muscular system; the integumentary system; or the eyes and ears. Each student should research his or her chosen body system, and describe its main parts or organs. Students should explain normal daily functions of the system, and should describe how the system functions under unusual circumstances, such as injury, fear, illness, or excitement.

Analysis (Answers will vary.)

- How many of the functions of each system are visible to the naked eye?

- How is the system essential to keeping a person alive?

- How is each system related to the other body systems being described?

- What noninfectious diseases can affect the proper functioning of your body system?

- What would happen if your body system ceased to function properly?

Chapter 15 • Activities   319F

CHAPTER 15

Overview
Tell students that this chapter will help them understand noninfectious diseases. Students will learn about the different organs and organ systems in the human body and how they can be affected by noninfectious diseases.

Assessing Prior Knowledge
Students should be familiar with the following topics:
- decision making
- risk factors
- infectious diseases

Question Box
Students may feel more comfortable asking questions if you set up a Question Box to collect their questions. Have students write and anonymously submit their questions about noninfectious diseases or the organs or body systems these diseases affect. Address these questions during class, or use these questions to introduce lessons that cover related topics.

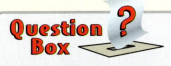

Check out *Current Health* articles and activities related to this chapter by visiting the HRW Web site at **go.hrw.com.** Just type in the keyword **HD4CH30T**.

Chapter Resource File
- Directed Reading **BASIC**
- Health Inventory **GENERAL**
- Parent Letter

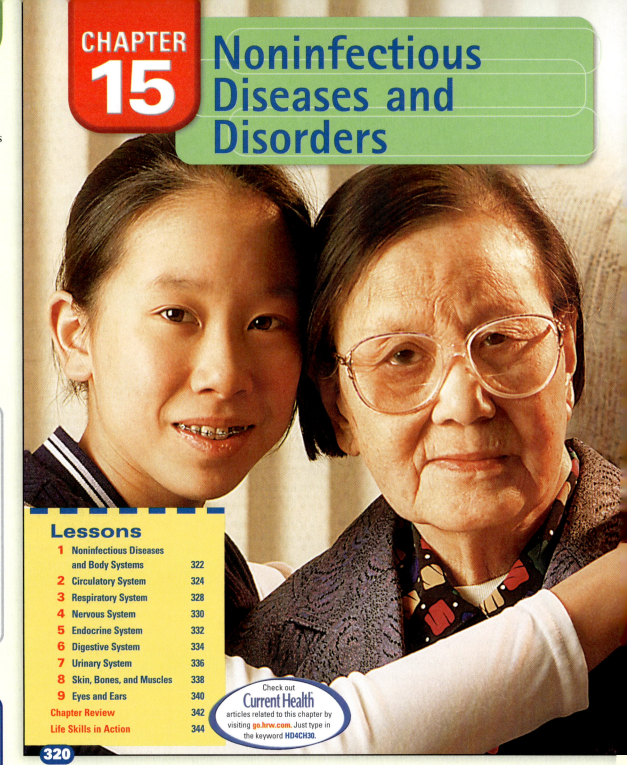

CHAPTER 15
Noninfectious Diseases and Disorders

Lessons
1. Noninfectious Diseases and Body Systems — 322
2. Circulatory System — 324
3. Respiratory System — 328
4. Nervous System — 330
5. Endocrine System — 332
6. Digestive System — 334
7. Urinary System — 336
8. Skin, Bones, and Muscles — 338
9. Eyes and Ears — 340

Chapter Review — 342
Life Skills in Action — 344

Check out **Current Health** articles related to this chapter by visiting **go.hrw.com.** Just type in the keyword **HD4CH30**.

Standards Correlations

National Health Education Standards

1.1 Explain the relationship between positive health behaviors and the prevention of injury, illness, disease and premature death. (Lessons 1–9)

1.3 Explain how health is influenced by the interaction of body systems. (Lessons 1–9)

1.5 Analyze how environment and personal health are interrelated. (Lessons 4–7)

1.6 Describe ways to reduce risks related to adolescent health problems. (Lessons 4, 6–7)

1.8 Describe how lifestyle, pathogens, family history, and other risk factors are related to the cause or prevention of disease and other health problems. (Lessons 1–9)

3.1 Explain the importance of assuming responsibility for personal health behaviors. (Lesson 4–7)

6.3 Predict how decisions regarding health behaviors have consequences for self and others. (Lessons 1–9)

" Usually, my grandmother is pretty **healthy.** She did **break** her left **hip** last year. It's OK now. She's never had a **medical emergency** or anything like that. I remember she had a really bad allergy attack once. The medicine she took made her feel a whole lot better. Now she's fine. "

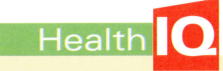

PRE-READING
Answer the following multiple-choice questions to find out what you already know about noninfectious diseases. When you've finished this chapter, you'll have the opportunity to change your answers based on what you've learned.

1. A body system is a group of ___ that work together.
   a. cells
   b. tissues
   c. organs
   d. hormones

2. Your heart is a muscular pump with ___ chambers
   a. two
   b. four
   c. six
   d. eight

3. ___ is a respiratory disease that causes parts of the lung to narrow.
   a. Appendicitis
   b. Cystic fibrosis
   c. Type 2 diabetes
   d. Asthma

4. The ___ is the main organ of the nervous system.
   a. brain
   b. spinal cord
   c. central nervous system
   d. peripheral nervous system

5. ___ is a disease in which the body produces no insulin.
   a. Type 2 diabetes
   b. Heart failure
   c. Hyperthyroidism
   d. Type 1 diabetes

6. Digestion of food begins in the
   a. large intestine.
   b. small intestine.
   c. stomach.
   d. mouth.

7. Most kidney disease results from diabetes and
   a. high blood pressure.
   b. cancer.
   c. drinking too little water.
   d. cataracts.

ANSWERS: 1. c; 2. b; 3. d; 4. a; 5. d; 6. d; 7. a

Using the Health IQ

Misconception Alert
Answers to the Health IQ questions may help you identify students' misconceptions.

Question 5: Students may not know that there is more than one type of diabetes. In type 1 diabetes, the body makes little or no insulin. In type 2 diabetes, the body produces insulin but cannot use it properly.

Question 6: Students may be surprised to learn that digestion begins in the mouth and not in the stomach.

Question 7: Students may know that high blood pressure is related to heart problems, but they may be surprised to know that it can be a factor in kidney disease as well.

Answers
1. c
2. b
3. d
4. a
5. d
6. d
7. a

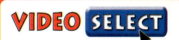

For information about videos related to this chapter, go to **go.hrw.com** and type in the keyword **HD4ND7V**.

Lesson 1 Focus

Overview
Before beginning this lesson, review with your students the objectives listed under the What You'll Do head in the Student Edition. This lesson defines noninfectious disease and lists some examples of noninfectious diseases and their causes. Students will also be introduced to some of the organs and organ systems of the human body.

Bellringer
Ask students to explain the difference between an infectious disease and a noninfectious disease. (An infectious disease is caused by a virus or a living organism. A noninfectious disease is not.)

Answer to Start Off Write
Accept all reasonable answers. Sample answer: A noninfectious disease is not caused by a virus or living organism but may result from heredity, an accident, or may be present at birth.

Motivate

Activity —————— GENERAL
Analyzing Lifestyle Have students make a list of five things they do that they think are good for them, and five things that they do that they think are not good for them. Ask them to write why they think these things are good or bad for them. Ask students if any of their activities put them at risk for a noninfectious disease. **LS Intrapersonal/Logical**

Lesson 1: Noninfectious Diseases and Body Systems

What You'll Do
- **Identify** three noninfectious causes of diseases.

Terms to Learn
- organ
- body system
- noninfectious disease

Start Off Write
What is a noninfectious disease?

In 1996, Lance Armstrong was told that he had a type of cancer. His cancer was treated, and in 1999, he won his first Tour de France, the world's toughest bicycle race.

Cancer is a serious disease that can attack any part of the body. But with proper support, the body has an amazing ability to fight diseases, such as cancer, and to heal.

Body Systems and Noninfectious Diseases
Your body is made up of cells, tissues, and organs. *Cells* are the simplest units of living organisms. A *tissue* is a group of similar cells that perform a single function. An **organ** is two or more tissues working together. Your heart, stomach, and brain are organs. A **body system** is a group of organs that work together. Different body systems work together to keep you healthy.

But sometimes, a disease can cause an organ or system not to work properly. A *disease* is any harmful change in your body's normal activities. A **noninfectious disease** is a disease that is not caused by a virus or living organism. Common noninfectious diseases include many kinds of cancer, most types of heart disease, and inherited disorders.

TABLE 1 Noninfectious Causes of Diseases

Cause of disease	Example	Organ or system affected
Congenital (present at birth)	cleft lip	mouth
Hereditary	cystic fibrosis	respiratory and digestive systems
Accident	brain injury	brain
Nutritional defect	iron deficiency (anemia)	blood and all systems
Metabolic disorder	diabetes	endocrine
Cancer	leukemia breast, lung, and stomach cancer	blood any organ or tissue
Immune defect (allergy)	asthma	respiratory system, eyes, and skin
Multiple causes	high blood pressure	heart and circulatory system

LIFE SCIENCE CONNECTION —————— GENERAL
Lifestyle Choices and Disease With an infectious disease, scientists can hunt for the disease-causing pathogen. With a noninfectious disease, scientists often don't know the cause. There are disorders of the immune system, the nervous system, and other body systems whose causes have yet to be discovered. But many noninfectious diseases—including some cancers, diabetes, and heart disease—can be traced directly to lifestyles and individual choices. Tobacco and alcohol use, lack of exercise, and poor diet all affect the health of the body.

Chapter Resource File
- Directed Reading BASIC
- Lesson Plan
- Lesson Quiz GENERAL

Transparencies
- TT Bellringer
- TT Body Organs and Systems

322 Chapter 15 • Noninfectious Diseases and Disorders

TABLE 2 Body Organs and Systems

Body organ or system	Importance to your body
Heart (organ)	pumps blood to every cell in the body; part of circulatory system
Circulatory system	carries blood and nutrients to every cell in the body; includes the heart, arteries, capillaries, and veins
Lungs	are used for breathing; part of the respiratory system
Respiratory system	takes oxygen into the body and releases carbon dioxide into the atmosphere; system includes the nose, trachea, bronchi, and lungs
Brain (organ)	controls and coordinates all mental and physical activity; part of the nervous system
Nervous system	controls the body's actions and reactions and the body's adjustments to the environment
Endocrine system	produces chemical messengers called *hormones*; includes the pituitary gland, thyroid gland, parathyroid glands, adrenal gland, pancreas, ovaries, and testes
Digestive system	provides the body with nutrients by acting on food and excretes digestive waste products; includes the mouth; esophagus, stomach, intestines, and anus
Urinary system	excretes urine, which is mostly water and waste products from cells; includes kidneys, ureters, urinary bladder, and urethra
Skin (organ)	encloses the body, protects the body from pathogens, insulates the body, and helps the body get rid of wastes
Skeletal system	provides structure and support for the body; protects organs such as the brain and the lungs
Muscular system	provides movement inside and outside of the body
Eyes	organs of sight
Ears	organs of hearing

Lesson Review

Using Vocabulary
1. Explain the difference between an organ and a body system.

Understanding Concepts
2. Give three noninfectious causes of diseases.
3. Explain how noninfectious diseases are different from infectious diseases.

Critical Thinking
4. **Analyzing Ideas** How may severe brain injuries be similar to a non-infectious disease?
5. **Making Inferences** Your body's immune system destroys most disease-causing organisms. Explain how being born with a disease of the immune system may affect a person's life.

internet connect
www.scilinks.org/health
Topic: Inherited Diseases
HealthLinks code: HD4062
Topic: Noninfectious Diseases
HealthLinks code: HD4070
HEALTH LINKS. Maintained by the National Science Teachers Association

Teach

Using the Figure — GENERAL
The table on this page lists the major organ systems of the human body and their importance. Have students copy the table and add a third column titled "Diseases." Have students research diseases of the body systems, and have them describe two major diseases that they learn about. Ask students whether each disease they described is an infectious disease or a noninfectious disease. **LS Visual/Verbal**

Close

Reteaching — BASIC
Body Organs and Systems Write the names of the organs listed in the table on this page on one set of index cards. You may also want to add organs that are not pictured. Write the names of the different body systems on another set of index cards. Give one card to each student and have them find an appropriate match. Each organ should pair up with the appropriate body system. **LS Kinesthetic**

Quiz — GENERAL
1. Explain the difference between cells and tissues. (Cells are the simplest units of living organisms. Tissues are made up of similar cells that perform a single function.)
2. Name a hereditary disease and a disease caused by nutritional deficiency. (Sample answer: Down syndrome and cystic fibrosis are hereditary; anemia is caused by nutritional deficiency.)
3. List the name and function of 3 organ systems in the human body. (Answers will vary, but should include information from the figure on this page.)

Answers to Lesson Review
1. An organ is two or more tissues working together, and a body system is a group of organs that work together.
2. Answers may include any of the causes in Table 1, such as congenital, heredity, nutrition, metabolism, cancer, or multiple causes.
3. An infectious disease is caused by a virus or a living organism, but a noninfectious disease is not.
4. Severe brain injury may damage the brain and prevent it from working properly, just as a noninfectious disease may prevent the brain from working properly.
5. A person born with a disease of the immune system may be unable to fight off infections that a person with a healthy immune system could. As a result, they would be much more likely to suffer serious health problems from things that a healthy person would be able to resist.

Lesson 1 • Noninfectious Diseases and Body Systems

Lesson 2

Focus

Overview
Before beginning this lesson, review with your students the objectives listed under the What You'll Do head in the Student Edition. This lesson describes the circulatory system, including the heart and blood. It also discusses circulatory system diseases and ways to avoid them.

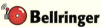

Have students write as many phrases as they can using the word *heart,* such as "have a heart" (be kind) or "broken heart" (very sad). Ask students to explain what each expression means.

Answer to Start Off Write
Sample answer: A heart attack is when part of the heart doesn't get enough blood and the heart can't pump blood properly.

Motivate

Activity — GENERAL
Heart Rate Students will work in pairs. Have one student in each pair record his or her heart rate for 15 seconds. Have the other student multiply this number by 4 and record it. The student whose pulse was recorded should walk around the room for one minute and then jog in place for one minute. Then the student should take his or her pulse again. Have the students switch roles. Discuss why the pulse increases and what the heart is doing during the activity. (Pulse will increase during and just after activity because the heart is circulating more oxygen to body tissues.) **LS Kinesthetic/Interpersonal**

Lesson 2 — Circulatory System

Tony had a physical exam when he tried out for the track team. His doctor found a heart murmur. Tony wants to know if he will be able to run track.

What You'll Do
- **Identify** the parts of the circulatory system.
- **Identify** two noninfectious diseases of the circulatory system.

Terms to Learn
- heart attack
- congenital disorder
- hypertension
- leukemia

Start Off Write
What is a heart attack?

Tony learned that there are many kinds of heart murmurs. Tony's doctor told him that his heart murmur is not unusual. The murmur is not dangerous, so Tony will be able to join the track team.

Your Heart

Your *circulatory system* is made up of your heart and blood vessels, through which blood circulates. The heart is a muscular pump that has four chambers. The two upper chambers hold the blood and are called the *atria* (singular, *atrium* [AY tree uhm]). The two lower chambers pump the blood and are called the *ventricles* (VEN tri kuhlz). Blood enters the right atrium from all parts of the body. This blood is low in oxygen. Blood goes into the right ventricle and is then pumped into the lungs. Between the atrium and the ventricle are valves that prevent blood from flowing backwards. In the lungs, blood picks up oxygen. The high-oxygen blood then returns to the left atrium and goes to the left ventricle. The left ventricle pumps the high-oxygen blood to the rest of the body, including to the heart itself. Like all muscles, the heart needs a constant supply of oxygen to keep beating.

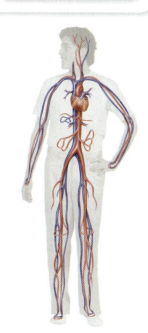

Figure 1 The circulatory system

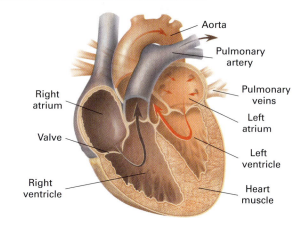

Figure 2 Diagram of a Healthy Heart

LIFE SCIENCE CONNECTION — GENERAL

Vessel Facts The largest blood vessel in the human body is the aorta, which, on average, has a diameter of about 2.5 cm. The smallest vessels are the capillaries, the smallest of which are about 4–6 microns (0.0004–0.0006 cm) in diameter. There's only one aorta, and there are millions of capillaries. Altogether, an adolescent's body holds between 25,000 and 60,000 miles of blood vessels. An adult's body may have up to 100,000 miles of blood vessels. If they were all laid end-to-end, they could circle the Earth at the equator almost 4 times!

Chapter Resource File
- Directed Reading **BASIC**
- Lesson Plan
- Datasheets for In-Text Activities **GENERAL**
- Lesson Quiz **GENERAL**

Transparencies
- TT Bellringer
- TT A Healthy Artery and a Blocked Artery

324 Chapter 15 • Noninfectious Diseases and Disorders

Heart Disease

Heart disease is any condition that affects the heart's ability to pump blood. There are many kinds of heart disease. For example, sometimes arteries are blocked and do not deliver as much blood to the heart as it needs. A **heart attack** happens when part of the heart does not receive enough blood and the heart does not pump well.

Heart failure is a condition that slowly develops as the heart muscle gets weaker. Having heart failure does not mean that your heart stops. During heart failure, the heart cannot pump enough blood to keep the body going. This condition may be caused by high blood pressure, a heart attack, or a congenital disorder. A **congenital disorder** is any disease, abnormality, or defect that is present at birth but is not inherited.

There are more than thirty kinds of congenital heart disease. For example, some babies are born with a hole between the two ventricles in their heart. This defect can be fixed with surgery. Tony's heart murmur is caused by a congenital defect that affects his heart valves. Some congenital defects are detected at birth, but some defects are not discovered for years.

Fighting Heart Disease

The best way to fight heart failure and heart attacks is to prevent them from happening at all. Good health habits can be started in middle school. These health habits are important for preventing heart disease later in life. Eating a nutritious diet, getting plenty of exercise, not being overweight, and not smoking can prevent most heart attacks. Some heart disease may be controlled with medicine, but some heart disease requires surgery. Surgery can also correct many congenital heart defects. But the best medicine for fighting heart disease is to make good health choices from the start.

Your Blood Vessels

There are three major types of blood vessels—arteries, veins, and capillaries. *Arteries* carry blood away from the heart to various organs. *Veins* carry blood from various parts of the body back to the heart. *Capillaries* (KAP uh LER eez) are very small tubes that connect arteries and veins. Some capillaries are so small that you need a microscope to see them.

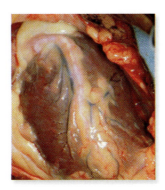

Figure 3 This heart has suffered a heart attack and part of the heart muscle was damaged.

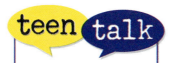

Teen: "I didn't know teens can have heart attacks. How would I know if I was having one?"

Expert: "Usually, a heart attack has warning signs such as the following:

- A sudden pressure, squeezing, or pain in the chest, possibly spreading to the arms, shoulders, neck, or jaw
- Sickness, nausea, or weakness
- Rapid, weak, or irregular pulse
- Sweating, fainting, shortness of breath, lightheadedness, or fear
- Pale or blue skin"

LIFE SCIENCE CONNECTION — ADVANCED

No Surgery Some people have a heart condition called *angina pectoris*, which is pain caused by the heart not getting enough blood. A new technique to correct this problem doesn't involve open-heart surgery. It is called *enhanced external counterpulsation* (EECP). One hour a day for seven weeks, inflatable cuffs wrapped around a patient's calf or thigh inflate and deflate in rhythm with the heart. The pulsating cuffs force blood through the blocked heart arteries, delivering more oxygen to the heart and reducing the pain. Have students research EECP and prepare a multimedia presentation or a poster explaining their findings. Students' presentations should also compare EECP with other treatments for angina. **LS Logical/Visual**

Teach

REAL-LIFE CONNECTION — BASIC

Family History Heredity is one factor leading to heart disease that we cannot control. Have students ask their parents or guardian about the history of heart disease in their family. Although heredity is a factor, taking steps such as a healthy diet and regular exercise can decrease the risk of heart disease. **LS Verbal/Interpersonal**

Life SKILL BUILDER — GENERAL

Assessing Your Health Have students make a list of all the food and drink they consume in a day, as well as the physical activity they engage in during the course of that day. Next to each item of food and drink, they should record a "plus" or a "minus" according to whether it was healthy (+) or unhealthy (–) for their heart. They should also add up the time spent engaging in physical activity. Ask students whether they eat more healthy or unhealthy foods, and whether they think they exercise enough. Use this information to point out that it's never too early to live a heart-healthy lifestyle. **LS Intrapersonal**

Activity

Writing Congestive heart failure is the heart's loss of its pumping ability accompanied by the accumulation of fluid in body tissues. Have students research congestive heart failure. Have students write a story for the newspaper that describes congestive heart failure and its symptoms. The article should also describe the damage it can cause and how to prevent it. Encourage students to illustrate their story.

Lesson 2 • Circulatory System

Teach, continued

Using the Figure — GENERAL
Hardening of the Arteries Use the pictures of the arteries to discuss how blocked arteries are the cause of most heart attacks. Arteries can become blocked by a buildup of fatty acids and other substances, such as cholesterol. When calcium deposits combine with the fatty buildup, the arteries harden. Both of these conditions make the heart work much harder to supply the body with blood, which can cause a heart attack. Ask students how these conditions can be prevented. (Not smoking, a healthy low-fat diet, and regular exercise can prevent these conditions.) **LS Visual**

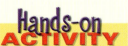

Answers
1. The chart will reflect a range of heart rates.
2. A graph or pie chart will reflect a range of heart rates, most in the range of 60 beats per minute to about 80 beats per minute.

LIFE SCIENCE CONNECTION — GENERAL
Someone who leads a largely sedentary lifestyle has a 35 to 52 percent greater risk of developing high blood pressure than someone who exercises regularly. And if that person is also overweight or obese, they have an even higher risk of developing high blood pressure. Have students research the relationship between weight, exercise, and high blood pressure. Students can present their results in a poster or other visual display. **LS Visual**

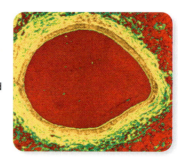 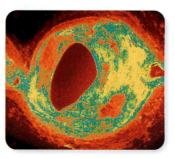

Figure 4 Healthy arteries, such as the one on the left, let blood flow freely to all parts of the body. Blood flow is reduced in a blocked or damaged artery, such as the one on the right.

Hands-on ACTIVITY

HEARTBEATS

1. Feel your pulse by placing two fingers at the pulse point on your neck or wrist.
2. Using a clock or stopwatch, count the number of beats you feel in 15 seconds.
3. Multiply this number by 4 to get the number of times your heart beats each minute. Record this number.

Analysis
1. Organize the data in step 3 into a data table.
2. Draw a bar graph to show what the range of heart rates for the class is and how often each rate happens.

Figure 5 High blood pressure can affect anyone. Some groups have higher rates of hypertension than others, but scientists do not know why.

Your Blood

Your heart pumps blood to the cells in your body. Blood has a liquid part, called *plasma*, and a solid part. Plasma is mostly water, but also includes other chemicals and nutrients.

The solid part of your blood is made up of two types of blood cells—red blood cells and white blood cells. *Red blood cells* carry oxygen to the cells of your body. Every cell in your body needs oxygen in order to keep working. *White blood cells* help fight infections. When you are sick, your white blood cell count may increase to help you fight the infection. Your blood also contains *platelets* (PLAYT lits) which are not true cells. Platelets help stop bleeding by plugging leaks in your arteries, veins, and capillaries.

When the heart tries to pump blood through a blocked artery, the result may be hypertension (HIE puhr TEN shuhn). **Hypertension** is a condition in which the pressure inside your large arteries is too high. Therefore, hypertension is also called *high blood pressure*. This disease can damage your arteries, heart, kidneys, and brain. High blood pressure can also be fatal.

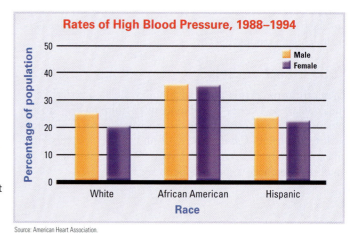

REAL-LIFE CONNECTION — ADVANCED
Blood Pressure Blood pressure is the force the blood exerts against the walls of a blood vessel. Blood pressure is usually measured by putting a cuff around a person's upper arm. Inflating the cuff temporarily stops the flow of blood through the artery in the arm. The doctor or technician slowly releases air from the cuff, listening closely to the artery with a stethoscope. The first sound of blood passing through the artery indicates that the heart is pumping with enough force to overcome the pressure of the cuff. This is the *systolic pressure*. As more pressure is released, the sound disappears and blood begins passing freely. This is *diastolic pressure*. Ask students to research what readings are considered normal blood pressure (90 systolic/60 diastolic to 140/90 is within normal range) and why high blood pressure is so dangerous. **LS Verbal**

326   Chapter 15 • Noninfectious Diseases and Disorders

Fighting Blood Diseases

Blood diseases may affect red blood cells, white blood cells, and platelets. *Anemia* (uh NEE mee uh) is a disease in which your body does not have enough red blood cells. Without these blood cells, your body cells cannot get enough oxygen. Anemia has several causes. For example, your body may not produce enough red blood cells because of a disease. Sometimes, severe blood loss from an accident or an injury can cause anemia. You may lose blood faster than your body can replace it, so you become anemic. You may also become anemic if your diet does not have enough iron. Eating foods high in iron, such as fish, lean meat, and green, leafy vegetables will help prevent anemia. Some diseases, such as sickle cell anemia, cause the body to make defective red blood cells. These defective blood cells cannot carry enough oxygen to the body cells.

White blood cells can be affected, too. For example, some medicines may affect your body's production of white blood cells and make your white cell count too low. And some diseases, such as leukemia (loo KEE mee uh), increase the number of white blood cells. **Leukemia** is cancer of the blood. It causes defective white cells to form in very large numbers.

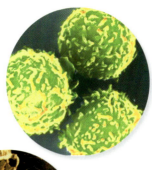

Figure 6 The top photo shows normal white blood cells. The bottom photo shows hairy cell leukemia white blood cells.

Platelet diseases happen when there are too few or too many platelets. With too few platelets, you may bruise easily or bleed too much. With too many platelets, your blood may clot too easily. Blood clots can be dangerous if they travel to your heart, lungs, or brain and stop the flow of blood to these vital organs. In some diseases, platelets do not form clots as they should.

Lesson Review

Using Vocabulary
1. Define *congenital disorder*.

Understanding Concepts
2. Identify the parts of the circulatory system.
3. Describe the flow of blood after it enters the right atrium. Draw a diagram if necessary.
4. Describe two noninfectious diseases of the circulatory system.

Critical Thinking
5. **Making Inferences** Aspirin reduces the clumping or clotting ability of platelets. Doctors sometimes tell patients who have had a heart attack caused by blood clots to take aspirin. Before the patient takes aspirin, what other problem should the doctor warn them about?

Lesson 3

Focus

Overview
Before beginning this lesson, review with your students the objectives listed under the What You'll Do head in the Student Edition. This lesson describes the different parts of the respiratory system and explains how it supplies oxygen to the body. Students will also learn about noninfectious respiratory diseases and how to avoid them.

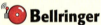 Bellringer
Ask students why it is so important to take care of their lungs. (Lungs supply oxygen to the body. Without adequate oxygen, the body cannot survive.)

Answer to Start Off Write
Accept all reasonable answers. Sample answer: Respiration, also known as breathing, is the process by which oxygen from the air enters your blood and carbon dioxide from your body goes into the air.

Motivate

Activity — GENERAL
Lung Cancer Poster Project
Organize students into groups. Have them research the topic of lung cancer, including the number of people afflicted with the disease, its causes, possible treatments, and ways to avoid it. Groups should organize their information into a poster that can be used to inform people about lung cancer. Have the groups present their findings to the class. **English Language Learners**
LS Visual/Logical

Lesson 3 — Respiratory System

Estebán's lungs sometimes fill with mucous and he feels as if he cannot breathe. Estebán loves soccer, but playing even part of a game makes him exhausted and weak.

What You'll Do
- **Describe** how the respiratory system works.
- **Identify** two noninfectious diseases of the respiratory system.

Terms to Learn
- asthma
- emphysema

Start Off Write
What is respiration?

Estebán has a disease called *cystic fibrosis* (SIS tik fie BROH sis), or CF. Cystic fibrosis impairs a person's breathing, or *respiration*. Respiration is the process by which a body takes in and uses oxygen and gets rid of carbon dioxide and water.

Your Respiratory System

Respiration is made possible by the respiratory system. The respiratory system consists of the nose, mouth, throat, voice box, trachea (TRAY kee uh), and lungs. Air enters the body through the nose and mouth and then enters the trachea. The trachea splits into two tubes called the *bronchi* (BRAHNG kie). Each of the bronchi attaches to a lung. In the lungs, the bronchi divide several times into very small tubes called *bronchioles*. Bronchioles end in small, thin air sacs called *alveoli* (al VEE uh LIE). In the alveoli, oxygen from the air enters your blood and carbon dioxide and water from your body go into the air.

Respiration is controlled by the brain. You don't even have to think about it. Muscles in the chest and between the chest and the abdomen move your chest and help you breathe. Some noninfectious diseases, such as CF, interfere with the airflow in the lungs. Other diseases affect the muscles that help you breathe.

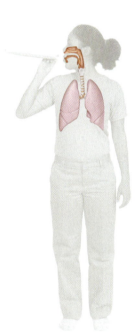

Figure 7 The respiratory system

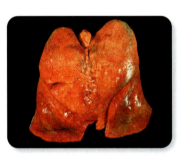
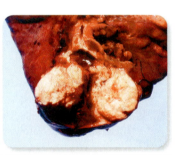

Figure 8 Healthy lungs, shown at left, provide oxygen to your body. A diseased lung, below, cannot provide the oxygen your body needs.

REAL-LIFE CONNECTION — ADVANCED
Lung Capacities Have students take as deep a breath as they can. Tell them that this is about 4.8 liters of air, known as the *vital capacity*. Ask them to take in a normal breath, and then let it out. Then, before breathing again, have them force more air out of their lungs. After a normal exhalation, they can forcefully expel about another liter of air, called the *expiratory reserve*. Have students research lung function, lung capacity, and the amount of air in their lungs. Have them make a poster showing their results.
LS Kinesthetic/Logical/Visual

Chapter Resource File
- Directed Reading **BASIC**
- Lesson Plan
- Lesson Quiz **GENERAL**

Transparencies
TT Bellringer

---

328 Chapter 15 • Noninfectious Diseases and Disorders

Respiratory Diseases

Estebán's CF is a respiratory disease. In CF, mucus in the lungs is thick and sticky, and it clogs the lungs. People with CF sometimes feel like they cannot breathe.

A common respiratory disease is asthma. **Asthma** causes the small bronchioles in the lung to narrow. Asthma causes shortness of breath, wheezing, or coughing. Allergies to smoke, dust, pollen, or other things in the environment may cause asthma attacks. Cold air, exercise, and respiratory infections may also trigger asthma attacks.

Emphysema is a respiratory disease that causes the alveoli to become thin and stretched. Oxygen and carbon dioxide cannot move through the damaged alveoli. As a result, a person with emphysema has difficulty breathing. Emphysema is strongly tied to cigarette smoking and is a disease mainly of adults.

Fighting Respiratory Diseases

Most noninfectious respiratory diseases cannot be cured, but they can be treated. For some respiratory diseases, such as CF and asthma, people take medicine to make breathing easier. People who have these diseases can often lead fairly normal lives. Emphysema, which is one of the worst respiratory diseases, cannot be cured or even treated very well. But emphysema can be almost completely prevented by not smoking cigarettes.

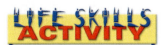

LIFE SKILLS ACTIVITY

MAKING GOOD DECISIONS

Suppose that a friend wants you to start smoking. What would you do? Use the steps for making decisions to show what you would decide. Explain why you would or would not choose to smoke.

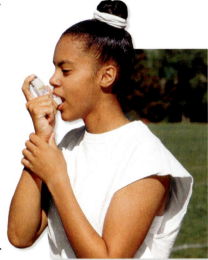

Figure 9 Some respiratory diseases, such as asthma, can be controlled with medication.

Lesson Review

Using Vocabulary

1. What is the difference between asthma and emphysema?

Understanding Concepts

2. Describe how the respiratory system works.

Critical Thinking

3. **Identifying Relationships** Air contains about 21 percent oxygen gas. If a person has trouble breathing because of an asthma attack or emphysema, what could a doctor do to help the person get more oxygen?

internet connect
www.scilinks.org/health
Topic: Asthma
HealthLinks code: HD4011
HEALTH LINKS. Maintained by the National Science Teachers Association

Teach

MATH CONNECTION — GENERAL

Breath of Life Tell students that, on average, a person at rest breathes in about 6 liters of air per minute. Because air is only 21 percent oxygen, a person breathes in about 1.26 liters of oxygen per minute. At this rate, ask students how many liters of oxygen they would breathe in during the course of an hour. Have them calculate the amount of oxygen a person breathes in during an entire day, during a year, and over the course of their lifetime (74 years for men, 80 years for women). (oxygen per hour: 75.6 liters; oxygen per day: 1,814.4 liters; oxygen per year: 662,256 liters; oxygen in a lifetime: 49,006,944 liters for men and 52,980,480 liters for women) **LS** Logical

Close

Reteaching — BASIC

Breathing Is Important The motto of the American Lung Association is "When you can't breathe, nothing else matters." Ask students what they think this means. (Sample answer: People breathe to provide their bodies with oxygen, and without oxygen, people cannot survive.) **LS** Logical/Verbal

Quiz — GENERAL

1. Which parts of the body make up the respiratory system? (nose, mouth, throat, voice box, trachea, and lungs)

2. What happens if the alveoli are damaged? (Oxygen from the air cannot enter your blood and carbon dioxide from your blood cannot go into the air. You could die.)

3. How can emphysema be almost completely prevented? (by not smoking cigarettes)

Answers to Lesson Review

1. Asthma causes the small bronchioles in the lung to narrow, and emphysema causes alveoli to become thin and stretched out.
2. Air enters the lungs through the nose and mouth and the trachea. In the alveoli, oxygen from the air enters the blood. At the same time, carbon dioxide from the body leaves the blood and is exhaled into the air.
3. A doctor could supply the person with air that is more than 21% oxygen from a tank through a mask.

LIFE SKILLS ACTIVITY

Answer
Answers will vary.

Extension: Have interested students make a list of all the dangerous substances in cigarettes and the effects they can have on the human body.

Lesson 4

Focus

Overview
Before beginning this lesson, review with your students the objectives listed under the What You'll Do head in the Student Edition. This lesson defines the parts of the central, peripheral, and autonomic nervous systems and explains how the nervous system controls the rest of the body systems. Students will learn about some noninfectious diseases that can affect the nervous system and how to avoid them.

🔔 Bellringer
Ask students to name the parts of the central nervous system. (brain and spinal cord)

Answer to Start Off Write
Accept all reasonable answers. Sample answer: If messages cannot get through, the body cannot respond properly.

Motivate

Activity — GENERAL
Using the Figure Have students examine the two brain scans in the figure on this page. Ask students what the different colors in the images mean. (Colors indicate levels of activity.) Ask them what differences they notice between the two images. How might these differences affect the body's normal activity? (When parts of the brain are injured or damaged, the brain cannot function normally. When parts of the brain don't function normally, a person is limited in the activities they can perform.)
LS Visual/Verbal

Lesson 4

What You'll Do
- Identify parts of the nervous system.
- Identify two noninfectious diseases of the nervous system.

Terms to Learn
- Alzheimer's disease
- central nervous system
- peripheral nervous system

Start Off Write
What happens if messages from your brain can't get through to your body?

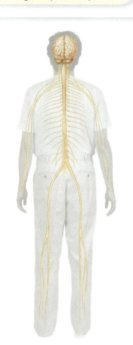

Figure 10 The nervous system

SOCIAL STUDIES CONNECTION — ADVANCED
A Full Life Although having a disease or disorder of the nervous system is a tragic and sometimes fatal condition, there are many people who not only live with these diseases, but rise above them. One example is Dr. Stephen Hawking, a British theoretical physicist who is one of the best-known scientists in the world and who has amyotrophic lateral sclerosis, or ALS, a disease that's better known as Lou Gehrig's disease. Have students research Dr. Hawking and how he uses a computer despite being almost completely unable to move or speak. **LS Verbal/Logical**

Nervous System

Gwen's aunt has Alzheimer's disease. Gwen has offered to help take care of her aunt as the disease worsens.

Gwen learned that **Alzheimer's disease** (AHLTS HIE muhrz di ZEEZ) is a disease of the brain that affects thinking, memory, and behavior. Eventually, her aunt will need almost constant care.

Your Brain and Nervous System

The *nervous system* is the command and control system for the body. It consists of several parts that connect to each other and that work together. The two main parts of the nervous system are the central nervous system (CNS) and the peripheral nervous system (PNS).

The **central nervous system** is made up of the *brain* and the *spinal cord*. The brain, located inside the skull, is the main organ of the nervous system. The *spinal cord* is the bundle of nerves that runs down the back, inside the backbone. The spinal cord is the main pathway for messages between the brain and the peripheral nervous system. The **peripheral nervous system** is made of all of the nerves outside the brain and the spinal cord. The PNS has two main parts, the *somatic* (so MAT ik) *nervous system* and the *autonomic* (ot uh NOM ik) *nervous system*. The somatic nervous system contains the nerves that send information between the CNS and bones, muscles, and skin. The autonomic nervous system controls body functions, such as digestion, breathing, blood pressure, and heart rate, which you do not usually control.

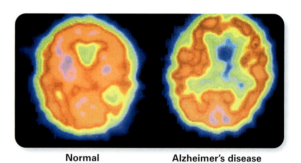

Normal | Alzheimer's disease

Figure 11 These photos show brain activity. The yellow and blue colors represent areas of reduced activity.

Chapter Resource File
- Directed Reading BASIC
- Lesson Plan
- Lesson Quiz GENERAL

Transparencies
TT Bellringer

330 Chapter 15 • Noninfectious Diseases and Disorders

TABLE 3 Examples of Nervous System Diseases

Disease	Description	Treatment or cure
Alzheimer's Disease	a degenerative disease of the brain that often causes loss of memory and changes in behavior	no known cure
Brain tumors	abnormal tissue growth in the brain; Brain tumors may be cancerous or noncancerous.	surgery, chemotherapy, radiation therapy, and medicine
Parkinson's disease	a degenerative disease of the nervous system that is usually associated with trembling of the arms, legs, and face, stiffness of the limbs, and slow movement	no known cure; Medicines may slow the progress of the disease.
Guillain-Barré syndrome	a disorder in which the body's immune system attacks part of the peripheral nervous system; first causes muscle weakness and a tingling sensation in the legs but then may cause paralysis and breathing difficulty	no known cure; The symptoms can be treated, and physical therapy may be used to keep the muscles flexible.

Noninfectious Nervous System Diseases

Some nervous system diseases, such as Alzheimer's disease and brain tumors, affect the brain. Other diseases, such as Guillain-Barré (ge LAN bah RAY) syndrome, affect nerves, or parts of nerves, outside the brain. Many diseases of the nervous system have no known cure, but the symptoms and effects of the diseases can be controlled and treated.

Injuries are another source of nervous system diseases. Head injuries may damage the brain and can affect your ability to think, move, remember, or speak. Spinal cord injuries can stop messages from traveling between your body and your brain. People who have spinal cord injuries may not be able to walk or use their hands. But many brain and spinal cord injuries can be prevented by wearing proper safety equipment and by being careful.

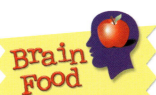

Brain Food

Young adults, in the 16- to 30-year-old age group, account for 55 percent of spinal cord injuries. The average age at injury is about 22.

Lesson Review

Using Vocabulary

1. Name the parts of the central nervous system.

Understanding Concepts

2. Describe two noninfectious diseases of the nervous system.

Critical Thinking

3. **Making Inferences** How might a disease affecting the spinal cord affect a musician or a dancer?

4. **Applying Concepts** Why are the symptoms of a serious brain injury likely to be similar to the symptoms of a serious brain disease?

Answers to Lesson Review

1. brain and spinal cord
2. Alzheimer's disease and Parkinson's disease
3. Sample answer: Nerve impulses back and forth between the person's brain and his or her hands or feet would be affected. A musician might not be able to move his or her hands and fingers to hold or play a musical instrument, and a dancer might not be able move his or her legs, feet, and toes to dance.
4. Both brain disease and brain injury can result in loss of control or use of muscles and damage to various mental functions. This is because both injury and disease can affect the same portions of the brain, producing similar symptoms.

Teach

INCLUSION Strategies — GENERAL
- Visually Impaired
- Learning Disabled

Give students with visual impairments a tactile description of the nervous system. With the student's permission, use a wooden spoon to trace a student's central nervous system gently from the top of his or her head to the base of his or her spine. Gently, run a hair pick with widely-spaced prongs along the student's back, arms, and legs to identify some of the functions of the peripheral nervous system. **LS Kinesthetic**

Close

Reteaching — BASIC

Teens and Safety Equipment Have students write a public service announcement that explains why it is necessary to protect the nervous system and urges teens to use safety equipment. The announcement should explain why most diseases and disorders of the nervous system result in a loss of control over the muscles in the body. (because the muscles are controlled by the nervous system) **LS Verbal**

Quiz — GENERAL

1. What are the three main parts of the nervous system? (central nervous system, peripheral nervous system, and autonomic nervous system)

2. Name one disease of the nervous system and list its symptoms. (Sample answer: Alzheimer's disease causes people to lose their memory, their ability to speak, and their ability to control their body.)

3. How can brain and spinal cord injuries often be prevented? (by wearing proper safety equipment when engaging in sports or leisure activities)

Lesson 5 Focus

Overview
Before beginning this lesson, review with your students the objectives listed under the What You'll Do head in the Student Edition. This lesson describes the endocrine system, the functions of several glands and hormones, and some diseases of the endocrine system.

Bellringer
Ask students to explain what a hormone is. (Hormones are chemicals released into your blood by endocrine glands.)

Answer to Start Off Write
Accept all reasonable answers. Sample answer: Hormones regulate your growth and nearly all body functions.

Motivate

Discussion — GENERAL
Life Changes Students at this age are involved in a very important phase of growing up. Many of them have begun or are about to begin going through puberty, often a time of overwhelming physical and mental change. Ask students to describe the various changes the human body goes through during puberty. Ask students how these physical and mental changes prepare people to function as adults. Discuss how the endocrine system is involved in these changes.
LS Intrapersonal

Lesson 5 — Endocrine System

What You'll Do
- **Describe** the function of the endocrine system.
- **Identify** three noninfectious diseases of the endocrine system.

Terms to Learn
- endocrine gland
- hormones
- type 1 diabetes
- type 2 diabetes

Start Off Write
What do hormones do?

Anthony's friend Sandra asked him to get ice cream with her. Anthony has diabetes and has to watch what he eats. But because he knows that his diabetes is under control, Anthony decides to go.

Diabetes is a disease that affects the body's ability to use sugar for energy. Anthony controls his diabetes by giving himself insulin shots every day. The insulin controls the level of sugar in Anthony's blood. By being careful, Anthony can eat a normal diet, including some ice cream occasionally.

Your Endocrine System
Diabetes is a disease of the endocrine system (EN doh krin SIS tuhm). The *endocrine system* is a network of glands throughout the body that produce chemicals that control many body functions. An **endocrine gland** is a group of cells or an organ that produces hormones. **Hormones** are the chemicals released directly into your blood by the endocrine system to regulate body functions.

Some hormones regulate your growth, and some help with digestion. Other hormones cause your body to change from being a child to being an adult. In fact, hormones affect nearly every body function, including your body's metabolism. *Metabolism* (muh TAB uh LIZ uhm) includes all the processes by which your body breaks down food and converts the energy in food into energy your body can use for growth and repair.

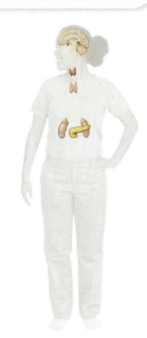

Figure 12 The endocrine system

TABLE 4 Glands of the Endocrine System

Pituitary gland	growth hormone
Thyroid gland	thyroid hormone (necessary for growth and metabolism)
Parathyroid gland	parathyroid hormone (necessary for calcium metabolism)
Pancreas	insulin (necessary for sugar metabolism)
Adrenal gland	sex hormones and hormones for salt metabolism
Testes	male sexual-development hormones
Ovaries	female sexual-development hormones

LIFE SCIENCE CONNECTION — ADVANCED
The Pituitary Gland The pituitary gland is sometimes called the master gland of the endocrine system because it controls all the other endocrine glands. Have students research the pituitary gland and the hormones it produces. [The pituitary gland produces a variety of hormones, including growth hormone, ACTH (which stimulates the adrenal glands), TSH (which stimulates the thyroid gland), FSH (which stimulates the ovaries and testes), and LH (which also stimulates the ovaries or testes).] **LS Logical**

Chapter Resource File
- Directed Reading **BASIC**
- Lesson Plan
- Lesson Quiz **GENERAL**

Transparencies
TT Bellringer

Chapter 15 • Noninfectious Diseases and Disorders

Endocrine System Diseases

There are two types of diabetes. Both types of diabetes may cause serious health problems, including blindness, heart disease, circulatory problems, stroke, and kidney disease. In **type 1 diabetes,** the body produces little or no insulin. *Insulin* is a hormone produced in the pancreas that helps your body store glucose, or sugar. Insulin also enables cells to use glucose for energy. Anthony controls his type 1 diabetes with daily insulin shots. In **type 2 diabetes,** the body makes insulin but cannot use it properly. Type 2 diabetes usually strikes people over age 40. Type 2 diabetes is linked to obesity and lack of exercise. A healthy diet and plenty of exercise help prevent or control type 2 diabetes.

Another endocrine system disease is hyperthyroidism (HIE puhr THIE royd IZ uhm). Hyperthyroidism causes the thyroid gland to produce too much thyroid hormone. Excess thyroid hormone speeds up metabolism and may cause weight loss and makes a person feel warm, sweaty, and nervous. At the end of the day, a person who has hyperthyroidism may feel very tired but may have trouble sleeping. Hyperthyroidism can usually be treated with medication.

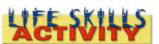

BEING A WISE CONSUMER

One of the main ingredients in fruit juices and regular soft drinks is sugar. Explain why these beverages may not be the best choice for someone with type 1 diabetes.

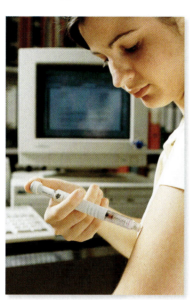

Figure 13 People who have type 1 diabetes can control their disease by taking insulin.

Lesson Review

Using Vocabulary
1. What is the endocrine system?
2. Write a sentence that correctly uses the terms *endocrine gland* and *hormone*.

Understanding Concepts
3. What are three noninfectious diseases of the endocrine system?

Critical Thinking
4. **Making Predictions** If someone takes too much insulin, what happens to the sugar level in his or her blood?
5. **Analyzing Ideas** Type 2 diabetes may be becoming more common among young children and teens. Explain why type 2 diabetes may be increasing in these age groups.

Lesson 6

Focus

Overview
Before beginning this lesson, review with your students the objectives listed under the What You'll Do head in the Student Edition. This lesson describes parts of the digestive system and how they work together. Students will also learn about digestive system diseases and how to avoid them.

Bellringer
Ask students to explain how food is digested. Tell them that they can write a paragraph or draw a picture explaining the process.

Answer to Start Off Write
Accept all reasonable answers. Sample answer: If you cannot absorb nutrients, you will become ill, and you may eventually die.

Motivate

Group Activity —— GENERAL
Digestive Health Organize students into groups and have them explore the best ways to maintain the health of their digestive system. One group may interview a gastroenterologist or other physician to learn about common digestive problems and how to avoid them. Other students may research over-the-counter medicines taken to relieve common digestive ailments. Still others may research which are the best foods to eat for a healthy digestive system. **LS Interpersonal** Co-op Learning

Lesson 6

Digestive System

Jasmine often has stomach cramps. She feels sick and is losing weight. Jasmine wants to know why she is sick.

What You'll Do
- **Identify** the parts of your digestive system.
- **Identify** two noninfectious disorders of the digestive system.

Terms to Learn
- celiac disease

Write
What happens if your intestines cannot absorb nutrients?

Jasmine's doctor ran a series of tests. The results show that Jasmine has a digestive system disease that keeps her body from absorbing nutrients from food.

Your Digestive System

Your *digestive system* is the body system that breaks down food so that it can be used by your body. Digestion of food begins in the mouth. Food passes from your mouth down your esophagus (i SAHF uh guhs) to the stomach. Your stomach holds food and partially digests it. From your stomach, food passes into the small intestine. In the small intestine, digestion of food is completed and nutrients from food are absorbed. The small intestine connects to the large intestine, where water from food is absorbed. The large intestine, or colon, ends at the rectum. Finally, the rectum ends at the anus. Solid waste—undigested and unabsorbed food—leaves the body through the anus.

Digestive enzymes are special proteins that help digestion. They are produced in the mouth, stomach, and small intestine. These enzymes break down food and make it usable. Your pancreas and liver are also involved in the digestive process. The liver produces *bile*, which helps digest fats. The pancreas produces a mixture of enzymes that help break down fats, proteins, and carbohydrates.

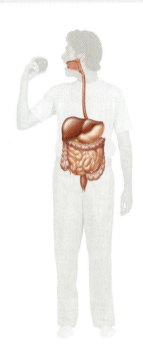

Figure 14 The digestive system

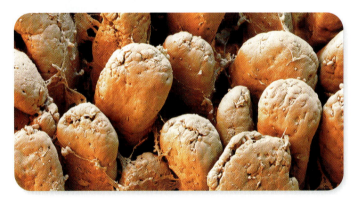

Figure 15 The small and large intestines are lined with villi, shown above. Villi absorb nutrients from food.

Career

Nutritionist Many advertisements for foods and beverages claim that one product is more nutritious than another product. Who studies whether something is nutritious or not? Nutritionists do. A nutritionist is a person who studies the materials that nourish the body and how the nutrients are used for cellular growth, repair, maintenance, and reproduction. Research about nutrients is important because some foods may strengthen the immune system or reduce the risk of certain kinds of cancer. Many nutritionists also educate the public about how good eating habits can help people lead healthy lives.

Chapter Resource File
- Directed Reading **BASIC**
- Lesson Plan
- Lesson Quiz **GENERAL**

Transparencies
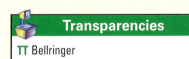
TT Bellringer

334 Chapter 15 • Noninfectious Diseases and Disorders

Noninfectious Digestive System Diseases

Jasmine has celiac disease (SEE lee AK di ZEEZ). **Celiac disease** is a disease that makes the body allergic to a protein called *gluten* (GLOOT n). Gluten is found in grains, such as wheat, rye, and barley. When someone who has celiac disease eats food with gluten, his or her immune system reacts by damaging the lining of the small intestine. This damage stops the person's intestine from absorbing the nutrients in his or her food. A person with celiac disease can live a normal life if he or she avoids food containing gluten.

Other digestive diseases include Crohn's disease, which attacks the lining of the intestines and causes diarrhea, cramps, and fever. Ulcerative colitis (UHL suhr AY tiv koh LIET is) is a similar disease that attacks the colon. These two diseases are often grouped together as inflammatory bowel disease (IBD). With proper medication and a healthy diet, people with IBD can usually live relatively normal lives.

Stomach cancer is another noninfectious disease of the digestive system. Stomach cancer has no known cause. Factors that may be related to stomach cancer include

- alcohol abuse
- tobacco abuse
- a diet that is high in smoked food and salted fish or meat
- a diet low in fiber and high in starch

Stomach cancer can be treated by surgery, radiation therapy, and chemotherapy. But it is better to avoid stomach cancer entirely. You can reduce your chances of getting stomach cancer by avoiding tobacco and alcohol and by eating a nutritious diet.

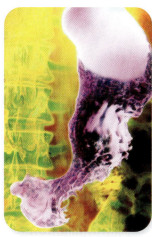

Figure 16 This colored x ray shows a stomach being destroyed by cancer. The pink area (upper right) is healthy stomach wall. The dark purple mass extending downward is the cancer that has attacked part of the stomach.

Lesson Review

Using Vocabulary
1. What is celiac disease?

Understanding Concepts
2. Describe two noninfectious diseases of the digestive system.
3. What are the parts of your digestive system?

Critical Thinking
4. **Identifying Relationships** Why would diseases such as celiac disease or Crohn's disease affect the health of the entire body even though they are diseases of the digestive system?

Answers to Lesson Review
1. Celiac disease is a disease of the digestive system that makes the body allergic to gluten.
2. Crohn's disease and stomach cancer
3. The digestive system includes the mouth, esophagus, stomach, small intestine, large intestine, rectum, and anus.
4. A disease that prevents nutrients from being absorbed by the body deprives all other body systems of the nutrition and energy they need to function properly.

Teach

REAL-LIFE CONNECTION — GENERAL

Small Intestine The small intestine is so named because it is only about 3–4 cm in diameter, which is narrow compared to the large intestine (about 6–8 cm in diameter). But the small intestine measures about 7 m long in the average adult. The *duodenum*, the first 25–30 cm of the small intestine, is where partially digested food is broken down further. The *jejunum*, the next 20 cm or so, is where many nutrients are absorbed. The *ileum*, the last 3–4 m of the small intestine, absorbs the remaining nutrients before digested material moves on to the large intestine. Have students research how food is moved through the intestines and how nutrients are absorbed. Ask students to illustrate their findings. **LS Logical/Visual**

Close

Reteaching — BASIC
Digestion Ask students to draw an outline of the human body. Have them draw or list, in order, the path that food travels as it's being digested. Remind students to label each part and explain its function. **LS Visual/Verbal**

Quiz — GENERAL
1. What is bile? (a substance produced by the liver that helps digest fats)
2. What are digestive enzymes and what role do they play in digestion? (Digestive enzymes are proteins produced in the mouth, stomach, and small intestine that break down food and make it usable.)

Lesson 7 Focus

Overview
Before beginning this lesson, review with your students the objectives listed under the What You'll Do head in the Student Edition. This lesson describes parts of the urinary system and its role in removing metabolic wastes from the body. The lesson also covers some noninfectious diseases of the urinary system.

Bellringer
Ask students what the purpose of the urinary system is. (The urinary system filters blood, removes metabolic wastes from the blood, and maintains salt and fluid levels in the body.)

Answer to Start Off Write
Accept all reasonable answers. Sample answer: The kidneys are organs that filter blood and remove wastes and water from the blood.

Motivate

Demonstration — GENERAL
How Kidneys Work Put some rice in a beaker of warm water. Pour the water through a strainer into another beaker. Show students that the strainer has caught the rice but has let the "starch water" pass. Discuss with students how this demonstration represents the way the kidneys work. Ask students why kidneys are important. (Kidneys remove wastes from the blood. Without kidneys, high blood pressure, kidney failure, and even death could result.)

Extension: Buy a beef kidney at a grocery store or butcher shop. Have students examine its structure.
LS Visual/Verbal — English Language Learners

Lesson 7

What You'll Do
- **Describe** the urinary system.
- **Identify** three noninfectious diseases that affect the urinary system.

Terms to Learn
- kidneys

Start Off Write
What do your kidneys do?

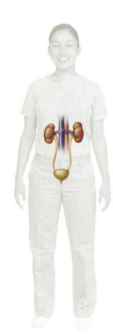

Figure 17 The urinary system

LIFE SCIENCE CONNECTION — ADVANCED
Vital Filters Your kidneys are very small—5 inches long by 2 or 3 inches wide and 1 inch thick (about the size of a small child's fist)—but they are very important. About once each hour, your kidneys filter every drop of blood in your body. At any moment, up to a quarter of the blood in your body is passing through your kidneys. Ask students to research how the urinary system and the kidneys help maintain salt and fluid balance in the body.
LS Verbal/Logical

Urinary System

Jackson's father has high blood pressure. His father's doctor said that high blood pressure can damage the kidneys.

Jackson is worried because he knows that kidney damage is serious. Jackson's father takes medicine to control his blood pressure. A doctor checks his father's kidneys every few months to make sure that they are healthy and are working properly.

Your Urinary System

Kidneys are organs that remove wastes and water from blood. Wastes removed by the kidneys are products of metabolism inside the cells. These wastes are not the same as digestive wastes. Kidneys are also important in maintaining the level of salt and fluid in the body. Maintaining this level helps control blood pressure.

Kidneys are part of the urinary system. The *urinary system* includes the two kidneys, two ureters (yoo REET uhrz), the urinary bladder, and the urethra (yoo REE thruh). As blood travels through your body, it collects the waste products from your cells. Your kidneys constantly clean your blood through more than a million tiny filters called *nephrons* (NEF RAHNZ). Nephrons collect waste products and water from the blood. Together, the waste products and water form *urine*. Urine leaves the kidneys through the *ureters*. It is transported by the ureters to the urinary bladder, where it is stored. Eventually, urine leaves the body through the *urethra*. The process of releasing urine from the body is called *urination*.

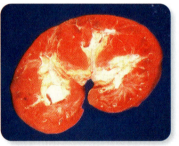

Figure 18 A healthy kidney is shown on the left. A kidney damaged by disease, such as the one shown on the right, cannot remove wastes from the body.

Chapter Resource File
- Directed Reading **BASIC**
- Lesson Plan
- Lesson Quiz **GENERAL**

Transparencies
- TT Bellringer

---

336 Chapter 15 • Noninfectious Diseases and Disorders

Noninfectious Urinary Diseases

Diabetes and hypertension cause most kidney disease. In diabetes, the body cannot use the sugar in the blood. This unused sugar damages small blood vessels and nephrons in the kidneys. In hypertension, the nephrons are damaged by the stress caused by high blood pressure. When nephrons are damaged, they are unable to filter blood and remove wastes.

In both diabetes and hypertension, wastes can build up in blood and organs and cause a variety of health problems, including complete kidney failure. If untreated, kidney disease can lead to death. Kidney disease can sometimes be treated with diet and medication. In other cases, dialysis is necessary.

Some kidney diseases are inherited. For example, polycystic (PAHL ee SIS tik) kidney disease (PKD) is hereditary. In PKD, hard growths, called *cysts* (SISTS) form in the kidneys. These cysts slowly replace large portions of the nephrons. PKD cannot be cured, but it can be treated with medication and a proper diet.

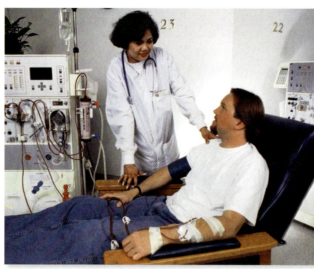

Figure 19 When a person's kidneys are severely diseased, a process called dialysis is used to filter wastes from the person's blood.

Lesson Review

Using Vocabulary
1. What are your kidneys?

Understanding Concepts
2. Draw a diagram showing the parts of the urinary system and the ways in which this system removes waste from the blood.
3. An older man has blockages in both his ureters. Will he be able to urinate?
4. What are three noninfectious diseases that affect the urinary system?

Critical Thinking
5. **Making Inferences** Some desert-dwelling animals, such as gerbils and some lizards, add little or no water to their cellular waste products. What advantage(s) may this system have for animals that use it?

Lesson 8

Focus

Overview
Before beginning this lesson, review with your students the objectives listed under the What You'll Do head in the Student Edition. In this lesson, students will learn about skin, bones, and muscles of the body. Students also learn about some noninfectious diseases that affect these tissues.

Bellringer
Ask students to imagine what a human body would be like without any one of the following: skin, bones, or muscles. Have them write a paragraph about the problems a person would have—besides just unpleasant appearance—without skin, bones, or muscles.

Answer to Start Off Write
Accept all reasonable answers. Sample answer: Bones are considered living tissue because bones are made of living bone cells.

Motivate

Activity — GENERAL
Prime Movers Have students hold an arm straight out, palm up, and then move their forearm up, bending at the elbow (i.e. flex their bicep). Ask students which muscles and bones work to perform this action. (bicep pulls and tricep relaxes; bones in forearm) Explain that muscles work in pairs and that they move body parts by pulling, not by pushing. Have students identify other muscle pairs that work this way. (muscles on the front and back of the thigh, muscles that flex and extend the foot)
LS Kinesthetic

Lesson 8 — Skin, Bones, and Muscles

Mohandas was hiking across a field when he stepped in a hole and fell. He broke his wrist while trying to break his fall. Now he has to wear a cast for 6 weeks!

What You'll Do
- **Describe** why your skin, bones, and muscles are important.
- **Describe** diseases of the skin, bones, and muscles.

Terms to Learn
- osteoporosis
- muscular dystrophy (MD)

Start Off Write
Why are bones considered living tissue?

Bones are made of connective tissue cells and minerals. Some people think that bones are lifeless. But bones, just like your brain or stomach, are living organs made of several different tissues.

Your Connective Tissues

You are made of more than just skin and bones. Your body has four basic kinds of tissue—epithelial tissue (EP i THEE lee uhl TISH oo), nervous tissue, muscle tissue, and connective tissue. Your skin and your stomach lining are made of epithelial tissue. Nervous tissue is found in your nerves, brain, and spinal cord. Your muscles are made of muscle tissue. And your bones, ligaments, and tendons are all made of connective tissue.

Your *skin* is a protective covering for your body. It receives signals from the environment, such as touch or pain. These signals travel to the brain along nervous tissue. *Bones* are solid structures made of proteins, minerals, and connective tissue. Blood vessels inside your bones deliver nutrients to the living bone cells. Your bones give you stability. They also protect important organs, such as the brain and the spinal cord. Bone marrow, located in the center of the bone, is where blood cells are formed. Your *muscles* are tissue that make it possible for your body to move. Your muscles are controlled by your nerves and your brain.

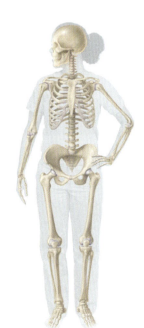

Figure 20 The skeletal system

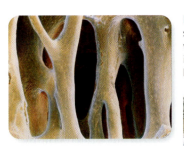
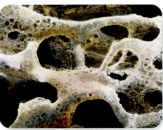

Figure 21 Healthy bone tissue is shown on the left. Bone tissue with osteoporosis, shown below, is weaker and more fragile than healthy bone tissue.

REAL-LIFE CONNECTION — BASIC
Skin Cancer Skin cancer is the most common form of cancer, and often results from overexposure of the skin to the sun's ultraviolet rays. Skin cancer develops from changes that happen slowly and cumulatively over many years. Some types of skin cancer are easily treated, but some can be fatal. Most forms of skin cancer are easy to detect. For people who are at risk for skin cancer, a thorough skin self-examination every month can help detect skin cancer early. Have students research why the rates of skin cancers in young people are increasing. **LS Verbal**

Chapter Resource File
- Directed Reading BASIC
- Lesson Plan
- Datasheets for In-Text Activities GENERAL
- Lesson Quiz GENERAL

Transparencies
TT Bellringer

---

338   Chapter 15 • Noninfectious Diseases and Disorders

Hands-on ACTIVITY

HOW MUCH SKIN DO YOU HAVE?

1. Use a cloth measuring tape or a piece of string to measure the average circumference and the length of each of the following body parts: head, torso, upper arm, lower arm, upper leg, and lower leg.
2. Multiply the average circumference by the length to get the amount of skin for each part.
3. Add together the amount of skin for each part to get your total amount of skin.

Analysis

1. Record the height, age, and total amount of skin for everyone in the class. Make graphs that show whether the amount of skin depends on height or age.
2. Does the amount of skin a person has depend on how old the person is? how tall the person is? Explain your answer.

Noninfectious Connective Tissue Diseases

There are many skin, bone, and muscle diseases. Some skin diseases, such as skin cancers, are caused by exposure to sunlight. Other skin diseases, such as eczema and psoriasis, have no known cause. Skin is your first line of defense against infection, so skin diseases and breaks in the skin should be treated quickly.

Osteoporosis is a bone disease that causes loss of bone density, so bones become brittle. Osteoporosis usually strikes older adults, especially women. It can be treated with calcium, vitamin D, and sometimes hormones. Another bone disease called *rickets* strikes young children. Rickets results from a lack of vitamin D, and can be treated with a proper diet.

Muscular dystrophy (MD) is a group of several inherited muscle diseases that cause muscles gradually to become weak and disabled. There are no cures for MD, but treatment and therapy can support people who have MD.

Myth & Fact

Myth: Cracking your knuckles makes your knuckles get bigger and will give you arthritis.

Fact: There is actually little scientific data available on this topic. One study concluded that there is no relation between knuckle cracking and damage to the finger joints.

Lesson Review

Using Vocabulary
1. What is osteoporosis?

Understanding Concepts
2. Why are bones, muscles, and skin important?
3. Identify a noninfectious bone disease.

Critical Thinking
4. **Making Inferences** Cancer is the uncontrolled growth of live cells. Can cancer attack bone tissue? Explain your answer.
5. **Making Inferences** Why is rickets rarely seen in this country?

Teach

Life SKILL BUILDER — GENERAL

Assessing Your Health Invite a nutritionist to speak to the class. Ask the nutritionist to help students assess their daily diet against recommended standards for strong bones and preventing osteoporosis. To prepare for the guest speaker, have students research foods or drinks that help in the development of healthy skin, bones, or muscles. Students may want to research diets or vitamin, mineral, and herbal supplements. Have students prepare questions to ask the nutritionist.
LS Interpersonal/Auditory

Close

Reteaching — BASIC

Skin, Bone, and Muscle Diseases Make a list of skin, muscle, and bone diseases on the board. Make a list of treatments or cures for these diseases, but not in order. Have students match the disease with the treatment. Also have students identify whether the disease is one of skin, muscle, or bone.
LS Verbal/Logical

Quiz — GENERAL

1. Name the four types of tissue in your body and give an example of each. (epithelial: skin; nervous: brain; muscle: muscles; connective: bones)
2. From where do living bone cells receive their nutrients? (blood vessels inside your bones)
3. What is muscular dystrophy? (a group of several hereditary muscle diseases that cause muscles to become weak and disabled.)

Answers to Lesson Review

1. a bone disease that causes loss of bone density so that bones become brittle or easily broken
2. Sample answer: Bones are important because they provide support and protection for body organs. Muscles are important because they help your body move. Skin is your body's first line of defense against infection.
3. rickets or osteoporosis
4. Cancer can attack bone tissue because bone tissue is living tissue.
5. Sample answer: Rickets is rare in this country because most children eat nutritious foods and get plenty of vitamin D.

Hands-on ACTIVITY

Answers

Analysis
Note: Some students may be very sensitive about their height and weight.
1. Answers will vary depending on the size and shape of the students.
2. Students should show their calculations. Sample answer: The amount of skin a person has does not depend on the person's age. The amount of skin depends more on a person's height.

Lesson 8 • Skin, Bones, and Muscles

Lesson 9

Focus

Overview
Before beginning this lesson, review with your students the objectives listed under the What You'll Do head in the Student Edition. In this lesson, students will learn about the structures of the eyes and ears, the functions that each performs, and noninfectious diseases that affect these organs.

Bellringer
Ask students to list ten things they would miss most if they could not see and ten things they would miss most if they could not hear. *(Answers will vary.)*

Answer to Start Off Write
Accept all reasonable answers. Sample answer: Your eyes and your ears convert information from the world around you into electrical impulses that are sent to your brain.

Motivate

Activity —— GENERAL

Binocular Vision Have pairs of students stand about two feet apart, facing each other. One student should extend his or her arm with the index finger pointed upward. The other student should cover one eye with one hand and, with the index finger of the other hand, attempt to touch his or her partner's fingertip. Ask students if this was easy to do. Ask them why it might have been difficult. *(Covering one eye disables binocular vision, which affects depth perception.)*
LS Kinesthetic

Lesson 9 — Eyes and Ears

Krishna sits at the front of the class. He still cannot see the board very clearly. He doesn't want to say anything because he is afraid that he will have to wear glasses.

What You'll Do
- **Describe** the function of eyes and ears.
- **Describe** three noninfectious diseases of the eyes and ears.

Terms to Learn
- cataract
- glaucoma
- deafness

Start Off Write
How do your eyes and ears give you information about your world?

Krishna may be right. He may have to get lenses to correct his vision. His vision is blurry, and he is missing important work on the board. But he thinks that glasses will make him look ugly.

Your Eyes and Ears

You are using your eyes to read this sentence. Your eyes are sensory organs that send information from the world around you to your brain. Light passes through the cornea, the pupil, and the lens of your eye. The lens focuses light on the retina. The *retina* is a layer of cells at the back of the eye. The cells of the retina send electrical impulses along the optic nerve to your brain. Your brain changes these electrical impulses into images. Usually, the parts of your eyes work together to make sure that you get this information. The images Krishna sees are blurred because his lenses don't focus light exactly on the retina.

Your ears are sensory organs used for hearing. They send information about sound to your brain. Each ear is divided into three parts—the outer, middle, and inner ears. Sound waves that reach the outer ear are funneled toward the eardrum and make the eardrum vibrate. These vibrations travel through the three small bones of the middle ear—the hammer, the anvil, and the stirrup—to the inner ear. The inner ear converts the vibrations into electrical impulses, which go to the brain. The inner ear also has a second function—maintaining your balance. People with a disease of the middle ear may feel dizzy and nauseated because the inner ear is sending incorrect messages to their brain.

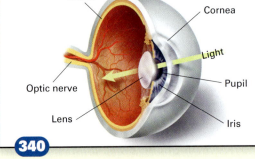
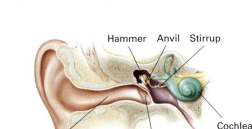

Figure 22 Your eyes and ears are sensory organs.

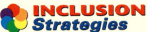

INCLUSION Strategies —— ADVANCED
- Gifted and Talented
- Behavior Control Issues

Ask students to prepare a presentation for the class (a chart, a poster, or a multimedia presentation) that combines information from the chapter. The presentation should show how body systems fit together in the body and how they work together to keep a body healthy. The presentation should also include common noninfectious diseases that affect each system. **LS** Verbal/Visual/Logical

Chapter Resource File
- Directed Reading BASIC
- Lesson Plan
- Lesson Quiz GENERAL

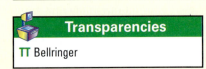

Transparencies
TT Bellringer

Noninfectious Diseases of the Eyes and Ears

Noninfectious eye diseases include cataracts and glaucoma (glaw KOH muh). A **cataract** is a clouding of the natural lens of the eye. Fortunately, the cloudy lens can be replaced with a plastic lens similar to a contact lens. **Glaucoma** is a disease that causes high pressure in the fluid inside the eye. This high pressure damages the optic nerve and causes a permanent loss of vision. Most cases of glaucoma cannot be cured, but glaucoma can be treated and vision can be saved. With regular eye exams, both cataracts and glaucoma can be detected early, and can be stopped or treated with medicine or surgery.

The most common hearing problem is deafness. **Deafness** is the partial or total loss of the ability to hear. There are many levels of hearing loss, from mild loss to total deafness. Deafness may be hereditary or may happen during the birth process. Infectious diseases, such as meningitis, may cause deafness. Noninfectious diseases, such as diabetes and leukemia, may also cause deafness. In teens, the most common cause of deafness is exposure to loud noise. Loud noise can cause damage to the inner ear, which may leave you unable to hear some sounds. You may be unable to hear parts of normal conversation. How can you tell if the noise is too loud? If you have to shout to be heard over the music, the music may be damaging your hearing.

Health Journal
Needing glasses to correct vision problems usually does not mean that you have an eye disease. Nevertheless, getting glasses is often very stressful for teens. What would you say to a friend to help relieve his or her stress about getting glasses?

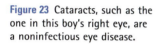

Figure 23 Cataracts, such as the one in this boy's right eye, are a noninfectious eye disease.

Lesson Review

Using Vocabulary
1. Define *deafness*.

Understanding Concepts
2. What is the function of your eyes and ears?
3. Describe three noninfectious diseases of the eyes and ears.

Critical Thinking
4. **Making Inferences** Your friend is suffering from a severe head cold. He also feels dizzy and sick. Is it possible that there is any connection between his cold and his dizziness? Explain your answer.

CHAPTER 15 CHAPTER REVIEW

Assignment Guide

Lesson	Review Question
1	1, 3, 9, 18
2	2, 10
3	11, 21
4	8, 13
5	5, 14, 19
6	15, 20
7	12, 17
8	4, 22–24
9	6–7, 16

ANSWERS

Using Vocabulary

1. body system
2. organ
3. noninfectious disease
4. Osteoporosis
5. Type 2 diabetes
6. cataract
7. glaucoma
8. The central nervous system is your brain and spinal cord. The peripheral nervous system is all the nerves outside of the central nervous system.
9. A noninfectious disease is a disease that is not caused by a living organism. A congenital disease is a disease that is present at birth but is not hereditary.
10. Hypertension is high blood pressure inside the arteries. A heart attack is when part of the heart does not get enough blood and the heart cannot pump properly.
11. Asthma causes the bronchioles in the lung to narrow. Emphysema causes the alveoli in the lungs to become stretched and thin.

Chapter Summary

- A noninfectious disease is a disease that is not caused by a virus or living organism.
- Noninfectious diseases can strike any organ or system in the body.
- Heart failure and heart attacks are two noninfectious diseases of the circulatory system.
- Asthma is a respiratory disease that makes breathing difficult.
- The nervous system has two main parts—the central nervous system and the peripheral nervous system.
- People with brain or spinal cord injuries may not be able to walk or use their hands.
- A person with diabetes cannot use glucose properly.
- The digestive system breaks down food so that it can by used by the body.
- Kidney disease damages the body's ability to remove waste products from the blood.
- Noninfectious diseases, such as cancer, can strike the skin, bones, and muscles.

Using Vocabulary

For each sentence, fill in the blank with the proper word from the word bank provided below.

organ   type 1 diabetes
osteoporosis   type 2 diabetes
noninfectious disease   body system
cataract   glaucoma

1. A(n) ___ is a group of organs that work together.
2. The heart is a(n) ___ that pumps blood throughout the body.
3. A(n) ___ is not caused by a virus or living organism.
4. ___ is a bone disease that causes bones to lose density.
5. ___ is a disease in which the body produces insulin but cannot use it properly.
6. A(n) ___ is clouding of the natural lens of the eye.
7. ___ is a disease that causes high fluid pressure inside the eye.

For each pair of terms, describe how the meanings of the terms differ.

8. central nervous system/peripheral nervous system
9. noninfectious disease/congenital disease
10. hypertension/heart attack
11. asthma/emphysema

Understanding Concepts

12. What is the relationship between kidneys and nephrons?
13. If a disease or injury seriously damaged the spinal cord, how might the body be affected?
14. What happens to the body if the thyroid gland produces too much hormone?
15. Describe the path of food through the digestive system, and explain why enzymes are important to digestion.
16. Explain why some airport workers wear protective headphones.
17. Why is it so important to avoid high blood pressure?

Understanding Concepts

12. Kidneys are organs that filter blood and remove wastes and water from it, and nephrons are tiny filters inside the kidneys that collect the wastes and water from the blood.
13. Damage to the spinal cord may cause paralysis, which can result in the inability to walk or to use the arms or hands.
14. The result is hyperthyroidism, which causes the metabolism to speed up, weight loss, a nervous feeling, and being very tired at the end of a day but unable to sleep.
15. Digestion begins in the mouth and continues through the esophagus, stomach, small intestine, and large intestine. Digestive wastes leave the body through the anus. Along the way, digestive enzymes break food down and make it usable for the rest of the body.
16. The noise of airplane engines can cause permanent damage to hearing.
17. High blood pressure can damage the heart, the kidneys, and the arteries. Damage to any of these body parts can cause illness or death.

Critical Thinking

Identifying Relationships

18. Why is it important to know whether a disease is infectious or noninfectious?

19. Type 2 diabetes usually strikes people in their 40s or 50s. But some studies show that type 2 diabetes is becoming more common in young children and teens. Why is it important for teens to develop good eating habits and get plenty of exercise?

20. Why is it important for the small intestine to be working properly?

21. Why is it important not to smoke cigarettes?

22. Describe how your nervous system is working with your skin, muscles, bones, eyes, and ears as you answer this question.

Making Good Decisions

23. Imagine that you have a family history of skin cancer. This type of cancer usually strikes people in their 20s or 30s. You have been offered a summer job working outside at a local swimming pool. Describe the steps you would take in deciding whether to accept the job.

24. Imagine that someone has discovered a drug that will make you 20 percent smarter than you are. Unfortunately, the drug has a side effect. The drug damages bone marrow. Would you take this new "smart pill" or not? Explain your answer.

Interpreting Graphics

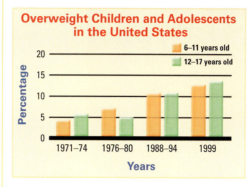

Overweight Children and Adolescents in the United States

Use the graph above to answer questions 25–28.

25. Between which two time periods did the prevalence of overweight adolescents from 12 to 17 years old show the greatest increase?

26. What general statement can you make about the percentage of overweight children in the years from 1988–1994 to 1999?

27. For 1999, what percentage of children ages 6 to 11 are overweight?

28. Being overweight is sometimes related to type 2 diabetes. Looking at the graph, what prediction would you make for the number of type 2 diabetes cases in the years after 2028?

Reading Checkup

Take a minute to review your answers to the Health IQ questions at the beginning of this chapter. How has reading this chapter improved your Health IQ?

Interpreting Graphics

25. Between 1976–1980 and 1988–1994
26. The percentage of overweight children for both age groups increased in those years.
27. approximately 13 percent
28. The number of type 2 diabetes cases will probably increase.

Chapter Resource File
- Concept Review GENERAL
- Concept Mapping GENERAL
- Performance-Based Assessment GENERAL
- Chapter Test GENERAL

Critical Thinking

18. Treatment for noninfectious diseases differs from treatment for infectious diseases. For example, noninfectious diseases do not spread from living thing to living thing and are often the result of heredity or lifestyle choices.

19. Poor diet and a sedentary lifestyle are major contributors to the development of type 2 diabetes. Young people should develop good eating and exercise habits in order to minimize their risk of developing type 2 diabetes later in life.

20. Nutrients are absorbed from food in the small intestine. If the small intestine does not absorb adequate nutrients, the rest of the body cannot function properly.

21. Cigarette smoking is the main cause of lung cancer and emphysema, two noninfectious diseases that destroy the lungs' ability to provide the body with the oxygen it needs to keep you alive. Not smoking will help keep your lungs healthy.

22. Your eyes, ears, skin, and muscles are all sending messages to your brain. Your brain sorts through all this information and tells your bones and muscles to move your pencil, and tells your eyes to read your answer again!

Making Good Decisions

23. Answers will vary, but should include inquiring about what hours the student would work, whether those hours are when the sun is at its most dangerous (usually noon to mid afternoon), and whether there is shelter from the sun during working hours.

24. Answers will vary, but most students would probably not take the drug, because healthy bone marrow is important for the production of red and white blood cells and for sound body structure.

Model

Introduce this activity by reminding students that using this Life Skill will help them take personal responsibility for their behavior. Then, review the scenario with the class.

Prepare students for this activity by modeling each of the steps of the skill. Make sure students understand each step before you move on to the next one.

Guided Practice: Practice with a Friend

Guided Practice is the stage in which you and the students analyze their approach to solving the problem given in the scenario and analyze their coping skills. Have students read Act 1. Discuss with the class the situation described and the way students are to act it out. Organize the class into groups of three. In each group, one person plays the role of Derek, another person plays Derek's brother, and the third person is the observer.

Proper pacing during the Guided Practice is important. The suggestions listed below will help you control the pace.

1. Stop after completing each step of coping.
2. Discuss with each group the observer's comments.
3. Ask the other members of each group to listen to the observer's suggestions and to suggest ways to improve their coping skills.
4. Instruct students to repeat the steps that need improvement and to include their modifications.
5. Check to make sure that students understand each step before they move on to the next step.
6. If time permits, repeat the exercise three times, switching roles each time. Each student should have the opportunity to play each role. `Co-op Learning`

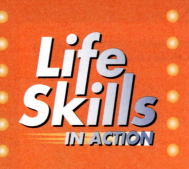

Life Skills IN ACTION

Coping

At times, everyone faces setbacks, disappointments, or other troubles. To deal with these problems, you have to learn how to cope. Coping is dealing with problems and emotions in an effective way. Complete the following activity to develop your coping skills.

Derek's Depression

ACT 1

Setting the Scene

Derek's mother has cancer. She has been receiving treatment for a year now. Sometimes, she seems to get better, but other times she seems to be very sick. Derek's mother remains hopeful that she will be cured and tries to keep Derek and his brother cheerful. But Derek is very worried about her. He has trouble sleeping at night and struggles with many different emotions.

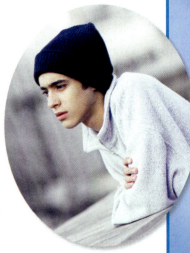

The 5 Steps of Coping

1. Identify the problem.
2. Identify your emotions.
3. Use positive self-talk.
4. Find ways to resolve the problem.
5. Talk to others to receive support.

Guided Practice

Practice with a Friend

Form a group of three. Have one person play the role of Derek and another person play the role of Derek's brother. Have the third person be an observer. Walking through each of the five steps of coping, role-play Derek dealing with his mother's illness. Derek can talk to his brother to receive support. The observer will take notes, which will include observations about what the person playing Derek did well and suggestions of ways to improve. Stop after each step to evaluate the process.

344 Chapter 15 • Life Skills in Action

Independent Practice

Check Yourself

After you have completed the guided practice, go through Act 1 again without stopping at each step. Answer the questions below to review what you did.

1. What are some emotions that Derek may be feeling?
2. How can positive self-talk help Derek cope with his problem?
3. Other than Derek's family members, who can Derek speak with to receive support?
4. Think about a time when you faced a difficult problem. How did you cope with the problem?

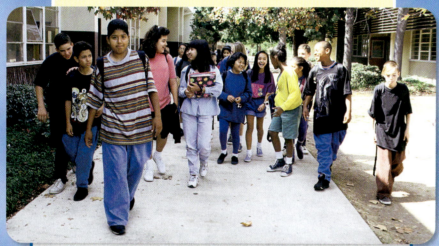

On Your Own

Derek's mother's health is getting worse. She needs to go to a cancer treatment center in another city, so the family moves there temporarily. Derek and his brother start attending school in the other city. Derek is having trouble fitting in at the new school. No one talks to him, and he is struggling with his schoolwork. Make a poster that shows how Derek could use the five steps of coping to cope with attending a new school.

Independent Practice: Check Yourself

Instruct students to repeat Act 1 without stopping at each step. Remind students to apply what they learned in the Guided Practice to the Independent Practice. Students do not have to use every step to cope successfully, nor do they have to follow steps 2–5 in order.

Encourage students to use the Check Yourself questions as a starting point for reviewing and analyzing their Independent Practice. Remind students that as they change roles, the answers to these questions may change for each actor. Encourage students to create additional questions for checking their coping skills. When students have finished the Independent Practice, have them answer the Check Yourself questions in writing. Use their answers to assess their understanding of the steps of coping and to assess their use of the steps to solve a problem.

Check Yourself Answers

1. Sample answer: Some emotions that Derek may be feeling include sadness, anger, and helplessness.
2. Sample answer: Derek can use positive self-talk to make himself feel better. A positive attitude will help him cope with his mother's illness.
3. Sample answer: Derek could talk to a school counselor or a teacher to receive support. He could also find a support group for relatives of cancer patients.
4. Sample answer: I coped with the death of my grandfather by thinking about the fun things that I used to do with him.

Act 2: On Your Own

This additional scenario gives students an opportunity to apply what they have learned in both the Guided Practice and the Independent Practice to a new situation.

Suggest to students that they use the Check Yourself questions as a starting point for coping in the new situation. Encourage students to be creative and to think of ways to improve their coping skills.

Assessment

Review the poster that students have created as part of the On Your Own activity. The posters should show that the students applied their coping skills in a realistic and effective manner. Display the posters around the room. If time permits, discuss some of the posters with the class.

Chapter 16 — Your Changing Body
Chapter Planning Guide

PACING	CLASSROOM RESOURCES	ACTIVITIES AND DEMONSTRATIONS
BLOCK 1 • 45 min pp. 346–349 **Chapter Opener**	CRF Health Inventory * ■ GENERAL CRF Parent Letter * ■	SE Health IQ, p. 347 CRF At-Home Activity * ■
Lesson 1 What Makes You You	CRF Lesson Plan * TT Bellringer *	TE Activities Travel Brochure of the Reproductive Systems, p. 345F TE Demonstration Tongue-Rolling Heredity, p. 348 GENERAL SE Hands-on Activity, p. 349 ♦ CRF Datasheets for In-Text Activities * GENERAL CRF Enrichment Activity * ADVANCED
BLOCK 2 • 45 min pp. 350–353 **Lesson 2** The Male Reproductive System	CRF Lesson Plan * TT Bellringer * TT The Male Reproductive System *	TE Group Activity Debate, p. 351 ♦ ADVANCED TE Group Activity Sexually Transmitted Diseases, p. 352 GENERAL CRF Life Skills Activity * ■ GENERAL CRF Enrichment Activity * ADVANCED
BLOCK 3 • 45 min pp. 354–359 **Lesson 3** The Female Reproductive System	CRF Lesson Plan * TT Bellringer * TT The Female Reproduction System * TT The Menstrual Cycle *	TE Activity Female Infertility, p. 356 ADVANCED CRF Enrichment Activity * ADVANCED
Lesson 4 The Endocrine System	CRF Lesson Plan * TT Bellringer *	TE Demonstration Surprise Quiz, p. 358 GENERAL CRF Enrichment Activity * ADVANCED
BLOCK 4 • 45 min pp. 360–363 **Lesson 5** Growing Up	CRF Lesson Plan * TT Bellringer * TT Pregnancy Timeline *	TE Activities Growth Scrapbook, p. 345F TE Activity Skit, p. 360 GENERAL TE Activity Trimester Fact Sheets, p. 361 ♦ GENERAL TE Group Activity Early Childhood Development, p. 362 ADVANCED TE Activity Practicing Wellness, p. 362 GENERAL SE Language Arts Activity, p. 363 CRF Enrichment Activity * ADVANCED
BLOCK 5 • 45 min pp. 364–367 **Lesson 6** Becoming an Adult	CRF Lesson Plan * TT Bellringer *	TE Activity Role-Playing, p. 364 GENERAL TE Demonstration Guest Speakers, p. 365 ♦ GENERAL TE Group Activity Course of Adulthood, p. 365 ADVANCED TE Demonstration Simulating Old Age, p. 366 ♦ BASIC SE Life Skills in Action Assessing Your Health, pp. 370–371 CRF Life Skills Activity * ■ GENERAL CRF Enrichment Activity * ADVANCED

BLOCKS 6 & 7 • 90 min Chapter Review and Assessment Resources

- SE Chapter Review, pp. 368–369
- CRF Concept Review * ■ GENERAL
- CRF Health Behavior Contract * ■ GENERAL
- CRF Chapter Test * ■ GENERAL
- CRF Performance-Based Assessment * GENERAL
- OSP Test Generator
- CRF Test Item Listing *

Online Resources

Visit go.hrw.com for a variety of free resources related to this textbook. Enter the keyword **HD4HR7**.

Students can access interactive problem solving help and active visual concept development with the *Decisions for Health* Online Edition available at **www.hrw.com**.

CNN student News
cnnstudentnews.com
Find the latest health news, lesson plans, and activities related to important scientific events.

Compression guide:
To shorten your instruction because of time limitations, omit Lessons 1 and 4.

KEY
- **TE** Teacher Edition
- **SE** Student Edition
- **OSP** One-Stop Planner
- **CRF** Chapter Resource File
- **TT** Teaching Transparency
- ***** Also on One-Stop Planner
- ■ Also Available in Spanish
- ♦ Requires Advance Prep

SKILLS DEVELOPMENT RESOURCES	LESSON REVIEW AND ASSESSMENT	STANDARDS CORRELATION
		National Health Education Standards
TE Inclusion Strategies, p. 348 BASIC **CRF** Cross-Disciplinary * GENERAL **CRF** Directed Reading * BASIC	**SE** Lesson Review, p. 349 **TE** Reteaching ♦, Quiz, p. 349 **CRF** Concept Mapping * GENERAL **CRF** Lesson Quiz * ■ GENERAL	
TE Reading Skill Builder Reading Hint, p. 351 BASIC **TE** Life Skill Builder Practicing Wellness, p. 352 GENERAL **SE** Life Skills Activity Assessing Your Health, p. 353 **CRF** Decision-Making * GENERAL **CRF** Directed Reading * BASIC	**SE** Lesson Review, p. 353 **TE** Reteaching ♦, Quiz, p. 353 **TE** Alternative Assessment, p. 353 GENERAL **CRF** Lesson Quiz * ■ GENERAL	1.1, 1.6, 1.7
CRF Decision-Making * GENERAL **CRF** Directed Reading * BASIC	**SE** Lesson Review, p. 357 **TE** Reteaching, Quiz, p. 357 **TE** Alternative Assessment, p. 357 GENERAL **CRF** Lesson Quiz * ■ GENERAL	1.1, 1.6, 1.7
SE Study Tip Organizing Information, p. 359 **TE** Reading Skill Builder Reading Organizer, p. 359 BASIC **CRF** Refusal Skills * GENERAL **CRF** Directed Reading * BASIC	**SE** Lesson Review, p. 359 **TE** Reteaching, Quiz, p. 359 **TE** Alternative Assessment, p. 359 ♦ GENERAL **CRF** Lesson Quiz * ■ GENERAL	1.3
TE Life Skill Builder Communicating Effectively, p. 361 GENERAL **CRF** Cross-Disciplinary * GENERAL **CRF** Directed Reading * BASIC	**SE** Lesson Review, p. 363 **TE** Reteaching, Quiz, p. 363 **TE** Alternative Assessment, p. 363 GENERAL **CRF** Concept Mapping * GENERAL **CRF** Lesson Quiz * ■ GENERAL	
SE Life Skills Activity Making Good Decisions, p. 365 **TE** Inclusion Strategies, p. 365 ♦ GENERAL **CRF** Refusal Skills * GENERAL **CRF** Directed Reading * BASIC	**SE** Lesson Review, p. 367 **TE** Reteaching ♦, Quiz, p. 367 **TE** Alternative Assessment, p. 367 GENERAL **CRF** Lesson Quiz * ■ GENERAL	1.2, 4.3

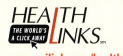

www.scilinks.org/health
Maintained by the **National Science Teachers Association**

Topic: Reproduction
HealthLinks code: HD4080

Topic: Growth and Development
HealthLinks code: HD4048

Topic: Pregnancy
HealthLinks code: HD4077

Technology Resources

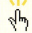 **One-Stop Planner**
All of your printable resources and the Test Generator are on this convenient CD-ROM.

 Guided Reading Audio CDs

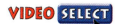
For information about videos related to this chapter, go to **go.hrw.com** and type in the keyword **HD4HR7V**.

Chapter 16 • Chapter Planning Guide **345B**

CHAPTER 16 — Your Changing Body
Chapter Resources

Teacher Resources

TEACHING TRANSPARENCIES

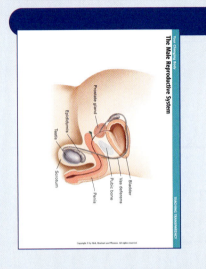
The Male Reproductive System

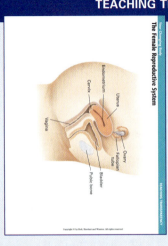
The Female Reproductive System

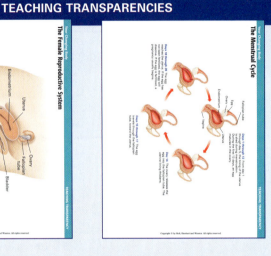
The Menstrual Cycle

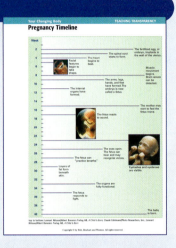
Pregnancy Timeline

LESSON PLANS
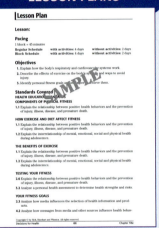

PARENT LETTER
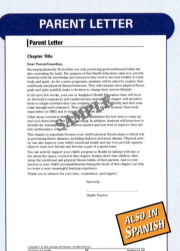
ALSO IN SPANISH

TEST ITEM LISTING
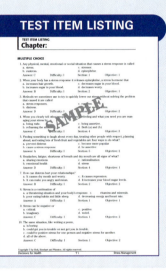

BELLRINGER TRANSPARENCIES
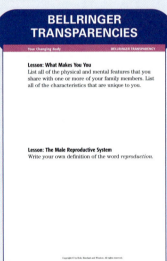

Meeting Individual Needs

DIRECTED READING
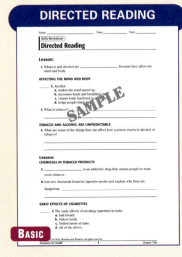
BASIC

CONCEPT MAPPING
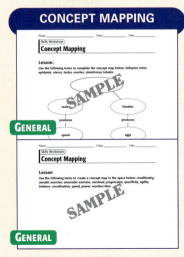
GENERAL

CONCEPT REVIEW
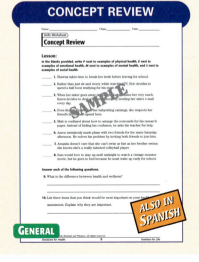
GENERAL · ALSO IN SPANISH

ENRICHMENT ACTIVITIES
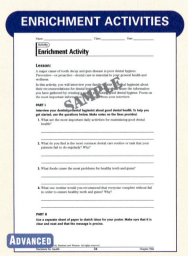
ADVANCED

345C Chapter 16 • Your Changing Body

Resources

These worksheet pages can be found in the Chapter Resource File and the One-Stop Planner. The transparencies can be found in the Teaching Transparencies binder and on the One-Stop Planner.

Activities

LIFE SKILLS ACTIVITIES
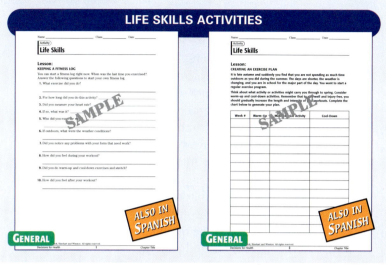

AT-HOME ACTIVITY
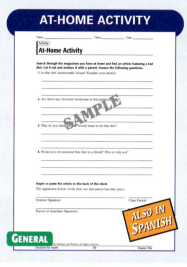

DATASHEETS FOR IN-TEXT ACTIVITIES
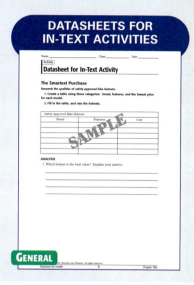

Applications

DECISION-MAKING
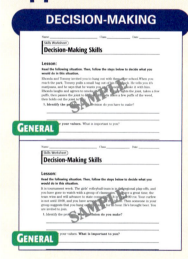

REFUSAL SKILLS
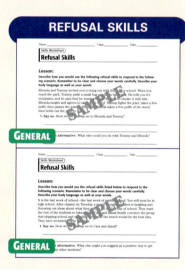

CROSS-DISCIPLINARY
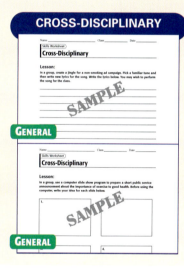

HEALTH BEHAVIOR CONTRACT
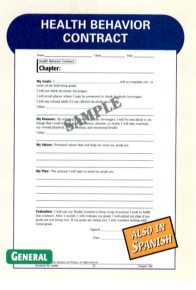

Assessments

HEALTH INVENTORY
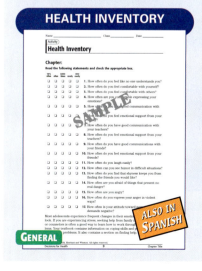

LESSON QUIZZES
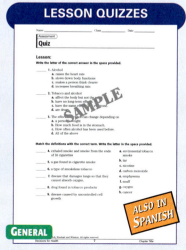

CHAPTER TEST
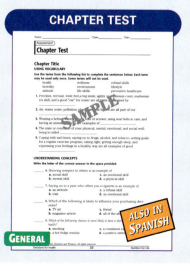

PERFORMANCE-BASED ASSESSMENT
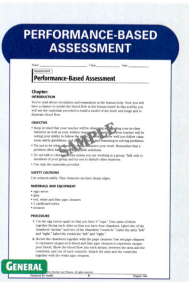

Chapter 16 • Chapter Resources and Worksheets 345D

CHAPTER 16 — Background Information

The following information focuses on facts about the male and female reproductive systems. This material will help prepare you for teaching the concepts in this chapter.

The Male Reproductive System

- For successful sperm production, testes must be kept at a lower temperature than the rest of the body. Muscles connected to the skin of the scrotum help regulate the testes' temperature. If the scrotum becomes too cold, these muscles contract and pull the testes closer to the body. However, if the scrotum becomes too hot, the muscles relax and allow the testes to hang farther from the body. The skin of the scrotum also contains many sweat glands to help cool the testes.

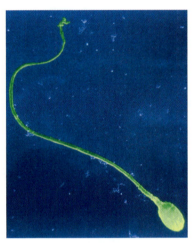

- About three percent of all full-term male babies are born with testes that have not descended. The testes will usually descend on their own before the child reaches the age of 1 year. Doctors will suggest surgery only if the child reaches age 2 or 3 and his testes still have not descended.

- During puberty, males start producing sperm. On average, a fully developed male reproductive system will produce over one billion sperm each day. Each sperm has a head that contains genetic material from the male. A membrane called the *acrosome*, which contains chemicals that will help the sperm penetrate the egg's outer membrane, covers the head. Behind the sperm's head is a midpiece that contains mitochondria. The mitochondria help provide the sperm with enough energy to swim. Powered by the mitochondria, the tail of the sperm moves back and forth to propel the sperm.

The Female Reproductive System

- Eggs start to develop within the female body long before a girl is born. Most females form approximately 2 million eggs before they are born, but by the time they are born, only around 700,000 eggs remain. Of the 700,000 eggs, only about 350,000 will still be viable once the reproductive system becomes fully developed during puberty. All of the surviving eggs are immature and will remain so until the girl reaches puberty. Despite the fact that the eggs are immature, they still age along with the girl. Some scientists believe that this aging is the reason that the risk of birth defects increases with the mother's age.

- The fallopian tubes have long finger-like projections that reach out over the ovaries but usually do not actually touch the ovaries. When an egg is released from the ovaries, it usually is drawn into the fallopian tube by currents created by the finger-like projections. Occasionally, the egg misses the fallopian tube and moves into the abdominal cavity, where it disintegrates.

- The inside of a fallopian tube is only about as thick as two human hairs. Many tiny hair-like structures inside the fallopian tubes propel the egg toward the uterus. The journey is only about 10 cm.

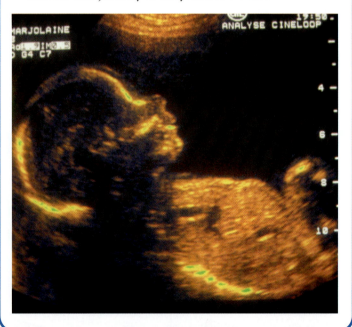

> For background information about teaching strategies and issues, refer to the *Professional Reference for Teachers.*

ACTIVITIES

CHAPTER 16

Consider using the activities on this page as students explore the lessons of this chapter. Look for other activities throughout the Student Edition chapter.

Travel Brochure of the Reproductive Systems

Procedure Organize students into small groups. Explain that each group belongs to a different "body travel agency." These travel agencies provide guided tours to all of the major body systems. The job of the group is to generate more business for their travel agency. The agencies have just started offering tours of the male and female reproductive systems and need attention-grabbing, high-quality advertisements for these new tours to attract more customers. Tell each group to choose one of the two reproductive systems and to create a brochure about it. The brochure should include maps, local sites, and possible dangers that the traveler should prepare for. Each group should split up into a writing team, an art team, and an editorial team. The three teams should work together to write and design the brochure. Students fluent in a language other than English should translate the brochures into their other language. When groups have finished their brochure, have them present their brochure to the class. Then, have the class vote on the best brochure (tell students that they are not allowed to vote for their own group).

Analysis After students have presented their brochures to the class, ask students to answer the following questions about the brochure they created:

- What information does your tour provide on the function of the reproductive system? (Answers may vary.)
- What are the most popular sites on the tour? (Answers may vary.)
- What are some of the possible dangers of the tour? (Answer will vary.)
- List three things you learned from the brochures of the other groups. (Answers may vary.)

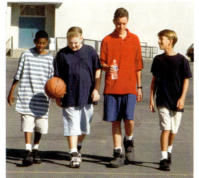

Growth Scrapbook

Procedure Ask students to collect pictures, letters, and other memorabilia from their life. With help from their parents or guardians, students should make copies of the memorabilia. Then, students should use the memorabilia to create a personal growth scrapbook. The scrapbook should contain information about their physical, social, and emotional development and accomplishments. Each entry should include a written description and an image that illustrates the development being discussed. Students may want to get a copy of their medical records to include statistics about their physical growth in the scrapbook. Suggest to students that they update their scrapbook throughout the rest of the semester.

Analysis Ask students the following questions when they have completed their scrapbooks:

- Describe how you have grown since birth. (Answers may vary.)
- How have you mentally and socially developed since you were a young child? (Answers may vary.)
- How have you grown this year? (Answers may vary.)
- How do you think you will develop in the future? (Answers may vary.)

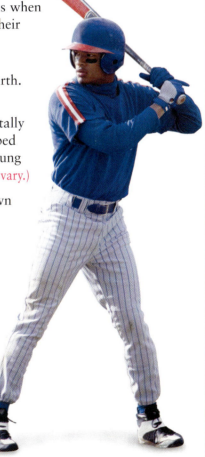

Chapter 16 • Activities 345F

CHAPTER 16

Overview
Tell students that this chapter describes heredity, the human reproductive systems, the endocrine system, and all of the stages of human development.

Assessing Prior Knowledge
Students should be familiar with the following topics:
- body systems
- hygiene and caring for the body
- infectious diseases

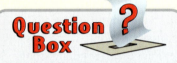

Students may feel more comfortable asking questions if you set up a Question Box to collect their questions. Have students write and anonymously submit their questions about human reproduction, growth, and development. Address these questions during class, or use these questions to introduce lessons that cover related topics.

Current Health

Check out *Current Health* articles and activities related to this chapter by visiting the HRW Web site at go.hrw.com. Just type in the keyword HD4CH31T.

Chapter Resource File
- Directed Reading BASIC
- Health Inventory GENERAL
- Parent Letter

CHAPTER 16 Your Changing Body

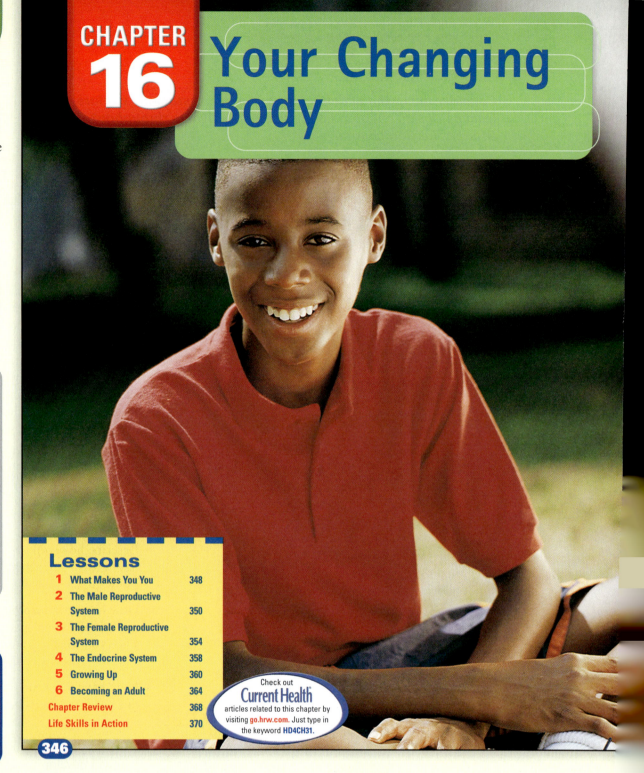

Lessons
1	What Makes You You	348
2	The Male Reproductive System	350
3	The Female Reproductive System	354
4	The Endocrine System	358
5	Growing Up	360
6	Becoming an Adult	364
	Chapter Review	368
	Life Skills in Action	370

Check out **Current Health** articles related to this chapter by visiting go.hrw.com. Just type in the keyword HD4CH31.

Standards Correlations

National Health Education Standards

1.1 (partial) Explain the relationship between positive health behaviors and the prevention of injury, illness, disease, and premature death. (Lessons 2–3)

1.2 Describe the interrelationship of mental, emotional, social, and physical health during adolescence. (Lesson 6)

1.3 Explain how health is influenced by the interaction of body systems. (Lesson 4)

1.6 Describe ways to reduce risks related to adolescent health problems. (Lessons 2–3)

1.7 (partial) Explain how appropriate health care can prevent premature death and disability. (Lessons 2–3)

> "So much has **changed** since last year. I look **different,** all of my classes are different, and I'm in a **new school.**
>
> I also have a lot of new responsibilities. This year, we get to join school sports teams. I'm really excited about joining the track team."

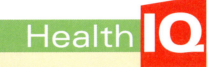

PRE-READING

Answer the following multiple-choice questions to find out what you already know about reproduction and development. When you've finished this chapter, you'll have the opportunity to change your answers based on what you've learned.

1. You may look like your brother or sister because
   a. you live in the same house.
   b. you share some of the same genes.
   c. you have the same last name.
   d. All of the above

2. How long does a human pregnancy last?
   a. 9 weeks
   b. 20 weeks
   c. 31 weeks
   d. 40 weeks

3. Which of the following substances can be harmful to the fetus if the mother uses the substance while she is pregnant?
   a. alcohol
   b. tobacco
   c. illegal drugs
   d. all of the above

4. Puberty is part of
   a. early childhood.
   b. adolescence.
   c. the menstrual cycle.
   d. adulthood.

5. Which of the following is a condition associated with aging?
   a. Alzheimer's disease
   b. endometriosis
   c. inguinal hernia
   d. all of the above

6. Which of the following is NOT a stage of grief?
   a. denial
   b. acceptance
   c. fear
   d. bargaining

7. Which of the following body systems helps control growth and development?
   a. skeletal system
   b. respiratory system
   c. endocrine system
   d. circulatory system

ANSWERS: 1. b; 2. d; 3. d; 4. b; 5. a; 6. c; 7. c

Using the Health IQ

Misconception Alert Answers to the Health IQ questions may help you identify students' misconceptions.

Question 3: Many students may not realize how dependent a fetus is on its mother's health habits. Explain to students that almost everything the mother eats, drinks, or breathes will be passed to the fetus. For this reason, even doctors must be very careful when deciding what medicines to prescribe to pregnant women.

Question 5: Students may think that most diseases are associated with old age. Tell students that diseases and disorders affect people of all ages. However, Alzheimer's disease is a disease that is typically associated only with people over the age of 65. In some rare cases, young adults have suffered from early onset Alzheimer's disease.

Question 6: Students may think that people who are grieving for a dead loved one are also dealing with their fear of death. Although many people fear dying, they generally do not face this fear as they are dealing with the loss of a loved one.

Answers
1. b
2. d
3. d
4. b
5. a
6. c
7. c

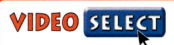

For information about videos related to this chapter, go to **go.hrw.com** and type in the keyword **HD4HR7V**.

Chapter 16 • Your Changing Body

Lesson 1 Focus

Overview
Before beginning this lesson, review with your students the objectives listed under the What You'll Do head in the Student Edition. In this lesson, students learn about how heredity and environment affect a person's development.

Bellringer
Ask students to list all of the physical and mental features that they share with one or more of their family members. Then, they should list all of the characteristics that are unique to them. Give adopted children the option to list their characteristics without comparing them. **LS Visual**

Answer to Start Off Write
Accept all reasonable answers. Sample answer: How you look is affected by where you live, the foods you eat, and how much exercise you get, all of which are part of your environment.

Motivate

Demonstration — GENERAL
Tongue-Rolling Heredity Have students determine whether they can roll their tongue. Inform them that this characteristic is a dominant trait that can be inherited. Have students find out which members of their immediate family can roll their tongues. Then, have students create a chart showing which family members can roll their tongue and which cannot. **LS Kinesthetic/Visual** **English Language Learners**

Lesson 1

What You'll Do
- **Explain** where your genes come from.
- **Describe** how your growth and development are affected by both heredity and environment.

Terms to Learn
- genes
- heredity
- sex cell
- environment

Start Off Write
How does your environment affect how you look?

What Makes You You

Jenny is going to the same school that her older brother, Sam, went to. The teachers always say things like "You must be Sam's sister" or "You look just like your brother Sam."

Have you ever wondered why some people look like a parent or a brother or a sister and why some people don't? What caused Sam and Jenny to look alike? The answer is in their genes (JEENZ).

From Two to You

The cells of every person carry a set of instructions called **genes** that describe how that person will look and grow. These instructions are passed from parents to children. The passing of traits from parents to children is called **heredity** (huh RED i tee). Each parent donates one-half of a set of instructions to the child through sexual reproduction. In sexual reproduction, a sex cell from the mother and a sex cell from the father join to form a new cell that has a full set of instructions for forming a new person. Over 9 months, this cell will develop into a baby. A **sex cell** is a cell that contains half of the genes of the parent. Because each parent's cell has one-half of the complete set of genes, a child will have some genes from the father and some genes from the mother. You may look like your parents or like your brother or sister because you share some of the same genes.

Your physical appearance isn't all you get from your parents. You also may have inherited some personality traits and some mental characteristics. But you are not only a sum of your genes. Other factors affect your development, too.

Figure 1 Your father's genes + your mother's genes = you

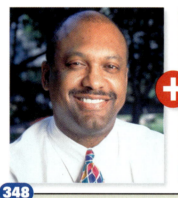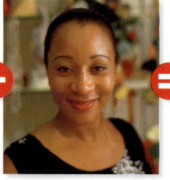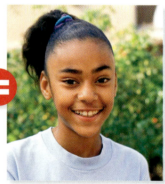

INCLUSION Strategies — BASIC
- Learning Disabled
- Attention Deficit Disorder
- Behavior Control Issues

Many students can better understand information when they can organize it and make it personal. Have students work in pairs to create Venn Diagrams to compare and contrast features of their environments. Tell students to consider components such as where they live, their parents' careers, whether they have siblings, what classes they are taking, what their hobbies are, and what their responsibilities are at home and in the community. **LS Visual**

Chapter Resource File
- Directed Reading BASIC
- Lesson Plan
- Datasheets for In-Text Activities GENERAL
- Lesson Quiz GENERAL

Transparencies
TT Bellringer

348 Chapter 16 • Your Changing Body

Why You Are Unique

Your growth and development are also influenced by your environment. Your **environment** is your surroundings, including people and places. Many factors affect your environment, including where you live and what your parents do. Your habits and personality are influenced by both people and opportunities. Education, nutritious foods, and a safe place to live all affect how you grow, think, and act. For example, if you live in a colder climate, you will probably dress differently than someone who lives in a warmer climate does. You may also enjoy activities associated with cold weather, such as hockey or ice skating.

No one knows exactly how much your heredity determines who you are and how much your environment does. But you are not a product of only one influence. By making good decisions, planning well, and working both smart and hard, you can have a happy and healthy life.

Hands-on ACTIVITY

THE EYES HAVE IT

1. Create a "family tree" of your immediate family and as much of your extended family as you can. Show the eye color of each family member.
2. Trace the trait of eye color from one generation to the next.

Analysis
1. What patterns do you see?

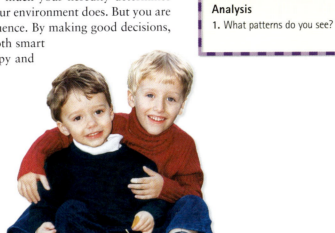

Figure 2 You and your brother or sister may look different because you inherited different genes from the same parents.

Lesson Review

Using Vocabulary
1. What are sex cells?
2. What is the difference between genes and heredity?

Understanding Concepts
3. Is your appearance determined by heredity, or is it determined by your environment?

Critical Thinking
4. **Identifying Relationships** How might nutrition affect your physical appearance?
5. **Analyzing Ideas** Which influence—heredity or environment—do you think is more important in shaping a person's appearance? in shaping a person's personality? Explain your answer.

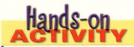

internet connect
www.scilinks.org/health
Topic: Reproduction
HealthLinks code: HD4080
HEALTH LINKS. Maintained by the National Science Teachers Association

Answers to Lesson Review

1. A sex cell is a cell that contains half the genes of the parent and that combines with another sex cell during reproduction.
2. Genes are the set of instructions in the cell that describes the person's traits. The passing of traits from parents to their children is called *heredity*.
3. Many physical traits, such as height and body shape, are determined by heredity, but these traits are also influenced by your environment.
4. Sample answer: Nutrition can affect how healthy your skin and hair are, how well your bones grow, and your overall body shape.
5. Answers may vary. Sample answer: I think heredity is more influential in shaping a person's appearance, because some traits cannot be changed by the environment. I think a person's personality is more influenced by his or her environment, because many people like things that their parent's don't like.

Teach

Sensitivity ALERT

Students who are adopted, have a family member suffering from a genetic disease, or are suffering from some sort of familial difficulty may be uncomfortable discussing genes and heredity. Make sure students realize that genes alone do not determine all of a person's characteristics—the environment is also very important in a person's development.

Hands-on ACTIVITY

Answer
Answers may vary.

Close

Reteaching — BASIC

Advice Letter Write the following letter on the board or overhead, and ask students to write a response:

Dear Doctor,

I have a twin brother. We are alike in so many ways. We have the same eyes, nose, and hair color. Plus, our voices sound almost exactly the same! However, we are interested in completely different things and excel at different subjects at school. How can we be so similar and so different at the same time?

Anonymous
LS Interpersonal/Verbal

Quiz — GENERAL

1. What two factors affect your characteristics? (heredity and environment)
2. Can a single human sex cell develop into a baby? Why or why not? (No, a sex cell only has half the total number of human genes. Two sex cells must combine to develop into a baby.)

Lesson 1 • What Makes You You   349

Lesson 2

Focus

Overview
Before beginning this lesson, review with your students the objectives listed under the What You'll Do head in the Student Edition. This lesson explains how the male reproductive system works, how sperm are made, and how to care for the male reproductive system.

Bellringer
Have students write their own definition of the word *reproduction*. (Students should include in their definition the idea of producing a copy of something, such as a copy of the parents.) Encourage students who are fluent in a language other than English to write a definition of the word *reproduction* in their native language. **LS Verbal** — English Language Learners

Answer to Start Off Write
Accept all reasonable answers. Sample answer: Males can protect their reproductive health by performing regular self-examinations and visiting a doctor regularly.

Motivate

Discussion — GENERAL
Body Systems Ask students to list some facts that they may already know about the male reproductive system. If students are embarrassed to talk about the topic, explain to students that, just like their other organ systems, it is important for them to learn about their reproductive system so that they know how to keep it in good health. **LS Verbal**

Lesson 2 — The Male Reproductive System

What You'll Do
- **Identify** the parts of the male reproductive system.
- **Describe** how sperm are made.
- **List** seven problems of the male reproductive system.
- **Explain** four ways to protect your reproductive system.

Terms to Learn
- sperm
- testes

Start Off Write
Describe one way that males can protect their reproductive health.

The father provides a sex cell that contains half the blueprint for forming a new person. Where in the man's body does this cell form?

In sexual reproduction, the man provides the sex cell called a **sperm**. Sperm is made in organs called **testes** (TES TEEZ). The testes (singular, *testis*), also called *testicles*, also make most of the man's primary sex hormone, *testosterone* (tes TAHS tuhr OHN).

The Male Anatomy
Figure 3 shows the organs of the male reproductive system. Some of these organs are outside the body, and some are inside the body. The outside organs are the penis and scrotum. The scrotum is a sack of skin that holds the two testes and the two epididymises. The reproductive organs inside a man's body are the vas deferens, the prostate gland, the seminal vesicles, the Cowper's glands, and the urethra.

Figure 3 The Male Reproductive System

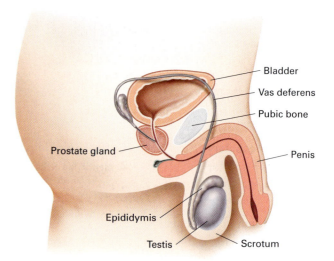

SOCIAL STUDIES CONNECTION
Homunculi or Genes? In medieval Europe, most doctors thought of sperm as being the seed for a baby and the woman's uterus as being similar to the soil that a seed must be planted in to grow. In the 1600s, many medical textbooks showed sperm as being a small sac with a tiny human inside. The tiny human was called a *homunculus*. This theory was not refuted until the 1800s, when scientists discovered that sperm contained cellular material, just like all the other cells in the body.

Chapter Resource File
- Directed Reading **BASIC**
- Lesson Plan
- Lesson Quiz **GENERAL**

Transparencies

TT Bellringer
TT The Male Reproductive System

350   Chapter 16 • Your Changing Body

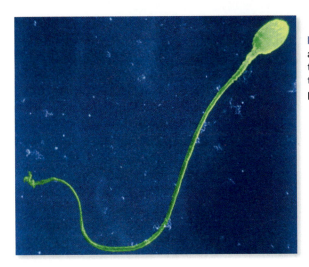

Figure 4 Sperm have a head and a tail. The head carries the genes of the father. The tail's swimming motion propels the sperm.

The Production of Sperm

Sperm are made in tightly coiled tubes inside the testes. The cells in these tubes make copies of their genes and then divide to make more cells. The new cells that form have one-half of the original number of genes. The sperm cells will carry the genes of the father into the mother's body, where the mother's sex cell, called an *egg*, can join with the sperm. But when they leave the testes, the sperm are immature and are not able to combine with a female egg. After about 70 days in the testes, the sperm pass to the epididymis.

Each testis continually releases immature sperm cells into an epididymis. In each epididymis, sperm mature and grow the tails that allow them to swim. Sperm's ability to swim is necessary for them to be able to reach an egg. When the sperm are fully grown, they move into the tubes called the *vas deferens*, each of which is attached to an epididymis. The vas deferens run from each epididymis out of the scrotum. Then, they widen to form a storage area for sperm located just above the prostate gland. Sperm pass through the prostate gland and past the Cowper's glands on their way from the storage area to the urethra. Those glands make a fluid that mixes with the sperm to form a fluid called *semen*. The semen passes to the outside of the body through the urethra, which is a tube that runs through the penis. After 2 weeks in the man's body, the sperm are broken down and reabsorbed by the body.

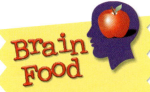

Brain Food

Sperm are kept 4°F (1°C to 2°C) cooler than the rest of the body. The temperature of the testes is controlled by a muscle that moves the scrotum closer to or farther from the body.

Attention Grabber

Seminiferous Tubules The tightly coiled tubes that sperm are made in are called the *seminiferous tubules*. These tubules account for 80 percent of the mass of each testis. If these tubules were uncoiled and placed end-to-end, they would stretch over 800 m, or about one-half mile, in length!

Teach

READING SKILL BUILDER — BASIC

Reading Hint Tell students that understanding this section requires students not only to read the text but also to study the accompanying figures. Tell students that the illustrations and captions will help them visualize and better understand the male reproductive system. **LS** Visual

Using the Figure — BASIC

Sperm Direct students' attention to the photo of the healthy sperm. Tell students that the average adult human male produces several hundred million sperm each day. Have students identify which part of the sperm they think carries the father's genes. (the head) **LS** Visual

Group Activity — ADVANCED

Debate Organize the class into several teams. Tell students the following information: A 40 percent decline in the average sperm count of men has been documented over the last 40 years. Some researchers blame environmental toxins, such as drugs, lead, and pesticides, for the decline in male fertility. Others claim that men who wear tight pants may decrease sperm production because the pants hold the testes too close to the body; the resultant increase in temperature causes sperm to die.

Have each team research a different possible cause for the decline in male fertility. Then, have teams provide an oral report to the class that describes the possible cause and explains how the risk posed by this factor can be reduced. **LS** Verbal

Lesson 2 • The Male Reproductive System

Teach, continued

Group Activity —— GENERAL

Sexually Transmitted Diseases Have students work in small groups to research sexually transmitted diseases that affect the male reproductive system. Students should focus on the incidence of the disease, risk factors, and methods of early detection. Have students use the information they gather to write a public-service brochure, complete with artwork, designed to educate the public about the diseases. It should emphasize the importance of prevention, early detection, and treatment. Encourage students who are fluent in a language other than English to translate their brochure into their native language. Allow time for students to view the brochures of other groups. **English Language Learners**
LS Visual

Life SKILL BUILDER —— GENERAL

Practicing Wellness In 1996, 25-year-old world-class cyclist Lance Armstrong was diagnosed with testicular cancer. Armstrong said that although he had annual physical exams and blood tests, his testicles were never examined. By the time of his diagnosis, the cancer had spread to his lymph nodes, lungs, and brain. Ask students how a routine monthly testicular examination might have affected Armstrong's health. (Routine self-examinations could have helped Armstrong identify and treat the cancer before it was able to spread.) Then, have students talk to their parent, guardian, or doctor about performing self-examinations.
LS Logical

Problems of the Male Reproductive System

Most men may not think about the possibility that something could go wrong with their reproductive system. As a result, boys and men often do not think of having checkups by a doctor unless they must do so for school or sports. But regular medical checkups can protect men's health in many ways. For example, during regular medical checkups, a doctor can identify potential problems and treat the problems before they get worse or cause permanent damage.

Some problems with the male reproductive system may produce a bump, a sore, or pain or discomfort in the testes or scrotum. Any bumps, pain, or uncomfortable rashes or sores require immediate medical attention. Other problems may have no visible symptoms. Table 1 describes some problems of the male reproductive system.

TABLE 1 Problems of the Male Reproductive System

Problem	Description	Treatment or prevention
Jock itch	an infection of the skin by a fungus; often happens when scrotum and groin skin stays hot and moist; symptoms are red, itchy, irritated skin	treated with medicated creams or ointments; prevented by keeping the area clean and dry
Sexually transmitted diseases (STDs)	diseases passed by sexual contact that involves the sex organs, the mouth, or the rectum; symptoms may include sores or discharge, but many STDs have no symptoms	medical treatment required; prevented by abstaining from sexual activity
Inguinal (ING gwi nuhl) hernia	a weakness in the lower abdominal wall that allows a small loop of the intestines to bulge through; causes a soft bulging area on the lower abdomen, just above where the legs join the body; may or may not be painful	medical treatment required; often surgery is required to repair a hernia
Trauma (injury)	injury to the scrotum or testicles; usually happens during athletic events, accidents, or falling on an object	treated by resting and by applying ice packs; requires medical care if swelling is massive or pain persists; prevented by wearing a protective cup
Urinary tract infections (UTIs)	infections in the urethra and bladder that cause frequency of and burning during urination, may cause urine to be bloody; relatively rare for men	medical care required; treated with antibiotics
Testicular cancer	uncontrolled growth of cells of the testes; usually does not cause pain; usually found as an enlargement of the testis or as a pea-sized lump on the testis	medical care, including surgery and chemotherapy, required; easily treatable when found early; detected by regular testicular exams
Testicular torsion	twisting of the testis around on the nerves and blood vessels attached to it; usually happens during athletic activity; produces swelling and pain	immediate medical care required

352

Attention Grabber

Testicular Cancer Male students may think that they don't have to worry about testicular cancer while they are young. Tell students that in the United States, testicular cancer accounts for only 1 percent of all cancers in males. However, testicular cancer is the most common abnormal growth in white males aged 15 to 34 years. Most deaths from testicular cancer occur among young adult men.

Staying Healthy

Some medical problems can damage your body for the rest of your life. Some tips for staying healthy are listed below.

- Bathe every day. Don't wear damp or tight clothing longer than you have to.
- Always wear protective gear when playing sports.
- Do regular testicular self-exams. Ask your doctor how to do these exams. See a doctor about any unusual pain, swelling, or tenderness or any unusual lumps or growths.
- To prevent STDs, do not have sex before marriage.

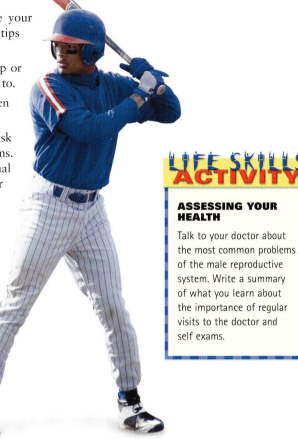

Figure 5 Wearing protective gear, such as a cup, when playing sports can help protect your reproductive system.

LIFE SKILLS ACTIVITY

ASSESSING YOUR HEALTH

Talk to your doctor about the most common problems of the male reproductive system. Write a summary of what you learn about the importance of regular visits to the doctor and self exams.

Lesson Review

Using Vocabulary
1. Name the male sex cell. Briefly describe how the cell is made.

Understanding Concepts
2. Which organs of the male reproductive system are outside the body? Which are inside the body?
3. List three problems of the male reproductive system, and describe how to prevent them.

Critical Thinking
4. **Identifying Relationships** How does wearing protective gear when playing sports help protect the male reproductive system?
5. **Analyzing Ideas** Why is it important that sperm cells contain only one-half of the man's genes?

Answers to Lesson Review

1. Sperm is the male sex cell. Cells in the testes make copies of themselves, then divide to make cells that have one-half of the original number of genes. These new cells mature into sperm.
2. The penis and scrotum are outside the body. The epididymis, vas deferens, prostate gland, Cowper's gland, seminal vesicles, and the urethra are inside the body.
3. Answers may vary. Sample answer: jock itch, keep the skin clean and dry; sexually transmitted diseases, abstain from sex before marriage; testicular cancer, perform regular self-examinations and go to the doctor regularly
4. Sample answer: Wearing protective gear when playing sports prevents trauma (injury) to the penis and testes. Preventing injury to these organs helps keep them working properly.
5. Sperm contain only one-half of the man's genes so that when the sperm combines with an egg that contains one-half of the mother's genes, a new cell with a complete set of genes is formed.

Teach, continued

LIFE SKILLS ACTIVITY

Extension: Testicular cancer is most frequently detected by men during self-examinations. Use this information to support your answer to this activity.
Answer
Answers may vary.

Close

Reteaching — BASIC

Quiz Cards Have each student write five questions about the male reproductive system on separate index cards. Collect all of the cards. Organize the class into two teams and give half the cards to each team. Have teams take turns asking each other questions. Then, have teams trade cards and repeat the activity. **LS Verbal**

Quiz — GENERAL

1. What is the scrotum? (the skin sac that hangs below the body and holds the testes)
2. List four ways to maintain the health of the male reproductive system (Bathe every day. Wear protective gear when playing sports. Do regular self-exams. Don't have sex before marriage.)
3. Name two glands of the male reproductive system. (prostate gland and Cowper's gland)

Alternative Assessment — GENERAL

Summarizing Table Have students design a table in which they list the major structures and functions of the male reproductive system. Have students include a column about the problems that affect each organ and possible ways to prevent the problems.
LS Visual

Lesson 2 • The Male Reproductive System

Lesson 3 Focus

Overview
Before beginning this lesson, review with your students the objectives listed under the What You'll Do head in the Student Edition. This lesson explains how the female reproductive system works, what the menstrual cycle is, and how to care for the female reproductive system.

🔔 Bellringer
Ask students to describe a cycle they have seen or learned about that takes place in nature. (Answers may vary. Accept all reasonable answers. Some possible natural cycles include the water cycle, the cycle of seasons, and the rock cycle.)
LS Visual

Answer to Start Off Write
Accept all reasonable answers. Sample answer: The menstrual cycle is the monthly cycle in which a mature egg is released from the ovary and the lining of the uterus is shed if a pregnancy does not begin.

Motivate

Discussion — GENERAL
Reproduction Lead a discussion about the similarities and differences among the ways that animals reproduce. For example, birds and ants lay eggs, but humans and sea stars don't. Females and males mate to reproduce in humans and birds, but not in sea stars. Help students understand that the end result of reproduction is the same for all animal species, but the means differ widely. **LS** Logical

Lesson 3

What You'll Do
- **Identify** the parts of the female reproductive system.
- **Describe** the typical menstrual cycle.
- **List** seven problems of the female reproductive system.
- **Explain** five ways to protect the female reproductive system.

Terms to Learn
- egg (ovum)
- ovulation
- menstruation

Write
What is the menstrual cycle?

Lesson 3
The Female Reproductive System

```
The father supplies the sex cell known
as sperm. Which sex cell does the mother
provide? Where in the woman's body does
this cell form?
```

In sexual reproduction, the woman provides the sex cell called the **egg,** or **ovum.** Women are born with all the eggs they will ever have; they do not make more. The eggs are stored in organs called *ovaries*. The ovaries make most of the woman's primary sex hormone, *estrogen* (ES truh juhn).

The Female Anatomy

Figure 6 shows the female reproductive system. A fallopian (fuh LOH pee uhn) tube runs between each ovary and the uterus. The fallopian tube does not actually connect to the ovary. The egg is drawn into the fallopian tube by sweeping movements of the ends of the fallopian tubes. The egg then travels through the tube to the uterus. The uterus is a muscular organ that holds a fetus during pregnancy. The uterus meets the vagina at the cervix. The vagina is the muscular organ that connects the outside of the body with the uterus. A woman's breasts are also a part of her reproductive system.

Figure 6 The Female Reproductive System

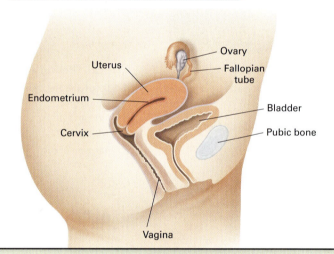

Background
Hymen The hymen is a thick fold of mucous membrane that partly or almost completely covers the vaginal opening. Traditionally, a ruptured hymen was considered a sign that a female had had sexual intercourse. However, hymens vary in thickness, and the hymen can be broken during vigorous physical activity, such as playing sports.

Chapter Resource File
- Directed Reading **BASIC**
- Lesson Plan
- Lesson Quiz **GENERAL**

Transparencies
TT Bellringer
TT The Female Reproductive System
TT The Menstrual Cycle

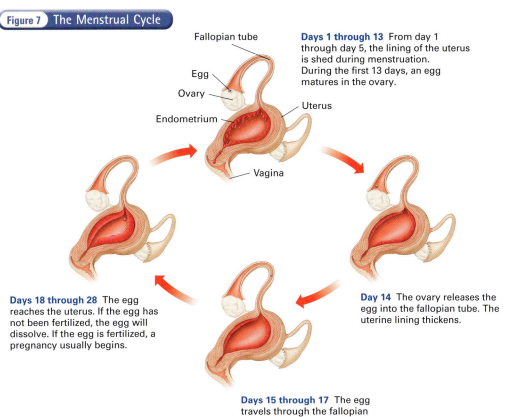

Figure 7 The Menstrual Cycle

Days 1 through 13 From day 1 through day 5, the lining of the uterus is shed during menstruation. During the first 13 days, an egg matures in the ovary.

Day 14 The ovary releases the egg into the fallopian tube. The uterine lining thickens.

Days 15 through 17 The egg travels through the fallopian tube, toward the uterus.

Days 18 through 28 The egg reaches the uterus. If the egg has not been fertilized, the egg will dissolve. If the egg is fertilized, a pregnancy usually begins.

The Menstrual Cycle

Every month, one of the ovaries releases a mature egg in a process called **ovulation** (AHV yoo LAY shuhn). During this time, the lining of the uterus thickens to prepare for a possible pregnancy. The uterine lining is called the *endometrium* (EN doh MEE tree uhm). If the egg is fertilized by a sperm cell in the fallopian tube, the fertilized egg will attach to the wall of the uterus and a pregnancy will begin. If the egg is not fertilized, the lining of the uterus will be shed. When the lining is shed, blood and tissue leave the body through the vagina. The monthly breakdown and shedding of the endometrium is called **menstruation** (MEN STRAY shuhn), or the menstrual period.

Ovulation and menstruation usually happen in a cycle, called the *menstrual cycle*, that lasts roughly 28 days. The typical menstrual cycle is shown in Figure 7. Girls often have their first menstrual period between the ages of 9 and 16.

Myth & Fact

Myth: Women always ovulate on the 14th day of the menstrual cycle.

Fact: The timing of ovulation can be irregular for every woman. Ovulation can happen at unusual times without a woman knowing it. However, ovulation generally happens toward the middle of the cycle.

Career

Gynecologists Physicians who have successfully completed specialized education and training in the health of the female reproductive system, including the diagnosis and treatment of disorders and diseases, are called *gynecologists*. An obstetrician/gynecologist, or ob/gyn, is a physician who provides medical and surgical care to women and has particular expertise in pregnancy, childbirth, and disorders of the reproductive system. This specialty includes knowledge of preventive care, prenatal care, detection of sexually transmitted diseases, Pap test screening, and family planning.

Lesson 3 • The Female Reproductive System

Teach, continued

Activity — ADVANCED

Female Infertility Tell students that blocked fallopian tubes and failure to ovulate are the two leading causes of female infertility. Have interested students research the underlying causes and the treatments for these two conditions. After students complete their research, they should form pairs and write informative pamphlets that explain to women the causes of infertility and what treatments are available. Students who are fluent in a language other than English should translate their pamphlet into their native language. Collect all the pamphlets and display them in the classroom. **English Language Learners**
LS Kinesthetic

Using the Figure — GENERAL

Reproductive Problems Draw students' attention to the table about female reproductive problems. Have students discuss ways to prevent and treat each of the listed diseases and disorders. Emphasize that not all of the listed maladies are preventable or 100 percent curable. Then have students make a list of things that women could do to protect themselves from having problems with their reproductive systems. **LS Visual**

Problems of the Female Reproductive System

Most healthy young women do not have any significant problems with their reproductive system. But the changes in the female reproductive system can cause young women a great deal of stress. Many of the health concerns of young women are related to the menstrual cycle and menstruation. Girls normally have irregular periods for the first few years after starting menstruation. Irregular periods vary in length and heaviness. Periods can come as often as every 3 weeks or as infrequently as every 6 weeks. Bleeding can last for only 1 day or for as long as 8 days. Both light and heavy bleeding are normal. Abdominal cramps that come with periods are also normal, unless the cramping is extremely severe.

Some female reproductive health problems are listed in Table 2. All of the problems listed in the table require medical care.

TABLE 2 Female Reproductive Problems

Problem	Description	Treatment or prevention
Urinary tract infections (UTIs)	infection of the urinary bladder, urethra, or kidneys that causes frequency of and burning during urination; may cause bloody urine	medical care required; usually treated with antibiotics and plenty of fluids
Vaginitis (VAJ uh NIET is)	infection of the vagina that causes itching, odor, and/or discharge from the vagina; caused by bacteria, fungi, or protozoans; sometimes called a *yeast infection*	medical care required; usually can be treated with antibiotics; may be prevented by keeping the area clean and dry and by not wearing damp clothes longer than is necessary
Endometriosis (EN doh MEE tree OH sis)	growth of tissue like that of the endometrium outside the uterus and inside a woman's body; during the menstrual period, bleeding inside the woman's body causes pain; may lead to infertility	medical care for severe cramps with periods may be required; treated with hormones and/or surgery
Sexually transmitted diseases (STDs)	diseases passed by sexual contact that involves the sex organs, the mouth, or the rectum; symptoms may include sores or discharge, but many STDs have no symptoms	medical treatment required; prevented by abstaining from sexual activity
Toxic shock syndrome	an infection by bacteria; most common in women who use tampons during menstruation; causes fever, chills, weakness, a rash, and many other symptoms	emergency medical care required; treated with hospitalization and antibiotics; may be prevented by changing tampons every 4 to 6 hours
Cervical, uterine, or ovarian cancer	uncontrolled growth of cells of the cervix, uterus, or ovaries; usually does not cause pain; is usually found by doctors during annual Pap smear tests and physical examinations	detected by annual pelvic exams and Pap-smear tests by a doctor; may be prevented by avoiding sexual activity to avoid contracting STDs that may increase the chance of cancer
Breast cancer	uncontrolled growth of cells of the breast; usually does not cause pain	can be detected during monthly self-examinations; your doctor can explain how to do these exams

Background

Ovarian Cysts Ovarian cysts often develop where a follicle has enlarged but has failed to break open and release an egg. Many are harmless and go away by themselves. Large cysts can cause pain, abdominal swelling, or even abnormal menstruation. In these cases, surgery may be required to remove the cysts from the ovary. Some studies indicate that obesity may be linked to having many cysts on the ovaries (polycystic ovary syndrome, or PCOS). PCOS is also associated with an inability to conceive.

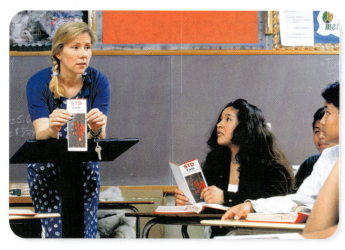

Figure 8 Learning about your reproductive health can help you make good decisions.

Staying Healthy

Some medical problems can damage your body for the rest of your life. Some tips for staying healthy are listed below.

- Bathe every day. Do not wear damp or tight clothing longer than is necessary.
- If you have questions about your health, talk to a parent or another trusted adult. See a doctor if necessary.
- Start going to a doctor for annual exams at age 18.
- Maintain good hygiene during menstrual periods. Bathe every day, and change sanitary pads or tampons every 4 to 6 hours.
- To protect yourself from STDs, do not have sex before marriage.

teen talk

Teen: I hear a lot about doing breast self-examinations and getting tested for cancer. How often should these tests be done?

Expert: Being tested regularly for different cancers of your reproductive system is very important. You can do breast self-examinations once a month. Once you reach age 18, you should start getting annual pelvic examinations and Pap tests. Ask your doctor for more information about these exams.

Lesson Review

Using Vocabulary

1. What is the female sex cell?
2. Describe the menstrual cycle.

Understanding Concepts

3. List the parts of the female reproductive system.
4. List six problems of the female reproductive system.
5. Describe five ways a woman can protect her reproductive health.

Critical Thinking

6. **Analyzing Ideas** Why do you think the endometrium is shed every month if a pregnancy does not begin?

Lesson 4 Focus

Overview
Before beginning this lesson, review with your students the objectives listed under the What You'll Do head in the Student Edition. In this lesson, students will learn about how hormones affect human development.

Bellringer
Write the following activity on the board or overhead projector:

Use your textbook to unscramble the following words.

nalgd (gland)

meornoh (hormone)

npoleevedmt (development)

LS Verbal

Answer to Start Off Write
Accept all reasonable answers. Sample answer: The endocrine system makes and releases hormones that control growth and development.

Motivate

Demonstration — GENERAL

Surprise Quiz Once students have been seated, tell them that you have decided to give a surprise quiz on what was covered in the last class. After they prepare to take the quiz, ask them to describe how their body reacted when they learned about the quiz. (increased heart rate, sweaty palms, heightened state of alert, etc.) Explain to students that they just had a stress reaction. All of the changes in their bodies were caused by a release of hormones into the bloodstream. Tell students that you will actually not be giving a quiz. **LS Kinesthetic**

Lesson 4 — The Endocrine System

Keeshawn grew 6 inches last year. His body is changing so quickly that his mom teases him about having to buy new clothes every month.

What You'll Do
- **Summarize** the role of hormones in growth and development.

Terms to Learn
- endocrine system
- gland
- hormone

Start Off Write
How does the endocrine system affect growth and development?

Keeshawn is growing so quickly because of his endocrine (EN doh KRIN) system. The **endocrine system** is a group of glands that release special chemicals that control much of how your body functions. A **gland** is a group of cells that make these chemicals for your body. The endocrine system is shown in Figure 9.

What Are Hormones?
Each gland produces its own specific type of hormone. **Hormones** are chemicals produced by the endocrine glands that travel through the bloodstream and cause changes in different parts of the body. Hormones regulate the growth and activity of the organs of your body. Hormones are responsible for how your body grows and changes. How you react to stress is also related to the release of hormones. The actions of hormones in the body are amazing: hormones are produced in tiny amounts but have a huge impact on the body's functions.

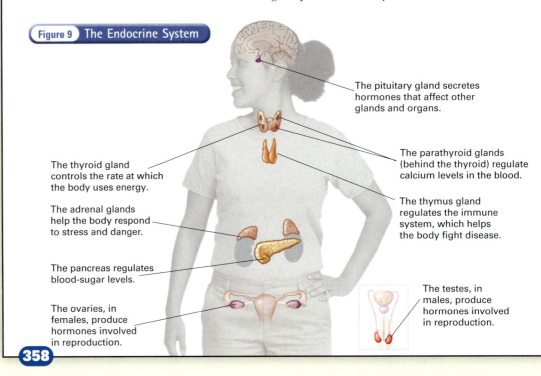

Figure 9 The Endocrine System

- The pituitary gland secretes hormones that affect other glands and organs.
- The thyroid gland controls the rate at which the body uses energy.
- The parathyroid glands (behind the thyroid) regulate calcium levels in the blood.
- The adrenal glands help the body respond to stress and danger.
- The thymus gland regulates the immune system, which helps the body fight disease.
- The pancreas regulates blood-sugar levels.
- The ovaries, in females, produce hormones involved in reproduction.
- The testes, in males, produce hormones involved in reproduction.

LIFE SCIENCE CONNECTION

Pituitary Hormones Choh Hao Li, a Chinese-American endocrinologist, isolated and identified five hormones of the pituitary gland. He discovered that the pituitary gland's growth hormone contains a chain of 256 amino acids. In 1970, he discovered a method for synthesizing the hormone and set the record for creating the largest synthesized protein molecule.

Chapter Resource File
- Directed Reading **BASIC**
- Lesson Plan
- Lesson Quiz **GENERAL**

Transparencies
TT Bellringer

358 Chapter 16 • Your Changing Body

TABLE 3 Human Endocrine Glands and Their Hormones

Gland	Hormone	Function
Ovary	estrogen, the primary female sex hormone	causes physical changes during puberty; essential for menstruation
	progesterone	prepares the lining of the uterus for pregnancy
Testis	testosterone, the primary male sex hormone	causes physical changes during puberty; essential for sperm production
Thyroid	thyroid hormones	regulate how the body stores and uses energy
Pituitary	human growth hormone	stimulates body growth

How Hormones Work

You may wonder how hormones affect some parts of your body and not others. Your body's organs and tissues chemically respond only to certain hormones. Hormones target certain organs and cause only the targeted organs to respond. When a hormone reaches the target organ, that organ responds to the hormone by reacting in a certain way. Although the amount of each hormone is very small, it must be precisely the right amount to cause the organ to respond correctly. For example, if you have too much of a given hormone, you will grow too much. If you have too little of that hormone, you will not grow enough. Table 3 describes how some hormones affect your body.

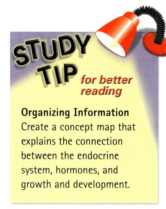

STUDY TIP for better reading

Organizing Information Create a concept map that explains the connection between the endocrine system, hormones, and growth and development.

Lesson Review

Using Vocabulary
1. What is a gland?
2. Define *hormone*. List two functions of hormones.

Understanding Concepts
3. How do hormones work in the body?
4. Why do hormones affect some parts of your body and not others?

Critical Thinking
5. **Making Inferences** Why might males and females have different primary sex hormones?
6. **Analyzing Ideas** Why is it important that hormones be released directly into the blood?

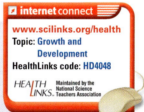

internet connect
www.scilinks.org/health
Topic: Growth and Development
HealthLinks code: HD4048
HEALTH LINKS. Maintained by the National Science Teachers Association

Answers to Lesson Review
1. A gland is a group of cells that make hormones.
2. Hormones are chemicals made by the endocrine glands that travel in the bloodstream and cause changes in different parts of the body. Hormones control growth and development. Hormones also control how the body stores and uses energy.
3. Hormones travel to specific organs and cause each organ to respond in a certain way.
4. Organs chemically respond only to certain hormones and not to others.
5. Males and females have different roles in reproduction, so they need different hormones to act on their body systems.
6. Hormones are released directly into the blood so that they can travel quickly to another place in the body.

Teach

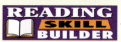 **BASIC**

Reading Organizer Have students practice taking notes as they read. Remind them that taking notes helps them learn as they read and also serves to transfer the information to long-term memory. Moreover, they will have information recorded in their own words that will be useful later when reviewing for a quiz or test. **LS Verbal**

Close

Reteaching — BASIC

Peer Reviews Ask students to write their own review questions and answers for this section. Afterwards, students can exchange review questions and try to answer the questions. They should then exchange their answers and grade each other. **LS Verbal**

Quiz — GENERAL

Ask students whether each statement below is true or false.

1. Estrogen is the primary female sex hormone. (true)
2. Glands are all concentrated in one place in the body. (false)
3. Hormones travel through the nervous system. (false)

Alternative Assessment — GENERAL

Model Have students build a model of how hormones work on body organs. Students may want to do this with clay, plastic foam, or cardboard. Some students may want to use liquids and food coloring to model how hormones travel through the bloodstream. Other students may want to build an electrical model. Encourage students to be creative. **LS Kinesthetic**

Lesson 4 • The Endocrine System

Lesson 5 Focus

Overview
Before beginning this lesson, review with your students the objectives listed under the What You'll Do head in the Student Edition. In this lesson, students learn about the stages of development from pregnancy to childhood.

🔔 Bellringer
Refer students to the ultrasound image on this page. Ask students to try to identify the fetus's head, nose, and spine. *(The head is at the left side of the photo. The nose is at the top and center of the photo. The spine is indicated by the yellow and green spots at the bottom of the photo.)* **LS Verbal**

Answer to Start Off Write
Accept all reasonable answers. Sample answer: During birth, the uterus contracts and the cervix expands until the mother can push the baby out of her body.

Motivate

Activity —— GENERAL
Skit Organize students into groups. Have each group write a skit that describes the stages of development they have gone through since their mother first became pregnant with them. Tell students that they can make the skit humorous or dramatic. Encourage students to add as many details about the different stages of development as possible. The groups can perform their skits for the rest of the class. **LS Kinesthetic**

360 Chapter 16 • Your Changing Body

Lesson 5

What You'll Do
- **Describe** the development of a fetus.
- **Summarize** the stages of childhood.

Terms to Learn
- pregnancy
- embryo
- fetus

Start Off Write
Describe what happens during birth.

Growing Up

> When the two separate sex cells combine, a new human cell is created. During pregnancy, this new cell grows into a baby.

The time when a woman is carrying a developing baby in her uterus is called **pregnancy.** Pregnancy begins with fertilization (FUHR t'l uh ZAY shuhn). Fertilization is the process by which the egg and sperm join and the genes of the mother and father combine. The new cell that forms during fertilization begins to grow based on the instructions from the parents' genes.

Pregnancy

From fertilization until the end of the eighth week of pregnancy, the developing cells are called an **embryo.** From the start of the ninth week until birth, the developing cells are called a **fetus.** The distinction between an embryo and a fetus is made because by the ninth week, all major organs have started to form. For the mother, the pregnancy is divided into three specific time periods called *trimesters*. Each trimester is about 3 months, or 13 weeks, long. Development during pregnancy is described in Figure 11.

While a fetus is inside its mother, it receives nutrition and oxygen through its umbilical cord. The umbilical cord is attached to what becomes the baby's "bellybutton." The other end of the umbilical cord is attached to the placenta. The *placenta* is a temporary organ attached to the inside wall of the mother's uterus during pregnancy. Nutrients and oxygen pass through the placenta from the mother's blood to the fetus. Waste products flow from the fetus's blood across the placenta to the mother.

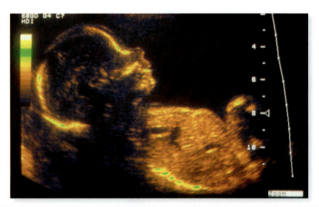

Figure 10 Ultrasound imagery uses soundwaves that bounce off of objects inside the body to produce a picture, such as the one shown here.

360

Background
Ultrasound Technology Ultrasound imaging, or sonography, is used to view objects inside the body. One common use of sonography is to look at developing fetuses in the uterus. Sound waves are transferred into the mother's abdomen. The waves bounce off of the fetus and back to a computer. The computer interprets the waves and shows an image of the fetus. These images allow doctors to identify potential problems and defects before the baby is born.

Chapter Resource File
- Directed Reading **BASIC**
- Lesson Plan
- Lesson Quiz **GENERAL**

Transparencies
TT Bellringer
TT Pregnancy Timeline

Figure 11 Pregnancy Timeline

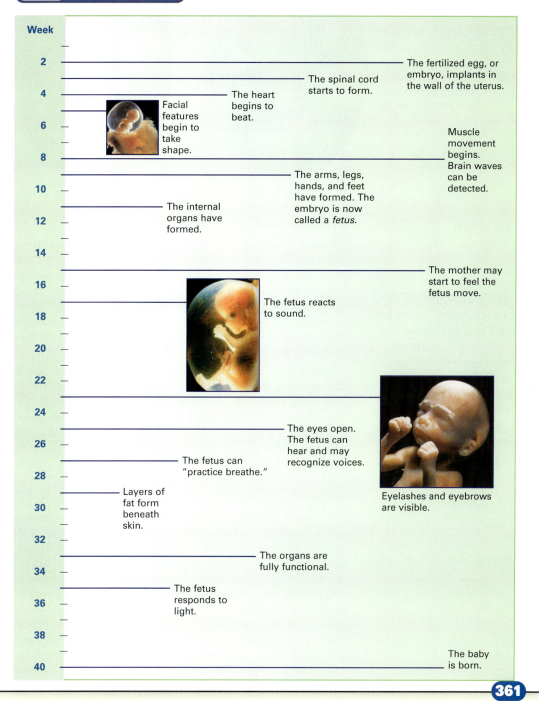

Week	
2	The fertilized egg, or embryo, implants in the wall of the uterus.
4	The spinal cord starts to form.
6	The heart begins to beat. Facial features begin to take shape.
8	Muscle movement begins. Brain waves can be detected.
10	The arms, legs, hands, and feet have formed. The embryo is now called a *fetus*.
12	The internal organs have formed.
16	The mother may start to feel the fetus move.
18	The fetus reacts to sound.
24	The eyes open. The fetus can hear and may recognize voices. Eyelashes and eyebrows are visible.
28	The fetus can "practice breathe."
30	Layers of fat form beneath skin.
34	The organs are fully functional.
36	The fetus responds to light.
40	The baby is born.

Teach

Life SKILL BUILDER — GENERAL

Communicating Effectively Tell students that the first few months of pregnancy are crucial for the healthy mental and physical development of the fetus. Drinking alcohol during a pregnancy can lead to birth defects and miscarriages. Have students research the causes and consequences of fetal alcohol syndrome (FAS). Students should create an educational poster to illustrate their findings. Encourage students who are fluent in a language other than English to design a bilingual poster. **LS** Visual **English Language Learners**

Using the Figure — BASIC

Pregnancy Timeline Direct students' attention to the pregnancy timeline on this page. Lead students through the figure so that they can see the dramatic changes that take place during fetal development. Emphasize that most of the structural features of a fetus form during the first trimester. During the second trimester, body structures become more refined. During the third trimester, most growth in body size takes place. **LS** Visual

Activity — GENERAL

Trimester Fact Sheets Organize students into small groups. Assign each group one of the three trimesters to research. The students should create an illustrated fact sheet about their assigned trimester. Hang the fact sheets around the room in sequential order, and have each group of students stand up and describe the changes that happen during their assigned trimester. **LS** Visual

Attention Grabber

Students may not understand just how astoundingly fast a fetus grows. Explain to these students that between fertilization and birth, the developing fetus increases in size from a single cell to 6 trillion cells!

Lesson 5 • Growing Up

Teach, continued

Answer to Health Journal
Answers may vary. This Health Journal may be especially appropriate for students who have an interest in the mental development of children.

Group Activity — ADVANCED
Early Childhood Development
Have groups of students research a child's growth and development stages during the first 18 months of life. This research could be organized in several ways. Groups could be assigned specific time periods, for example, the first three months after birth. Or they could be assigned to research specific behaviors, for example, changes in facial expressions, recognition of people and objects in the environment, or physical movements. Have each group make a presentation to the class that includes visuals such as photographs, drawings, computer animations, or graphs. **LS Verbal**

Activity — GENERAL
Practicing Wellness Have students read about the changes a child goes through during childhood. Then, have students make a list of the mental, physical, and emotional needs they think children of each age group would have. Tell students to use the list to create a chart. In the chart, students should write down ways that a parent provides for these needs. **LS Interpersonal**

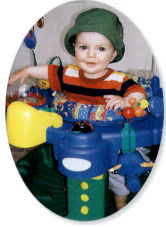
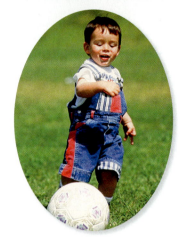

Figure 12 Children of different ages have different abilities, as these four children do.

Infancy Early Childhood

Health Journal
Spend some time with younger children of varying ages. What types of differences do you see in how they move and communicate? How do they communicate with others around them? How does communication change as children get older?

Infancy and Early Childhood
When a baby first arrives, the baby is totally dependent on someone else. The baby needs to be fed, to have his or her diapers changed, and to be protected from injury and disease. During the first year of life, called *infancy*, the baby grows quickly and learns to do a number of new things. By 9 or 10 months, most babies can sit up, crawl, and pull up to a standing position. Within another 3 to 6 months, most babies can walk and say a few words.

At age 1, early childhood begins. This stage lasts until age 3. During early childhood, children are often called *toddlers*. In this stage, children learn to feed themselves, throw a ball, run, climb, and turn doorknobs. They also learn to say several words. They improve in almost all physical skills. A child at this age can learn to pedal a small tricycle, kick a ball, and slide down a small slide.

Middle Childhood
After age 3, children enter middle childhood. This stage lasts until about age 6. During this stage, children learn to draw with a pencil or crayon and put together simple jigsaw puzzles. They run and jump more gracefully than before. Children in this stage begin to ask many questions. Because of the development of the brain, children start to understand and remember the answers to their questions. During these years, most children begin to learn to read. They also start to imitate adults, friends, and brothers and sisters. During this time, children begin to develop their identity and personality and to make and play with friends.

REAL-LIFE CONNECTION — ADVANCED
Skull Growth and Forensic Science
Several bones of a baby's skull are not fused as they are in adults. These bones are not fused because they must allow the child's brain to grow. Forensic scientists can use the skulls of unidentified bodies to determine the age of a victim based on the extent of fusion along sutures in the skull. Have interested students research the practice of identifying age by cranial characteristics. **LS Logical**

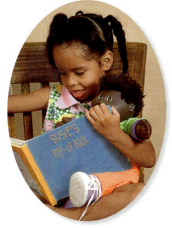
Middle Childhood

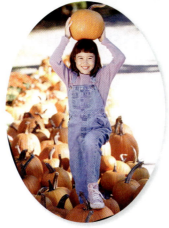
Late Childhood

Late Childhood

Late childhood lasts from age 6 until about age 11. During these years, physical ability dramatically improves, and physical size increases. Growth during this time takes place in spurts. These rapid physical changes sometimes make children feel awkward and self-conscious.

Children in this stage need to be active physically, mentally, and socially. Participating in physical activity can help children stay strong and healthy. Exploring skills and interests helps older children develop mentally. Late childhood is also a time of increased social development. Forming friendships with others of the same age becomes important and allows children to develop new social skills. At the end of late childhood, children are prepared to enter adolescence.

LANGUAGE ARTS ACTIVITY

Write a short story about a child who is in one of the stages between infancy and late childhood. Write the story in the first person. The language in the story should reflect the age of the child who is telling the story.

Lesson Review

Using Vocabulary

1. Define *pregnancy*.
2. What is the difference between an embryo and a fetus?

Understanding Concepts

3. Summarize the development of a fetus.
4. Summarize the development of children between birth and age 11.

Critical Thinking

5. **Making Inferences** Why is it important for infants and toddlers to receive a lot of physical and emotional care?
6. **Analyzing Ideas** The mother passes nutrients to the fetus through the placenta. Why is it important for the mother to avoid alcohol, tobacco, and other drugs?

internet connect
www.scilinks.org/health
Topic: Pregnancy
HealthLinks code: HD4077
HEALTH LINKS. Maintained by the National Science Teachers Association

---

Answer to Language Arts Activity

Answers may vary. You may need to remind students that first person perspective uses I, me, and my.

Close

Reteaching — BASIC

Development Timeline Have students draw a complete timeline of the development of a human from fertilization to late childhood. Have students who are fluent in a language other than English translate their timeline into their native language. **LS** Verbal — English Language Learners

Quiz — GENERAL

1. What is an embryo? (the human cells that develop from a fertilized egg until the eighth week of pregnancy)
2. What is the purpose of the placenta? (The placenta supplies the developing fetus with oxygen and nutrients.)
3. In what week of pregnancy does the spinal cord form? (week 3)

Alternative Assessment — GENERAL

Screenplay Have students write a screenplay that dramatizes the stages of human development from fertilization to late childhood. The screenplay can be a documentary or a fictional story. Have students provide illustrated storyboards of some of the scenes. **LS** Verbal

---

Answers to Lesson Review

1. Pregnancy is the time when a woman is carrying a developing baby in her uterus.
2. An embryo is the developing human between fertilization and the 8th week of pregnancy. A fetus is the developing human between the 9th week of pregnancy and birth.
3. Answers may vary, but should follow the timeline in this lesson.
4. During infancy, a baby grows quickly and learns to perform simple physical tasks. During early childhood, most children improve their physical skills and learn to talk. During middle childhood, children learn to move more gracefully and start asking many questions. During late childhood, physical and mental abilities improve dramatically and children begin to be more social.
5. Sample answer: Children of this age are not able to take care of themselves and need a lot of care to develop properly.
6. Alcohol, drugs, and other substances can be passed to the developing fetus through the placenta. These substances can harm the fetus and cause it to develop abnormally.

Lesson 5 • Growing Up   363

Lesson 6 Focus

Overview
Before beginning this lesson, review with your students the objectives listed under the What You'll Do head in the Student Edition. This lesson describes the changes that take place during adolescence and how these changes help prepare adolescents for adulthood. Students also explore what happens to their bodies as they age and about the stages of grief.

🔔 Bellringer
Have students draw pictures of all the stages they will go through throughout their lives. (The pictures may have a baby, a toddler, an adolescent, a young adult, a middle-aged adult, and then an older adult.)
LS Visual

Answer to Start Off Write
Accept all reasonable answers. Sample answer: Adults are people who are physically mature and who are required to take care of themselves.

Motivate

Activity —————— GENERAL
Role-Playing Have students role-play different situations that people might face as adults, such as interviewing for a job or dealing with the affects of aging. **LS** Kinesthetic

---

Lesson 6 — Becoming an Adult

What You'll Do
- **Explain** how the physical, mental, social, and emotional changes of adolescence prepare you for adulthood.
- **Describe** what happens to the body during aging.
- **List** the five stages of grief.

Terms to Learn
- adolescence
- puberty
- adulthood
- grief

Start Off Write
What does *being an adult* mean?

> Hassan noticed that he looked different in the mirror. He was getting taller, and the shape of his body was changing. His shoulders were getting wider, and hair was starting to grow on his face.

Your body changes as you get older. The changes Hassan is seeing are only the beginning of the changes he will go through as he becomes an adult.

Adolescence
The time in life when a person matures from a child to an adult is called **adolescence.** Adolescence begins with puberty and lasts until the person is physically mature. **Puberty** is the stage of development when the reproductive organs mature and the person becomes able to reproduce. Puberty begins at different times for different people. In general, puberty starts earlier for girls than it does for boys. This growth from childhood to maturity involves mental, emotional, physical, and social growth.

The physical changes of adolescence are caused by increased amounts of hormones in the body. High levels of hormones cause girls to have a menstrual cycle and to develop breasts. Different hormones cause boys to start making sperm. Both boys and girls have growth spurts and begin to grow body hair.

Both boys and girls go through mental, social, and emotional changes, too. These changes prepare them for adulthood. Adolescents must learn how to interact with others and how to perform tasks of adults, such as taking care of a family and holding a steady job.

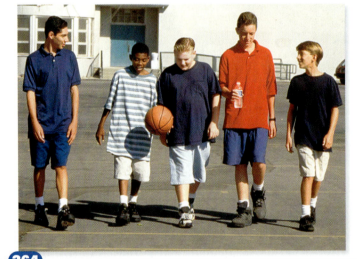

Figure 13 All of these boys are normal. Growth spurts during adolescence happen at different times for different people.

364

Background
Developmental Differences Adolescents develop at different rates, and making students aware that these differences are normal is important. Girls usually begin to mature before boys. Many boys do not reach their full height until after they graduate from high school. Among students in the same grade level, height differences of a foot or more are not unusual. This height increase requires so much of the body's energy that some adolescent boys appear quite thin because their body has not yet added muscle mass. Girls may have the opposite problem. As they mature and develop more body fat, many girls become overly concerned about staying thin.

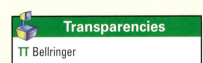

Chapter Resource File
- Directed Reading BASIC
- Lesson Plan
- Lesson Quiz GENERAL

Transparencies
TT Bellringer

364 Chapter 16 • Your Changing Body

Preparing for Adult Roles

During adolescence, you grow mentally as your brain matures. You learn to understand more-complex concepts. You learn the importance of making good decisions and accepting the consequences of your decisions and actions. These mental changes prepare you for adult tasks, such as getting a job.

The sex hormones your body produces may make you interested in romantic relationships with others. Friendships and dating relationships help you prepare for adult relationships. Learning to be more independent and more responsible prepares you for having a job or a family.

All of the changes of adolescence can be confusing and even scary. Sometimes, adolescents are tempted to engage in risky behaviors as a way of dealing with these changes. Parents and other trusted adults can help you deal with the changes you are experiencing and can help you prepare to take on adult roles.

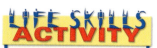

MAKING GOOD DECISIONS

Form a group discussion in which the topic of debate is how intensely teens should begin planning for future goals while they are still in middle school and high school.

Adulthood

An adult is a person who is fully grown physically and mentally. **Adulthood** is the stage of life that follows adolescence and lasts until the end of life. During adulthood, many people fulfill personal and vocational goals. Adulthood is the time in life when people establish careers. Many adults get married and have children. Many adults find fulfillment in participating in community events and in continuing to learn.

Adults must be responsible for their own health and safety. They must pay their bills and provide food, shelter, and clothing for themselves and, if they have a family, for their spouse and children. These responsibilities can be stressful for adults.

Adults who have developed physically, mentally, emotionally, and socially are best able to cope with the demands of adulthood. Emotional and mental development during adolescence helps adults maintain stable home and work lives. This stability allows them to work well with others and provide for the needs of their families.

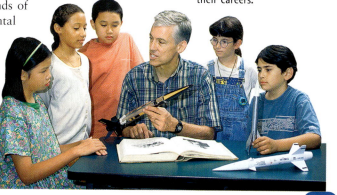

Figure 14 Many adults achieve personal and vocational goals through their careers.

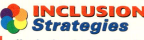

- Hearing Impaired
- Developmentally Delayed
- Learning Disabled

A visual demonstration can help students understand the aging process. On the board, create a graph with a y-axis that has the following intervals: high, medium, and low. On the x-axis, place these age groups: 0–1, 1–3, 3–6, 6–11, 11–18, 18–40, 40–70, and 70+. Subdivide each age group into two categories: Walking speed and Amount eaten. Have students agree on how each age group performs each category. Then, place Xs on the lines marked high, medium and low for each category. Connect the Xs with a curved line to reveal a bell-shaped curve that shows that as you grow from an infant to an adult, you walk faster and eat more; then, as you age, you begin to walk slower and eat less. **LS Visual**

Teach

LIFE SKILLS ACTIVITY

Answer
Answers may vary.

Extension: Do you know what career you would like to have as an adult? What education or training do you need for that career?

Demonstration — GENERAL

Guest Speakers Invite a selection of professionals who deal with adolescent problems to visit your class. Possible visitors might include a physician or nurse, a psychotherapist, a drug or eating-disorder counselor, and a social worker. Ask each visitor to tell the class about his or her work with adolescents. Students may want to ask questions, such as what are the most common problems the speaker sees and what approaches the speaker finds most effective in helping struggling adolescents. **LS Verbal**

Group Activity — ADVANCED

Course of Adulthood Organize students into pairs. Have each pair design a timeline that tracks general psychological, social, and physical development through adulthood. After groups have completed the timeline, have them create a fictional adult character and plot important life events and developmental changes for that person on the timeline. Students may want to speak with parents or other older adults to generate ideas for their character's life. Tell students that the progress of the fictional character through life should approximate the developmental patterns shown on the timeline. Ask the pairs to display their timelines and discuss them with the class. Have the class determine whether each fictional character's progression through adulthood is realistic.
LS Interpersonal Co-op Learning

Lesson 6 • Becoming an Adult   **365**

Teach, continued

Answer to Health Journal
Answers may vary. This Health Journal can be used to begin a class discussion on the roles of older adults in communities and society. Remember that some students may be uncomfortable sharing personal information.

Debate — ADVANCED

Stereotypes Tell students that many Americans have stereotypical views of older adults. Invite students to suggest what some of these stereotypes might be. Have the class debate where these stereotypes may have originated and whether they are valid. **LS Interpersonal**

Demonstration — BASIC

Simulating Old Age To help students understand some of the physical changes that occur during the aging process, have them simulate some of the experiences of some aging adults. Have students carefully place cotton balls in their ears to experience hearing loss. Have them remove their own corrective eyeglasses or wear an old pair of scratched sunglasses to experience vision loss. Have them try to take coins out of a change purse while wearing gloves to simulate loss of manual dexterity. Have students discuss the experience. **LS Kinesthetic**

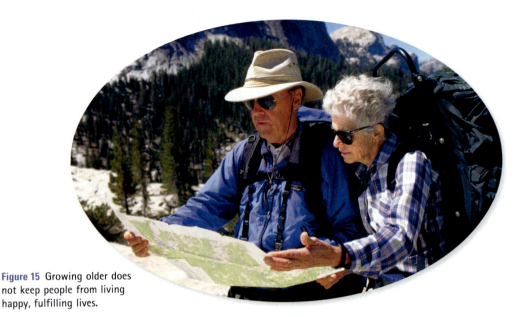

Figure 15 Growing older does not keep people from living happy, fulfilling lives.

Health Journal
Interview someone whom you consider a role model. This person can be anyone you admire. In what ways can you be like that person? In what ways do you not want to be like that person? Explain your answers.

Aging

Part of adulthood is growing older, or *aging*. Even during adulthood, our bodies continue to change. Over time, our bodies begin to wear down, and eventually they work less efficiently. One way to stay as healthy as possible for as long as possible is to take good care of yourself now. Taking good care of yourself includes eating nutritious foods and exercising regularly. It also means avoiding many risky behaviors, such as using tobacco, alcohol, and other drugs, and avoiding unnecessary physical risks, such as not wearing protective gear and seat belts.

As people age, health problems such as arthritis, Alzheimer's disease, heart disease, and cancer may arise. While each condition can be treated, many have no cure. Some of these conditions can be prevented by maintaining good health habits for an entire lifetime. Other conditions are related to heredity or environmental factors that are beyond your control. Many conditions can be managed because of advances in medical technology. These advances have improved the quality of life for many people and have increased the length of time that people live.

Even as they get older, most adults find ways to be fulfilled. Many older adults retire and begin to spend more time with their families and friends. They have more time to travel and work on their hobbies. Most adults stay healthy and active for most of their lives.

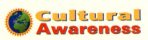

Multigenerational Households In some cultures, grandparents traditionally live with their children and grandchildren in a multigenerational household, regardless of health or economic circumstances. If any students live in a multigenerational household, ask them to share their experiences. While some of these cultural traditions have faded in American society, some U.S. families are once again living in multigenerational households because of economic necessity. In fact, about 5 percent of U.S. children live in a household that includes their grandparents.

Preparing for Adult Roles

During adolescence, you grow mentally as your brain matures. You learn to understand more-complex concepts. You learn the importance of making good decisions and accepting the consequences of your decisions and actions. These mental changes prepare you for adult tasks, such as getting a job.

The sex hormones your body produces may make you interested in romantic relationships with others. Friendships and dating relationships help you prepare for adult relationships. Learning to be more independent and more responsible prepares you for having a job or a family.

All of the changes of adolescence can be confusing and even scary. Sometimes, adolescents are tempted to engage in risky behaviors as a way of dealing with these changes. Parents and other trusted adults can help you deal with the changes you are experiencing and can help you prepare to take on adult roles.

Adulthood

An adult is a person who is fully grown physically and mentally. **Adulthood** is the stage of life that follows adolescence and lasts until the end of life. During adulthood, many people fulfill personal and vocational goals. Adulthood is the time in life when people establish careers. Many adults get married and have children. Many adults find fulfillment in participating in community events and in continuing to learn.

Adults must be responsible for their own health and safety. They must pay their bills and provide food, shelter, and clothing for themselves and, if they have a family, for their spouse and children. These responsibilities can be stressful for adults.

Adults who have developed physically, mentally, emotionally, and socially are best able to cope with the demands of adulthood. Emotional and mental development during adolescence helps adults maintain stable home and work lives. This stability allows them to work well with others and provide for the needs of their families.

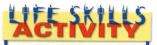

MAKING GOOD DECISIONS

Form a group discussion in which the topic of debate is how intensely teens should begin planning for future goals while they are still in middle school and high school.

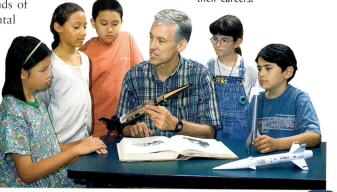

Figure 14 Many adults achieve personal and vocational goals through their careers.

Teach, continued

Answer to Health Journal
Answers may vary. This Health Journal can be used to begin a class discussion on the roles of older adults in communities and society. Remember that some students may be uncomfortable sharing personal information.

Debate — ADVANCED
Stereotypes Tell students that many Americans have stereotypical views of older adults. Invite students to suggest what some of these stereotypes might be. Have the class debate where these stereotypes may have originated and whether they are valid. **LS Interpersonal**

Demonstration — BASIC
Simulating Old Age To help students understand some of the physical changes that occur during the aging process, have them simulate some of the experiences of some aging adults. Have students carefully place cotton balls in their ears to experience hearing loss. Have them remove their own corrective eyeglasses or wear an old pair of scratched sunglasses to experience vision loss. Have them try to take coins out of a change purse while wearing gloves to simulate loss of manual dexterity. Have students discuss the experience. **LS Kinesthetic**

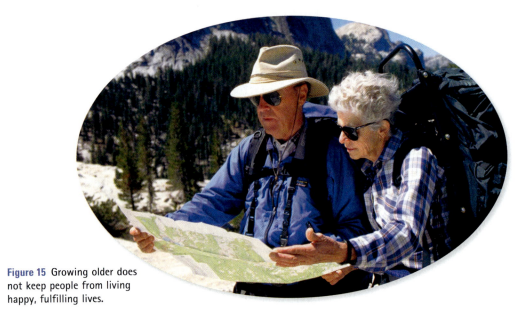

Figure 15 Growing older does not keep people from living happy, fulfilling lives.

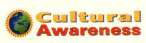

Interview someone whom you consider a role model. This person can be anyone you admire. In what ways can you be like that person? In what ways do you not want to be like that person? Explain your answers.

Aging

Part of adulthood is growing older, or *aging*. Even during adulthood, our bodies continue to change. Over time, our bodies begin to wear down, and eventually they work less efficiently. One way to stay as healthy as possible for as long as possible is to take good care of yourself now. Taking good care of yourself includes eating nutritious foods and exercising regularly. It also means avoiding many risky behaviors, such as using tobacco, alcohol, and other drugs, and avoiding unnecessary physical risks, such as not wearing protective gear and seat belts.

As people age, health problems such as arthritis, Alzheimer's disease, heart disease, and cancer may arise. While each condition can be treated, many have no cure. Some of these conditions can be prevented by maintaining good health habits for an entire lifetime. Other conditions are related to heredity or environmental factors that are beyond your control. Many conditions can be managed because of advances in medical technology. These advances have improved the quality of life for many people and have increased the length of time that people live.

Even as they get older, most adults find ways to be fulfilled. Many older adults retire and begin to spend more time with their families and friends. They have more time to travel and work on their hobbies. Most adults stay healthy and active for most of their lives.

Cultural Awareness

Multigenerational Households In some cultures, grandparents traditionally live with their children and grandchildren in a multigenerational household, regardless of health or economic circumstances. If any students live in a multigenerational household, ask them to share their experiences. While some of these cultural traditions have faded in American society, some U.S. families are once again living in multigenerational households because of economic necessity. In fact, about 5 percent of U.S. children live in a household that includes their grandparents.

366 Chapter 16 • Your Changing Body

Death

Life expectancy for both men and women in the United States is the highest it has ever been. *Life expectancy* is the average number of years that people are expected to live. People are living longer because medical advances are keeping people healthy longer. Everyone eventually dies. *Death* is the end of life. At death, all of the body functions that are necessary for life stop.

Dealing with death will always be difficult. When someone you love dies, you will probably feel grief. **Grief** is a deep sadness about a loss. Many people go through five stages when dealing with death: denial, anger, bargaining, despair, and acceptance. Going through these stages helps people come to terms with their loss and prepare to live their lives without the person who has died.

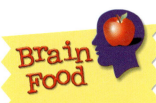

Brain Food

The average life expectancy in the United States for a man is 74 years. The average life expectancy for a woman in the United States is 80 years.

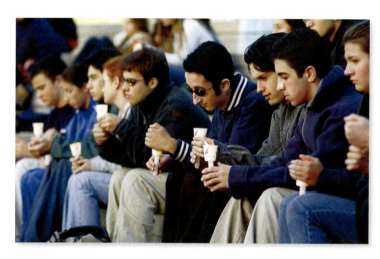

Figure 16 Many people rely on their family or friends for comfort when they grieve.

Lesson Review

Using Vocabulary
1. What is the difference between adolescence and puberty?

Understanding Concepts
2. How do changes during adolescence prepare you for adult roles?
3. Describe what happens to the body during aging.
4. List the five stages of grief.

Critical Thinking
5. **Making Inferences** Why might your health habits as a young person influence your health as you grow older? Give two examples of health habits that can have negative effects on your long-term health. Explain your answer.

Answers to Lesson Review

1. Adolescence is the stage of development between childhood and adulthood. Puberty is the time during adolescence when the reproductive system becomes mature.
2. Sample answer: The physical changes during adolescence prepare your body to produce children. The mental, emotional, and social changes during adolescence prepare you for the roles and responsibilities that you will have as an adult.
3. As you age, your body begins to wear down and work less efficiently.
4. denial, anger, bargaining, despair, and acceptance
5. Sample answer: If you start healthy habits early, your body will stay healthy longer. For example, not exercising and not eating a healthy diet will weaken your body and make you more susceptible to disease.

Close

Reteaching — BASIC

Development Flashcards Give each student three index cards, and ask students to write a different physical, emotional, and social change that occurs during adolescence or adulthood on each card. Have students mix their cards together. From the mixed stack of cards, have each student randomly chose three cards. When students have their cards, they should read the change aloud, identify the stage of development, and describe one effect of the change.
LS Interpersonal

Quiz — GENERAL

1. What is the main physical development that happens during puberty? (The reproductive organs mature.)
2. Name four health problems that may arise in late adulthood. (Alzheimer's disease, arthritis, heart disease, and cancer)
3. What is grief? (a deep sadness caused by loss)

Alternative Assessment — GENERAL

Instruction Manual Have students write an instruction manual for life. The instruction manual should tell a young person what to expect as they go through the stages of life. Students may choose to give advice about how to handle some of the changes that will take place as they get older. Encourage students to illustrate their manuals. Students who are fluent in a language other than English should translate their manual into their native language. **English Language Learners**
LS Verbal

Lesson 6 • Becoming an Adult

CHAPTER 16 REVIEW

Assignment Guide

Lesson	Review Questions
1	1, 4, 11, 24
2	2, 12
3	3, 7, 16, 23
4	6, 15, 25–26
5	5, 8, 18–19, 22, 27
6	9, 17, 20–21, 28–31
1 and 5	10
2 and 3	13–14

ANSWERS

Using Vocabulary

1. heredity
2. testes
3. ovaries
4. environment
5. uterus
6. Hormones are chemicals that cause changes in the body. Hormones are made and released by glands.
7. Menstruation is the monthly breakdown and shedding of the endometrium. Ovulation is the monthly release of a mature egg from the ovary.
8. An embryo is the developing human between fertilization and the 8th week of pregnancy. A fetus is the developing human between the 9th week of pregnancy and birth.
9. Adolescence is the stage of development between childhood and adulthood. Puberty is the time during adolescence when the reproductive system becomes mature.

16 CHAPTER REVIEW

Chapter Summary

■ The passing of genes from parent to child is called *heredity*. ■ The male sex cell is called *sperm*. ■ The female sex cell is called the *egg*, or *ovum*. ■ Hormones are chemicals that control the growth and activity of the body. ■ When egg and sperm combine, a new human cell forms and develops into a fetus. ■ Pregnancy is divided into three trimesters; each trimester is about 3 months long. ■ During infancy and childhood, people grow rapidly both physically and mentally. ■ Adolescence is the stage of development from the start of puberty to adulthood. ■ An adult is a person who is fully developed physically and mentally. ■ Aging is a natural part of life. ■ Death is the end of life. People experience grief when someone dies.

Using Vocabulary

For each sentence, fill in the blank with the proper word from the word bank provided below.

testes   uterus
penis   ovaries
heredity environment

1. The passing of characteristics from parent to child is called ___.
2. The ___ are the male reproductive organs that make sperm and testosterone.
3. The organs that release eggs are called the ___.
4. Your surroundings, including your home and your family, are your ___.
5. During pregnancy, the fetus develops inside the mother's ___.

For each pair of terms, describe how the meanings of the terms differ.

6. hormone/gland
7. menstruation/ovulation
8. embryo/fetus
9. adolescence/puberty

Understanding Concepts

10. Briefly describe how sex cells combine to pass on the genes of both mother and father.
11. How are growth and development affected by heredity and environment?
12. What are sperm, and how are they made?
13. List and describe two problems of the male reproductive system and two problems of the female reproductive system.
14. Identify four ways to protect your reproductive system from harm.
15. What role does the endocrine system play in growth and development?
16. Summarize the typical menstrual cycle.
17. Describe what happens to the body during aging.
18. Describe human development from fertilization to birth.
19. Summarize the stages of childhood.
20. Explain how changes that happen during adolescence prepare people for adult roles.
21. What are the five stages of grief?

Understanding Concepts

10. Sex cells have half of the total amount of genetic material. When these cells combine, they form a single cell with the total amount of genetic material, half from the mother and half from the father.
11. Heredity gives your body instructions on how to develop and what to look like. Environment also influences your development through your nutrition, activities, and social interactions.
12. Sperm are male sex cells. They are made by cell division in small tubules inside the testes.
13. Sample answer: male, jock itch—an itchy infection of the skin in the groin area; testicular cancer—abnormal cell growth in the testes; female, vaginitis—infection of the vagina; breast cancer—abnormal cell growth in the breasts
14. Sample answer: Maintain good hygiene. Wear protective gear during sports. Perform regular self-examinations. Talk to trusted adults about your reproductive health.
15. The endocrine system releases hormones that control growth and development.
16. The endometrium is shed through menstruation. The endometrium begins to thicken to prepare for pregnancy. The ovum is released from the ovary and is carried toward the uterus. If the ovum is not fertilized, the cycle begins again as the endometrium is shed.

Critical Thinking

Analyzing Ideas

22. A fetus in the uterus receives all of its nourishment from its mother. Why should expectant mothers avoid using alcohol and other drugs?

23. Having the sexually transmitted disease human papillomavirus, HPV, increases the chances that a woman will get cervical cancer. Explain how abstaining from sexual activity can reduce a woman's chance of getting cervical cancer later in life.

24. Two identical twins share the same genes and grew up in the same house with the same parents. Explain why their personalities and likes and dislikes can be different.

25. What are some health problems that you could have if your body produced too much or too little of the thyroid hormone that regulates how your body stores fat and uses energy?

Using Refusal Skills

26. Some students on your sports team have been taking hormones called *steroids* to make their muscles grow bigger and faster. One day, they offer you some steroids. What reasons would you give for refusing the steroids?

27. Imagine that you are baby-sitting for an infant. After you have been baby-sitting for about an hour, your friend calls and invites you to go with him to the movies. He says that you'll be gone for only two hours and that the baby will be all right alone for that long. How do you explain to him that you can't leave the baby alone?

Interpreting Graphics

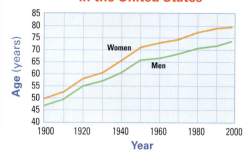

Average Life Expectancy in the United States

Use the figure above to answer questions 28–31.

28. The graph above shows average life expectancy in the United States from 1900 to 1997. What was life expectancy for men in 1940? What was life expectancy for women in 1930?

29. By how many years did life expectancy for men increase between 1900 and 1997? By how many years did life expectancy change for women between 1900 and 1997?

30. What was the difference (in years) between life expectancy for men and life expectancy for women in 1980?

31. What may have caused the increase in life expectancy over the last 100 years?

Reading Checkup

Take a minute to review your answers to the Health IQ questions at the beginning of this chapter. How has reading this chapter improved your Health IQ?

---

17. The body begins to wear down and becomes less efficient.
18. Sample answer: The fertilized egg implants on the uterus wall. A placenta and umbilical cord form. The embryo develops into a fetus. The body organs develop and begin to function. Then, the baby is born.
19. Answers may vary. Accept all reasonable responses.
20. Sample answer: The physical changes during adolescence prepare your body to produce children. The mental, emotional, and social changes during adolescence prepare you for the roles and responsibilities that you will have as an adult.
21. denial, anger, bargaining, despair, and acceptance

Critical Thinking

Analyzing Ideas

22. Alcohol and other drugs that a mother takes will be passed to the fetus. Alcohol and other drugs can cause developmental problems for the fetus.
23. By abstaining from sex, a woman will not put herself at risk for catching an STD, such as HPV. Staying free of STDs will reduce a woman's chance of developing cervical cancer.
24. Sample answer: The twins responded differently to their environment.
25. Sample answer: You could gain too much weight if your body does not burn enough energy. You could lose too much weight if your body burns too much energy.

Using Refusal Skills

26. Sample answer: "No thanks, my body will develop properly on its own. If I take steroids now, I will be putting the wrong level of hormones into my body and I could cause problems in how I grow."
27. Sample answer: "I'm sorry, I can't go. Babies can't take care of themselves and can't be left alone. They need constant care and attention. We'll have to go to the movies another time."

Interpreting Graphics

28. men, 1940: 62 years; women, 1930: 61 years
29. men: 26 years; women: 28 years
30. about 8 years
31. Better living and working conditions and advancement in medical technology may have contributed to the increase in life expectancy.

Chapter Resource File

- Concept Review GENERAL
- Concept Mapping GENERAL
- Performance-Based Assessment GENERAL
- Chapter Test GENERAL

Chapter 16 • Chapter Review

Model

Introduce this activity by reminding students that using this Life Skill will help them take personal responsibility for their behavior. Then, review the scenario with the class.

Prepare students for this activity by modeling each of the steps of the skill. Make sure students understand each step before you move on to the next one.

Guided Practice: Practice with a Friend

Guided Practice is the stage in which you and the students analyze their approach to solving the problem given in the scenario and analyze their ability to assess their health. Have students read Act 1. Discuss with the class the situation described and the way students are to act it out. Organize the class into groups of two. In each group, one person plays the role of Maura, and the second person is the observer.

Proper pacing during the Guided Practice is important. The suggestions listed below will help you control the pace.

1. Stop after completing each step of assessing your health.
2. Discuss with each group the observer's comments.
3. Ask the other members of each group to listen to the observer's suggestions and to suggest ways to improve the way they assess their health.
4. Instruct students to repeat the steps that need improvement and to include their modifications.

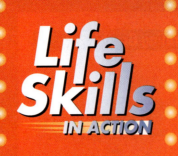

Life Skills IN ACTION

Assessing Your Health

Assessing your health means evaluating each of the four parts of your health and examining your behaviors. By assessing your health regularly, you will know what your strengths and weaknesses are and will be able to take steps to improve your health. Complete the following activity to improve your ability to assess your health.

Puberty Blues

ACT 1

Setting the Scene

Maura is going through puberty, and she doesn't like it. She grew several inches over the last half year and her body seems to change shape daily. None of Maura's clothes fit well any more, and she feels awkward just walking down the hallway at school. Maura used to be a cheerful person, but now her mood changes very often and very rapidly.

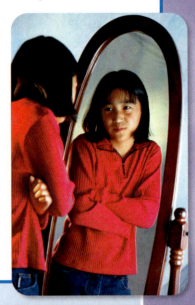

The 4 Steps of Assessing Your Health

1. Choose the part of your health you want to assess.
2. List your strengths and weaknesses.
3. Describe how your behaviors may contribute to your weaknesses.
4. Develop a plan to address your weaknesses.

Guided Practice

Practice with a Friend

Form a group of two. Have one person play the role of Maura, and have the second person be an observer. Walking through each of the four steps of assessing your health, role-play Maura analyzing one of the four parts of her health. The observer will take notes, which will include observations about what the person playing Maura did well and suggestions of ways to improve. Stop after each step to evaluate the process.

5. Check to make sure that students understand each step before they move on to the next step.
6. If time permits, repeat the exercise and have students switch roles. Each student should have the opportunity to play each role.
   Co-op Learning

Independent Practice

Check Yourself

After you have completed the guided practice, go through Act 1 again without stopping at each step. Answer the questions below to review what you did.

1. Which part of her health did Maura assess? Why did you choose that part?
2. What are Maura's strengths and weaknesses?
3. What plan did Maura develop to address her weaknesses?
4. Name a weakness in one of your health behaviors. What can you do to improve this health behavior?

On Your Own

Over the last few months, Maura has felt like spending more and more time alone. She doesn't hang out with her friends as much as she used to, and she prefers staying in her room when she is home with her family. When Maura is alone, she reads and writes in her journal. Yesterday, Maura's best friend called and asked why Maura didn't like her anymore. Make a flowchart showing how Maura could use the four steps of assessing your health to assess her social health.

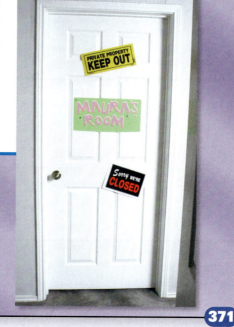

Independent Practice: Check Yourself

Instruct students to repeat Act 1 without stopping at each step. Remind students to apply what they learned in the Guided Practice to the Independent Practice.

Encourage students to use the Check Yourself questions as a starting point for reviewing and analyzing their Independent Practice. Remind students that as they change roles, the answers to these questions may change for each actor. Encourage students to create additional questions for checking their ability to assess their health. When students have finished the Independent Practice, have them answer the Check Yourself questions in writing. Use their answers to assess their understanding of the steps of assessing their health and to assess their use of the steps to solve a problem.

Check Yourself Answers

1. Sample answer: Maura assessed her emotional health. I chose that part of her part of her health because Maura was having a hard time dealing emotionally with puberty.
2. Sample answer: One of Maura's strengths is that she used to be a cheerful person. She could probably be cheerful again. One of Maura's weaknesses is that she feels awkward.
3. Sample answer: Maura planned to buy new clothes. She believed that new clothes would fit her better, which would help her feel less awkward.
4. Sample answer: A weakness in my health behaviors is that I don't get enough sleep every night and I become cranky when I am tired. I could improve this health behavior by starting my homework earlier in the evening so that I can go to bed earlier.

Act 2: On Your Own

This additional scenario gives students an opportunity to apply what they have learned in both the Guided Practice and the Independent Practice to a new situation.

Suggest to students that they use the Check Yourself questions as a starting point for assessing their health in the new situation. Encourage students to be creative and to think of ways to improve their ability to assess their health.

Assessment

Review the flowcharts that students have made as part of the On Your Own activity. The flowcharts should show that the students followed the steps of assessing their health in a realistic and effective manner. If time permits, ask student volunteers to draw one or more of their flowcharts on the blackboard. Discuss the flowcharts and the way the students used the steps of assessing their health.

Chapter 17 — Your Personal Safety
Chapter Planning Guide

PACING	CLASSROOM RESOURCES	ACTIVITIES AND DEMONSTRATIONS
BLOCK 1 • 45 min pp. 372–377 **Chapter Opener**	CRF Health Inventory * ■ GENERAL CRF Parent Letter * ■	SE Health IQ, p. 373 CRF At-Home Activity * ■
Lesson 1 Injury Prevention at Home and at School	CRF Lesson Plan * TT Bellringer * TT Home Safety Tips *	TE Group Activity Skit, p. 374 GENERAL TE Activity Positive Reinforcement, p. 375 BASIC TE Demonstration Police Officer, p. 376 ◆ BASIC CRF Enrichment Activity * ADVANCED
BLOCK 2 • 45 min pp. 378–383 **Lesson 2** Fire Safety	CRF Lesson Plan * TT Bellringer *	TE Group Activity Poster Project, p. 379 GENERAL CRF Life Skills Activity * ■ GENERAL CRF Enrichment Activity * ADVANCED
Lesson 3 Safety on the Road	CRF Lesson Plan * TT Bellringer *	TE Group Activity, pp. 380, 382 ◆ SE Hands-on Activity, p. 382 CRF Datasheets for In-Text Activities * GENERAL TE Demonstration Seat Belts, p. 382 ◆ BASIC SE Life Skills in Action Being a Wise Consumer, pp. 404–405 CRF Enrichment Activity * ADVANCED
BLOCK 3 • 45 min pp. 384–387 **Lesson 4** Safety Outdoors	CRF Lesson Plan * TT Bellringer *	TE Activities Comparing Sunscreens, p. 371F ◆ TE Group Activity Dark and Light Clothing, p. 385 GENERAL CRF Enrichment Activity * ADVANCED
BLOCK 4 • 45 min pp. 388–393 **Lesson 5** Natural Disasters	CRF Lesson Plan * TT Bellringer *	TE Activities Building a Hurricane-Proof House, p. 371F ◆ TE Group Activity, pp. 388, 390 GENERAL TE Activity Emergency Kit, p. 391 ◆ GENERAL CRF Life Skills Activity * ■ GENERAL CRF Enrichment Activity * ADVANCED
Lesson 6 Deciding to Give First Aid	CRF Lesson Plan * TT Bellringer *	TE Activity Skit, p. 392 GENERAL CRF Enrichment Activity * ADVANCED
BLOCK 5 • 45 min pp. 394–397 **Lesson 7** Abdominal Thrusts and Rescue Breathing	CRF Lesson Plan * TT Bellringer * TT Rescue Breathing for Adults * TT Rescue Breathing for Small Children *	TE Activity Abdominal Thrust Poster, p. 395 GENERAL CRF Enrichment Activity * ADVANCED
BLOCK 6 • 45 min pp. 398–401 **Lesson 8** First Aid for Injuries	CRF Lesson Plan * TT Bellringer *	TE Activity Role-Play, p. 398 ◆ GENERAL TE Demonstration, pp. 399 ◆, 401 ◆ SE Science Activity, p. 400 TE Group Activity Poster Project, p. 400 GENERAL CRF Enrichment Activity * ADVANCED

BLOCKS 7 & 8 • 90 min Chapter Review and Assessment Resources

- SE Chapter Review, pp. 402–403
- CRF Concept Review * ■ GENERAL
- CRF Health Behavior Contract * ■ GENERAL
- CRF Chapter Test * ■ GENERAL
- CRF Performance Based Assessment * GENERAL
- OSP Test Generator
- CRF Test Item Listing *

Online Resources

Visit **go.hrw.com** for a variety of free resources related to this textbook. Enter the keyword **HD4SA7**.

Holt Online Learning

Students can access interactive problem solving help and active visual concept development with the *Decisions for Health* Online Edition available at **www.hrw.com**.

CNN Student News

cnnstudentnews.com

Find the latest health news, lesson plans, and activities related to important scientific events.

Compression guide:
To shorten your instruction because of time limitations, omit Lessons 2, 4 and 5.

KEY
- **TE** Teacher Edition
- **SE** Student Edition
- **OSP** One-Stop Planner
- **CRF** Chapter Resource File
- **TT** Teaching Transparency
- * Also on One-Stop Planner
- ■ Also Available in Spanish
- ♦ Requires Advance Prep

SKILLS DEVELOPMENT RESOURCES	LESSON REVIEW AND ASSESSMENT	STANDARDS CORRELATION
		National Health Education Standards
TE Life Skill Builder, pp. 375, 376 `GENERAL` TE Inclusions Strategies, p. 377 `BASIC` CRF Cross-Disciplinary * `GENERAL` CRF Directed Reading * `BASIC`	SE Lesson Review, p. 377 TE Reteaching, Quiz, p. 377 CRF Lesson Quiz * ■ `GENERAL`	1.1, 3.4, 3.5, 3.6, 5.6, 5.7
CRF Cross-Disciplinary * `GENERAL` CRF Directed Reading * `BASIC`	SE Lesson Review, p. 379 TE Reteaching, Quiz, p. 379 CRF Lesson Quiz * ■ `GENERAL`	1.1, 3.4, 3.5
SE Life Skills Activity Communicating Effectively, p. 381 TE Reading Skill Builder Paired Summarizing, p. 381 `BASIC` TE Life Skill Builder Practicing Wellness, p. 381 CRF Refusal Skills * `GENERAL` CRF Directed Reading * `BASIC`	SE Lesson Review, p. 383 TE Reteaching, Quiz, p. 383 TE Alternative Assessment, p. 383 `GENERAL` CRF Lesson Quiz * ■ `GENERAL`	1.1, 3.4, 3.5
TE Life Skill Builder Practicing Wellness, p. 385 TE Life Skill Builder Being a Wise Consumer, p. 386 `GENERAL` CRF Refusal Skills * `GENERAL` CRF Directed Reading * `BASIC`	SE Lesson Review, p. 387 TE Reteaching, Quiz, p. 387 TE Alternative Assessment, p. 387 `GENERAL` CRF Concept Mapping * `GENERAL` CRF Lesson Quiz * ■ `GENERAL`	1.1, 3.4, 3.5
SE Life Skills Activity Communicating Effectively, p. 390 CRF Directed Reading * `BASIC`	SE Lesson Review, p. 391 TE Reteaching, Quiz, p. 391 CRF Lesson Quiz * ■ `GENERAL`	1.1, 3.4, 3.5
SE Life Skills Activity Practicing Wellness, p. 393 TE Inclusion Strategies, p. 393 ♦ `BASIC` CRF Decision-Making * `GENERAL` CRF Directed Reading * `BASIC`	SE Lesson Review, p. 393 TE Reteaching, Quiz, p. 393 CRF Concept Mapping * `GENERAL` CRF Lesson Quiz * ■ `GENERAL`	1.1, 3.4, 3.5
TE Reading Skill Builder Reading Organizer, p. 395 `BASIC` TE Life Skill Builder, pp. 395, 396 `ADVANCED` CRF Decision-Making * `GENERAL` CRF Directed Reading * `BASIC`	SE Lesson Review, p. 397 TE Reteaching, Quiz, p. 397 TE Alternative Assessment, p. 397 `GENERAL` CRF Lesson Quiz * ■ `GENERAL`	1.7, 2.6, 3.5
TE Life Skill Builder Making Good Decisions, p. 399 `GENERAL` CRF Directed Reading * `BASIC`	SE Lesson Review, p. 401 TE Reteaching, Quiz, p. 401 CRF Lesson Quiz * ■ `GENERAL`	1.7, 2.6, 3.5

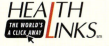

www.scilinks.org/health

Maintained by the **National Science Teachers Association**

Topic: Air Bags
HealthLinks code: HD4006

Topic: First Aid
HealthLinks code: HD4042

Topic: Fires
HealthLinks code: HD4041

Topic: Safety
HealthLinks code: HD4084

Technology Resources

One-Stop Planner
All of your printable resources and the Test Generator are on this convenient CD-ROM.

 Guided Reading Audio CDs

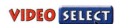

For information about videos related to this chapter, go to **go.hrw.com** and type in the keyword **HD4SA7V**.

Chapter 17 • Chapter Planning Guide **371B**

Chapter 17: Your Personal Safety
Chapter Resources

Teacher Resources

TEACHING TRANSPARENCIES

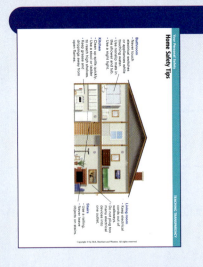
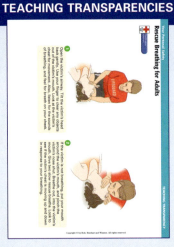
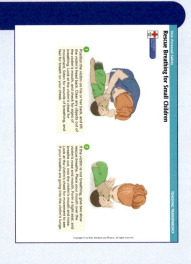

BELLRINGER TRANSPARENCIES

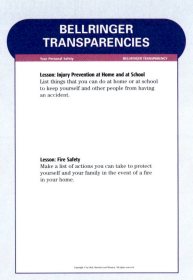

LESSON PLANS
PARENT LETTER
TEST ITEM LISTING

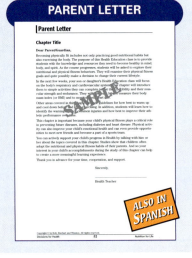
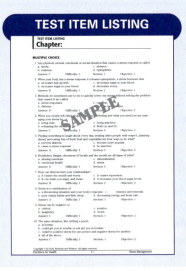

Meeting Individual Needs

DIRECTED READING
CONCEPT MAPPING
CONCEPT REVIEW
ENRICHMENT ACTIVITIES

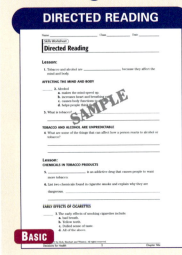
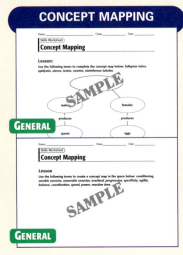
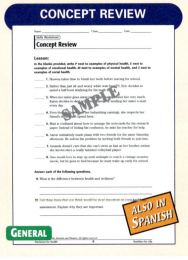
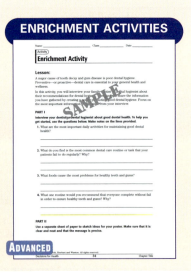

Resources

These worksheet pages can be found in the Chapter Resource File and the One-Stop Planner. The transparencies can be found in the Teaching Transparencies binder and on the One-Stop Planner.

Activities

LIFE SKILLS ACTIVITIES
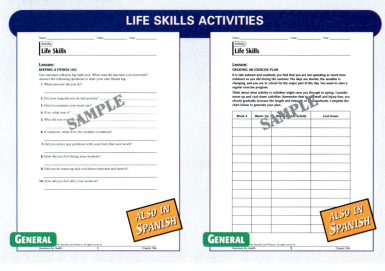

AT-HOME ACTIVITY
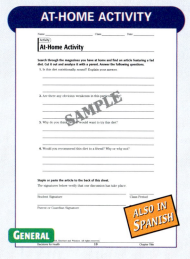

DATASHEETS FOR IN-TEXT ACTIVITIES
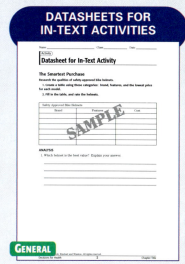

Applications

DECISION-MAKING
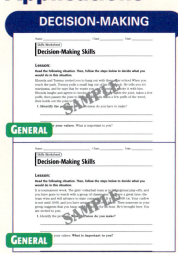

REFUSAL SKILLS
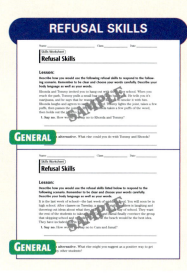

CROSS-DISCIPLINARY
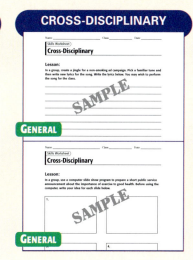

HEALTH BEHAVIOR CONTRACT
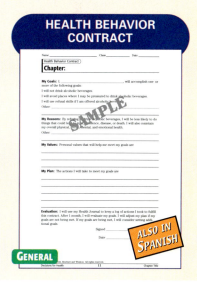

Assessments

HEALTH INVENTORY
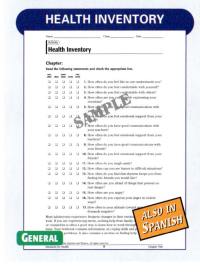

LESSON QUIZZES
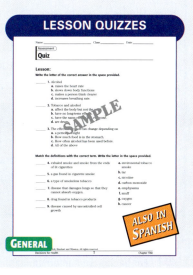

CHAPTER TEST
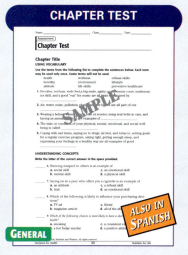

PERFORMANCE-BASED ASSESSMENT
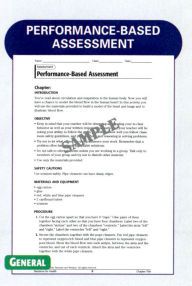

Chapter 17 • Chapter Resources and Worksheets   371D

CHAPTER 17 — Background Information

The following information focuses on fires, tornadoes, and hurricanes. This material will help prepare you for teaching the concepts in this chapter.

Fires

- Fires in the home can be caused by overheated or overloaded electrical wires, open flames, improper disposal of smoking materials, unattended outdoor and fireplace fires, damaged appliances, and accidents when cooking. Some fires are caused by unsupervised children playing with matches.

- Fires in the home are more likely to occur in the winter months. Many of these fires occur when portable heaters, kerosene heaters, fireplaces, and wood stoves are used improperly or malfunction.

- Most residential fires start in the kitchen. Some fires start when all the liquid boils out of a pan and the remaining food burns. A grease fire starts when oily or greasy foods are cooked at too high a temperature. Water will cause grease to splatter and spread. So, a fire extinguisher, salt, baking soda, or a pan lid should be used to smother a grease fire. An oven fire usually remains contained if the oven is not opened. In a closed oven, a fire will run out of oxygen and stop burning.

- About 600 children under the age of 14 die in residential fires each year. Nearly 40,000 children are injured. The majority of these injuries and deaths are caused by smoke inhalation. Many of the rest are caused by burns.

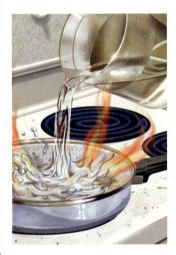 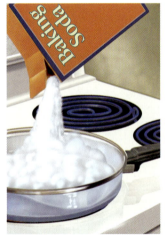

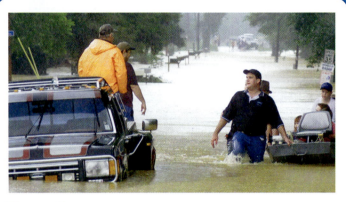

Tornadoes

- In most tornadoes, wind speeds are less than 112 miles per hour. Tornadoes are usually about 400 to 500 feet wide. Rarely, tornadoes reach the width of 1 mile. The average tornado lasts less than 10 minutes. Some may last a few seconds, and others last over an hour.

- Tornadoes are given a rating based on the Fujita scale, or the F-scale. In theory, tornadoes can have ratings between F1 and F12. However, in practice, tornadoes are rated from F1 to F5, F5 being the most severe. A tornado's rating on the F-scale is based on wind speed and the damage the tornado causes. However, because tornado wind speeds are often unknown and damage assessment is often subjective, the F-scale is flawed. But it remains the only way to rate tornadoes until scientists have the ability to accurately measure ground-level wind speeds of tornadoes.

Hurricanes

- The rising ocean water ahead of a hurricane is called the *storm surge*. Storm surges often cause coastal flooding. Hurricanes often also cause heavy rainfall. This rainfall can cause inland flooding hundreds of miles from the coast.

- The strength of a hurricane is expressed by categories that relate wind speeds and potential damage. A Category 1 hurricane has slower wind speeds than storms in higher categories. A Category 4 hurricane has wind speeds between 131 and 155 miles per hour. A Category 4 hurricane will cause 100 times more damage than a Category 1 storm.

For background information about teaching strategies and issues, refer to the *Professional Reference for Teachers*.

ACTIVITIES

CHAPTER 17

Consider using the activities on this page as students explore the lessons of this chapter. Look for other activities throughout the Student Edition chapter.

Comparing Sunscreens

Procedure Have students work in groups of four. Provide each group with a different bottle of sunscreen. Tell students that the products that protect the best block long and short wavelengths of UV light, or UVA and UVB wavelengths. Also, an effective sunscreen will have an SPF, or sun protection factor, of 15 or higher.

Have groups examine the label on their bottle of sunscreen. Students should describe the product. Then, students should identify whether the sunscreen protects against UVA and UVB wavelengths. They should also identify the SPF of the sunscreen, whether it is waterproof, and whether it is sweatproof. Have students smell and feel the sunscreen and rate how they like it. Finally, have the students compile their findings in a consumer report.

Safety Caution: Students with sensitive skin may be allergic to some sunscreens. Exempt these students from the testing portion of the activity.

Analysis Ask the following questions:

- What does SPF stand for? (sun protection factor)
- What is the range of SPFs? (Answers may vary, but most products have SPFs ranging from 4 to 45.)
- If a higher SPF offers more protection, who should use a sunscreen with a very high SPF? (Sample answer: People who burn easily or are in areas with bright sunlight should use a higher SPF.)
- Under what conditions might you need to apply sunscreen more often? (Sample answer: If you are outside for a long time, in the water for a long time, or sweating a lot, you may want to reapply your sunscreen.)

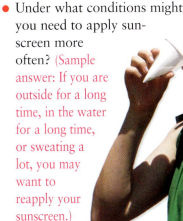

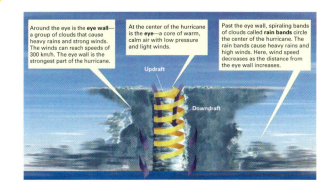

Building a Hurricane-Proof House

Procedure Tell students that thousands of homes are damaged by hurricanes each year. Tell students that their job is to design and build the most wind-resistant building they can. It should be able to withstand a hurricane.

Have students work in groups of four. Give each group construction paper, straws, a glue stick, and cellophane tape. Give each team a plastic foam tray, which they can use as a base. Then, have students design and build their homes. Have them draw a top and side view on the construction paper.

To test the homes, have students take their homes outside. Secure the base of each home, and use a leaf blower to test it. From ten feet away, the leaf blower can model a tropical storm. Up close, it models a high-category hurricane. Turn the leaf blower on every side of the home to see if it can withstand the winds of a hurricane.

Analysis Ask the following questions:

- How did you decide how to build your home? (Accept all reasonable answers.)
- What type of construction resulted in a more wind-resistant home? (Sample answer: More rounded, or domelike homes were more wind-resistant.)
- Should extra money be spent to make new homes in coastal areas more wind resistant? Why or why not? (Accept all reasonable answers. Sample answer: Yes, because then there would be less damage to homes during a hurricane.)

CHAPTER 17

Overview
Tell students that this chapter will help them learn about preventing accidents at home, at school, on the road, and outdoors. Students will also learn about fire safety and natural disasters. Finally, students will learn about emergencies and first aid.

Assessing Prior Knowledge
Students should be familiar with the following topics:
- decision making
- refusal skills
- conflict management

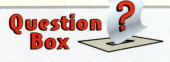

Students may feel more comfortable asking questions if you set up a Question Box to collect their questions. Have students write and anonymously submit their questions about safety, natural disasters, and first aid. Address these questions during class, or use these questions to introduce lessons that cover related topics.

Current Health
Check out *Current Health* articles and activities related to this chapter by visiting the HRW Web site at **go.hrw.com.** Just type in the keyword **HD4CH32T**.

Chapter Resource File
- Directed Reading BASIC
- Health Inventory GENERAL
- Parent Letter

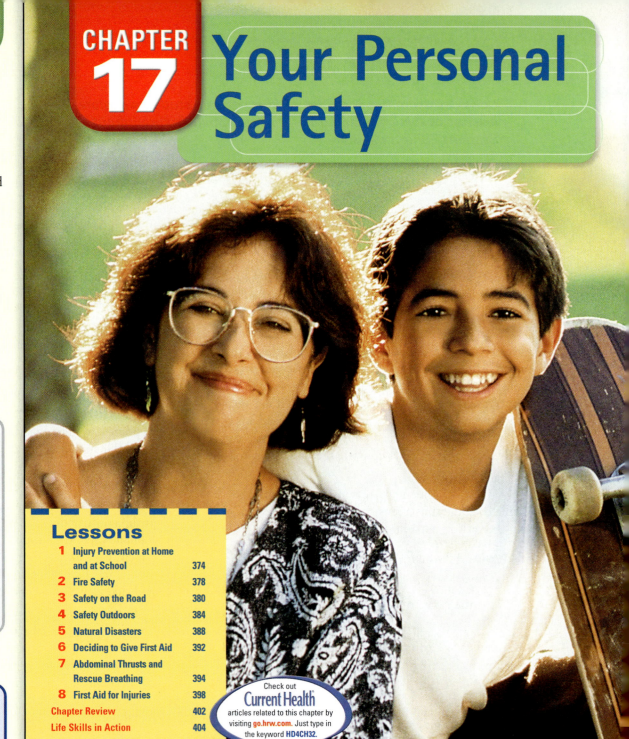

CHAPTER 17 Your Personal Safety

Lessons
1	Injury Prevention at Home and at School	374
2	Fire Safety	378
3	Safety on the Road	380
4	Safety Outdoors	384
5	Natural Disasters	388
6	Deciding to Give First Aid	392
7	Abdominal Thrusts and Rescue Breathing	394
8	First Aid for Injuries	398
	Chapter Review	402
	Life Skills in Action	404

Check out *Current Health* articles related to this chapter by visiting **go.hrw.com.** Just type in the keyword **HD4CH32**.

Standards Correlations

National Health Education Standards

1.1 (partial) Explain the relationship between positive health behaviors and the prevention of injury, illness, disease, and premature death. (Lessons 1–6)

1.7 (partial) Explain how appropriate health care can prevent premature death and disability. (Lessons 7–8)

2.6 Describe situations requiring professional health services. (Lessons 7–8)

3.4 Demonstrate strategies to improve or maintain personal and family health. (Lessons 1–6)

3.5 Develop injury prevention and management strategies for personal and family health. (Lessons 1–8)

3.6 Demonstrate ways to avoid and reduce threatening situations. (Lesson 1)

5.6 (partial) Demonstrate refusal and negotiation skills to enhance health. (Lesson 1)

5.7 Analyze the possible causes of conflict among youth in schools and communities. (Lesson 1)

" My mom **worries** about me when I go **skateboarding.**

So, I make sure I skateboard **safely.** I always use my helmet, elbow pads, knee pads, and wrist guards. And I always go with a group of my friends. Mom also worries less when I tell her where I'll be. "

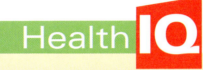

PRE-READING
Answer the following multiple-choice questions to find out what you already know about safety. When you've finished this chapter, you'll have the opportunity to change your answers based on what you've learned.

1. What can you do to avoid violence at school?
   a. walk away
   b. use conflict management skills
   c. tell an adult
   d. all of the above

2. To give first aid for a cut, you should
   a. use sterile gloves.
   b. remove soaked gauze.
   c. always elevate the injured limb.
   d. None of the above

3. Which of the following should NOT be used on a grease fire?
   a. fire extinguisher
   b. salt
   c. water
   d. baking soda

4. A second-degree burn
   a. affects all layers of skin.
   b. forms blisters.
   c. looks dark or dry and white.
   d. affects the top layer of skin.

5. Which of the following should NOT be done to save a choking infant?
   a. firm blows to the infant's back with the heel of your hand
   b. thrusts to the breastbone
   c. removing the object from the infant's mouth using your fingers
   d. none of the above

6. A below-normal body temperature is called
   a. frostbite.
   b. heat exhaustion.
   c. hypothermia.
   d. heatstroke.

ANSWERS: 1. d; 2. a; 3. c; 4. b; 5. c; 6. c

Using the Health IQ

Misconception Alert
Answers to the Health IQ questions may help you identify students' misconceptions.

Question 2: Some students may think that they should remove soaked gauze from a cut. However, if blood has stopped flowing or if it has slowed, removing the gauze could make the cut bleed more. Also, a limb should not be elevated if doing so makes the injury worse.

Question 3: Some students may think that they can use water to put out a grease fire. However, using water on a grease fire can cause it to spread. To put out a grease fire, students should use a fire extinguisher, salt, or baking soda.

Question 5: Some students may not realize that using their fingers to remove an object from an infant's mouth can push the object further into the infant's throat. Be sure to emphasize that students should not use their fingers to remove an object from an infant's mouth.

Answers
1. d
2. a
3. c
4. b
5. c
6. c

For information about videos related to this chapter, go to **go.hrw.com** and type in the keyword **HD4SA7V**.

Lesson 1 Focus

Overview
Before beginning this lesson, review with your students the objectives listed under the What You'll Do head in the Student Edition. In this lesson, students will learn about accidents and injuries that can happen at home and at school. They will also learn about gun safety and seven ways to protect themselves from injury.

Bellringer
Ask students to list things that they can do at home or at school to keep themselves and other people from having an accident. (Accept all reasonable answers. Sample answers: I can pick up my things. I can wipe up spills. I can tell an adult if there is a dangerous situation.) **LS** Verbal

Answer to Start Off Write
Accept all reasonable answers. Sample answer: I can stay away from violent people and violent places. I can also tell an adult if I am having trouble avoiding violence.

Motivate

Group Activity —— GENERAL
Skit Have students work in groups of four. Ask groups to write and perform a skit about safety at school. Skits should address lab and shop safety or violence in school. Consider asking students to perform their skits for a school assembly. **LS** Interpersonal/Kinesthetic

---

Lesson 1 — Injury Prevention at Home and at School

What You'll Do
- **Identify** four accidents that happen at home.
- **Describe** two risks at school.
- **List** five ways to avoid violence.
- **Describe** what you should do if you find a gun.
- **List** seven ways to protect yourself from injury.

Terms to Learn
- accident
- violence

Start Off Write
How can you avoid violent situations at school?

Yuli has a 2-year-old brother. Yuli and his family do a lot to make sure that Yuli's brother doesn't get hurt. They're careful to pick up anything he might choke on and to close cabinet doors.

Yuli and his family are trying to make sure that Yuli's brother doesn't have an accident. An **accident** is an unexpected event that may lead to injury.

Accidents at Home
Many accidents can happen at home. The following are four common types:

- **Falls** The most common accidents are falls. Move objects out of walkways, and wipe up spills to prevent falls.
- **Fires** Burns and smoke inhalation from fires can lead to death. Open flames, unattended stoves, and some chemicals can cause fires.
- **Electrocution** (ee LEK truh KYOO shuhn) Bare wires and overloaded outlets can cause electrocution. Also, using electrical appliances near water can lead to electrocution.
- **Poisoning** Household chemicals can cause poisoning if they are mistaken for something that is safe to eat or drink. Medicines can poison someone if taken incorrectly.

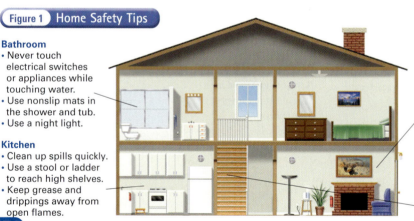

Figure 1 Home Safety Tips

Bathroom
- Never touch electrical switches or appliances while touching water.
- Use nonslip mats in the shower and tub.
- Use a night light.

Kitchen
- Clean up spills quickly.
- Use a stool or ladder to reach high shelves.
- Keep grease and drippings away from open flames.

Living room
- Keep electrical cords out of walkways.
- Do not plug too many electrical devices into one outlet.

Stairs
- Use a railing.
- Never leave objects on stairs.

REAL-LIFE CONNECTION —— BASIC
Home-Safety Survey Ask students to survey the potential accidents in their homes. Students should identify the most common type of potential accident. Then, students should write a proposal addressed to their families. Their proposals should describe potential accidents and what the members of the family can do to ensure that everyone is safe. **LS** Verbal/Interpersonal

Chapter Resource File
- Directed Reading BASIC
- Lesson Plan
- Lesson Quiz GENERAL

Transparencies
TT Bellringer
TT Home Safety Tips

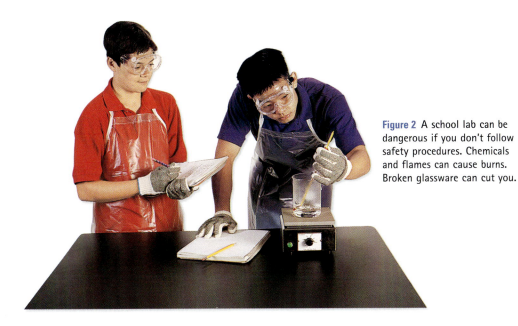

Figure 2 A school lab can be dangerous if you don't follow safety procedures. Chemicals and flames can cause burns. Broken glassware can cut you.

Safety in Class

Many of the injuries that happen at home can also happen at school. But some accidents are more likely to happen only at school. For example, injuries can happen during a lab class or in the wood shop. Glass containers, Bunsen burners, and chemicals can cause injury during a lab class. A shop class has dangerous equipment, such as saws. You should follow your teacher's instructions to avoid injury. You should also wear safety equipment, such as goggles, aprons, and gloves, to avoid injury.

Violence at School

Using physical force to hurt someone or to cause damage is called **violence**. Anger, stress, illegal drugs, prejudice, and peer pressure may make someone act violently. *Gangs* are groups of people who often use violence.

The best way to avoid violence or gangs is to walk away from any situation that could become violent. You can also use your refusal skills and your conflict management skills to avoid violence. Some situations are hard to handle on your own. If you don't think you can avoid violence, talk to your parents or a school counselor. One of the best ways to avoid violence and gangs is to look for positive alternatives. Join the school band or a sports team. Start a new club. Volunteer at the local nursing home or food bank.

Health Journal
Write about a time when you or someone you know got hurt accidentally at home or in class. Describe how the accident could have been avoided.

LIFE SCIENCE CONNECTION — ADVANCED

Poisons Different poisons enter the body in different ways. For example, a poison may be eaten, drunk, inhaled, or absorbed through the skin. Ask interested students to list some common poisons that enter the body in each of these ways. Students should also identify the recommended care for a victim of each poison. Have students create a table to present their findings. **LS Verbal**

Teach

Discussion — GENERAL
Classroom Safety Ask students which school classes have more safety requirements than others. (Accept all reasonable answers. Students will likely mention laboratory and shop classes. Some students may mention home economics or physical education classes.) Ask students to describe some of the precautions they need to take in a science classroom during a laboratory experiment. (Sample answer: I need to wear goggles to protect my eyes. Also, I wear gloves to protect my hands. Sometimes, I wear an apron over my clothes to protect my body.) **LS Verbal**

Activity — BASIC
Positive Reinforcement Have students work in pairs. Ask students to take turns telling each other what they will do to avoid violence. Students should provide each other with positive encouragement. **LS Intrapersonal/Interpersonal**

Life SKILL BUILDER — GENERAL
Communicating Effectively Ask students to interview a lab teacher, shop teacher, or school guidance counselor about school safety. Students should identify the steps they can take to ensure their personal safety and what the person they are interviewing is responsible for when ensuring the safety of students. Ask students to write a magazine article about their findings.
LS Interpersonal/Verbal

Answer to Health Journal
Answers may vary. This Health Journal can be used to begin a class discussion on accidents in school. Remember that some students may be uncomfortable sharing personal information.

Lesson 1 • Injury Prevention at Home and at School

Teach, continued

Sensitivity ALERT

Some students may be uncomfortable talking about guns. This is especially true if students have experienced gun violence. Consider inviting a school guidance counselor to take part in the class discussion regarding gun safety.

Demonstration — BASIC

Police Officer Ask a local police officer to come to the classroom and give a presentation about gun safety. The presentation should address what students should do if they ever find a gun and what they should do if their parents keep guns in the home. **LS Verbal**

Life SKILL BUILDER — GENERAL

Making Good Decisions Ask students to apply their decision-making skills to the following scenario: "Stephanie, Angela, Clay, and Gabe usually walk home from school together. Sometimes, they take a short cut through the park. One day, they found a gun on the ground behind one of the trash cans in the park. What should they do?" (Sample answer: Stephanie, Angela, Clay, and Gabe should not touch the gun. They should find a trusted adult and tell him or her about the gun right away.) **LS Verbal**

Gun Safety

Maybe you've seen articles or news reports about school shootings. School shootings don't happen very often. In fact, many gun-related injuries are accidental. Guns are dangerous. But you can do the following to stay safer:

- Avoid guns. If you find a gun, walk away and tell an adult right away. Don't touch the gun.
- Lock up guns in the home. If your parents have a gun, ask them to keep it locked up. Also, ask your parents to keep the gun unloaded.
- Many families hunt or shoot together. Before you go hunting, take a class in gun safety. A shooting range or local organization may offer these classes.
- Always hunt or shoot with an experienced adult. You should never use a gun without supervision.

Guns have no place in school. School shootings are frightening reminders of the harm that guns can do. Maybe you know about a student carrying a gun to school. If so, let an adult know. You should also tell an adult if you hear a student talking about hurting others. The student may just be joking. He or she may not actually want to hurt someone else. But don't take the risk. When you tell an adult, you're not just protecting yourself. You're also protecting other people.

Brain Food

In 1999, about 4 percent of unintentional deaths of 10- to 14-year-olds in the United States were caused by gunshot wounds.

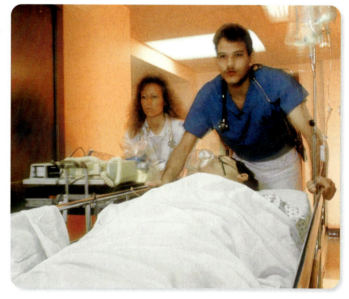

Figure 3 Each year, thousands of people visit the hospital with gunshot wounds.

376

LANGUAGE ARTS CONNECTION — GENERAL

Poetry Have students write a poem to express their feelings about the violence in their school or community or in the world. Have volunteers share their poems with the class. Invite discussion about the usefulness of poetry for expressing feelings about difficult subjects. Remember that some students may be uncomfortable sharing personal information. **LS Verbal/Intrapersonal**

Seven Ways to Protect Yourself

Many accidents don't cause an injury. But some accidents can be very serious. People have accidents every day, but you can avoid many accidents. The following are seven things you can do to stay safer:

1. **Think before you act.** Think about the consequences of your actions. Don't do something you know is dangerous.
2. **Pay attention.** Be aware of your surroundings. Look out for dangers around you.
3. **Know your limits.** Some things are safe only if you know what you're doing. Don't do something you know you aren't ready to do.
4. **Practice refusal skills.** Learn to say no when something is not safe.
5. **Use safety equipment.** Safety equipment helps keep you from getting hurt.
6. **Change risky behavior.** Change bad habits that put you or anyone else at risk.
7. **Change risky situations.** If you see a risky situation, try to fix it. Or, if you can't fix it, tell an adult about it.

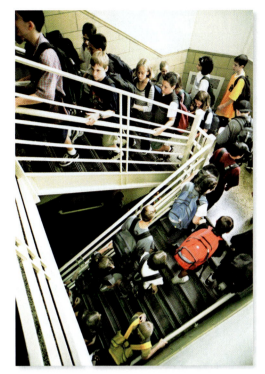

Figure 4 A busy school hallway provides plenty of opportunities for a person to have an accident.

Lesson Review

Using Vocabulary
1. What is an accident?
2. Define *violence*.

Understanding Concepts
3. Describe four common accidents.
4. What are two risky places at school? What could cause injuries in these two places?
5. List seven ways to avoid accidents.

Critical Thinking
6. **Making Good Decisions** Teddy's family goes hunting in the fall. Teddy has taken a gun safety class. If he finds an unlocked gun, what should he do?
7. **Applying Concepts** Identify the possible accidents in the following scenario: Fred's brother left his robe on the bathroom floor and the hairdryer next to the tub. Also, Fred's brother didn't wipe off the floor after he took a shower.

internet connect
www.scilinks.org/health
Topic: Safety
HealthLinks code: HD4084
HEALTH LINKS. Maintained by the National Science Teachers Association

Lesson 2

Focus

Overview
Before beginning this lesson, review with your students the objectives listed under the What You'll Do head in the Student Edition. In this lesson, students will learn about fire safety. They will also learn about putting out small fires.

Bellringer
Have students write down what they can do to protect themselves and their families in the event of a fire in their homes. **Verbal**

Answer to Start Off Write
Accept all reasonable answers. Sample answer: Use baking soda, salt, or a pan lid to smother the fire.

Motivate

Discussion — GENERAL
Fire Drills Ask students what they should do if there is a fire at school. (Sample answers: If the fire has not been reported, I should report it to an adult. If the fire alarm goes off, I should follow the school's fire drill procedures.) Ask students where they are supposed to go from the classroom if the fire alarm goes off. (Answers may vary, but make sure students understand the proper escape route from the classroom.) Find out if students know where to go from each of their other classrooms. Discuss what they should do if they do not know the escape routes. (Students may suggest asking the teacher in each room. They may also mention that fire drill procedures should be posted in every room.) **Verbal**

Lesson 2 — Fire Safety

What You'll Do
- **Describe** two devices that protect you from fire.
- **List** four ways to put out small fires.

Terms to Learn
- smoke detector
- fire extinguisher

Start Off Write
How should you put out a grease fire?

Tori and her family sat down one evening and made a family evacuation plan. They drew a map of the house with ways to escape in case of a fire. They even started practicing their evacuation plan once a month.

Many people don't understand how dangerous fire is. Fire can spread quickly and cause a lot of damage.

Fire Prevention and Detection
Many things can cause fires. Open flames, unattended stoves, overloaded circuits, and even a large pile of newspaper can start a fire. Avoiding these situations can help you stay safe.

Not all fires can be avoided. But if you have smoke detectors in your home, you will know about fires when they happen. A **smoke detector** is an alarm that detects smoke from a fire. Ask your parents to install smoke detectors in every major room of your house. Check the smoke detectors monthly to make sure they still work. Replace the batteries once a year or as needed.

What do you do when the smoke detector goes off? You need to get out of the building right away! Your family should make a family evacuation plan and practice it. This plan will help you get out of the building faster during a fire. Never go back into the building once you've left.

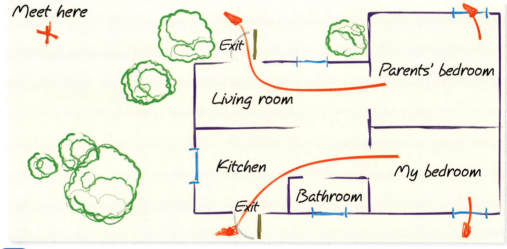

Figure 5 A fire evacuation plan can save your life.

MATH CONNECTION — GENERAL
Fire Department Activity Tell students that in the United States, fire departments respond to almost four fires each minute. Have students calculate about how many fires firefighters respond to in:

- one hour (240 fires; 4 fires × 60 minutes)
- one day (5,760 fires; 240 fires × 24 hours)
- one 30-day month (172,800 fires; 5,760 fires × 30 days)
- one year (2,102,400 fires; 5,760 fires × 365 days)

Logical

Chapter Resource File
- Directed Reading BASIC
- Lesson Plan
- Lesson Quiz GENERAL

Transparencies
TT Bellringer

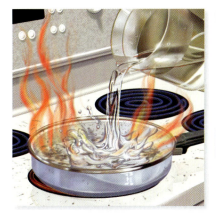
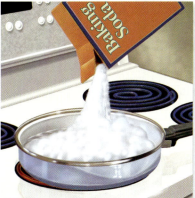

Figure 6 Grease floats on water. So, if you try to put out a grease fire by using water, the fire will spread. Instead, use baking soda or salt to smother the fire. You can also put the lid over the pan.

How to Put Out Small Fires

Some fires are small enough to be put out with a fire extinguisher. A **fire extinguisher** is a device that releases chemicals to put out a fire. You should put fire extinguishers in areas where fires are likely to start, such as the kitchen. Read the instructions on the fire extinguisher. Then, you'll know how to use it. Also, have your fire extinguisher checked each year to make sure it still works.

You can use the fire extinguisher to put out a small fire. You can also use water, baking soda, or salt to smother a fire. But don't use water on a grease fire. The figure above discusses how to put out a grease fire.

Putting out a fire can be dangerous. If you have any doubts about whether you can put a fire out, leave the building. Call for help from a neighbor's home. Do not go back into the building.

Health Journal
Walk through your home. Make a list of some fire hazards that you see. Describe ways you can fix them.

Lesson Review

Using Vocabulary
1. How do a smoke detector and fire extinguisher protect you?

Understanding Concepts
2. List four ways to put out small fires.

3. Why should you have a family evacuation plan?

Critical Thinking
4. **Applying Concepts** Kira is cooking some bacon when it catches on fire. The fire is not a very big fire. What should Kira do?

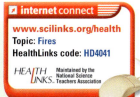

internet connect
www.scilinks.org/health
Topic: Fires
HealthLinks code: HD4041
HEALTH LINKS. Maintained by the National Science Teachers Association

Lesson 3

Focus

Overview
Before beginning this lesson, review with your students the objectives listed under the What You'll Do head in the Student Edition. In this lesson, students will learn about walking, cycling, and skating safety. They will also learn about safety in automobiles and buses.

Bellringer
Have students list ways they stay safe when they are walking home from school, cycling, skating, and riding in a car or bus. (Sample answers: I always look both ways. I wear a helmet. I wear bright clothes. I always use my seat belt. I don't distract the driver.) **LS Verbal**

Answer to Start Off Write
Accept all reasonable answers. Sample answer: A bicycle helmet protects your head if you have an accident.

Motivate

Group Activity — GENERAL
Teaching Others Have students work in groups of four. Ask groups to write newsletters for younger children. The newsletters should include articles, puzzles, comic strips, coloring pages, poems, and other materials about staying safe while walking to school. Ask students who speak other languages to translate the newsletters. **LS Visual/Verbal** Co-op Learning   English Language Learners

---

Lesson 3 — Safety on the Road

Donnie has been teaching his younger sister, Katy, about road safety. He wants to make sure she is safe when she walks to school. He showed Katy how to use the crosswalk.

What You'll Do
- **Describe** seven ways to protect yourself while walking.
- **Explain** why you should use a helmet while cycling and skating.
- **Describe** how seat belts and air bags protect you.
- **List** four bus safety practices.

Start Off Write
Why do you think it is important to wear a bicycle helmet every time you ride your bike?

Donnie is teaching Katy how to stay safe near a road. Roadways are some of the most dangerous areas. People can get hurt while walking, riding a bike, skating, or riding in a car.

Safety While Walking
Walking down the street may not seem like a risky activity. But if you don't pay attention, you could get hurt. By paying attention, you'll know when it is safe to cross the street. You'll also be aware of automobile drivers who may not be paying attention to you. Follow these tips to stay safer:

- Use sidewalks when they are available.
- Walk facing the traffic.
- Cross the street only at crosswalks.
- Always look both ways before crossing the street, even if you're in a crosswalk. Before crossing, look for traffic to the left, to the right, and to the left again.
- Make sure the driver can see you if you're crossing in front of a vehicle.
- Try to avoid walking at night. If you must walk somewhere in the dark, wear bright or reflective clothing.
- Don't wear headphones when you're walking. Headphones may keep you from hearing approaching danger.

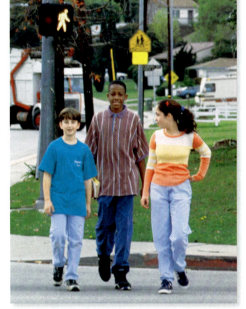
Figure 7 Using the crosswalk reduces your chances of injury.

REAL-LIFE CONNECTION — ADVANCED
Pedestrian Accidents Ask interested students to research the incidence of automobile accidents involving pedestrians and cyclists. Students should identify how often these accidents happen and the incidence per age group. Have students make charts and graphs describing their findings. **LS Visual**

Chapter Resource File
- Directed Reading **BASIC**
- Lesson Plan
- Datasheets for In-Text Activities **GENERAL**
- Lesson Quiz **GENERAL**

Transparencies
TT Bellringer

380   Chapter 17 • Your Personal Safety

Safety on Wheels

Cycling and skating are fun ways to exercise. But more than 300,000 people get hurt each year in cycling accidents. People also get hurt when they are in-line skating or skateboarding.

Head injuries are the most serious type of cycling and skating injury. You should wear a helmet every time you ride or skate, even if you're just going down the street. In fact, many states and cities have laws requiring teens to wear helmets while riding their bikes. Helmets aren't the only way to protect yourself. You should also remember the following safety tips:

- Wear your safety equipment. In addition to helmets, you can use knee and elbow pads to prevent injury. Skaters can also use wrist guards to protect their wrists if they fall.
- Pay attention to traffic. Watch out for busy intersections. If you are riding a bike, walk it through the intersection.
- Follow the rules of the road. For example, cyclists should ride with traffic and follow the same rules as cars do.
- Wear the right clothes. Baggy clothes may get caught in bicycle chains. Wear brightly-colored clothes so that you are visible to traffic.
- Ride and skate only in designated areas. Cyclists should stay to the side of the road. Also, many communities have parks and trails set aside for cyclists and skaters to enjoy.
- Always ride and skate with friends. Friends can help you if you have an accident or if you have a problem with your equipment.
- Avoid riding and skating at night. If you have to ride at night, make sure you have a headlight and blinking taillight on your bike. If you're skating, you should also use a light. Wear bright, reflective clothing.

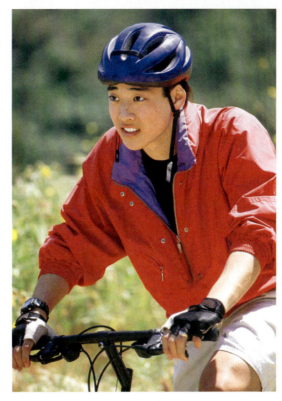

Figure 8 Helmets can keep you from getting seriously hurt if you fall while riding your bike.

LIFE SKILLS ACTIVITY

COMMUNICATING EFFECTIVELY

Imagine that you work for a bicycle, in-line skate, or skateboard company. Design an advertisement for your product that promotes the safe use of your product. Show your ad to your classmates. Does your ad inspire them to use your product safely? If not, how could you improve your ad?

Life SKILL BUILDER

Practicing Wellness A bicycle helmet protects the head in the event of an accident. But if it doesn't fit correctly, the helmet may not provide much protection. Remind students of the following tips about correctly wearing a bicycle helmet:

- Wear the helmet flat on top of your head. It should not be tilted backwards.
- The helmet should fit snuggly. When you move your head, the helmet should not slip.
- The helmet should not block your view. It should not slip forward over your eyes.
- Be sure that the chin-strap buckle is securely fastened.

Teach, continued

Demonstration — BASIC

Seat Belts Put a small doll in a toy car or truck. The doll should not fit too snugly. Place the vehicle at the top of a ramp about 30 cm above the tabletop. Secure a book or another solid object at the bottom of the ramp. Release the toy car. Ask students, "What happened to the doll?" (Sample answer: The doll was thrown out of the car.) Ask how this demonstrates how seat belts can protect people during accidents. (Sample answer: Seat belts can keep you from being thrown out of a car during an accident.) **LS Visual** English Language Learners

Group Activity — ADVANCED

Egg Car Have students work in groups of four. Have students imagine that they are designing a safety device for a new vehicle. The new vehicle must be able to roll down a ramp and into an obstacle without injuring the passenger, a raw egg. Provide students with a toy car and a variety of materials, such as rubber bands, foam peanuts, plastic bags, bubble wrap, and cotton balls. Also provide wood or plastic eggs for practice runs and raw eggs for their final test run. Have groups create an egg-safe vehicle and test it.

Safety Caution: Raw eggs can carry salmonella. Make sure students wash their hands with soap and warm water after the experiment. **LS Kinesthetic**

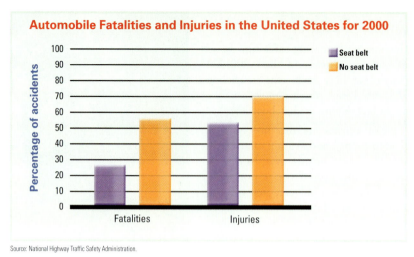

Figure 9 Many people die or get hurt in auto accidents because they are not wearing seat belts.

Vehicle Safety

Did you know that automobile accidents are a leading cause of death for people under age 14? Many of these people weren't wearing their seat belts. Seat belts keep you from being thrown around in a car. They also keep you from being thrown out of the vehicle. You should wear your seat belt every time you ride in a car, truck, or SUV.

Air bags inflate during an accident. Air bags, along with seat belts, keep passengers from hitting the dashboard or windshield. But air bags are made to protect larger people. They may hurt a smaller person. For the best protection, anyone under age 12 should ride in the back seat. Also, infants and smaller children should ride in child safety seats or booster seats until they are big enough to use a seat belt correctly.

Hands-on ACTIVITY

CAR HABITS

1. For 1 week, watch the members of your family when you ride in the car. Write down where each member of your family sits in the car.
2. Write down how often everyone uses a seat belt. Record the length of each trip.

Analysis

1. Did everyone use seat belts? If not, do you think the length of your trip was the reason?
2. Did anyone in your family sit in an unsafe position in the car?
3. How can you promote vehicle safety in your family?

Attention Grabber

Sleep and Driving The following information about sleep and vehicle safety in the United States may interest students:

Each year, about 100,000 automobile crashes, 40,000 injuries, and 1,550 fatalities result from a driver falling asleep between midnight and 6 A.M. These figures do not include accidents that happened during the day, those that involved more than one car or passengers, or those that also involved alcohol.

###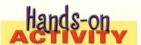

Answer

Accept all reasonable answers.

Extension: Ask students to write a public safety announcement about automobile safety.

Bus Safety

Many teens travel to and from school on a bus. Follow these tips to stay safer.

- Don't distract the driver. He or she needs to concentrate on the road.
- Sit down while the bus is moving. This way you won't fall if the bus goes over a bump or stops suddenly.
- Make sure the driver can see you when you get off the bus. Don't cross the street behind the bus or bend over while in front of the bus.
- Learn where the emergency exits are located. If there is an emergency, follow the driver's instructions.

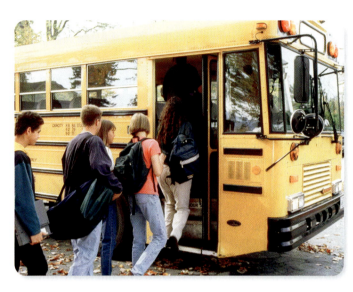

Figure 10 A bus is a convenient way to get to school. By following the safety tips, you can make sure it is a safe trip!

Lesson Review

Understanding Concepts

1. List seven ways to stay safe while walking down the street.
2. Why should you wear a helmet while cycling and skating?
3. How do seat belts and air bags protect you?
4. What are four ways to stay safe when riding the bus?

Critical Thinking

5. **Applying Concepts** Eduardo's parents have a car with air bags. If Eduardo is 11 years old, where in the car should he sit? Eduardo has a 3-year-old sister. Where should she sit?

internet connect
www.scilinks.org/health
Topic: Air Bags
HealthLinks code: HD4006
HEALTH LINKS. Maintained by the National Science Teachers Association

Answers to Lesson Review

1. use sidewalks when they are available, walk facing the traffic, cross the street only at crosswalks, always look both ways before crossing the street, make sure the driver can see you if you cross in front of a vehicle, avoid walking at night, and don't wear headphones when walking
2. Sample answer: Head injuries are the most serious type of cycling and skating injury, so you should wear a helmet to protect your head.
3. Sample answer: Seat belts keep you from being thrown around in a car or being thrown out of a car. Air bags keep you from hitting the dashboard or windshield.
4. don't distract the driver, sit down while the bus is moving, make sure the driver can see you when you get off the bus, and learn where the emergency exits are located
5. Sample answer: Eduardo should sit in the back seat because he is less than 12 years old. Eduardo's 3-year-old sister is probably too small to use a seat belt correctly, so she should sit in a child safety seat or booster seat in the back seat of the car.

REAL-LIFE CONNECTION — BASIC

Bus Rules School bus drivers often post rules that riders are asked to follow. Ask students to make note of the rules the next time they ride the bus. Have them record the rules and then explain how these rules keep bus passengers safe. **LS Visual/Verbal**

Close

Reteaching — BASIC

Chapter Outline Ask students to use the heads in the chapter to write an outline of the material covered. Students should include in their outlines the safety tips described in the chapter. **LS Verbal**

Quiz — GENERAL

1. When riding your bicycle on the street, where should you ride? (Sample answer: You should ride with the traffic and to the side of the road.)
2. Where should you cross a street when walking? (Sample answer: You should cross at a crosswalk.)
3. Where should you cross the street after getting off a school bus? (Sample answer: You should cross in front of the bus so that the bus driver can see you.)
4. Why are air bags risky for children? (Sample answer: Air bags are designed for bigger people. So, they may hurt a smaller person.)

Alternative Assessment — GENERAL

Drawing Cartoons Have students draw a cartoon about two teens riding their bikes. Students should make sure that their cartoons describe the cycling safety tips outlined in the chapter. **LS Visual**

Lesson 3 • Safety on the Road

Lesson 4

Focus

Overview
Before beginning this lesson, review with your students the objectives listed under the What You'll Do head in the Student Edition. In this lesson, students will learn how to stay safe outdoors. They will also learn about safety for cold and hot weather.

Bellringer
Ask students to identify the safety hazards in the following scenario: "Four friends are going camping in Alaska. They are going to an isolated area of Denali National Park. It should be warm during the day, but the temperatures may drop below freezing at night." (Students will likely recognize that going to an isolated area can be risky. Students should also recognize that nighttime temperatures may cause hypothermia.) **LS** Verbal

Answer to Start Off Write
Accept all reasonable answers. Sample answer: I can drink plenty of water and stop to rest in the shade to avoid heat injuries on a hot day.

Motivate

Discussion — GENERAL
Safety Outdoors Ask volunteers to relate some of the risks they have encountered outdoors. Also, ask students to relate some of the injuries they have had while outdoors. Have students relate ways to avoid or deal with some of the situations mentioned. Remember that some students may be uncomfortable sharing personal information. **LS** Verbal

---

Lesson 4 — Safety Outdoors

Jenny was watching a special on TV about climbers on Mount Everest. Some of the climbers died because of the extreme cold.

What You'll Do
- **List** two injuries caused by cold weather.
- **Identify** two injuries caused by hot weather.
- **Describe** three ways to protect yourself while doing outdoor activities.

Terms to Learn
- hypothermia
- frostbite
- heat exhaustion
- heatstroke

Start Off Write
How can you avoid heat-related injuries when you exercise on a hot day?

Winter weather may look pretty in pictures, but it can be dangerous. Hot weather can be dangerous, too.

Safety on a Cold Day

You may have noticed that you shiver when you get cold. Shivering helps keep you warm. But people who are cold for a long time or who get wet on a cold day may develop hypothermia (HIE poh THUHR mee uh). **Hypothermia** is a below-normal body temperature. People who have hypothermia shiver uncontrollably. They also feel sleepy, have slurred speech, and seem confused. A hypothermia victim should be kept warm. Remove any wet clothes, and wrap the victim in dry blankets. Call for help.

Cold weather can also cause frostbite. **Frostbite** is damage to skin and other tissues that is caused by extreme cold. Frostbite usually affects the fingers, toes, ears, or nose. Frostbitten skin is pale, stiff, and numb. If someone has frostbite, call for help. Put the affected area in lukewarm water until help arrives.

You can avoid hypothermia and frostbite by dressing in layers on cold days. Also, wear gloves and a hat to protect your hands and ears. Avoid going outside on extremely cold days. Go inside if you start shivering.

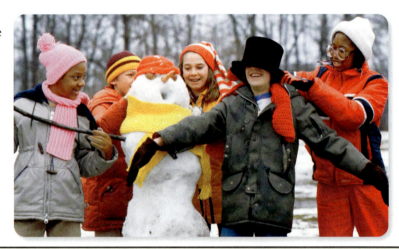

Figure 11 Dressing for the weather can keep you warm on chilly days.

EARTH SCIENCE CONNECTION — ADVANCED
Wind Chill and Heat Index Sometimes, wind and humidity can make a difference in how cold or how hot it feels outside. When it is windy, it feels colder outside. On hot days, higher humidity can make people feel hotter. Ask interested students to research the wind chill factor and the heat index. Students should identify how each relative temperature is calculated. **LS** Verbal

Chapter Resource File
- Directed Reading BASIC
- Lesson Plan
- Lesson Quiz GENERAL

Transparencies
TT Bellringer

384   Chapter 17 • Your Personal Safety

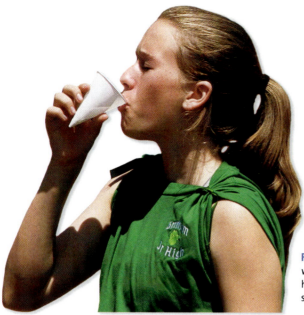

Figure 12 Drinking plenty of water is one way to avoid heat injuries. Also, try to stay in the shade.

Safety on a Hot Day

Summer is a great time to go outside and enjoy exercise. But did you know that summer weather can cause injury? Sometimes, it gets so hot that your body can't keep cool. If you can't stay cool, you can develop heat exhaustion (eg ZAWS chuhn) or heatstroke.

Heat exhaustion is a condition caused by too much water loss through sweating on a hot day. On hot days, your body absorbs heat from the sun and the air. Exercising makes you even warmer. Sweating helps your body cool down. But if you don't drink enough water to replace the water you lose as sweat, you may get heat exhaustion. Signs of heat exhaustion include headache, dizziness, nausea, and clammy skin. The best way to treat heat exhaustion is to stop exercising. Go inside, and drink cool fluids. If the symptoms do not improve, call for help.

Heatstroke is an injury that happens when the body cannot control its temperature. A person who has heatstroke can't sweat. His or her body temperature rises. The signs of heatstroke are high fever and dry skin. Sometimes, a victim may collapse and have convulsions. Someone with heatstroke should be taken to a doctor right away. Heatstroke can be life threatening.

The best way to avoid heat injuries is to drink plenty of water. Take plenty of breaks in the shade. If you're outside for a long time, you may also want to eat. Water and food help your body keep you cool.

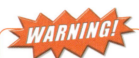

Heatstroke

Adolescents are more likely to get heatstroke than adults are. Your body is still developing, so your body's cooling system is not as advanced as an adult's system is. Because your body doesn't cool as efficiently as an adult's body does, you should be very careful on hot days.

Life SKILL BUILDER

Practicing Wellness Traveling during a snowstorm can be dangerous. Suggest the following tips for winter safety:

- Ask your parents to keep a winter emergency kit in the car. It should include warm blankets, gloves, hats, signal flares, water, and some nonperishable food.
- If you're stuck in the car, wrap yourself in blankets. Wear a hat and gloves to protect your head and hands. If there are other people in the car, sit close together to conserve body warmth.
- If you're stuck in the car, don't sleep.
- If you're stuck in the car, run the motor and heater for 10 minutes each hour. Open the window a crack when the heater is on.
- If you're stuck in the car, move your arms and legs to improve circulation and stay warmer.

Teach

Group Activity —— GENERAL

Dark and Light Clothing Have students work in groups of four. Ask students to fill two beakers with the same volume of water. Then, students should put a thermometer in each beaker and record the temperature. Have groups cover one beaker with black construction paper and the other beaker with white construction paper. Students should then place the beakers in bright sunlight. Have them record the temperature in the beakers every five minutes for half an hour. After students finish the activity, ask them the following:

- Did one beaker have a higher temperature than the other? If so, which one? (Sample answer: The beaker that was covered in black paper had a higher temperature.)
- Why do you think there was a temperature difference between the beakers? (Sample answer: Black objects absorb sunlight while white objects reflect it.)
- How does this information affect the clothing you will chose to wear on a hot day? (Sample answer: I will wear light-colored clothing on a hot day because it will help keep me cooler than dark clothing.)

LS Kinesthetic/Logical

LIFE SCIENCE CONNECTION —— ADVANCED

Water and Temperature Regulation Ask interested students to research how water is important to the function of the body. In particular, have students focus on the role of water in regulating the temperature of the body. Have students create a visual presentation to share with the class. **LS** Visual/Verbal

Lesson 4 • Safety Outdoors **385**

Teach, continued

Using the Figure — BASIC

Skit Organize the class into four groups. Assign each group one of the lists of safety tips in the figure on these pages. Have groups write and perform a skit based on their assigned safety tips. Students' skits should address a situation in which someone has done something unsafe while outdoors.
LS Verbal/Interpersonal
Co-op Learning

LIFE SCIENCE CONNECTION — ADVANCED

Fluid Intake Ask interested students to research the fluid needs of the body. Students should identify how much fluid people need to consume to replace fluid lost through exertion or sweating. For example, students could examine the fluid needs of someone who is hiking, someone who is cycling, or someone who is skiing. Have students create a table showing their findings. **LS** Verbal

REAL-LIFE CONNECTION — GENERAL

Dangerous Wildlife Ask interested students to identify the dangerous wildlife that people may encounter when they are hiking locally. Students should also identify what people should do if they encounter these animals. Have students make a poster about their findings. **LS** Visual

---

Figure 13 Playing It Safe Outdoors

Hiking and Camping Safety

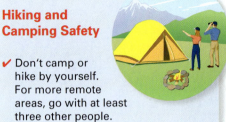

- ✓ Don't camp or hike by yourself. For more remote areas, go with at least three other people.
- ✓ Leave a plan of your activities with friends and park headquarters.
- ✓ Plan for emergencies. Carry emergency signal devices. Know where you can find ranger stations or telephones along your route.
- ✓ Carry a first-aid kit.
- ✓ Carry plenty of food and water.
- ✓ Carry bug repellant and sunscreen.
- ✓ Become familiar with the area. Carry a map and compass.
- ✓ Be aware of dangerous wildlife.
- ✓ Make sure all campfires are properly contained and extinguished.

Water Safety

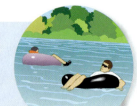

- ✓ Learn to swim.
- ✓ Swim with a buddy.
- ✓ Swim in designated areas. Avoid areas that aren't supervised.
- ✓ Obey posted warning signs.
- ✓ Don't run near water.
- ✓ Don't dive into unfamiliar bodies of water.
- ✓ Swim parallel to shore instead of away from shore.
- ✓ When at the beach, check surf conditions before getting in the water.
- ✓ Watch out for water plants and animals that may be dangerous.
- ✓ Wear a life jacket when boating.

Playing Safe

Outdoor adventures are exciting and fun. But they can be risky, too. The figure above provides some tips for hiking and camping, water safety, skiing and snowboarding, and mountain biking. Remember the following tips whenever you go outside:

- Drink plenty of water. Drinking water is important in both hot and cold weather. Water helps your body regulate its temperature.
- Use sunscreen, even on cold or cloudy days. This will prevent sunburn. Sunscreen can also prevent skin cancer. Wear a hat and sunglasses to protect your head and eyes.
- Watch the weather. Be ready for weather changes. Dress warmly on cold days. Wear light-colored, cool clothes on hot days.

Life SKILL BUILDER — GENERAL

Being a Wise Consumer Bring catalogs for camping clothing to class. Have students examine the catalogs. Ask students, "Did you notice any similarities in the different kinds of camping clothing?" (Students may notice that construction of clothing is similar and designed for comfort. They may also notice that most of the clothing is nylon or another synthetic material.) "Why do you think camping clothing is often made of quick-drying materials?" (Sample answers: These materials may be more comfortable. Also, on a cold day, quick-drying clothes can prevent hypothermia. Some students may note that wearing quick-drying clothes on a hot day helps keep them cooler.) **LS** Verbal

---

386 Chapter 17 • Your Personal Safety

Skiing and Snowboarding Safety

✔ Learn how to use skis and a snowboard.

✔ Ski and snowboard on slopes within your skill level.

✔ Ski and snowboard in designated areas.

✔ Control your speed.

✔ Pay attention to fellow skiers and snowboarders.

✔ When you stop on the trail, move to the side. Avoid blocking the trail.

✔ Use safety equipment such as wrist guards and goggles.

✔ Make sure equipment is in good shape and fits correctly.

✔ Wear warm clothes. Dress in layers, and wear a hat and gloves.

Mountain Biking Safety

✔ Wear a helmet. Make sure it fits correctly.

✔ Don't ride alone.

✔ Don't ride trails that are too difficult for you.

✔ Develop your bike-handling skills.

✔ Watch where you're going.

✔ Learn safe riding practices. Watch out for other cyclists and hikers on the trail.

✔ Carry plenty of water.

✔ Make sure your bike is the right size for you.

✔ Tune up your bike regularly. Make sure brakes work correctly and tires are inflated.

Lesson Review

Using Vocabulary

1. What are hypothermia and frostbite?

2. Compare heat exhaustion and heatstroke.

Understanding Concepts

3. What are three ways to stay safe whenever you're outside?

Critical Thinking

4. **Making Inferences** According to the weather report, the temperature outside is 60°F right now. Later, the temperature will be close to 90°F. If you and your friends want to play soccer in the park, what should you wear? What should you bring?

Close

Reteaching — BASIC

Safety Tips Write the following in columns on the board: *hot weather, cold weather, hiking and camping, water, skiing and snowboarding,* and *mountain biking.* Then, ask student volunteers to write safety tips under each head.
LS Verbal

Quiz — GENERAL

1. How can sunscreen help you stay safe? (Sunscreen helps prevent sunburn. It can also prevent skin cancer.)

2. How can you avoid heat injuries? (Sample answer: The best way to avoid heat injuries is to drink plenty of water. You can also take breaks in the shade. If you're outside for a long time, you may also want to eat. Water and food will help your body stay cool.)

3. How can you prevent cold-weather injuries? (Sample answer: You can dress in layers. You can also wear gloves and a hat to protect your hands and ears. Avoid going outside on extremely cold days, and go inside if you start shivering.)

Alternative Assessment — GENERAL

Safety Story Have students write a story that describes safety tips for the following scenario: "A group of teenagers is taking a week-long canoe trip on a remote river. There is little shade on the river, and the temperature will be hot during the day."
LS Verbal

Answers to Lesson Review

1. Hypothermia is a below-normal body temperature. Frostbite is damage to skin and other tissues that is caused by extreme cold.

2. Heat exhaustion is a condition caused by too much water loss through sweating on a hot day. Signs of heat exhaustion include headache, dizziness, nausea, and clammy skin. Heatstroke is an injury that happens when the body cannot control its temperature. A person who has heatstroke cannot sweat and his or her body temperature rises. Sometimes, a victim may collapse or have convulsions.

3. Sample answer: Use sunscreen, even on cloudy days, and wear a hat and sunglasses. Drink plenty of water. Watch the weather and be prepared for weather changes.

4. Sample answer: Dress in layers, but make sure you have cool, light-colored clothing for when it gets warmer. Take plenty of water and some food. Wear sunscreen.

Lesson 5

Focus

Overview
Before beginning this lesson, review with your students the objectives listed under the What You'll Do head in the Student Edition. In this lesson, students will learn about natural disasters and how they can stay safe.

Bellringer
Have students name a type of natural disaster and how to protect themselves during it. **LS Verbal**

Answer to Start Off Write
Accept all reasonable answers. Sample answer: My family can keep an emergency kit. We should keep flashlights, a radio, batteries, food, and water in our kit. We should also have clothes and first-aid supplies.

Motivate

Group Activity —— GENERAL
Role-Play Have students work in groups of four. Ask groups to role-play a scenario in which they are a family who just heard a tornado warning on the radio. Then, have students discuss how they think they would react to an actual tornado. **LS Interpersonal/Intrapersonal**

Lesson 5 — Natural Disasters

Ryo goes to school in southern California. His school sometimes has earthquake drills. Students get under their desks during the drills.

What You'll Do
- **Describe** four types of natural disasters.
- **Describe** how you can prepare for natural disasters.

Terms to Learn
- earthquake
- tornado
- hurricane
- flood

Start Off Write
What can you and your family do to prepare for a natural disaster?

Have you ever been in an earthquake? An **earthquake** is a shaking of the Earth's surface caused by movement along a break in the Earth's crust. One way to stay safe during an earthquake is to hide under a table or a desk. Because earthquakes are common in southern California, many schools there have earthquake drills.

Earthquakes

Sometimes, earthquakes cause a lot of damage. In fact, some earthquakes are called natural disasters. *Natural disasters* are natural events that cause widespread injury, death, and property damage. Severe earthquakes damage buildings and roads. Earthquakes can cause landslides. Earthquakes may start fires by breaking gas lines.

During an earthquake, stay away from windows and glass. If you are outside, move away from any tall structures. Avoid power lines and trees. If you are in a car, ask the driver to pull over in an open area. Stay in the car until the earthquake is over.

After an earthquake is over, you may not have electricity or water. Watch out for broken glass and debris. Avoid downed power lines. If you think your building has been damaged, go outside until you're sure it is safe.

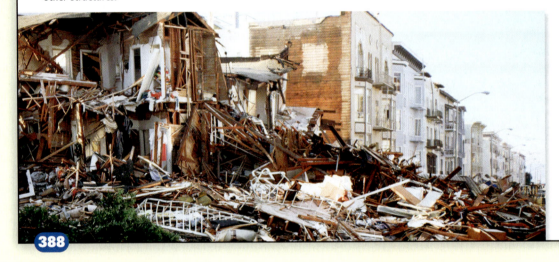

Figure 14 This earthquake in San Francisco destroyed homes, businesses, and other structures.

PHYSICAL SCIENCE CONNECTION — ADVANCED
Richter Scale The Richter scale describes the magnitude of an earthquake. Ask interested students to research how the Richter scale works. Have students identify the strengths of some major earthquakes based on the Richter scale. Then, have students make a poster and present their findings to the class. **LS Verbal/Visual**

Chapter Resource File
- Directed Reading **BASIC**
- Lesson Plan
- Lesson Quiz **GENERAL**

Transparencies
TT Bellringer

---

388 Chapter 17 • Your Personal Safety

Figure 15 The Anatomy of a Hurricane

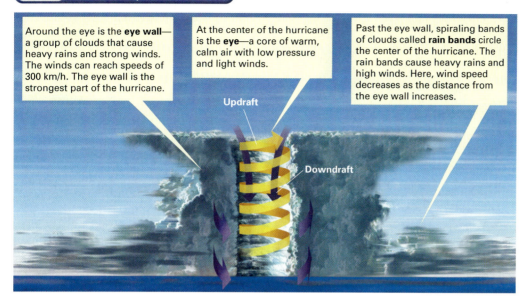

Around the eye is the **eye wall**—a group of clouds that cause heavy rains and strong winds. The winds can reach speeds of 300 km/h. The eye wall is the strongest part of the hurricane.

At the center of the hurricane is the **eye**—a core of warm, calm air with low pressure and light winds.

Past the eye wall, spiraling bands of clouds called **rain bands** circle the center of the hurricane. The rain bands cause heavy rains and high winds. Here, wind speed decreases as the distance from the eye wall increases.

Tornadoes and Hurricanes

A **tornado** is a spinning column of air that has a high wind speed and touches the ground. Tornadoes can pick up objects, such as trees, cars, and houses. Most tornadoes are short lived and travel only a few miles. If there is a tornado in your area, go to the basement or the cellar. If you don't have a basement or cellar, go to the bathroom or a closet in the center of your house. If you are outside when a tornado approaches, go indoors. If you can't go indoors, lie down in a large open field or deep ditch.

A **hurricane** is a large, spinning tropical weather system with wind speeds of at least 74 miles per hour. The figure above shows the structure of a hurricane. These storms usually form over warm tropical waters in the Gulf of Mexico or Caribbean Sea. Hurricanes can last for a few days. They often produce high winds, heavy rains, and high surf. Areas near the coast are often evacuated during a hurricane.

New technology has made storm prediction more accurate. There are two kinds of weather alerts. A *watch* is a forecast that alerts people that severe weather may happen. A *warning* is a forecast that tells people that severe weather has developed. Watches and warnings alert people about tornadoes, hurricanes, thunderstorms, floods, and winter storms.

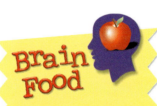

Brain Food

Hurricanes that occur in the northwestern part of the Pacific Ocean near the South China Sea are called *typhoons* (tie FOONZ). Hurricanes that occur in the Indian Ocean are called *cyclones* (SIE KLOHNZ).

Teach

Using the Figure — BASIC

The Anatomy of a Hurricane Ask students to study the illustration on this page. Then, ask them to describe the parts of a hurricane in their own words. Ask students, "Which part of a hurricane most likely causes high surf?" (Sample answer: The eye wall probably causes high surf because of high winds. Also, the rain bands may also cause high surf because of high winds.) "If a hurricane sometimes causes flooding, which part of a hurricane is likely the cause?" (Sample answer: The eye wall and rain bands both cause heavy rains. Also, they cause high winds which may cause heavy surf. So they are likely the cause of flooding.)
LS Verbal/Visual/Logical

Debate — ADVANCED

Development and Natural Disasters Have interested students research and debate whether new housing developments should be built in areas that are prone to natural disasters, such as earthquakes or floods. **LS** Logical

SOCIAL STUDIES CONNECTION — GENERAL

Naming Hurricanes Ask interested students to research how hurricanes, tropical storms, and tropical depressions are named in the Atlantic and Pacific. Have students write a magazine article about their findings. **LS** Verbal

REAL-LIFE CONNECTION — GENERAL

Hurricane Mitch Have interested students investigate Hurricane Mitch. Students should identify how long it lasted and the amount of damage it did. Also, have students locate the areas most affected by Hurricane Mitch. Ask students to share their findings with the class. (The weather system known as Hurricane Mitch started as a tropical depression on October 21 and ended on November 4, 1998, after becoming too weak to be classified as a tropical depression. Hurricane Mitch struck Honduras and Nicaragua, but caused widespread flooding throughout Central America, including El Salvador, Guatemala, and Mexico. About 11,000 people died as a result of the storm. Hurricane Mitch caused more than $5 billion in damage.) **LS** Verbal

Lesson 5 • Natural Disasters

Teach, continued

Group Activity — GENERAL

Poster Project Have students work in groups of four. Ask students to create a poster with tips on how to prepare for a flood and how to stay safe during a flood. Ask students who speak other languages to translate their poster. **LS Visual** — English Language Learners

LANGUAGE ARTS CONNECTION — BASIC

Water Words Have students brainstorm words and phrases that are related to floods and flooding, such as *floodwater*, *high-water mark*, and *crest*. Have students look up the words in the dictionary, write a definition, and then write an original sentence using the word or phrase. **LS Verbal**

REAL-LIFE CONNECTION — ADVANCED

Flood Control Ask interested students to identify ways that floods are controlled. For example, students could focus on dams, floodplains, and sand bags. Ask students to write a report about their findings. **LS Verbal**

LIFE SKILLS ACTIVITY

Answer
Accept all reasonable answers.

Extension: Ask students to research contemporary emergency alert systems and compare them to the system they designed.

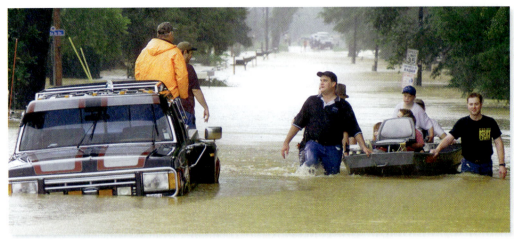

Figure 16 This flood caused a lot of damage around the Mississippi River. Many homes, businesses, and vehicles were caught in its path.

Floods

Storms often produce a lot of rain, hail, or snow. Storms can also cause large waves along the coast. Where does all of this water go? Sometimes, an area gets so much rain that the ground can't absorb any more moisture. So, the area begins to flood. A **flood** is an overflowing of water into areas that are normally dry. Floods tend to occur near rivers or creeks. Some flooding also occurs around lakes and oceans.

Usually, floods can be predicted. But sometimes a flash flood occurs. A *flash flood* is a flood that rises and falls with little or no warning. Flash floods usually happen because of a sudden, intense rainfall, a failed dam, or melting ice.

Floodwater can move very quickly. The water doesn't have to be very deep to pick up a vehicle. People should not drive through floodwater. Many people die each year because they try to drive through a flooded section of road. The best thing to do during a flood is to find high ground and wait until the water goes down.

LIFE SKILLS ACTIVITY

COMMUNICATING EFFECTIVELY

Design an emergency warning system. You can use radio, TV, or emergency sirens. Describe a way you can warn people about different kinds of weather emergencies. Include watches and warnings in your emergency warning system. Share your ideas with the class.

Attention Grabber

Mississippi River Flood Students may find the following facts about the Mississippi River flood of 1993 interesting:

- The Mississippi and its tributaries (the Missouri, Kansas, Illinois, Des Moines, and Wisconsin rivers) all flooded.
- In St. Louis, Missouri, the Mississippi River was above flood stage for more than 2 months.
- Downstream from St. Louis, about 3 billion cubic meters of water overflowed onto floodplains.
- About 17,000 square miles of land were flooded in North Dakota, South Dakota, Nebraska, Kansas, Missouri, Iowa, Wisconsin, Minnesota, and Illinois.

Be Prepared

The best way to stay safe during a storm or natural disaster is to be prepared. Your family should have an emergency kit. Include the following in your kit:

- a battery-operated radio, a flashlight, and batteries
- a first-aid kit and medicine
- canned or freeze-dried food and bottled water
- clothes, shoes, and bedding for everyone

Store your kit in the place where you will seek shelter during an emergency. And remember to stay calm during an emergency.

Myth & Fact

Myth: You don't have to replace anything in your emergency kit except when you use it.

Fact: Food, batteries, medicine, and water can go bad after a long period of time. You should replace most of these items after their expiration dates. Water should be replaced every 6 months.

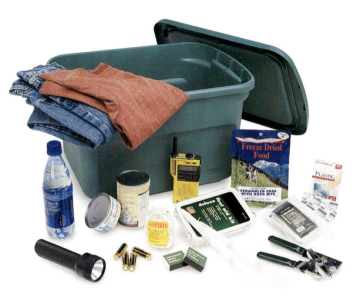

Figure 17 An emergency kit can keep you safe during a natural disaster.

Lesson Review

Using Vocabulary

1. Describe four kinds of natural disasters.

Understanding Concepts

2. What is a natural disaster?
3. Compare a watch and a warning.
4. What should you include in your emergency kit?

Critical Thinking

5. **Applying Concepts** Are all earthquakes, tornadoes, hurricanes, and floods considered natural disasters? Explain your answer.
6. **Making Inferences** Why should emergency kits include a battery-operated radio and a flashlight?

Answers to Lesson Review

1. An earthquake is a shaking of the Earth's surface caused by movement along a break in the Earth's crust. A tornado is a spinning column of air that has a high wind speed and touches the ground. A hurricane is a large, spinning tropical weather system with wind speeds of at least 74 miles per hour. A flood is an overflowing of water into areas that are normally dry.
2. a natural event that causes widespread injury, death, and property damage
3. A watch is a forecast that alerts people that severe weather may happen. A warning is a forecast that tells people that severe weather has developed.
4. a battery-operated radio, a flashlight, batteries, a first-aid kit and medicine, canned or freeze-dried food and bottled water, and a change of clothes and shoes for everyone
5. Sample answer: No, not all earthquakes, tornadoes, hurricanes, and floods are natural disasters. For example, there are many small earthquakes in California each year that cause little to no damage.
6. Sample answer: You may lose power during a storm or earthquake. So, you won't have any lights. A flashlight can provide light. A battery-operated radio can help you know about an emergency when the power is out.

Activity — GENERAL

Emergency Kit Bring an emergency kit to class. Ask students to examine the items in the kit. Then, ask the following questions: "Why are a flashlight, battery-powered radio, and batteries so important?" (Sample answer: A flashlight gives you light if the power goes out. A radio can keep you informed about an emergency and what to do to stay safe. You should have extra batteries in case you need to replace them.) "Why do you need a change of clothing?" (Sample answer: Your clothes may be damaged. Also, extra clothes can keep you warm if your clothes get wet or if the temperature drops.)

Close

Reteaching — BASIC

Have students divide a sheet of paper into four sections and write the name of a type of natural disaster in each section. Then, have them describe how to prepare for and stay safe during each type of disaster. **LS** Verbal

Quiz — GENERAL

1. What is a flash flood? (A flash flood is a flood that rises and falls with little or no warning.)
2. What should you do during a flood? (Sample answer: You should move to higher ground and wait until the water goes down.)
3. If you don't have a basement or cellar, where should you go during a tornado? (a bathroom or closet at the center of the house)

Lesson 6

Focus

Overview
Before beginning this lesson, review with your students the objectives listed under the What You'll Do head in the Student Edition. In this lesson, students will learn how to handle an emergency and how to make an emergency phone call.

Bellringer
Ask students to list the three steps of handling an emergency situation. (check out the situation, call for help, and care for the victim)
LS Verbal

Answer to Start Off Write
Accept all reasonable answers. Sample answer: I will need to tell the operator my name and where I am. I will also need to tell the operator what happened and if anyone is hurt.

Motivate

Activity — GENERAL
Skit Have students work in groups of four. Have groups write a skit to show how they would respond if one of them was babysitting and the child had an accident. Skits should show how the baby-sitter would handle the accident and what the baby-sitter would do if he or she had to make an emergency phone call.
LS Verbal/Kinesthetic

Lesson 6 Deciding to Give First Aid

What You'll Do
- **Describe** the three steps of handling an emergency.
- **List** four things you need to say during an emergency phone call.

Terms to Learn
- emergency
- first aid

Start Off Write
What information do you need to provide when you make an emergency phone call?

Maggie's parents posted an emergency phone-number list next to the phone. Maggie's parents included 911, local emergency numbers, and their work numbers on the emergency phone-number list.

An **emergency** is a sudden event that demands immediate action. Maggie's parents keep an emergency phone-number list near the phone so that Maggie knows whom to call during an emergency.

Handling an Emergency
Do you know what to do in an emergency? Follow these steps:

1. **Check out the situation.** Make sure you're safe. If you're not sure you're safe, leave the area. If someone is hurt, try to find out what's wrong. Stay calm, and don't panic.

2. **Call for help.** Yell for help, or use the phone to call for emergency services.

3. **Care for the victim.** During some emergencies, someone may be hurt. You may need to give first aid until help arrives. **First aid** is emergency medical care for someone who has been hurt or who is sick. If you have training, give the victim first aid. You should not give first aid if you haven't taken a first-aid class. Taking a class helps you act quickly and correctly when someone is hurt.

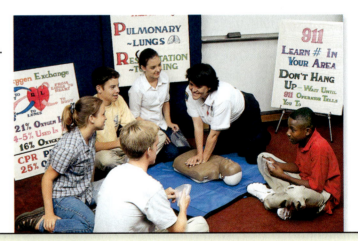

Figure 18 Taking a first-aid class can help you take care of people when they are hurt.

MISCONCEPTION ALERT
911 Students may not understand that 911 is for emergencies only. Help students understand that if they are not in danger or the victim of an accident is not in immediate need of medical care, they should not call 911. Explain that students should call their parents, a trusted neighbor, or a relative instead. Also, if your area offers it, tell students about 311, a phone number for non-emergency situations requiring professional assistance.

Chapter Resource File
- Directed Reading **BASIC**
- Lesson Plan
- Lesson Quiz **GENERAL**

Transparencies
TT Bellringer

---

392   Chapter 17 • Your Personal Safety

Making an Emergency Phone Call

In most areas of the United States, dialing 911 will get you help during an emergency. If your area doesn't have 911, be sure to know your local emergency number. The operator will need the following information when you call:

- your name and location
- the type of emergency
- the condition of anyone who is hurt
- what you've done to help the victim

Stay as calm as possible. Don't hang up until the operator does. He or she may have special instructions for you.

Your family should keep an emergency phone-number list next to every phone in the house. That way, everyone knows whom to call during an emergency. The table below lists some of the numbers that should be on an emergency phone-number list.

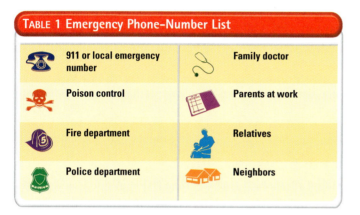

TABLE 1 Emergency Phone-Number List

☎	911 or local emergency number	🩺	Family doctor
☠	Poison control	📓	Parents at work
🧑‍🚒	Fire department	👤	Relatives
🛡	Police department	🏘	Neighbors

LIFE SKILLS ACTIVITY

PRACTICING WELLNESS

In pairs, practice making an emergency phone call. One person should act as the operator. The other should give information.

Lesson Review

Using Vocabulary

1. What is first aid?

Understanding Concepts

2. What are the three steps of handling emergencies?
3. What four things should you tell an operator during an emergency phone call?

Critical Thinking

4. **Making Inferences** Why is it a good idea to include your neighbors' phone numbers and your relatives' phone numbers on your emergency phone-number list?

Lesson 7 Focus

Overview
Before beginning this lesson, review with your students the objectives listed under the What You'll Do head in the Student Edition. In this lesson, students will learn about abdominal thrusts and rescue breathing.

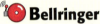 **Bellringer**
Ask students to describe how they can help someone who is not breathing. **LS Verbal**

Answer to Start Off Write
Accept all reasonable answers. Sample answer: If I have training, I can give the victim abdominal thrusts.

Motivate

Discussion — GENERAL
Choking Invite students to relate personal experiences involving choking. Remember that some students may be uncomfortable sharing personal information. Ask students to describe what happens when a person chokes. (Sample answer: The victim can't breathe. He or she will probably grab his or her throat.) Ask students what they think their first reaction will be if they see someone choking. (Answers may vary. Some students will likely state that they want to hit the victim on the back. Explain to students this may actually make the situation worse by lodging the object on which the victim is choking deeper into the throat.) **LS Verbal**

Lesson 7: Abdominal Thrusts and Rescue Breathing

What You'll Do
- Describe how to give abdominal thrusts to adults and to infants.
- Explain how to give rescue breathing to adults and to small children.

Terms to Learn
- abdominal thrusts
- rescue breathing
- cardiopulmonary resuscitation (CPR)

 Start Off Write
How do you save someone who is choking?

Rashid went out to dinner with his parents. While they were eating, Rashid saw a waiter save a choking man's life. The waiter gave the choking man abdominal thrusts (ab DAHM uh nuhl THRUHSTS).

Abdominal thrusts are actions that apply pressure to a choking person's stomach to force an object out of his or her throat.

First Aid for Choking Infants
You can easily tell when an adult is choking. Adults usually grab their throats. But you may have a hard time telling when an infant is choking. A choking infant won't make any noise and may turn blue. Call for help if an infant appears to be choking. Do not put your fingers in the infant's mouth to remove the object. This could push the object farther into the throat.

Your first instinct may be to give the infant back blows or to turn the infant upside down. But be careful. You may hurt the infant. The figure below describes the steps you need to take to save a choking infant.

 Figure 19 Saving a Choking Infant — Certification required

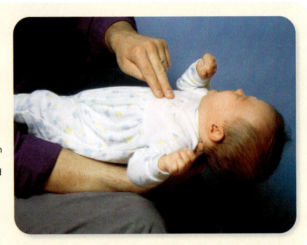

1. Put the infant face up on your forearm. Place your other arm over the infant, and hold his or her jaw. Turn the infant over.

2. Support your arm on your thigh or knee so the infant's head is lower than his or her chest. Give the infant five firm back blows with the heel of your hand.

3. If the object doesn't come loose, turn the infant over. Place two fingers on the infant's breastbone, between and just below the infant's nipples. Push the breastbone in five times.

4. Repeat back blows and chest thrusts until the object comes loose.

REAL-LIFE CONNECTION — BASIC
First-Aid Certification Reinforce the idea that students should not give first aid unless they have been trained to do so. Then, ask interested students to locate first-aid courses in your community. Have students make a pamphlet describing the courses they find. **LS Visual/Verbal**

Chapter Resource File
- Directed Reading **BASIC**
- Lesson Plan
- Lesson Quiz **GENERAL**

Transparencies
- TT Bellringer
- TT Rescue Breathing for Adults
- TT Rescue Breathing for Small Children

First Aid for Choking Adults

Sometimes, someone who seems to be choking may not be in danger. If the victim can speak, breathe, or cough, do not give abdominal thrusts. Let the victim cough until the object comes out.

If the choking person cannot speak or breathe, call for help. Begin abdominal thrusts. Abdominal thrusts compress the victim's abdomen. This increases the pressure in the victim's lungs. This pressure forces the object out of the victim's airway. You can even do abdominal thrusts on yourself. Take a look at the figure below to learn how to give abdominal thrusts to adults and to yourself.

Myth & Fact

Myth: You should slap a choking person on the back.

Fact: Slapping a person on the back can lodge an object deeper in the throat, making the object more difficult to remove.

Figure 20 Saving an Adult Choking Victim Certification required

▶ **How to Give Abdominal Thrusts to Another Person**

1. The victim may be standing or sitting. Stand or kneel behind the victim. Wrap your arms around the victim.
2. Make one hand into a fist. Place the thumb side of your fist against the victim's stomach, between the belly button and the end of the breastbone.
3. Cover your fist with your other hand. Give five quick upward thrusts into the victim's stomach.
4. Repeat thrusts until the object comes loose.

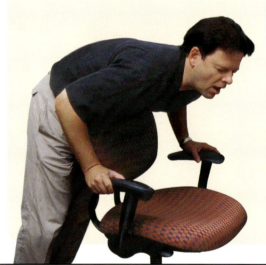

◀ **How to Give Abdominal Thrusts to Yourself**

1. If other people are around, let them know that you need help.
2. Use a chair back, counter, or any other high, solid object. Lean forward and press your stomach against the object.
3. You can also make your hand into a fist. Place it against your stomach, between your belly button and your breastbone. Cover your fist with your other hand. Quickly pull in and upward.

Attention Grabber

Choking and Infants The following information about choking and small children may interest students:

Most choking deaths in small children and infants are not caused by food. They are caused by toys and household items. According to one study, almost 70 percent of choking deaths among children three years old or younger were the result of choking on toys and other products made for children.

Teach

READING SKILL BUILDER — BASIC

Reading Organizer As they read the lesson, ask students to create an outline to organize the material that is covered. **LS** Verbal

Activity — GENERAL

Abdominal Thrust Poster Explain to students that many restaurants post signs informing people about what to do if someone is choking. Then, ask students to create their own posters about first aid for choking. Posters should illustrate the proper way to give abdominal thrusts. Ask students who speak other languages to translate their posters. Consider hanging the posters in the school cafeteria. **LS** Verbal/Visual — English Language Learners

LIFE SCIENCE CONNECTION — GENERAL

Eating and Breathing People are able to eat and breath at the same time. Ask interested students to identify the structures in the human body that make this possible. Then, have students identify what actions make people more likely to choke. Have students write a report based on their findings. **LS** Verbal

Life SKILL BUILDER — ADVANCED

Evaluating Media Messages Have interested students watch fictional medical and emergency TV shows. Then, have them write a paper discussing how accurately the shows depict first aid for medical emergencies involving choking and cessation of breathing. If students find any inaccuracies, ask them to discuss why they think the inaccuracies happen. **LS** Visual

Lesson 7 • Abdominal Thrusts and Rescue Breathing

Teach, continued

Life SKILL BUILDER — Advanced

Practicing Wellness Have students who are first-aid certified share their experience with their classmates. Students should relate why they took the class and what they learned in the class. **LS Verbal**

Discussion — GENERAL

Comprehension Check Write the phrase *cardiopulmonary resuscitation* on the board. Ask students, "What does this mean?" (Sample answer: Cardiopulmonary resuscitation, or CPR, is an emergency technique used to save a victim who isn't breathing and who doesn't have a heart beat.) "How is it different from rescue breathing?" (Sample answer: CPR is used to save someone who is not breathing and doesn't have a heart beat. Rescue breathing is used for someone who isn't breathing.) **LS Verbal**

LANGUAGE ARTS CONNECTION — Advanced

Roots Have students find the origins and roots of the words "cardiopulmonary" and "resuscitation." Have students present their findings to the class. Then, ask the class to brainstorm other words with some of the same roots. (Sample answers: *cardiac, cardiorespiratory, pulmonary,* and *resuscitate*) **LS Verbal**

Breathing Mask
If you have a breathing mask, you should use it while giving rescue breathing. A breathing mask can protect you and the victim from disease.

Rescue Breathing for Adults

Sometimes, a person stops breathing. You should act quickly when you find someone who isn't breathing. When someone doesn't breathe for several minutes, permanent injuries or even death can happen. A person who isn't breathing needs rescue breathing. **Rescue breathing** is an emergency technique in which a rescuer gives air to someone who is not breathing.

Don't move the victim unless you're sure doing so is safe. Lay the victim on his or her back. See if the victim is breathing. Tilt the victim's head back. Clear any objects out of the victim's mouth. Look, listen, and feel for breathing. Never give rescue breathing to someone who can still breathe. Before you give rescue breathing, call for help. The figure below shows you how to give rescue breathing.

Sometimes, a victim needs CPR. CPR stands for cardiopulmonary resuscitation (KAHR dee oh PUL muh NER ee ri SUHS uh TAY shuhn). **Cardiopulmonary resuscitation** is an emergency technique used to save a victim who isn't breathing and who doesn't have a heart beat.

CPR and rescue breathing require special training. You shouldn't give either unless you have been trained. The YMCA and the Red Cross offer first-aid and CPR training.

Figure 21 Rescue Breathing for Adults — Certification required / FIRST AID

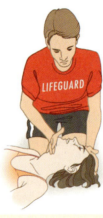
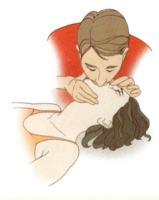

1 Open the victim's airway. Tilt the victim's head back gently. Use your finger to clear any objects out of the victim's mouth. Look at the victim's chest for movement. Also, listen for the sounds of breathing, and feel for breath on your cheek.

2 If the victim is not breathing, put your mouth around the victim's mouth, and pinch the victim's nose shut. Breathe out, into the victim's mouth. Give two slow rescue breaths. Look to see if the victim's chest is moving up and down in response to your breathing.

REAL-LIFE CONNECTION — GENERAL

CPR for Pets Students may be interested to know that CPR can be performed on house pets as well as on human beings. Ask interested students to research rescue breathing and CPR techniques for pets. Have students present their findings to the class. **LS Verbal**

LIFE SCIENCE CONNECTION — Advanced

Illustrating CPR Ask interested students to research how CPR works. Have students make a poster of the human body showing how CPR affects the various organs of the body and how each organ is affected by a lack of oxygen. **English Language Learners** **LS Visual**

Figure 22 Rescue Breathing for Small Children Certification required

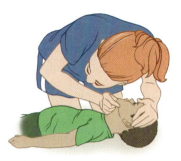

1 Position the victim on his or her back, and tilt the victim's head back. Clear any objects out of the victim's mouth, and check for signs of breathing. Look at the victim's chest for movement, listen for sounds of breathing, and feel for breath on your cheek.

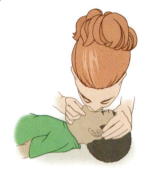

2 If the victim is not breathing, give two slow rescue breaths. Place your mouth over the victim's nose and mouth. Form a tight seal, and breathe out, into the victim's mouth and nose. Look at the victim's chest for movement to see if your breaths are going into the victim's lungs.

Rescue Breathing for Small Children

Rescue breathing is different for adults and small children. First, you don't breathe only into a small child's mouth. You need to breathe into both the child's nose and the child's mouth. Second, you need to remember that small children have smaller lungs than an adult. When giving a small child air, you should give him or her less air than you would give an adult. The figure above shows rescue breathing for small children. The same techniques can be used for an infant. You should get special training before giving rescue breathing to a small child or infant.

Lesson Review

Using Vocabulary
1. What are abdominal thrusts?
2. What does CPR stand for?

Understanding Concepts
3. Describe how to give abdominal thrusts to infants and to adults.
4. Describe how to give rescue breathing to small children and to adults.

Critical Thinking
5. **Applying Concepts** Explain why you need to breathe into an infant's nose as well as into his or her mouth when you perform rescue breathing.
6. **Making Inferences** Why is it so important to take a class before giving abdominal thrusts or rescue breathing?

Close

Reteaching — BASIC

Rescue Illustrations Show students pictures of abdominal thrusts and rescue breathing steps. Include pictures of procedures for adults, small children, and infants. Ask students to describe what is happening in each picture. **LS** Verbal/Visual

Quiz — GENERAL

1. What is rescue breathing? (an emergency technique in which a rescuer gives air to someone who is not breathing)
2. How do you give abdominal thrusts to yourself? (Sample answer: If other people are around, let them know you are choking. Use a chair back, counter or other high, solid object to give yourself abdominal thrusts. Lean forward against the object and press your stomach against it. You can also make your hand into a fist, place it against your stomach, and use your other hand to pull your fist in and upward against your stomach.)
3. How do abdominal thrusts work? (Sample answer: Abdominal thrusts compress the abdomen, which increases the pressure in the lungs. This pressure forces the object out of the airway.)

Alternative Assessment — GENERAL

Interview Have students work in pairs and interview each other about what to do when someone is choking or not breathing. Students should differentiate between infants and adults. Have students write articles based on their interviews. **LS** Verbal/Interpersonal

Answers to Lesson Review

1. actions that apply pressure to a choking person's stomach to force an object out of his or her throat
2. *cardiopulmonary resuscitation*
3. Turn the infant over, and give the infant five firm back blows. If the object doesn't come loose, turn the infant back over, and give five chest thrusts. For adults, wrap your arms around the victim, and place the thumb side of your fist against the victim's stomach, between the belly button and the end of the breastbone. Cover your fist with your other hand and give five thrusts.
4. For adults, tilt the victim's head back and clear any objects out of the victim's mouth. Look, listen, and feel for breathing. If the victim isn't breathing, seal your mouth over the victim's mouth, pinch the nose shut, and give rescue breaths. For small children, seal your mouth over the victim's mouth and nose to give rescue breaths. Also, give small children less air than you give adults.
5. An infant face is smaller, so it is harder to seal your mouth over the infant's mouth alone.
6. Sample answer: If you don't learn how to give abdominal thrusts or rescue breathing properly, you may hurt the victim more.

Lesson 8

Focus

Overview
Before beginning this lesson, review with your students the objectives listed under the What You'll Do head in the Student Edition. In this lesson, students will learn about first aid for bleeding, burns, poisoning, fractures, dislocations, and head, back, and neck injuries.

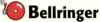 Bellringer
Have students list some injuries that could that should be treated with first aid. (Sample answers: bleeding, burns, poisoning, and broken bones) **LS** Verbal

Answer to Start Off Write
Accept all reasonable answers. Sample answer: I should call for help. Then, I should cover the burn with a clean, wet cloth. I shouldn't remove any clothing that is stuck to the burn.

Motivate

Activity —— GENERAL
Role-Play Bring gauze, bandages, and antiseptic to class. Have students brainstorm a scenario involving a person who gets cut and begins to bleed. Have students use the gauze, bandages, and antiseptic to role-play this scene to show how they would respond.
LS Kinesthetic

Lesson 8

What You'll Do
- **Describe** the treatment for bleeding.
- **Explain** how to care for burns.
- **Describe** how to care for a poisoning victim.
- **Describe** how to care for broken bones and dislocations.
- **Explain** how to care for someone who has a head, neck, or back injury.

Terms to Learn
- fracture
- dislocation

Start Off Write
What is the proper first aid for a third-degree burn?

First Aid for Injuries

Paz cut her arm when she crashed her bike. Her mother took her to the emergency room. She had to get 10 stitches to close the cut!

Most cuts and scrapes aren't as serious as Paz's was. But you still need to clean and take care of your small cuts.

Bleeding

Most cuts and scrapes only need to be washed with soap and water. But deep cuts can be very dangerous. If someone gets a cut, stop the bleeding right away. Put a piece of sterile gauze over the cut. Use your hand to put pressure on the cut. If the cut is on an arm or a leg, elevate the limb above the heart. But don't elevate the limb if doing so may cause more injury. Don't remove the gauze if it is soaked. Just add more gauze and apply more pressure. If the bleeding doesn't stop within a few minutes, or if the wound is very large, call for help. You should visit the emergency room for a deep cut, even if the bleeding has stopped. The cut may need stitches.

If you need to help someone who has a cut, use sterile gloves. The gloves will protect you from diseases carried in the blood. They will also protect the victim from any diseases you have. If you don't have gloves, be sure to wash exposed areas with soap and water as soon as you can.

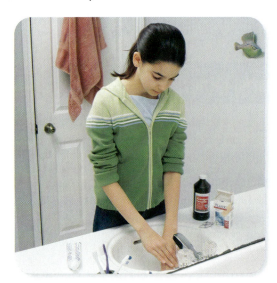

Figure 23 If you cut your hand, wash it with soap and water. Put pressure on the cut until it stops bleeding. Tell your parents about your injury.

398

Career

Emergency Nurse An emergency nurse assists medical doctors in the emergency room. Emergency nurses are also responsible for monitoring emergency room patients. An emergency nurse completes a 4-year bachelor's degree or 2-year associate's degree and takes an exam to become a registered nurse. Many emergency nurses also take a certified emergency nurse, or CEN, exam.

Chapter Resource File
- Directed Reading **BASIC**
- Lesson Plan
- Lesson Quiz **GENERAL**

Transparencies
TT Bellringer

TABLE 2 Treating Burns

Type of burn	Description	Treatment
First-degree burns	The burned area is red. Only the top layer of skin is affected.	Run cool water over the burn. Use antibiotic cream on the burn until it heals. If the burn covers most of the body, call a doctor.
Second-degree burns	The top two layers of skin are affected. The skin blisters. The burns are very painful.	Run cool water over the skin or use a wet cold compress. Cover the burn with a sterile bandage. If the burn is larger than 2 inches, go to the emergency room.
Third-degree burns	All three layers of skin are affected. Some muscle and bone may also be burned. Skin will look dark, dry, and leathery. There may be little pain because nerve endings have been damaged.	Call for help immediately. Cover the burn with a clean, wet cloth. Do not remove any clothing stuck to the burn.

Burns

Have you ever burned your hand on the stove? Most burns are caused by heat. Open flames, hot objects, or boiling liquids can cause burns. Some chemicals also cause burns. There are three types of burns. The table above describes each type of burn.

The severity and location of a burn determine whether you should go to the hospital. You should see a doctor if you have a large burn. Also, if you have a burn on your face, hands, feet, or groin, you should see a doctor, even if the burn is small. If a burn isn't cared for properly, it could become infected or leave a scar. Some burns will leave scars anyway. But getting proper care may ensure that scars are smaller and less severe.

Poisoning

Poisons can be eaten, drunk, inhaled, or absorbed through the skin. Many poisonings are accidental. Some poisons are obvious. Pesticides, cleaning products, and automobile fluids all have warning labels. Some substances don't seem so harmful. But some medicines, such as aspirin, can cause poisoning if you take too much of them.

If you find someone who has been poisoned, try to find out what the poison is. Ask the victim or look for bottles and packages in the area. How a victim is cared for depends on the poison. Call 911. Then, call your local poison control center. The operator at the poison control center can tell you what to do for the victim until help arrives.

Myth & Fact

Myth: You can use butter to treat a burn.

Fact: Butter and other oil-based products can retain heat and cause an infection. You should use water and a sterile bandage to treat a burn.

Teach

Demonstration — GENERAL

First-Aid Instructor Ask a first-aid instructor to visit the classroom. Ask the instructor to demonstrate various first-aid procedures. If possible, have student volunteers take part in the demonstration. Consider asking the instructor to teach an actual first-aid certification course so that students may become certified in first aid. **LS** Visual/Kinesthetic

Life SKILL BUILDER — GENERAL

Making Good Decisions Give students the following scenario: "Sasha is babysitting for a neighbor when she notices that several poisonous cleaning products are accessible to the children." Have students list and discuss ways Sasha could respond to this situation. **LS** Verbal

Using the Figure — BASIC

Treating Burns The table on this page describes three different kinds of burns. Ask students to relate a time when they were burned or when they helped with the treatment of a burn. Students should relate the type of burn and what they did to take care of it. Remember that some students may be uncomfortable sharing personal information. **LS** Verbal

---

Cultural Awareness — ADVANCED

Traditional Chinese Medicine Ask interested students to research traditional Chinese medicine. Students should identify the differences between traditional Chinese medicine and Western medicine. Students should also examine the effectiveness of Chinese practices. Have students draw a table comparing Chinese medicine and Western medicine. **LS** Verbal

Lesson 8 • First Aid for Injuries

Teach, continued

Answer to Science Activity
Accept all reasonable answers.

Extension: Ask students to interview X-ray technicians and other imaging technicians about diagnosing injuries.

Group Activity — GENERAL

Poster Project Have students work in six groups. Assign each group a type of injury described in the lesson. Ask students to make posters describing the type of injury and basic first aid for the injury. Students can use magazine clippings and cartoons to make their posters exciting. Display the posters in the classroom.
LS Visual — English Language Learners

Discussion — GENERAL

Comprehension Check Some students may have difficulty differentiating between fractures and dislocations. Ask students the following questions: "What is a fracture?" (an injury in which a bone has been cracked or broken) "What is a dislocation?" (an injury in which a bone has been forced out of its normal position in a joint) "What is the major difference between the two injuries?" (Sample answer: In a dislocation, the bone itself is not actually injured.) "How do you care for fractures and dislocations?" (Sample answer: Avoid moving the hurt limb. Call for help or ask an adult to take the victim to the emergency room. For a broken bone, you can use a splint to keep the injured area from moving.) **LS Verbal**

SCIENCE ACTIVITY

An X-ray machine is often used to diagnose fractures and dislocations. However, there are other machines that can be used to create an image of an injured limb. Research X-ray machines and other imaging machines. Create a poster that compares how each machine works, the type of image each produces, and the specific injuries that each can be used to diagnose.

Fractures

Your bones are very strong. But they can be broken in an accident. A **fracture** is a broken or cracked bone. Falls, rough sports, and car accidents all cause fractures. The area around a fractured bone swells and is painful. An injured limb may also look odd or be hard to move.

If you find someone who has a fracture, call for help. In the meantime, avoid moving the injured bone. Moving a broken bone can make the injury worse. Don't try to straighten the fracture. You can use ice to reduce swelling, but be careful. For some fractures, you can use a splint. A splint is a stiff object, such as a stick or a board, that you can use to keep the injured area from moving.

Dislocations

Elbows, fingers, and shoulders are common areas for dislocations. A **dislocation** is an injury in which a bone has been forced out of its normal position in a joint. Dislocations happen when a person falls or runs into something. Dislocations are painful. A dislocated joint may swell and bruise. The injured joint may look unusual.

Victims who have dislocations should go to the emergency room. Call for help, or ask an adult to take the victim to the hospital. Don't move the dislocated limb. Make sure the victim is as comfortable as possible. Stay calm, and wait for help to arrive.

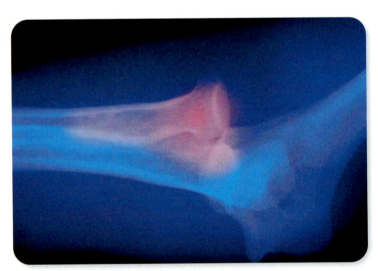

Figure 24 This X ray shows a dislocated elbow.

400

LIFE SCIENCE CONNECTION — ADVANCED

Skeletal System Have students draw and label the major bones of the skeletal system. Then, have students research the most commonly fractured bones or dislocated joints. Students should label these bones and joints on their diagrams. Ask students to indicate how long it takes for these injuries to heal.
LS Visual

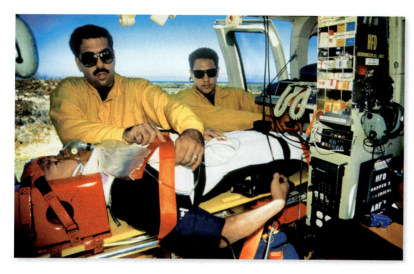

Figure 25 Special equipment keeps a victim's head and neck still after an accident.

Head, Neck, and Back Injuries

Maybe you've bumped your head. You probably had a lump that went away pretty quickly. But some head, neck, and back injuries are very serious. Your brain and nerves in your neck and back control how you move and breathe. If these areas are injured, the damage may not be reversible. Some people who hurt their heads, necks, or backs never recover.

So what do you do for someone who has hurt his or her head, neck, or back? First, don't move the victim. Moving a victim can make the injury worse. The victim may be unconscious. Check to make sure the victim is breathing. Call for help. Keep the victim warm. If the victim is conscious, do your best to keep him or her awake until help arrives. Tell the victim not to move.

Lesson Review

Using Vocabulary

1. Compare fractures and dislocations.

Understanding Concepts

2. What should you do for someone who has a cut?
3. Describe how to take care of burns.
4. What should you do for a poisoning victim?

Critical Thinking

5. **Making Good Decisions** Imagine you found someone unconscious on the floor. There is a bruise on the victim's forehead. What should you do?

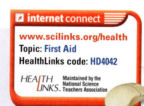

www.scilinks.org/health
Topic: First Aid
HealthLinks code: HD4042

17 CHAPTER REVIEW

Assignment Guide

Lesson	Review Questions
1	8, 10–12, 28
2	1, 13
3	14, 19, 21
4	2–3, 15, 26
5	4, 16, 22
6	7, 17
7	5, 9
8	6, 18, 20, 23, 25, 27, 29–32
1 and 3	24

ANSWERS

Using Vocabulary

1. A smoke detector is an alarm that detects smoke from a fire. A fire extinguisher is a device that releases chemicals to put out a fire.
2. Hypothermia is a below-normal body temperature. Frostbite is damage to skin and other tissues caused by extreme cold.
3. Heat exhaustion is a condition caused by too much water loss through sweating. Heatstroke is an injury in which the body can't control its temperature.
4. A tornado is a spinning column of air that has a high wind speed and touches the ground. A hurricane is a large, spinning tropical weather system with wind speeds of at least 74 miles per hour.
5. Rescue breathing is an emergency technique in which a rescuer gives air to someone who is not breathing. CPR is an emergency technique used to save a victim who isn't breathing and who doesn't have a heart beat.
6. dislocation
7. First aid
8. Violence
9. abdominal thrusts

Chapter Summary

- An accident is an unexpected event that may lead to injury.
- Violence is using physical force to hurt someone or cause damage.
- A smoke detector is an alarm that detects smoke from a fire.
- A fire extinguisher is a device that releases chemicals to put out a fire.
- Helmets protect cyclists and skaters from head injuries.
- Seat belts and air bags protect people travelling in a car.
- Hypothermia and frostbite are injuries caused by cold weather.
- Heat exhaustion and heatstroke are injuries caused by hot weather.
- One way to be prepared for a natural disaster is to have an emergency kit.
- The first thing to do during an emergency is to make sure you're safe.
- You should not give first aid unless you have had special training.

Using Vocabulary

For each pair of terms, describe how the meanings of the terms differ.

1. smoke detector/fire extinguisher
2. hypothermia/frostbite
3. heat exhaustion/heatstroke
4. tornado/hurricane
5. rescue breathing/CPR

For each sentence, fill in the blank with the proper word from the word bank provided below.

fracture   emergency
first aid   dislocation
violence   abdominal thrust

6. An injury in which a bone has been forced out of joint is called a(n) ___.
7. ___ is emergency medical care for someone who is hurt or sick.
8. ___ is using physical force to hurt someone.
9. Actions that apply pressure to a person's stomach to force an object out of the throat are called ___.

Understanding Concepts

10. List four common accidents and ways to avoid them.
11. What are five ways to avoid violence?
12. What should you do if you find a gun?
13. How should you put out a grease fire?
14. If you are walking, riding your bike, or skating after dark, what should you do to stay safe?
15. How does drinking plenty of water keep you safe when you're outside?
16. List four types of natural disasters. How can you prepare for a natural disaster?
17. Arrange the following steps of handling an emergency in the correct order.
    a. Care for the victim.
    b. Check out the situation.
    c. Call for help.
18. What should you do for someone who has a head, neck, or back injury?
19. How can you stay safe in a car? on the bus?
20. What is the first aid for the three types of burns?

Understanding Concepts

10. Sample answer: You can avoid falls by moving objects out of walkways and wiping up spills. You can prevent fires by not leaving flames and stoves unattended. You can also keep a fire extinguisher. You can avoid electrocution by avoiding bare wires and overloaded outlets and by not using electrical appliances near water. You can avoid poisoning by storing poisonous chemicals properly and by following the directions on medicine labels.
11. walk away, use refusal skills, use conflict management skills, tell an adult, and look for positive alternatives
12. Sample answer: Do not touch the gun. Walk away and tell an adult right away.
13. Sample answer: Use a fire extinguisher or use a pan lid, salt, or baking soda to smother the fire. Do not use water on a grease fire.

Chapter Resource File
- Concept Review GENERAL
- Concept Mapping GENERAL
- Performance-Based Assessment GENERAL
- Chapter Test GENERAL

Critical Thinking

Applying Concepts

21. Your friend just bought in-line skates and wants to know what kind of safety equipment to get. What would you recommend?

22. Imagine that you are listening to the radio when you hear that a tornado warning has been issued for your area. What should you do?

23. You should see a doctor if you have a burn on your hands, feet, or face. Why is it important to see a doctor for these burns?

24. Sam walks to school in the morning. His first class is wood shop. Then he has a lab class. After school, he goes skateboarding with his friends. They like to try some pretty hard tricks. How can Sam use some of the seven ways to stay safe to make sure that he doesn't have an accident?

Making Good Decisions

25. Imagine that you are at a friend's house. You go into the kitchen and find your friend's younger brother unconscious on the floor. You notice that there is an empty bottle of antifreeze on the floor. What should you do?

26. It is a cold winter day. Maria and Sarah are hiking when Maria notices that Sarah is shivering. Maria asks Sarah if she is OK. Sarah seems confused and her speech is slurred. What should Maria do?

27. George and several friends are at his friend Ben's house. Ben wants to show everyone his parents' gun. George's friends want to see it. What should George do?

28. Imagine that you and a friend are out riding bikes. You're both wearing your helmets. Your friend has an accident. Your friend has several cuts that are bleeding, and his arm is twisted at an odd angle. How should you help your friend?

Interpreting Graphics

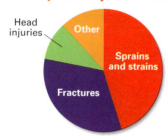

Trampoline Injuries Each Year

Use figure above to answer questions 29–32.

29. What is the most common type of trampoline-related injury each year?

30. Which injury is the least common type of trampoline-related injury each year?

31. About what percentage of the injuries are strains and sprains?

32. What two types of injuries make up more than 75 percent of all trampoline-related injuries each year?

Reading Checkup

Take a minute to review your answers to the Health IQ questions at the beginning of this chapter. How has reading this chapter improved your Health IQ?

---

14. Sample answer: I should wear bright or reflective clothes and use lights.
15. Sample answer: Drinking water can prevent heat exhaustion and heatstroke.
16. Sample answer: earthquakes, hurricanes, tornadoes, and floods; You can prepare an emergency kit and keep it where you will seek shelter.
17. b, c, a
18. Sample answer: I should not move the victim. I should call for help. If the victim is awake, I should tell him or her not to move and keep him or her awake until help arrives. I should keep the victim warm until help arrives.
19. Sample answer: In a car, I can wear my seatbelt. I can also sit in the back seat. On the bus, I can avoid distracting the driver, sit down while the bus is moving, and learn where the emergency exits are.
20. For a first-degree burn, run cool water over the burn and use antibiotic cream on it while it heals. For a second-degree burn, run cool water over the burn or use a wet cold compress. See a doctor if the burn is larger than 2 inches. For a third-degree burn, cover the burn with a clean, wet cloth and call for help.

Critical Thinking

Applying Concepts

21. Sample answer: a helmet, knee pads, elbow pads, and wrist guards
22. Sample answer: I should go to the basement or cellar. If I don't have one, I should go to a bathroom or closet in the center of my home.
23. Sample answer: Burns can leave scars. If there are scars on your hands and feet, they can make it difficult to walk or use your hands. On your face, they can be disfiguring. A doctor can help prevent scarring.
24. Sample answer: In shop and lab class, Sam should use his safety equipment and pay attention. While skateboarding, Sam should use his safety equipment, pay attention, think before he acts, and know his limits.

Making Good Decisions

25. Sample answer: I should call 911. Then, I should call poison control and tell the operator that my friend's brother probably drank antifreeze. Then, I should follow the operator's instructions.
26. Sample answer: Sarah has hypothermia. So, Maria should take Sarah someplace warm right away. Maria should wrap Sarah in a blanket, and call for help.
27. Sample answer: George should use his refusal skills to tell Ben that he doesn't want to see the gun. If Ben still plans on showing everyone the gun, George should leave.
28. Sample answer: My friend's arm may be broken. I should not move it. I should call for help and take care of my friend's cuts.

Interpreting Graphics

29. sprains and strains
30. head injuries
31. about 45%
32. fractures and sprains and strains

Model

Introduce this activity by reminding students that using this Life Skill will help them take personal responsibility for their behavior. Then, review the scenario with the class.

Prepare students for this activity by modeling each of the steps of the skill. Make sure students understand each step before you move on to the next one.

Guided Practice: Practice with a Friend

Guided Practice is the stage in which you and the students analyze their approach to solving the problem given in the scenario and analyze their ability to be a wise consumer. Have students read Act 1. Discuss with the class the situation described and the way students are to act it out. Organize the class into groups of two. In each group, one person plays the role of Beth, and the second person is the observer.

Proper pacing during the Guided Practice is important. The suggestions listed below will help you control the pace.

1. Stop after completing each step of being a wise consumer.
2. Discuss with each group the observer's comments.
3. Ask the other members of each group to listen to the observer's suggestions and to suggest ways to become a wiser consumer.
4. Instruct students to repeat the steps that need improvement and to include their modifications.

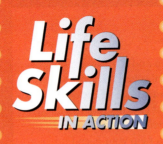

Life Skills IN ACTION

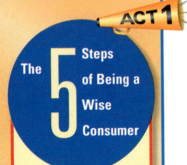

ACT 1

The 5 Steps of Being a Wise Consumer

1. List what you need and want from a product or a service.
2. Find several products or services that may fit your needs.
3. Research and compare information about the products or services.
4. Use the product or the service of your choice.
5. Evaluate your choice.

Being a Wise Consumer

Going shopping for products and services can be fun, but it can be confusing, too. Sometimes, there are so many options to choose from that finding the right one for you can be difficult. Being a wise consumer means evaluating different products and services for value and quality. Complete the following activity to learn how to be a wise consumer.

The Best Baby Seat

Setting the Scene

Beth's mother is having a baby. Beth is very excited and wants to help her mother get ready for the baby. Her mother asked Beth to help her research a baby seat to use in the car. Beth wants to find the best baby seat possible because she knows that the baby's safety is very important. She decides to start researching baby seats on the Internet.

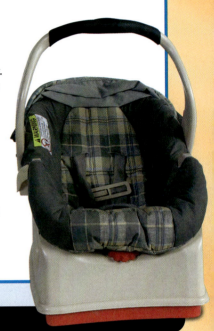

Guided Practice

Practice with a Friend

Form a group of two. Have one person play the role of Beth, and have the second person be an observer. Walking through each of the five steps of being a wise consumer, role-play Beth selecting and evaluating a baby seat for her mother's baby. The observer will take notes, which will include observations about what the person playing Beth did well and suggestions of ways to improve. Stop after each step to evaluate the process.

5. Check to make sure that students understand each step before they move on to the next step.
6. If time permits, repeat the exercise and have the students switch roles. Each student should have the opportunity to play each role. `Co-op Learning`

Independent Practice

Check Yourself

After you have completed the guided practice, go through Act 1 again without stopping at each step. Answer the questions below to review what you did.

1. What are some things that Beth may look for in a baby seat?
2. Other than the Internet, where can Beth find information about baby seats?
3. What are some ways Beth can evaluate the baby seat she selects?
4. When you are looking for safety equipment, why is it important to research several products before buying one?

ACT 2

On Your Own

Beth's mother loves the baby seat Beth selected and is impressed that Beth put a lot of effort in picking a good one. She takes Beth out to buy her a present as a thank you for finding the baby seat. Beth decides that she wants a camera so that she can take pictures of the baby when it arrives. Draw a comic strip that shows how Beth can use the five steps of being a wise consumer to find a good camera.

Independent Practice: Check Yourself

Instruct students to repeat Act 1 without stopping at each step. Remind students to apply what they learned in the Guided Practice to the Independent Practice.

Encourage students to use the Check Yourself questions as a starting point for reviewing and analyzing their Independent Practice. Remind students that as they change roles, the answers to these questions may change for each actor. Encourage students to create additional questions for checking their ability to be a wise consumer. When students have finished the Independent Practice, have them answer the Check Yourself questions in writing. Use their answers to assess their understanding of the steps of being a wise consumer and to assess their use of the steps to solve a problem.

Check Yourself Answers

1. Sample answer: Beth may want to know if a baby seat provides enough protection for the baby, if the seat is comfortable, and if the seat is easy to use.
2. Sample answer: Beth could read a consumer magazine or could talk to a salesperson at a store that sells baby seats.
3. Sample answer: Beth can evaluate how easy the seat is to use by trying to install it in a car and by trying to fasten a doll into the seat.
4. Sample answer: It is important to research several safety products before buying one because some products provide more protection than others do. Also, some safety products can only be used in certain situations. For example, some baby seats can only be used in certain kinds of cars.

Act 2: On Your Own

This additional scenario gives students an opportunity to apply what they have learned in both the Guided Practice and the Independent Practice to a new situation.

Suggest to students that they use the Check Yourself questions as a starting point for being a wise consumer in the new situation. Encourage students to be creative and to think of ways to improve their ability to be a wise consumer.

Assessment

Review the comic strips that students have created as part of the On Your Own activity. The comic strips should show a realistic conversation and should show that the students followed the steps of being a wise consumer in a realistic and effective manner. Display the comic strips around the room. If time permits, ask student volunteers to act out the dialogues of one or more of the comic strips. Discuss the comic strip's dialogue and the use of the steps of being a wise consumer.

Appendix

The Food Guide Pyramid

Do you know which foods you need to eat to stay healthy? How much of each food do you need to eat? The Food Guide Pyramid is a tool you can use to make sure you're eating healthfully. Each of the major food groups has its own block on the pyramid. The larger the block, the more you need to eat from that food group. The smaller the block, the less you need to eat from that food group. Use the Food Guide Pyramid as a guide for choosing a healthy diet!

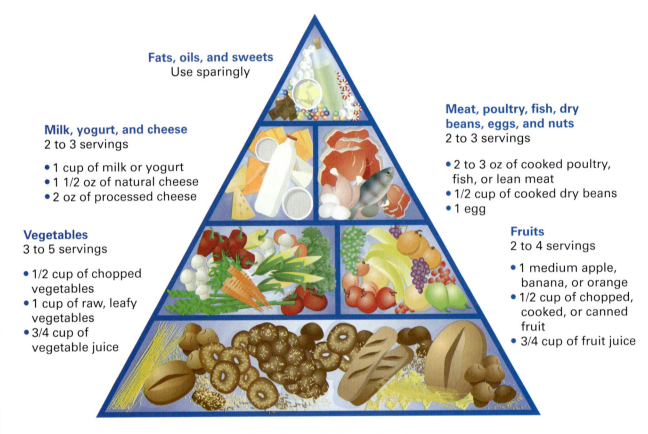

Fats, oils, and sweets
Use sparingly

Meat, poultry, fish, dry beans, eggs, and nuts
2 to 3 servings
- 2 to 3 oz of cooked poultry, fish, or lean meat
- 1/2 cup of cooked dry beans
- 1 egg

Milk, yogurt, and cheese
2 to 3 servings
- 1 cup of milk or yogurt
- 1 1/2 oz of natural cheese
- 2 oz of processed cheese

Vegetables
3 to 5 servings
- 1/2 cup of chopped vegetables
- 1 cup of raw, leafy vegetables
- 3/4 cup of vegetable juice

Fruits
2 to 4 servings
- 1 medium apple, banana, or orange
- 1/2 cup of chopped, cooked, or canned fruit
- 3/4 cup of fruit juice

Bread, cereal, rice, and pasta
6 to 11 servings
- 1 slice of bread
- 1 oz of ready-to-eat cereal
- 1/2 cup of rice or pasta
- 1/2 cup of cooked cereal

Alternative Food Guide Pyramids

The Vegetarian Food Guide Pyramid

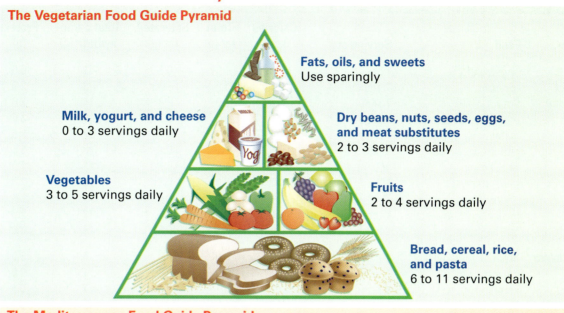

Fats, oils, and sweets
Use sparingly

Milk, yogurt, and cheese
0 to 3 servings daily

Dry beans, nuts, seeds, eggs, and meat substitutes
2 to 3 servings daily

Vegetables
3 to 5 servings daily

Fruits
2 to 4 servings daily

Bread, cereal, rice, and pasta
6 to 11 servings daily

The Mediterranean Food Guide Pyramid

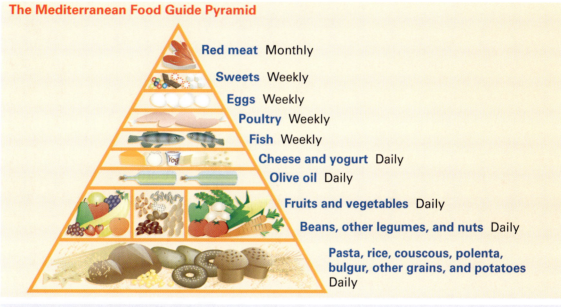

Red meat Monthly
Sweets Weekly
Eggs Weekly
Poultry Weekly
Fish Weekly
Cheese and yogurt Daily
Olive oil Daily
Fruits and vegetables Daily
Beans, other legumes, and nuts Daily
Pasta, rice, couscous, polenta, bulgur, other grains, and potatoes Daily

The Asian Food Guide Pyramid

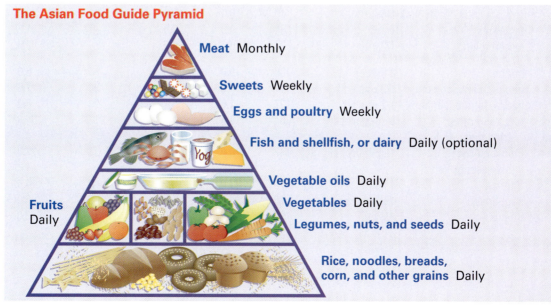

Meat Monthly
Sweets Weekly
Eggs and poultry Weekly
Fish and shellfish, or dairy Daily (optional)
Vegetable oils Daily
Fruits Daily
Vegetables Daily
Legumes, nuts, and seeds Daily
Rice, noodles, breads, corn, and other grains Daily

TABLE 1 Calorie and Nutrient Content of Common Foods

Food group	Food	Serving size	Calories (kcal)	Total fat (g)	Saturated fat (g)	Total carbo-hydrate (g)	Protein (g)
Bread, cereal, rice and pasta	bagel, plain	1 bagel	314	1.8	0.3	51	10.0
	biscuit	1 biscuit	101	5.0	1.2	13	2.0
	bread, white	1 slice	76	1.0	0.4	14	2.0
	bread, whole wheat	1 slice	86	1.0	0.3	16	3.0
	matzo	1 matzo	111	0.2	0.0	22	3.5
	pita bread, wheat	1 pita	165	1.0	0.1	33	5.0
	rice, brown	1/2 cup	110	1.0	0.2	23	2.0
	rice, white and enriched	1/2 cup	133	0.0	0.1	29	2.0
	tortilla, corn and plain	1 tortilla, 6 in.	58	0.7	0.1	12	2.0
	tortilla, flour	1 tortilla, 8 in.	104	2.3	0.6	18	3.0
Vegetables	broccoli, cooked	1 cup	27	0.0	0.0	5	3.0
	carrots, raw	1 baby carrot	4	0.0	0.0	1	0.0
	celery, raw	4 small stalks	10	0.1	0.0	2	0.5
	corn, cooked	1 ear	83	1.0	0.0	19	2.6
	cucumber, raw with peel	1/8 cup	25	0.1	0.0	6	0.6
	green beans, cooked	1 cup	44	0.4	0.0	10	2.4
	onions, raw, sliced	1/4 cup	11	0.0	0.0	3	0.3
	potatoes, baked with skin	1/2 cup	66	0.1	0.0	15	1.0
	salad, mixed green, no dressing	1 cup	10	1.0	0.0	2	1.4
	spinach, fresh	1 cup	7	0.1	0.0	1	0.9
Fruits	apple, raw, with skin	1 medium apple	81	0.1	0.1	21	0.2
	banana, fresh	1 medium banana	114	1.0	0.2	27	1.0
	cherries, sweet, fresh	1 cup, with pits	84	0.3	0.0	19	1.4
	grapes	1/2 cup	62	0.1	0.0	16	0.6
	orange, fresh	1 large orange	85	0.0	0.0	21	1.7
	peach, fresh	1 medium peach	37	0.0	0.0	9	1.0
	pear, fresh	1 medium pear	123	1.0	0.0	32	0.8
	raisins, seedless, dry	1 cup	495	0.2	0.0	131	5.3
	strawberries, fresh	1 cup	46	0.0	0.0	11	0.9
	tomatoes, raw	1 cup	31	0.5	0.0	7	1.3
	watermelon	1/2 cup	26	0.0	0.0	6	0.0
Meat, poultry, fish, dry beans, eggs, and nuts	bacon	3 pieces	109	9.0	3.3	0	6.0
	beans, black, cooked	1/2 cup	114	0.0	0.1	20	7.6
	beans, refried, canned	1/2 cup	127	1.0	0.1	23	8.0
	chicken breast, fried meat and skin	1 split breast	364	18.5	4.9	13	34.8
	chicken breast, skinless, grilled	1 split breast	142	3.0	0.9	73	27.0
	chorizo	1 link	273	23.0	8.6	1	14.5
	egg, boiled	1 large egg	78	5.3	1.0	0	6.0
	humus	1/4 cup	106	5.2	0.0	13	3.0

TABLE 1 Calorie and Nutrient Content of Common Foods (continued)

Food group	Food	Serving size	Calories (kcal)	Total fat (g)	Saturated fat (g)	Total carbohydrate (g)	Protein (g)
Meat, poultry, fish, dry beans, eggs, and nuts (continued)	peanut butter	2 Tbsp	190	16.0	3.0	7	8.0
	pork chop	3 oz	300	24.0	9.7	0	19.7
	roast beef	3 oz	179	6.5	2.3	0	28.1
	shrimp, breaded and fried	4 large shrimp	73	3.5	0.6	3	6.4
	steak, beef, broiled	6 oz	344	14.0	5.2	0	52.0
	sunflower seeds	1/4 cup	208	19.0	2.0	5	7.0
	tofu	1/2 cup	97	5.6	0.8	4	10.1
	tuna, canned in water	3 oz	109	2.5	0.7	0	20.1
	turkey, roasted	3 oz	145	4.2	1.4	0	24.9
Milk, yogurt, and cheese	cheese, American, prepackaged	1 slice	70	5.0	2.0	2	4.0
	cheese, cheddar	1 oz	114	9.0	6.0	0	7.1
	cheese, cottage, lowfat	1/2 cup	102	1.4	0.9	4	7.0
	cheese, cream	1 Tbsp	51	5.0	3.2	0	1.1
	milk, chocolate, reduced fat (2%)	1 cup	179	5.0	3.1	26	8.0
	milk, lowfat (1%)	1 cup	102	3.0	1.6	12	8.0
	milk, reduced fat (2%)	1 cup	122	5.0	2.9	12	8.1
	milk, skim, fat free	1 cup	91	0.0	0.0	12	8.0
	milk, whole	1 cup	149	8.0	5.1	11	8.0
	yogurt, lowfat, fruit flavored	1 cup	231	3.0	2.0	47	12.0
Fats, oils, and sweets	brownie	1 square	227	10.0	2.0	30	1.5
	butter	1 tsp	36	3.7	2.4	0	0.0
	candy, chocolate bar	1.3 oz	226	14.0	8.1	26	3.0
	soda, no ice	12 oz	184	0.0	0.0	38	0.0
	cheesecake	1 piece	660	46.0	28.0	52	11.0
	cookies, chocolate chip	1 cookie	59	2.5	0.8	8	0.6
	cookies, oatmeal	1 cookie	113	3.0	0.8	20	1.0
	gelatin dessert, flavored	1/2 cup	80	0.0	0.0	19	2.0
	ice-cream cone, one scoop regular ice cream	1 cone	178	8.0	4.9	22	3.0
	margarine, stick	1 tsp	34	3.8	0.7	0	0.0
	mayonnaise, regular	1 Tbsp	57	4.9	0.7	4	0.1
	pie, apple, double crust	1 piece	411	18.0	4.0	58	3.7
	popcorn, microwave, with butter	1/3 bag	170	12.0	2.5	26	2.0
	potato chips	1 oz	150	10.0	3.0	10	1.0
	pretzels	10 twists	229	2.1	0.5	48	5.5
	tortilla chips, plain	1 oz	140	7.3	1.4	18	2.0

Food Safety Tips

Few things taste better than a hot, home-cooked meal. It looks good and it smells good, but how do you know if it is safe to eat? Food doesn't have to look or smell bad to make you ill. To protect yourself from food-related illnesses, follow the food safety tips listed below.

Tips for Preparing Food

- Wash your hands with hot, soapy water before, during, and after you prepare food.
- Do not defrost food at room temperature. Always defrost food in the refrigerator or in the microwave.
- Always use a clean cutting board. If possible, use two cutting boards when preparing food. Use one cutting board for fruits and vegetables and the other cutting board for raw meat, poultry, and seafood.
- Wash cutting boards and other utensils with soap and hot water, especially those that come in contact with raw meat, poultry, and seafood.
- Keep raw meat, poultry, seafood, and their juices away from other foods.
- Marinate food in the refrigerator. Do not use leftover marinade sauce on cooked foods unless it has been boiled.

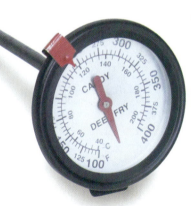

Tips for Cooking Food

- Use a food thermometer when cooking to ensure that food is cooked to a proper temperature.
- Red meats should be cooked to a temperature of 160°F.
- Poultry should be cooked to a temperature of 180°F.
- When cooked completely, fish flakes easily with a fork.
- Eggs should be cooked until the yolk and the white are firm.

Tips for Cleaning the Kitchen

- Wash all dishes, utensils, cutting boards, and pots and pans with hot, soapy water.
- Clean countertops with a disinfectant, such as a household cleaner that contains bleach. Wipe the countertop with paper towels, which can be thrown away. If you use a cloth towel, put it in the wash after using it.
- Refrigerate or freeze leftovers within 2 hours of cooking. Leftovers should be stored in small, shallow containers.

The Physical Activity Pyramid

How often do you exercise during the week? Do you think you get enough exercise to stay fit? Take a look at the Physical Activity Pyramid to find out if you're exercising enough to stay fit!

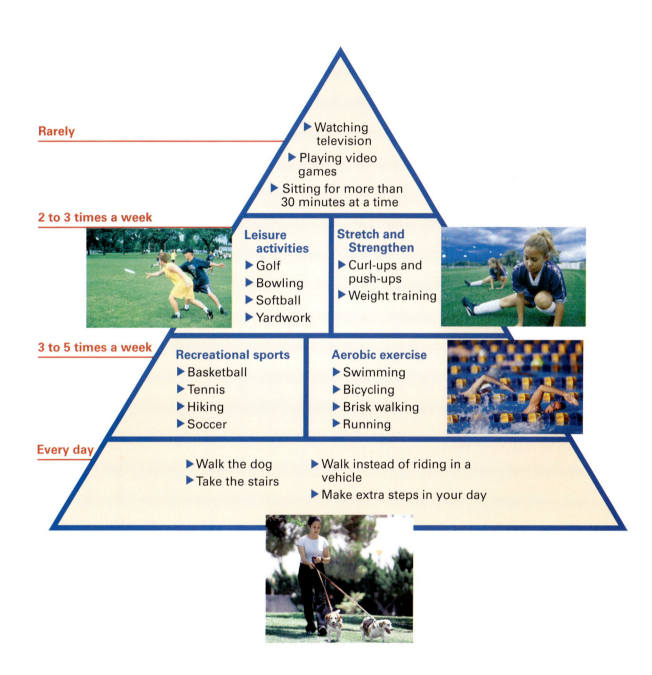

Rarely
- Watching television
- Playing video games
- Sitting for more than 30 minutes at a time

2 to 3 times a week

Leisure activities
- Golf
- Bowling
- Softball
- Yardwork

Stretch and Strengthen
- Curl-ups and push-ups
- Weight training

3 to 5 times a week

Recreational sports
- Basketball
- Tennis
- Hiking
- Soccer

Aerobic exercise
- Swimming
- Bicycling
- Brisk walking
- Running

Every day
- Walk the dog
- Take the stairs
- Walk instead of riding in a vehicle
- Make extra steps in your day

Water Safety

Water activities can be refreshing, fun, and exciting. But water can also be dangerous. Thousands of people drown each year. In fact, drowning is the second-leading cause of accidental death for people under the age of 15. But you can make sure you're safe around water. Keep the following tips in mind.

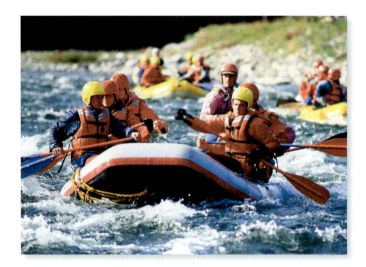

Swimming

- One of the best ways to stay safe in the water is to learn how to swim.
- Always swim with other people.
- Obey posted safety warnings. Signs around swimming areas let you know about safety risks.
- Swim in designated areas.
- Avoid areas that don't have a lifeguard on duty.
- Watch out for boats. Boaters often can't see swimmers.
- Don't swim away from shore. Swim parallel to shore. That way you can get back to shore more easily if you get tired.
- Avoid swimming in rough water and bad weather.

Diving

- Don't dive into unfamiliar bodies of water. If the water is shallow, you could injure your head, neck, or back.
- Get into water feet first until you know the water is deep enough to dive safely.
- Lower yourself into the water. Jumping feet first into shallow water could lead to foot, leg, and spine injuries.

Boating

- Always wear a life jacket. A life jacket can keep your head above water if you have an accident while boating.
- Always go boating with an experienced person.
- Don't stand in the boat. The boat may tip over, or you may fall out.
- Avoid boating in bad weather.
- Avoid rough water unless you know how to handle it. If you are white-water rafting, wear your life jacket and wear a helmet to protect your head.

Staying Home Alone

It is not unusual for teens to spend time home alone after school. Their parents may still be at work. Or they may be running errands. If you spend time at home alone, remember the following safety tips:

- Lock the doors and make sure your windows are locked.
- Never let anyone who calls or comes to your door know that you are home alone.
- Don't open the door for anyone you don't know or for anyone that isn't supposed to be at your home. If the visitor is delivering a package, ask him or her to leave it at the door. If the visitor wants to use the phone, send him or her to a phone booth. If the visitor is selling something, you can tell him or her through the door, "We're not interested."
- If a visitor doesn't leave or you see someone hanging around your home, call a trusted neighbor or the police for help.
- If you answer the phone, don't tell the caller anything personal. Offer to take a message without revealing you're alone. If the call becomes uncomfortable or mean, hang up the phone and tell your parents about it when they get home. You can also avoid answering the phone altogether when you're alone. Then, the caller can leave a message on the answering machine.
- Keep an emergency phone number list next to every phone in your home. If there is an emergency, call 911. Don't panic. Follow the operator's instructions. If the emergency is a fire, immediately leave the building and go to a trusted neighbor's home to call for help.
- Find an interesting way to spend your time. Time passes more quickly when you're not bored. Get a head start on your homework, read a book or magazine, clean your room, or work on a hobby. Avoid watching television unless your parents have given you permission to watch a specific program.
- Consider having a friend stay with you. But do so only if your parents have given you permission to have your friend over. That way, you won't be alone and you will have someone to pass the time with you.
- Remember your safety behaviors. By practicing them, you can make sure you stay safe.

☑ Think before you act.
☑ Pay attention.
☑ Know your limits.
☑ Practice refusal skills.
☑ Use safety equipment.
☑ Change risky behavior.
☑ Change risky situations.

Emergency Kit

A disaster can happen anytime and anywhere. During a disaster, people lose power, gas, and water. Sometimes, people are not able to get help for a few days. You can prepare for disasters by making an emergency kit. There are six basic things you should keep stocked in your emergency kit.

1. **Water** Store water in plastic containers. You'll need water for drinking, food preparation, and cleaning. Store a gallon of water per person per day. Have at least three days' worth of water in your kit.

2. **Food** Store at least three days' worth of nonperishable food. These foods include canned foods, freeze-dried foods, canned juices, and high-energy foods, such as nutrition bars. You should also keep vitamins in your emergency kit.

3. **First-Aid Kit** Someone may get hurt, so you'll want to have plenty of first-aid supplies. Include the following supplies in your first-aid kit:
   - self-adhesive bandages
   - gauze pads
   - rolled gauze
   - adhesive tape
   - antibacterial ointment and cleansers
   - thermometer
   - scissors, tweezers, and razor blades
   - sterile gloves and breathing mask
   - over-the-counter medicines

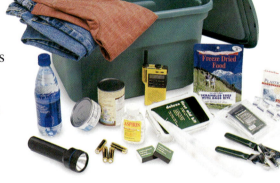

4. **Clothing and Bedding** An emergency kit should include at least one complete change of clothing and shoes per person. You should also store blankets or sleeping bags, rain gear, and thermal underwear.

5. **Tools and Supplies** Always keep your emergency kit stocked with a flashlight, battery-operated radio, and extra batteries. Also, include a can opener, cooking supplies, candles, waterproof matches, fire extinguisher, tape, and hardware tools. You should also store emergency signal supplies, such as signal flares, whistles, and signal mirrors.

6. **Special Items** Be sure to remember family members who have special needs. For example, store formula, baby food, and diapers for infants. For adults, you might keep contact lens supplies, special medications, and extra eyeglasses in your emergency kit.

Internet Safety

The Internet is a wonderful tool. It allows you to communicate with people, access information, and educate yourself. You can also use it to have fun. But when using any tool, there are certain precautions or safety measures you must take. Using the Internet is no different. Listed below are some rules to follow to make sure you stay safe when you are using the Internet.

Rules for Internet Safety

- Set up rules with your parents or another trusted adult about what time of day you can use the Internet, how long you can use the Internet, and what sites you can visit on the Internet. Follow the rules that have been set.

- Do not give out personal information, such as your address, telephone number, or the name and location of your school.

- If you find any information that makes you uncomfortable, tell a parent or another trusted adult immediately.

- Do not respond to any messages that make you uncomfortable. If you receive such a message, tell your parents or another trusted adult immediately.

- Never agree to meet with anyone before talking to your parents or another trusted adult. If your parents give you permission to meet someone, make sure you do so in a public place. Have an adult come with you.

- Do not send a picture of yourself or any other information without first checking with your parents or a trusted adult.

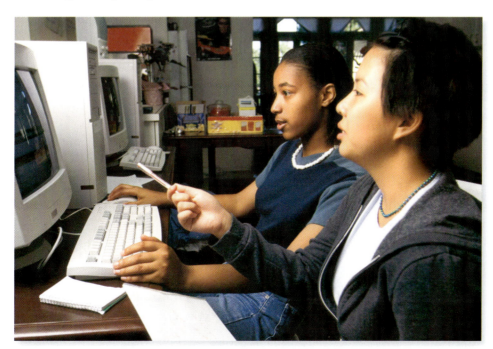

Baby Sitter Safety

Baby-sitting is an important job. You're responsible for taking care of another person's children. You have to make decisions not only for yourself but also for other people. So, you have to make good decisions. Keep the following tips in mind when you baby-sit.

Before you Baby-Sit

- Take a baby-sitting course or first-aid class.
- Find out what time you should arrive and arrange for your transportation to and from the home.
- Ask the parents how long they plan to be away.
- Find out how many children you will be caring for and what your responsibilities are.
- Settle on how much the parents will pay you for your work.
- Consider visiting the family while the parents are home so you can get to know the children a few days before you baby-sit.

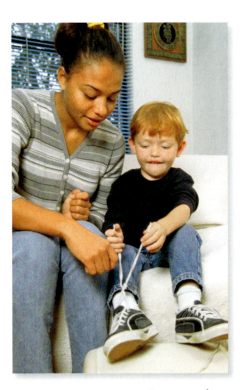

When You Arrive

- Arrive early so the parents can give you information about caring for the children. Ask the parents about the children's eating habits, TV habits, and bedtime routine.
- Find out where the parents are going. Write down the address and phone number for where they will be and put it next to the phone. Find out when they plan to return. If the parents have a cellular phone, be sure to get that number, too.
- Know where the emergency numbers are posted. Also, make sure you have the address for the home so that you can give it to an operator in the event of an emergency.
- If you are watching toddlers or infants, find out where their formula and diaper supplies are stored.
- Learn where the family keeps their first-aid supplies. If the children need any medicine while you care for them, make sure you know how to give it to them. Remember that you shouldn't give children medicine unless you have the parents' permission to do so.
- Ask if the children have any special needs. For example, some children are diabetic or asthmatic. Make sure you know what to do if they have any trouble.

While You Are Baby-Sitting

- Never leave a child alone, even for a short time.
- Don't leave an infant alone on a changing table, sofa, or bed.
- Check on the children often, even when they're sleeping.
- Don't leave children alone in the bathtub or near a pool.
- Keep breakable and dangerous objects out of the reach of children.
- Keep the doors locked. Unless the parents have given you permission, do not open the door for anyone.
- If the phone rings, take a message. Do not let the caller know that you are the baby sitter and that the parents are not home.
- If the child gets hurt or sick, call the parents. Don't try to take care of it yourself. In case of a serious emergency, call 911. Then, call the parents.

FUN THINGS YOU CAN DO WHILE YOU BABY-SIT

Baby-sitting is a huge responsibility. But it is also very rewarding. Children love it when you pay attention to them and when you play with them. Don't be afraid to get down on the floor with them. They like you to play at their level. Consider doing the following fun activities, but remember to always get the parents' permission, first!

- Take children outside or to a local park to play.
- Read stories to each other. Let the children pick their favorite story.
- Go to story time at the local library.
- Draw pictures, or color in coloring books. Take this a step further by pretending there is an art gallery in the house. Hang up the pictures, and pretend to be visiting the gallery.
- Pretend you are at a restaurant during mealtimes. Have the children make up menus and pretend to be waiters.
- Plan a scavenger hunt.
- Bring some simple craft items for the children, and let them get creative.
- Play board games or card games.

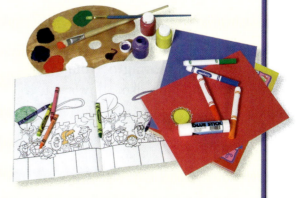

The Body Systems

The Nervous System

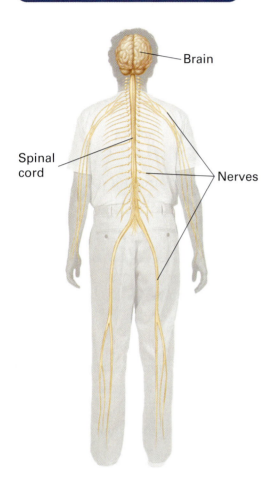

The Endocrine System

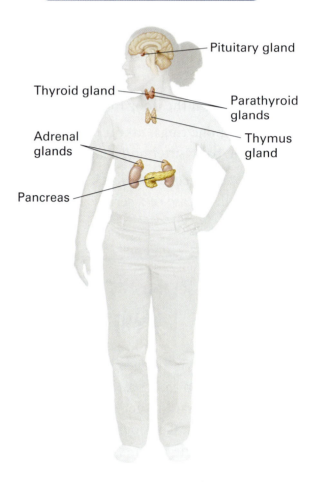

The Nervous System

The nervous system controls all of your body's functions. The nervous system is composed of the brain, the spinal cord, nerves, and sensory organs, such as your eyes, ears, and taste buds. The nervous system controls voluntary activities, such as walking, and involuntary activities, such as the beating of your heart. The nervous system also allows you to hear, see, smell, taste, and detect pain and pressure.

The Endocrine System

The endocrine system helps the nervous system control your body's functions. The endocrine system also helps regulate growth. The endocrine system is a network of tissues and organs that make and release hormones. Hormones are chemicals that cause changes in the body. Some hormones control how your body grows. Other hormones control how your body responds to stress.

The Skeletal System

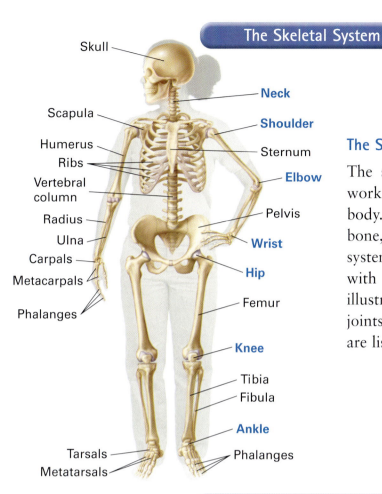

The Skeletal System

The skeletal system provides a framework that supports and protects your body. The skeletal system is made up of bone, cartilage, and joints. The skeletal system also stores minerals and works with muscles to help you move. The illustration at left lists the bones and joints of your skeletal system. The joints are listed in blue.

The Muscular System

The Muscular System

The muscular system works with the skeletal system to allow you to move. The muscular system is made up of muscles, or tissue composed of cells that contract and expand to cause movement. There are three types of muscle in the body. Smooth muscle is found in the digestive tract, blood vessels, and reproductive organs. Cardiac muscle is found in the heart. Skeletal muscle attaches to bones. The illustration at right shows the skeletal muscles of the muscular system.

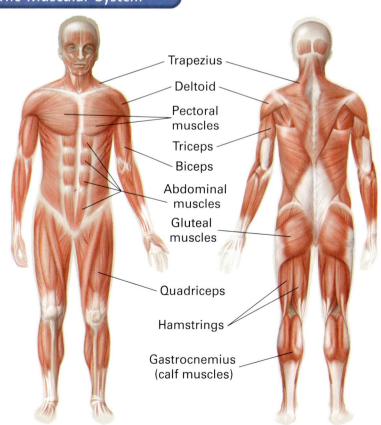

Appendix 419

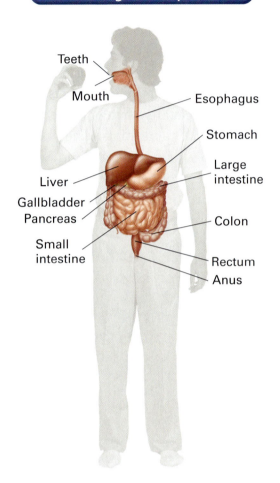

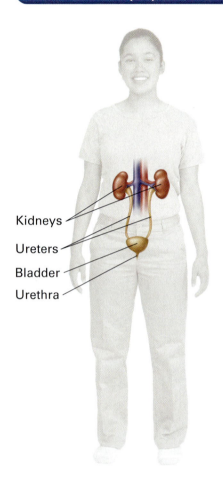

The Digestive System

The digestive system breaks down food into simpler substances, transfers nutrients to the blood, and removes solid waste from your body. The digestive system is composed of organs, such as the stomach and intestines, and glands, such as the liver and gallbladder, that work together to digest food.

The Urinary System

The urinary system filters liquid waste products from the blood and eliminates them from your body. Waste products are filtered from the blood by the kidneys. The waste products are moved from the kidneys to the bladder. Wastes are then eliminated from the body through urination.

The Circulatory System

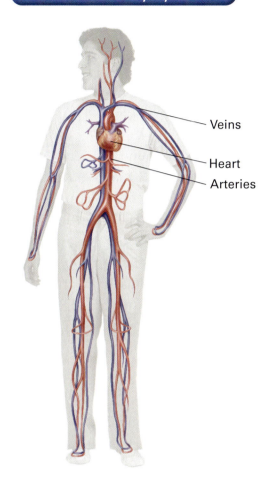

The Respiratory System

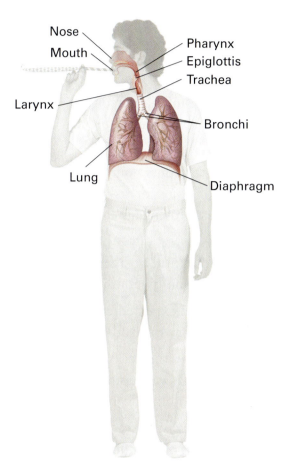

The Circulatory System

The circulatory system is responsible for transporting and distributing gases, nutrients, and hormones throughout your body. The circulatory system also collects and transports waste products for elimination from your body and protects your body from disease. The circulatory system is made up of your heart, blood vessels, and blood.

The Respiratory System

The respiratory system transfers oxygen from the air into your body and removes carbon dioxide from your body. The gases move into and out of the body through the action of breathing. Air enters the body through the mouth and nose. The air moves through the throat and into the lungs. In the lungs, oxygen and carbon dioxide are exchanged between the blood and the lungs.

Glossary

abdominal thrusts (ab DAHM uh nuhl THRUHSTS) the act of applying pressure to a choking person's stomach to force an object out of the throat (394)

abstinence the refusal to take part in an activity that puts your health or the health of others at risk; in particular the refusal to engage in sexual activity (314)

abuse the harmful or offensive treatment of one person by another person (182)

accident an unexpected event that may lead to injury or death (374)

active listening the act of hearing and showing that you understand what a person is communicating (138)

active rest a way to recover from exercise by reducing the amount of activity you do (86)

acute injury (uh KYOOT IN juh ree) an injury that happens suddenly (82)

additives the chemicals that help tobacco stay moist, burn longer, and taste better (220)

adolescence the stage of development during which humans grow from childhood to adulthood (364)

adulthood the period of life that follows adolescence and that ends at death (365)

aerobic exercise (er OH bik EK suhr SIEZ) exercise that lasts a long time and uses oxygen to get energy (72)

aggression any action or behavior that is hostile or threatening to another person (210)

AIDS acquired immune deficiency syndrome (uh KWIERD im MYOON dee FISH uhn see SIN DROHM), an illness that is caused by HIV infection and that makes an infected person more likely to get unusual forms of cancer and infection because HIV attacks the body's immune system (312)

alcohol abuse the inability to drink in moderation or at appropriate times (251)

alcoholism a disease caused by addiction to alcohol; a physical and emotional addiction to alcohol (258)

Alzheimer's disease (AHLTS HIE muhrz di ZEEZ) a brain disease that affects thinking, memory, and behavior; people who have Alzheimer's may lose their ability to speak and to control their bodies (330)

anaerobic exercise (an er OH bik EK suhr SIEZ) exercise that does not use oxygen to get energy and that lasts a very short time (72)

anorexia nervosa (AN uh REKS ee uh nuhr VOH suh) an eating disorder that involves self-starvation, an unhealthy body image, and extreme weight loss (122)

antibiotic a drug that kills bacteria or slows the growth of bacteria (309)

asthma a respiratory disorder that causes the small bronchioles in the lung to narrow; asthma causes shortness of breath, wheezing, coughing, or breathing with a whistling sound (329)

attitude the way in which you act, think, or feel that causes you to make particular choices (10)

bacteria (bak TIR ee uh) extremely small, single-celled organisms that do not have a nucleus; single-celled microorganisms that are found everywhere (306)

behavior the way that a person chooses to respond or act (179)

binge drinking for men, drinking five or more drinks in one sitting; for women, drinking four or more drinks in one sitting (253)

binge eating disorder an eating disorder in which a person has difficulty controlling how much food he or she eats (123)

blood alcohol concentration (BAC) the percentage of alcohol in a person's blood (249)

body image the way that you see yourself and imagine your body (116)

body language a way of communicating by using facial expressions, hand gestures, and posture (138, 178, 203)

body system a group of organs that work together to complete a specific task in the body (322)

brainstorming the act of thinking of all of the ways to carry out a decision (25)

bulimia nervosa (boo LEE mee uh nuhr VOH suh) an eating disorder in which a person eats a large amount of food and then tries to remove the food from his or her body (122)

bullying scaring or controlling another person by using threats or physical force (200)

carbohydrate (KAHR boh HIE drayt) a chemical composed of one or more simple sugars; includes sugars, starches, and fiber (99)

carcinogen any chemical or agent that causes cancer (226)

cardiopulmonary resuscitation (CPR) (KAHR dee oh PUL muh NER ee ri SUHS uh TAY shuhn) a life-saving technique that combines rescue breathing and chest compressions (396)

cardiovascular disease a disorder of the circulatory system (225)

cataract a clouding of the natural lens of the eye (341)

celiac disease (SEE lee AK di ZEEZ) a disease of the digestive system that makes the body allergic to the protein gluten (335)

central nervous system (CNS) the brain and spinal cord (330)

chronic injury an injury that develops over a long period of time (83)

collaboration a solution to a conflict in which both parties get what they want without having to give up anything important (205)

communication the ability to exchange information and the ability to express one's thoughts and feelings clearly (40)

community a group of people who have a common background or location or who share similar interests, beliefs, or goals (184)

competition a contest between two or more individuals or teams (74)

compromise a solution to a conflict in which both sides give up things to come to an agreement (205)

conflict any situation in which ideas or interests go against one another (198)

congenital disorder any disease, abnormality, or disorder that is present at birth but that is not inherited (325)

consequence a result of one's actions and decisions (23)

coping dealing with problems and troubles in an effective way (39)

creative expression the use of an art to express emotion (139)

deafness the partial or total loss of the ability to hear (341)

defense mechanism an automatic, short-term behavior to cope with distress (141, 164)

depressant (dee PREHS uhnt) any drug that decreases activity in the body (248, 285)

depression a mood disorder in which a person is extremely sad and hopeless for a long period of time (145)

diet a pattern of eating that includes what a person eats, how much a person eats, and how often a person eats (96)

Dietary Guidelines for Americans a set of suggestions designed to help people develop healthy eating habits and increase physical activity levels (102)

digestion the process of breaking down food into a form that the body can use (95)

dislocation an injury in which a bone has been forced out of its normal position in a joint (400)

distress any stress response that keeps you from reaching your goals or that makes you sick; the negative physical, mental, or emotional strain in response to a stressor (159)

driving under the influence (DUI) the driving of a motor vehicle by a person who is legally intoxicated or who is using illegal drugs (256)

drug any chemical substance that causes a change in a person's physical or psychological state (248, 270)

drug abuse the purposeful misuse of a legal drug or the use of an illegal drug (277)

drug addiction the condition in which a person can no longer control his or her need or desire for a drug (230, 278)

drug misuse use of a drug that differs from the intended use (276)

earthquake a shaking of the Earth's surface that is caused by movement along a break in the Earth's crust (388)

eating disorder a disease in which a person has an unhealthy concern for his or her body weight and shape (121)

egg the sex cell made by females (354)

embryo a developing human, from fertilization until the end of the eighth week of pregnancy (360)

emergency a sudden event that demands immediate action (392)

emotion a feeling that is produced in response to a life event (134)

emotional health the way that a person experiences and deals with feelings (135)

emphysema a respiratory disease in which oxygen and carbon dioxide have difficulty moving through the alveoli because the alveoli are thin and stretched out or have been destroyed (329)

endocrine gland a group of cells or an organ that produces hormones (332)

endocrine system (EN doh krin SIS tuhm) a network of tissues and organs that release chemicals that control certain body functions (358)

endurance (en DOOR uhns) the ability to do activities for more than a few minutes (66)

environment all of the living and nonliving things around you (9, 349)

environmental tobacco smoke (ETS) the mixture of exhaled smoke and smoke from the ends of burning cigarettes (223)

exercise any physical activity that maintains or improves your physical fitness (68)

fad diet a diet that promises quick weight loss with little effort (120)

fatigue physical or mental exhaustion; a feeling of extreme tiredness (162)

fats an energy-storage nutrient that helps the body store some vitamins (99)

fetal alcohol syndrome (FAS) a group of birth defects that affect an unborn baby that has been exposed to alcohol (255)

fetus the developing human in a woman's uterus, from the start of the ninth week of pregnancy until birth (360)

fire extinguisher a device that releases chemicals to put out a fire (379)

first aid emergency medical care for someone who has been hurt or who is sick (392)

flexibility (FLEKS uh BIL uh tee) the ability to bend and twist joints easily (67)

flood an overflowing of water into areas that are normally dry (390)

Food Guide Pyramid a tool for choosing what kinds of foods to eat and how much of each food to eat every day (103)

fracture a crack or break in a bone (400)

friendship a relationship between people who enjoy being together, who care about each other and who often have similar interests (186)

frostbite damage to skin and other tissues caused by extreme cold (384)

genes (JEENZ) a set of instructions found in every cell of a person's body that describe how that person's body will look, grow, and function (348)

gland a tissue or group of tissues that makes and releases chemicals such as hormones (332, 358)

glaucoma a disease that causes pressure in the fluid inside the eye; the high pressure damages the optic nerve and causes a permanent loss of vision (341)

goal something that someone works toward and hopes to achieve (32)

good decision a decision in which a person carefully considers the outcome of each choice (22)

grief a feeling of deep sadness about a loss (367)

hallucinogen (huh LOO si nuh juhn) any drug that causes a person to hallucinate (288)

health a condition of physical, emotional, mental, and social well-being (4)

healthy weight range an estimate of how much one should weigh depending on one's height and body frame (124)

heart attack a condition in which the heart does not receive enough blood and the heart tissue is damaged or killed, which causes the heart not to pump well (325)

heat exhaustion (HEET eg ZAWS chuhn) a condition caused by losing too much water through sweating on a hot day (385)

heatstroke a failure of the body's heat-regulation systems (385)

heredity (huh RED i tee) the passing down of traits from parents to their biological child (8, 348)

HIV human immunodeficiency virus (HYOO muhn IM myoo NOH dee FISH uhn see VIE ruhs), a virus that attacks the human immune system and that causes AIDS (312)

hobby something that you like to do or to study in your spare time (262)

hormone a chemical made in one part of the body that is released into the blood, that is carried through the bloodstream, and that causes a change in another part of the body; controls growth and development and many other body functions (134, 332, 358)

hurricane a large, spinning tropical weather system that has wind speeds of at least 74 miles per hour (389)

hypertension (HIE puhr TEN shuhn) a condition in which the pressure inside the large arteries is too high; also called *high blood pressure* (326)

hypothermia (HIE poh THUHR mee uh) a below-normal body temperature (384)

infectious disease (in FEK shuhs dih ZEEZ) any disease that is caused by an agent or pathogen that invades the body (304)

inhalant (in HAY luhnt) any drug that is inhaled and that is absorbed into the bloodstream through the lungs (289)

interest something that one enjoys and wants to know more about (33)

intoxication (in TAHKS i KAY SHUHN) the physical and mental changes produced by drinking alcohol (250)

kidneys organs that filter blood and remove liquid wastes and extra water from the blood (336)

leukemia (loo KEE mee uh) cancer of the tissues of the body that make white blood cells (327)

life skills tools that help you deal with situations that can affect your health (12)

lifestyle a set of behaviors by which you live your life (10)

marijuana (mar uh WAH nuh) the dried flowers and leaves of the *Cannabis* plant (286)

mediation a process in which a third party, called a *mediator,* becomes involved in a conflict, listens to both sides of the conflict, and then offers solutions to the conflict (207)

medicine a drug that is used to cure, prevent, or treat pain, disease, or illness (274)

menstruation (MEN STRAY shuhn) the monthly breakdown and shedding of the lining of the uterus during which blood and tissue leave the woman's body through the vagina (355)

mental health the way that people think about and respond to events in their lives (134)

mental illness a disorder that affects a person's thoughts, emotions, and behaviors (144)

mineral (MIN uhr uhlz) an element that is essential for good health (100)

muscular dystrophy a group of hereditary muscle diseases that cause muscles to become weak and disabled gradually (339)

negative thinking focusing on the bad parts of a situation (140)

neglect the failure of a parent or other responsible adult to provide for basic needs, such as food, clothing, or love (182)

negotiation discussion of a conflict to reach an agreement (204)

nicotine a highly addictive drug that is found in all tobacco products (221)

nicotine replacement therapy (NRT) a form of medicine that contains safe amounts of nicotine (235)

noninfectious disease a disease that is not caused by a pathogen (322)

nurturing (NUR chuhr ing) providing the care and other basic things that people need in order to grow (181)

nutrient a substance in food that the body needs in order to work properly (95)

Nutrition Facts label a label that is found on the outside packages of food and that states the number of servings in the container, the number of Calories in each serving, and the amount of nutrients in each serving (104)

option a choice that you can make (25)

organ two or more tissues that work together to perform a special function (322)

osteoporosis a bone disease that causes loss of bone density (339)

over-the-counter (OTC) medicine any medicine that can be bought without a prescription (275)

overtraining a condition caused by too much exercise (81)

ovulation (AHV yoo LAY shuhn) the process in which the ovaries release a mature ovum every month (355)

peer pressure a feeling that you should do something because your friends want you to (29, 232, 246)

peripheral nervous system (PNS) the nerves that connect the brain and spinal cord to all other parts of the body (330)

persistence the commitment to keep working toward a goal even when things make a person want to quit (37)

phobia (FOH bee uh) a strong, abnormal fear of something (147)

physical dependence a state in which the body chemically needs a drug in order to function normally (279)

physical fitness the ability to perform daily physical activities without becoming short of breath, sore, or overly tired (66)

positive self-talk thinking about the good parts of a bad situation (140)

positive stress stress response that makes a person feel good; the stress response that happens when a person wins, succeeds, and achieves (169)

pregnancy the time when a woman carries a developing fetus in her uterus (360)

prescription medicine (pree SKRIP shuhn MED i suhn) a medicine that can be bought only with a written order from a doctor (274)

preventive healthcare taking steps to prevent illness and accidents before they happen (11)

protein (PROH TEEN) a nutrient that supplies the body with energy for building and repairing tissues and cells (99)

psychiatrist (sie KIE uh trist) a medical doctor who specializes in how illnesses of the brain and body are related to emotions and behavior (150)

psychological dependence (SIE kuh LAHJ it kuhl dee PEN duhns) the state of emotionally or mentally needing a drug in order to function (279)

puberty the period of time during adolescence when the reproductive system becomes mature (364)

R

reaction time the amount of time that passes from the instant when the brain detects an external stimulus until the moment a person responds (250)

recovery the process of learning to live without alcohol (259)

redirection taking energy from your stress response and directing it into an activity that is not stressful (167)

reframing looking at a situation from another point of view and changing one's emotional response to the situation (167)

refusal skill a strategy to avoid doing something that you don't want to do (42)

relationship an emotional or social connection between two or more people (176)

relaxation the state of doing something to take one's mind off a problem and to focus on something else that is not stressful (167)

rescue breathing an emergency technique in which a rescuer gives air to someone who is not breathing (396)

resting heart rate (RHR) the number of times that the heart beats per minute while the body is at rest (71)

S

self-concept a measure of how you see and imagine yourself as a person (54)

self-esteem a measure of how much you value, respect, and feel confident about yourself (32, 50)

sex cell a parent cell that joins with another sex cell to create a new cell that contains all of the information needed to develop into a new human being (348)

sexual abstinence (SEK shoo uhl AB stuh nuhns) the refusal to take part in sexual activity (190)

sexually transmitted disease (STD) any of a number of infections that are spread from one person to another by sexual contact (314)

smoke detector a small, battery-operated alarm that detects smoke from a fire (378)

social strain the awkwardness of a situation or the tension among family members and friends because of the use of tobacco (229)

sperm the sex cell made by males (350)

sportsmanship the ability to treat all players, officials, and fans fairly during competition (74)

stimulant (STIM yoo luhnt) any drug that increases the body's activity (284)

strength the amount of force that muscles can apply when they are used (66)

stress the combination of a new or possibly threatening situation and the body's natural response to the situation (158)

GLOSSARY

stress management the ability to handle stress in healthy ways (167)

stress response a set of physical changes that prepare your body to act in response to a stressor; the body's response to a stressor (162)

stressor anything that triggers a stress response (158)

success the achievement of one's goals (36)

suicide the act of killing oneself (145)

targeted marketing advertising aimed at a particular group of people (233)

testes (TES TEEZ) the male reproductive organs that make sperm and the hormone testosterone (350)

THC tetrahydrocannabinol, the active substance in marijuana (286)

therapist a professional who is trained to treat emotional problems by talking about them (150)

tobacco a plant whose leaves can be dried and mixed with chemicals to make products such as cigarettes, smokeless tobacco, and cigars (231)

tolerance (TAHL uhr uhns) the ability to overlook differences and to accept people for who they are (184); a condition in which a person needs more of a drug to feel the original effects of the drug (231)

tornado a spinning column of air that has high wind speed and that touches the ground (389)

trigger a person, situation, or event that influences emotions (142)

type 1 diabetes a disease of the endocrine system in which the body makes little or no insulin (333)

type 2 diabetes a disease of the endocrine system in which the body makes insulin but cannot use insulin properly (333)

vaccine a substance that is used to make a person immune to a certain disease (311)

values beliefs that one considers to be of great importance (25)

verbal communication the act of expressing and understanding thoughts and emotions by talking (138)

violence physical force that is used to harm people or damage property (208, 375)

virus a tiny, disease-causing particle that consists of genetic material and a protein coat and that invades a healthy cell and instructs that cell to make more viruses (310)

vitamin (VIET uh minz) an organic compound that controls many body functions and that is needed in small amounts to maintain health and allow growth (100)

weight training the use of weight to make muscles stronger or bigger (76)

wellness a state of good health that is achieved by balancing physical, emotional, mental, and social health (7)

withdrawal uncomfortable physical and psychological symptoms produced when a person who is physically dependent on drugs stops using drugs (231, 278)

Spanish Glossary

abdominal thrusts/empujes abdominal acción de aplicar presión al estómago de una persona atragantada para lograr que un objeto salga por la garganta (394)

abstinence/abstinencia decisión de no participar en una actividad que ponga en riesgo la salud propia o la de otros; especialmente la decisión de no participar en actividades sexuales (314)

abuse/abuso tratamiento dañino u ofensivo de una persona hacia otra (182)

accident/accidente acontecimiento inesperado que puede provocar lesión o muerte (374)

active listening/escuchar activamente acción de escuchar y demostrar que comprendes lo que una persona intenta comunicar (138)

active rest/descanso activo forma de recuperarse del ejercicio reduciendo la cantidad de actividad que realizas (86)

acute injury/lesión aguda lesión que se produce de manera repentina (82)

additives/aditivos sustancias químicas que permiten que el tabaco se mantenga húmedo, permanezca encendido por más tiempo y tenga un mejor sabor (220)

adolescence/adolescencia etapa del desarrollo en la que los seres humanos pasan de la infancia a la edad adulta (364)

adulthood/edad adulta período de la vida que sigue a la adolescencia y termina con la muerte (365)

aerobic exercise/ejercicio aeróbico ejercicio que se realiza durante un período de tiempo prolongado y utiliza el oxígeno para obtener energía (72)

aggression/agresión toda acción o conducta hostil o amenazante hacia otra persona (210)

AIDS/SIDA síndrome de inmunodeficiencia adquirida, enfermedad producida por la infección del VIH que hace que una persona infectada tenga más posibilidades de contraer formas poco comunes de cáncer e infecciones debido a que el VIH ataca al sistema inmunológico del cuerpo (312)

alcohol abuse/abuso de alcohol incapacidad de beber con moderación o en los horarios adecuados (251)

alcoholism/alcoholismo enfermedad ocasionada por la adicción al alcohol; adicción física y emocional al alcohol (258)

Alzheimer's disease/enfermedad de Alzheimer enfermedad del cerebro que afecta el pensamiento, la memoria y la conducta; las personas con la enfermedad de Alzheimer pueden perder la capacidad de hablar y controlar el cuerpo (330)

anaerobic exercise/ejercicio anaeróbico ejercicio que no utiliza el oxígeno para obtener energía y que se realiza durante un período de tiempo corto (72)

anorexia nervosa/anorexia nerviosa trastorno alimenticio en el que la persona deja de comer, tiene una percepción enferma de su cuerpo y sufre una pérdida de peso extrema (122)

antibiotic/antibiótico droga que mata a las bacterias o demora su crecimiento (309)

asthma/asma trastorno respiratorio que hace que los bronquiolos pequeños en los pulmones se estrechen; el asma produce dificultad para respirar, jadeo, tos o un silbido al respirar (329)

attitude/actitud forma particular de actuar, pensar o sentir de una persona (10)

bacteria/bacteria organismos unicelulares extremadamente pequeños que no tienen núcleo; microorganismos de una sola célula que se encuentran en todas partes (306)

behavior/conducta la forma en la que una persona decide reaccionar o actuar (179)

binge drinking/beber compulsivamente en el caso de los hombres, beber cinco o más bebidas en una misma ocasión; en el caso de las mujeres, beber cuatro o más bebidas en una misma ocasión (253)

binge eating/disorder trastorno alimenticio compulsivo trastorno alimenticio en el que una persona tiene dificultad para controlar cuánto come (123)

blood alcohol concentration (BAC)/ concentración de alcohol en la sangre (CAS) porcentaje de alcohol en la sangre de una persona (249)

body image/imagen corporal forma en que piensas en ti mismo y en tu cuerpo (116)

body language/lenguaje corporal forma de comunicarse utilizando expresiones de la cara, gestos con la mano y la postura del cuerpo (138, 178, 203)

body system/sistema corporal grupo de órganos que trabajan juntos para cumplir una función específica en el cuerpo (322)

brainstorming/lluvia de ideas acción de pensar en todas las maneras posibles de llevar a cabo una decisión (25)

bulimia nervosa/bulimia nerviosa trastorno alimenticio en el que una persona come una gran cantidad de alimentos y luego intenta eliminar la comida del cuerpo (122)

bullying/gandallismo acción de asustar o manipular a otra persona mediante amenazas o la fuerza física (200)

carbohydrate/carbohidratos sustancia química compuesta por uno o más azúcares simples; incluye azúcares, féculas y fibras (99)

carcinogen/carcinógeno toda sustancia química o agente que causa cáncer (226)

cardiopulmonary resuscitation (CPR)/ resucitación cardiopulmonar (RCP) técnica para salvar la vida que combina la recuperación de la respiración y compresiones en el pecho (396)

cardiovascular disease/enfermedad cardiovascular enfermedades y trastornos originados por el daño progresivo al corazón y los vasos sanguíneos (225)

cataract/catarata opacidad del cristalino natural del ojo (341)

celiac disease/enfermedad celíaca enfermedad del aparato digestivo que hace que el cuerpo se vuelva alérgico a la proteína de gluten (335)

central nervous system (CNS)/sistema nervioso central (SNC) el cerebro y la médula espinal (330)

chronic injury/lesión crónica lesión que se desarrolla durante un largo período de tiempo (83)

collaboration/colaboración solución a un problema en el que ambas partes obtienen lo que desean sin tener que renunciar a nada importante (205)

communication/comunicación capacidad de intercambiar información y de expresar los pensamientos y los sentimientos propios con claridad (40)

community/comunidad grupo de personas que tienen un origen común, residen en la misma zona o comparten intereses, creencias u objetivos similares (184)

competition/competencia enfrentamiento entre dos o más personas o equipos (74)

compromise/convenio solución a un problema en el que ambas partes renuncian a ciertas cosas para lograr un acuerdo (205)

conflict/conflicto toda situación en la que las ideas o los intereses se enfrentan (198)

congenital disorder/trastorno congénito toda enfermedad, anormalidad o trastorno presente al nacer pero no hereditario (325)

consequence/consecuencia resultado de las acciones y las decisiones de una persona (23)

coping/sobrellevar manejar los problemas y los inconvenientes de manera eficaz (39)

creative expression/expresión creativa uso de una actividad artística para expresar emociones (139)

deafness/sordera pérdida total o parcial de la capacidad de oír (341)

defense mechanism/mecanismo de defensa conducta automática que se mantiene durante un período de tiempo corto para sobrellevar dificultades (141, 164)

depressant/depresivo droga que disminuye la velocidad del funcionamiento del cuerpo y el cerebro (248, 285)

depression/depresión tristeza y desesperanza que impiden a una persona realizar las actividades diarias (145)

diet/dieta plan de alimentos que incluye lo que una persona come, cuánto come y cada cuánto come (96)

Dietary Guidelines for Americans/Guía alimenticia para los Estadounidenses conjunto de sugerencias diseñado para ayudar a las personas a crear hábitos alimenticios sanos y aumentar los niveles de actividad física (102)

digestion/digestión proceso de descomponer los alimentos de manera que el cuerpo pueda utilizarlos (95)

dislocation/dislocación lesión en la que un hueso sale de su posición normal en una articulación (400)

distress/alteración toda respuesta nerviosa que hace que una persona no logre alcanzar una meta o se enferme; tensión física, mental o emocional negativa que se manifiesta como respuesta a un factor estresante (159)

driving under the influence (DUI)/conducir bajo efectos (CBE) situación en la que una persona que legalmente está intoxicada o ha consumido drogas ilegales conduce un vehículo motorizado (256)

drug/droga toda sustancia química que provoca un cambio en el estado físico o psicológico de una persona (248, 270)

drug abuse/abuso de drogas uso incorrecto o inseguro de una droga (277)

drug addiction/drogadicción estado en el que una persona ya no puede controlar el consumo de una droga (230, 278)

drug misuse/uso indebido de drogas uso de una droga distinto al uso adecuado (276)

earthquake/terremoto temblor de la superficie de la Tierra producido por un movimiento a lo largo de una ruptura en la corteza terrestre (388)

eating disorder/trastorno alimenticio enfermedad en la que una persona se preocupa de manera negativa por su silueta y su peso corporal (121)

egg/óvulo célula sexual elaborada por las mujeres (354)

embryo/embrión ser humano en desarrollo, desde el momento de la fecundación hasta la octava semana del embarazo (360)

emergency/emergencia hecho repentino que requiere acción inmediata (392)

emotion abuso/emocional uso repetido de acciones y palabras que implican que una persona no tiene valor ni poder (134)

emotional health/intimidad emocional condición de estar emocionalmente relacionado con otra persona (135)

emphysema/enfisema enfermedad respiratoria en la que el oxígeno y el dióxido de carbono no se pueden desplazar fácilmente a través de los alvéolos dado que éstos se afinaron, se distendieron o se han destruido (329)

endocrine gland/glándula endocrina órgano que libera hormonas en el torrente sanguíneo o en el líquido que rodea las células (332)

endocrine system/sistema endocrino red de tejidos y órganos que liberan sustancias químicas que controlan ciertas funciones corporales (358)

endurance/resistencia capacidad de realizar actividades durante más de unos pocos minutos (66)

environment/medio ambiente todos los seres vivos y elementos sin vida que rodean a una persona (9, 349)

environmental tobacco smoke (ETS)/ humo de tabaco ambiental (HTA) mezcla del humo exhalado por los fumadores y el humo de los cigarrillos al consumirse (223)

exercise/ejercicio toda actividad física que mantiene o mejora el estado físico (68)

fad diet/dieta de moda dieta que permite bajar de peso rápidamente con poco esfuerzo (120)

fatigue/fatiga agotamiento físico o mental; sensación de mucho cansancio (162)

fats/grasas nutriente que almacena energía y permite al cuerpo almacenar algunas vitaminas (99)

fetal alcohol syndrome (FAS)/síndrome de alcohol fetal (SAF) grupo de defectos de nacimiento que afectan a un bebé que estuvo expuesto al alcohol durante la gestación (255)

fetus/feto ser humano en desarrollo en el útero de la madre, desde el inicio de la novena semana de embarazo hasta el nacimiento (360)

fire extinguisher/extintor dispositivo que libera sustancias químicas para apagar un incendio (379)

first aid/primeros auxilios atención médica de emergencia para una persona que se lastimó o está enferma (392)

flexibility/flexibilidad capacidad de doblar y girar las articulaciones con facilidad (67)

flood/inundación exceso de agua en zonas normalmente secas (390)

Food Guide Pyramid/Pirámide alimenticia herramienta para escoger qué tipos de alimentos se deben comer y qué cantidad de cada alimento se debe comer cada día (103)

fracture/fractura fisura o rotura de un hueso (400)

friendship/amistad relación entre personas que disfrutan de estar juntas, se cuidan entre sí y suelen tener intereses similares (186)

frostbite/congelación daño a la piel y a otros tejidos provocado por un frío intenso (384)

genes/genes conjunto de instrucciones que se encuentran en todas las células del cuerpo de una persona y proporcionan una descripción del cuerpo: qué aspecto tendrá, cómo crecerá y cómo funcionará (348)

gland/glándula tejido o grupo de tejidos que elaboran y liberan sustancias químicas; por ejemplo, las hormonas (332, 358)

glaucoma/glaucoma enfermedad que produce presión en el líquido dentro del ojo; la alta presión daña el nervio óptico y provoca la pérdida permanente de la visión (341)

goal/meta algo por lo que una persona se esfuerza y que espera alcanzar (32)

good decision/buena decisión decisión que toma una persona luego de analizar sus consecuencias detenidamente (22)

grief/duelo sentimiento de profunda tristeza por una pérdida (367)

hallucinogen/alucinógeno toda droga que produce alucinaciones en una persona (288)

health/salud condición de bienestar físico, emocional, mental y social (4)

healthy weight range/rango de peso saludable cálculo del peso que debería tener una persona según su altura y su estructura corporal (124)

heart attack/ataque al corazón daño y pérdida de la función de una zona del músculo del corazón debido a la falta de suministro de sangre (325)

heat exhaustion/agotamiento por calor condición causada por la pérdida excesiva de agua a través de la transpiración en un día de calor (385)

heatstroke/insolación falla del sistema de regulación de calor del cuerpo (385)

heredity/herencia transmisión de rasgos de padres a hijos (8, 348)

HIV/VIH virus de inmunodeficiencia humana, un virus que ataca al sistema inmunológico del ser humano y causa el SIDA (312)

hobby/prueba de anticuerpo del VIH algo que te gusta hacer o estudiar en el tiempo libre (262)

hormone/hormona sustancia química elaborada en una parte del cuerpo que se libera dentro de la sangre, se transporta a través del torrente sanguíneo y produce un cambio en otra parte del cuerpo; controla el crecimiento y el desarrollo y muchas otras funciones del cuerpo (134, 332, 358)

hurricane/huracán fenómeno del clima tropical que produce una masa grande y giratoria de vientos que se desplazan por lo menos a aproximadamente 74 millas por hora (389)

hypertension/hipertensión condición en la que la presión dentro de las arterias grandes es demasiado alta; también se llama *presión arterial alta* (326)

hypothermia/hipotermia temperatura corporal inferior al valor normal (384)

infectious disease/enfermedad infecciosa toda enfermedad causada por un agente o un patógeno que invade el cuerpo (304)

inhalant/inhalantes drogas que se inhalan en forma de vapor y se absorben en el torrente sanguíneo a través de los pulmones (289)

interest/interés algo que uno disfruta y desea conocer mejor (33)

intoxication/intoxicación cambios físicos y mentales producidos por beber alcohol (250)

kidneys/riñones órganos que filtran la sangre y eliminan los desechos líquidos y la cantidad adicional de agua de la sangre (336)

leukemia/leucemia cáncer de los tejidos del cuerpo que producen glóbulos blancos (327)

life skills/destrezas para la vida herramientas que te ayudan a manejarse en situaciones que pueden afectar tu salud (12)

lifestyle/estilo de vida conjunto de conductas que marcan tu forma de vivir (10)

marijuana/marihuana flores y hojas secas de la planta *Cannabis* (286)

mediation/mediación proceso en el que un tercero, llamado *mediador*, participa en un conflicto, escucha a ambas partes y, luego, ofrece soluciones al conflicto (207)

medicine/medicamento toda droga utilizada para curar, prevenir o tratar enfermedades o molestias (274)

menstruation/menstruación proceso mensual de desprendimiento del recubrimiento interior de la matriz durante el que la sangre y los tejidos salen del cuerpo de la mujer a través de la vagina (355)

mental health/salud mental forma en la que una persona piensa y responde a hechos de su vida (134)

mental illness/enfermedad mental trasforno que afecta los pensamientos, las emociones y la conducta de una persona (144)

mineral/mineral elemento esencial para una buena salud (100)

muscular dystrophy/distrofia muscular grupo de enfermedades musculares hereditarias que hacen que los músculos se debiliten y atrofien poco a poco (339)

negative thinking/pensamiento negativo concentración en los aspectos malos de una situación (140)

neglect/negligencia incumplimiento de un padre u otro adulto responsable en su deber de satisfacer las necesidades básicas, tales como comida, ropa o amor (182)

negotiation/negociación debate sobre un conflicto para llegar a un acuerdo (204)

nicotine/nicotina droga altamente adictiva que se encuentra en todos los productos con tabaco (221)

nicotine replacement therapy (NRT)/ terapia de reemplazo de nicotina (TRN) tratamiento con medicamentos que contienen cantidades seguras de nicotina (235)

noninfectious disease/enfermedad no infecciosa enfermedad que no es causada por un agente patógeno (322)

nurturing/nutrir proporcionar los cuidados y otros elementos básicos que las personas necesitan para crecer (181)

nutrient/nutriente sustancia en los alimentos que el cuerpo necesita para funcionar correctamente (95)

Nutrition Facts label/etiqueta de Valores nutricionales etiqueta que se encuentra en el exterior de los envases de alimentos y en la que se informa el número de porciones que incluye el envase, el número de calorías que contiene cada porción y la cantidad de nutrientes que aporta cada porción (104)

option/opción elección que puedes realizar (25)

organ/órgano dos o más tejidos que trabajan juntos para llevar a cabo una función especial (322)

osteoporosis/osteoporosis enfermedad que produce la pérdida de la densidad de los huesos (339)

over-the-counter (OTC) medicine/ medicamentos de venta sin receta (VSR) todo medicamento que se puede comprar sin receta médica (275)

overtraining/sobreentrenamiento condición causada por el exceso de ejercicio (81)

ovulation/ovulación proceso mensual mediante el cual los ovarios liberan un óvulo maduro (355)

peer pressure/presión de pares sensación de que debes hacer algo que tus amigos quieren que hagas (29, 232, 246)

peripheral nervous system (PNS)/sistema nervioso periférico (SNP) nervios que conectan al cerebro y la médula espinal con todas las demás partes del cuerpo (330)

persistence/persistencia compromiso a seguir trabajando para alcanzar una meta aun cuando las situaciones hacen que se quiera renunciar (37)

phobia/fobia miedo fuerte y anormal a algo (147)

physical dependence/dependencia física condición en la que el cuerpo depende de una droga determinada para funcionar (279)

physical fitness/buen estado físico capacidad de realizar actividades físicas todos los días sin sentir falta de aire, dolor o cansancio extremos (66)

positive self-talk/lenguaje interno positivo pensar sobre los aspectos buenos de una situación mala (140)

positive stress/estrés positivo respuesta de estrés que hace que una persona se sienta bien; respuesta de estrés que se produce cuando una persona experimenta triunfos y logros (169)

pregnancy/embarazo período durante el cual una mujer lleva a un feto en desarrollo dentro de la matriz (360)

prescription medicine/medicamento recetado medicamento que se puede comprar sólo con una orden escrita del médico (274)

preventive healthcare/cuidado preventivo de la salud medidas para prevenir enfermedades y accidentes antes de que ocurran (11)

protein/proteína nutriente que suministra energía al cuerpo para construir y reparar tejidos y células (99)

psychiatrist/psiquiatra médico que se especializa en estudiar cómo se relacionan las enfermedades del cerebro y el cuerpo con las emociones y la conducta (150)

psychological dependence/dependencia psicológica estado de necesidad mental o emocional de una droga para poder funcionar (279)

puberty/pubertad período de tiempo durante la adolescencia en el que se produce la maduración del aparato reproductor (364)

R

reaction time/tiempo de reacción cantidad de tiempo que transcurre desde el instante en el que el cerebro detecta un estímulo externo hasta el momento de respuesta de la persona (250)

recovery/recuperación proceso de aprender a vivir sin alcohol (259)

redirection/redireccionamiento desviar energía de una respuesta de estrés a una actividad no estresante (167)

reframing/reenfocar analizar una situación desde otro punto de vista y cambiar la respuesta emocional a esa situación (167)

refusal skill/habilidad de negación estrategia para evitar hacer algo que no quieres hacer (42)

relationship/relación conexión emocional o social entre dos o más personas (176)

relaxation/relajación estado de hacer algo para despejar un problema de la mente y concentrarse en otra cosa que no sea estresante (167)

rescue breathing/respiración de rescate técnica de emergencia mediante la cual una persona le proporciona aire a la que no respira (396)

resting heart rate (RHR)/índice de pulsaciones en reposo (IPR) número de veces que el corazón late por minuto mientras el cuerpo está en reposo (71)

S

self-concept/autoconcepto medición de cómo una persona se ve y se imagina a sí misma como individuo (54)

self-esteem/autoestima medición de cuánto se valora, respeta y cuánta confianza en sí misma tiene una persona (32, 50)

sex cell/célula sexual célula paterna o materna que se une con otra célula sexual para crear una célula nueva que contiene toda la información necesaria para desarrollar un nuevo ser humano (348)

sexual abstinence/abstinencia sexual negación de participar en actividades sexuales (190)

sexually transmitted disease (STD)/enfermedad de transmisión sexual (ETS) cualquiera de un número de infecciones que se transmiten de una persona a otra a través del contacto sexual (314)

smoke detector/detector de humo
alarma pequeña que funciona con pilas utilizada para detectar el humo de un incendio (378)

social strain/tensión social incomodidad de una situación o la tensión entre integrantes de una familia y amigos por el consumo de tabaco (229)

sperm/espermatozoide célula sexual elaborada por los hombres (350)

sportsmanship/actitud deportiva capacidad de tratar a todos los jugadores, funcionarios y espectadores de manera justa durante una competencia (74)

stimulant/estimulante toda droga que aumente la actividad del cuerpo (284)

strength/fuerza cantidad de fuerza empleada por los músculos al utilizarlos (66)

stress/estrés combinación de una situación nueva o posiblemente amenazante y la respuesta natural del cuerpo a esa situación (158)

stress management/control del estrés capacidad de manejar el estrés de forma sana (167)

stress response/respuesta de estrés conjunto de cambios físicos que preparan el cuerpo para actuar en respuesta a un factor estresante; respuesta del cuerpo a un factor estresante (162)

stressor factor/estresante cualquier factor que origine una respuesta de estrés (158)

success/éxito logro de las metas propuestas (36)

suicide/suicidio acción de matarse a uno mismo (145)

targeted marketing/comercialización dirigida publicidad que apunta a un grupo de personas en particular (233)

testes/testículos órganos reproductores masculinos que producen espermatozoides y la hormona testosterona (350)

THC/THC tetrahidrocanabinol, sustancia activa en la marihuana (286)

therapist/terapeuta profesional capacitado en el tratamiento de problemas emocionales a través de charlas (150)

tobacco/tabaco planta cuyas hojas se secan y mezclan con sustancias químicas para hacer productos tales como cigarrillos, tabaco rapé y puros (231)

tolerance/tolerancia capacidad de aceptar a las personas por lo que son a pesar de las diferencias (184); condición en la que una persona necesita más cantidad de una droga para sentir sus efectos originales (231)

tornado/tornado columna giratoria de aire que tiene vientos de alta velocidad y cuyo extremo toca el suelo (389)

trigger/disparador persona, situación o acontecimiento que afecta a las emociones (142)

type 1 diabetes/diabetes tipo 1 enfermedad del sistema endocrino en la que el cuerpo produce poca cantidad o nada de insulina (333)

type 2 diabetes/diabetes tipo 2 enfermedad del sistema endocrino en la que el cuerpo produce insulina pero no puede utilizarla correctamente (333)

V

vaccine/vacuna sustancia que generalmente se prepara a partir de patógenos débiles o sin vida o material genético y se introduce en un cuerpo para proporcionar inmunidad (311)

values/valores creencias que uno considera de mucha importancia (25)

verbal communication/comunicación verbal acción de expresarse y comprender los pensamientos y las emociones mediante el habla (138)

violence/violencia fuerza física que se utiliza para dañar a una persona o una propiedad (208, 375)

virus/virus partícula pequeña, capaz de causar enfermedades, formada por material genético y un revestimiento de proteína que invade a una célula sana y le indica que produzca más virus (310)

vitamin/vitamina compuesto orgánico que controla muchas funciones del cuerpo y que es necesario en pequeñas cantidades para mantener la salud y permitir el crecimiento (100)

W

weight training/entrenamiento con pesas uso de pesas para fortalecer y agrandar los músculos (76)

wellness/bienestar estado de buena salud que se logra mediante el equilibrio de la salud física, emocional, mental y social (7)

withdrawal/supresión síntomas psicológicos y físicos molestos que se producen cuando una persona que tiene dependencia a una droga deja de consumirla (231, 278)

Index

Note: Page numbers followed by *f* refer to figures. Page numbers followed by *t* refer to tables. Boldface page numbers refer to the main discussions.

911 calls, 393

abdominal thrusts, 394–395, 394*f*, 395*f*
abstinence, sexual, **190–191,** 191*t*, 310
abuse, 182–183, 182*t*
academic self-concept, 55
accidents, 374, 374*f*, 382*f*. *See also* **injuries**
acquired immune deficiency syndrome (AIDS), 271, 282, **312–313**
active listening, 138
active rest, 86
acute injuries, 82
addiction
   to alcohol, 258–259
   definition, 230
   to drugs, 278–279
   to tobacco, 230, 230*f*
   tolerance, dependence, and withdrawal, 231, 234, 259, 278
additives, in tobacco, 220
adolescence, 364–365
adrenal glands, 332*t*, 358*f*
adulthood, 365

advertisements
   for alcohol, 260–261
   body image and, 118
   influences on decisions, 30–31
   self-esteem and, 53
   for smoking, 31, 233
aerobic exercise, 72–73
affection, 188, 188*t*
aggression, 210
AIDS (acquired immune deficiency syndrome), 271, 282, **312–313**
air bags, 382
alcohol, 246–267
   advertisements for, 260–261
   alcohol abuse, 251
   alcoholism, 258–259, 267
   alternatives to, 262–263
   binge drinking, 253, 267
   decision making and, 252–253
   drunk driving and, 256–257, 257*f*, 267
   effects on body, 248, 267, 285
   fatal dose, 249
   harmful effects on teens, 247
   intoxication, 249–250, 249*f*, 250*f*
   liquor vs. beer and wine, 253
   long-term effects, 251
   poisoning, 248, 267
   pregnancy and, 255
   pressures to drink, 260
   quitting, 259
   reasons teens drink, 246
   resources for help with, 263
   violence and, 254, 267
alcoholism, 258–259, 267
alcohol poisoning, 248, 267

alternative Food Guide Pyramids, 407, 407*f*
alveoli, 328
Alzheimer's disease, 330, 330*f*, 331*t*. *See also* **diseases**
ammonia, 220
amputation, 225
anaerobic exercise, 72–73
anemia, 327
anger. *See also* **violence**
   controlling, 212
   misdirection of, 136
   usefulness of, 136
   violence and, 209
anorexia nervosa, 122, 122*t*. *See also* **eating disorders**
anxiety disorders, 147. *See also* **mental illness**
art, expressing emotions through, 139, 212
arteries, 225, 325, 325*f*, 326*f*
Asian diets, 407, 407*f*
assertiveness, 56, 179
asthma
   inhalers for, 272, 272*f*
   symptoms of, 329
atrium (plural, *atria*), 324, 325*f*
attitudes, healthy, 10
automobile safety, 382, 382*f*
autonomic nervous system, 330

babies, 360, 361*f*, 362
baby-sitting, 416–417
BAC (blood alcohol concentration), 249, 249*f*, 250, 256
back injuries, 401. *See also* **injuries**

Index **441**

INDEX

bacteria, 302–303, 302f
bacterial infections, 302–305
   antibiotics and, 305
   avoiding, 304
   sinus infections, 303
   strep throat, 303
   tuberculosis, 304, 304f
behavior, definition of, 179
bench press, 78f
biceps curl, 78f
bicycle safety, 381, 387f
bidis, 222
binge drinking, 253. *See also* **alcohol**
binge eating disorder, 123. *See also* **eating disorders**
bipolar mood disorder, 146. *See also* **mental illness**
birth defects, 255
bleeding, first aid for, 398
blended families, 180
blood
   clots, 327
   diseases, 327
   transfusions, 312
   vessels, 325, 325f
blood alcohol concentration (BAC), **249,** 249f, 250, 256
blood pressure
   drug abuse and, 282f
   high, 326, 326f
   kidney disease and, 337
BMI (body mass index), 124
boating safety, 412
bodies, 348–367
   female reproductive system, 354–357, 354f
   heredity, 348
   male reproductive system, 350–353, 350f
   uniqueness of, 349
bodybuilding, 76–79
body composition, 67

body image, 116–119
   definition, 116
   family and friends as influences on, 119
   healthy and unhealthy, 117
   "I" statements, 119
   media influences on, 118
   self-esteem and, 53
body language
   during conflicts, 203, 203f
   expressing emotions, 138, 178, 178f
   violence and, 209
   while listening, 41
body mass index (BMI), 124
body systems, 322–341
   circulatory system, 324–327, 324f, 325f, 421
   digestive system, 334–335, 334f, 420
   endocrine system, 332–333, 332f, 332t, 358–359, 418
   eyes and ears, 340–341, 340f
   nervous system, 330–331, 330f, 331t
   overview, 322, 323f
   reproductive system, 348–367
   respiratory system, 328–329, 328f
   skin, bones, and muscles, 338–339, 338f, 419
   urinary system, 336–337, 336f, 420
bones, 338, 338f, 419
boys
   problems of the reproductive system and, 352, 352t
   reproductive system of, 350–353, 350f
   self care, 353
   sperm, 351, 351f
brain, 330, 330f

brainstorming, 25
brain tumors, 331t. *See also* **cancer**
breakfasts, healthy, 106
breast cancer, 356t. *See also* **cancer**
breast self-examinations, 357
breathing, rescue, 396–397, 396f, 397f
breathing masks, 396
bronchi, 328
bronchioles, 328
bulimia nervosa, 122, 122t. *See also* **eating disorders**
bullying, 200
burns, first aid for, 399, 399t
bus safety, 383

caffeine, 270, 284t
calcium, 100, 104
Calories, 104, 127, 408–409t
camping safety, 386, 386f
cancer
   breast, 356t
   diet and, 15
   female reproductive system, 356
   leukemia, 327, 327f
   lung, 9, 226
   male reproductive system, 352t
   skin, 339
   stomach, 335, 335f
   tobacco use and, 226
cannabis, 286–287
capillaries, 325, 325f
capsules, 271
carbohydrates, 99
carbon monoxide, 220, 272
cardiopulmonary resuscitation (CPR), 396
carriers, disease, 304

cataracts, 341
celiac disease, 335. See also **diseases**
central nervous system (CNS), 249, 330
cervical cancer, 356t. See also **cancer**
cervix, 354f. See also **female reproductive system**
character, 25
child abuse, 182–183, 182t
chlamydia, 311t. See also **sexually transmitted diseases**
choices, 22, 27. See also **decisions**
choking, first aid for, 394–395, 394f, 395f
chronic bronchitis, 224
chronic diseases, 224. See also **noninfectious diseases**
chronic injuries, 83. See also **injuries**
Churchill, Winston, 146
cigarettes. See also **tobacco**
   addiction to, 230, 230f
   advertising, 233
   breaking rules, 228
   early effects of, 221
   flavored, 222
   harmful effects of, 227
   litter from, 235
   quitting, 234–239
   reasons for using, 232–233, 232t
   reasons not to start smoking, 239
   social strain, 229
   types of, 222
cigars, 222. See also **tobacco**
circulatory system, 324–327
   blood, 326–327, 326f
   heart, 324–325, 325f
   overview, 324, 421
clothing, for exercise, 86
CNS (central nervous system), 249, 330
cocaine, 284t, 272
colds, 307, 307t
cold weather safety, 384
collaboration, 205
communication, 40–41. See also **body language**
   during conflicts, 202–205, 209
   creative expression, 139
   definition, 40
   of emotions, 138–139
   listening skills, 41, 138
   in relationships, 178
   skills, 40
   using refusal skills, 42–43
communities, 184–185
competition, in sports, 74
compromise, 205
conflicts, 198–207. See also **violence**
   body language, 203, 203f
   choosing the right words during, 203
   compromise and collaboration, 205
   definition, 198
   expressing yourself during, 202
   at home, 199
   listening, 204
   mediation, 207
   negotiation, 204
   out of control, 206, 206t
   with peers, 200
   reasons for, 199
   recognizing, 198
   at school, 201
   turning into violence, 209
congenital disorders, 325
congenital heart disease, 325. See also **diseases**
consequences of decisions, 23, 26
consumer skills, 13, 233
contagious diseases, 300. See also **infectious diseases**
controlled-release capsules, 271
cool-downs, 84
coping, 39, 141, 164–165
coughing, 301, 315
CPR (cardiopulmonary resuscitation), 396
cramps (menstrual), 356
creative expression, 139, 212
cremaster muscle, 351
Crohn's disease, 335. See also **diseases**
crystal meth, 284t. See also **drugs**
cyclones, 389
cystic fibrosis, 328. See also **diseases**
cysts, 337

Daily Values, 104
daydreaming, 165t
deafness, 341
deaths
   alcohol-related, 257f, 267
   from automobiles, 382f
   drug-related, 283
   grief over, 367
   from gunshot wounds, 376
decisions
   alcohol use and, 252–253
   changing your mind, 26
   consequences of, 23, 26
   definition, 22
   effect of new information on, 31
   evaluating choices, 27

decisions *(continued)*
family influences on, 28
good, 22
learning from mistakes, 37
media influences on, 30
peer pressure and, 29
reaching goals through, 36
steps in making, 24–27
values, 25
defense mechanisms, 141, **164–165,** 165*t*
dehydration, 101
delusions, 146. *See also* **mental illness**
denial, 165, 165*t*
dental exams, 11*f*
dependence, on drugs, 231, 258, 278
depressants, 248, 249, 285. *See also* **drugs**
depression, 145–146, 150, 150*f*. *See also* **mental illness**
devaluation, 141
diabetes, 332–333, 337, 341. *See also* **diseases**
diet. *See also* **nutrition**
anemia and, 327
breakfasts, 106
Calorie and nutrient contents, 408–409*t*
cancer and, 15
Dietary Guidelines for Americans, 102, 102*t*
eating at home, 109
eating disorders, 120–123
eating out, 108
fad diets, 120
food choices, 96
Food Guide Pyramid, 103, 103*f*
Nutrition Facts label, 104, 104*f*
reasons for eating, 126
serving sizes and portions, 105

snacks, 107, 107*f*
vegetarian, 407, 407*f*
Dietary Guidelines for Americans, 102, 102*t*
digestion, 95, 248
digestive system, 334–335, 334*f*, 420
disasters, 388–391. *See also* **natural disasters**
diseases. *See also* **infectious diseases; noninfectious diseases; sexually transmitted diseases;** *specific diseases*
effect of environment on, 9
food-related, 410, 410*t*
inherited, 8
stress and, 161
vitamins and minerals and, 100
dislocations, 400. *See also* **injuries**
distress, 166–169. *See also* **stress**
avoiding, 168, 168*f*
definition, 159
preventing, 169
warning signs of, 166
diving safety, 412
driving under the influence (DUI), 256–257, 257*f*, 283. *See also* **alcohol**
drug abuse, 277–283. *See also* **drugs**
addiction, 278–279, 279*f*
health problems from, 282, 282*f*
HIV and AIDS, 312
legal problems, 283
money problems, 281
problems with family and friends, 280
psychological dependence, 279

reasons to be drug free, 290
refusing drugs, 292, 293*t*
school problems, 281, 281*f*
ways to stay drug free, 291
drugs, 270–295. *See also* **drug abuse**
addiction to, 278–279, 279*f*
definition, 270
depressants, 285
hallucinogens, 288
inhalants, 272, 289
marijuana, 272, 286–287
misuse of, 276
needle-sharing, 271
over-the-counter medicines, 275, 275*f*
prescription medicines, 274, 274*f*
psychological dependence, 279
reasons to be free of, 290
refusing, 292, 293*t*
stimulants, 284, 284*t*
taken by injection, 271
taken by smoking, 272
taken by transdermal patch, 273
taken orally, 271
ways to stay free of, 291
drunk driving, 256–257, 257*f*, 267
drunken behavior, 247, 249*f*, 249–250
DUI (driving under the influence), **256–257,** 257*f*, 283

ears, 340–341, 340*f*
earthquake safety, 388
eating at home, 109. *See also* **diet**

eating disorders, 120–123
  anorexia nervosa, 122, 122*t*
  binge eating disorder, 123
  bulimia nervosa, 122, 122*t*
  causes, 121*t*
  definition, 121
  getting and giving help for, 123
  overexercising, 121
  unhealthy eating behaviors, 120
eating journals, 126
eating out, 108. *See also* **diet**
EBV (Epstein-Barr virus), 308. *See also* **diseases**
eggs, human, 351, 354, 354*f*, 355*f*
electrocution, 374
embryo, 360
emergencies, 392–393. *See also* **first aid; natural disasters**
emergency kits, 391, **414**
emergency phone calls, 393, 393*f*
emotional abuse, 182*t*
emotional health, 5, **135**
emotional spectrum, 135, 135*f*
emotions, 134–143
  alcohol use and, 247
  anger, 136
  body language, 138
  communication and, 138
  during conflict, 198–199
  definition, 134
  drug abuse and, 282
  emotional health, 5, 135
  emotional spectrum, 135, 135*f*
  expression of, 139
  food choices and, 97, 126
  getting help for, 148–151
  hormones and, 134

  love and hate, 136
  physical effects of, 137, 137*t*
  resources for help, 263
  self-talk and, 140
  triggers for, 142
emphysema, 224, 329. *See also* **tobacco**
endocrine system, 332–333
  anatomy, 332, 332*f*
  diseases of, 333
  hormones from, 332, 332*t*, 358–359, 358*f*, 359*t*
  overview, 418
endometriosis, 356*t*. *See also* **female reproductive system**
endometrium, 354*f*, 355, 355*f*. *See also* **female reproductive system**
endurance, 66, 69
environment, 9, 349
environmental tobacco smoke (ETS), 223
enzymes, 334
epididymis, 350*f*. *See also* **male reproductive system**
epinephrine, 162, 164
Epstein-Barr virus (EBV), 308. *See also* **diseases**
essential nutrients, 98–100
estrogen, 359*t*. *See also* **female reproductive system**
ETS (environmental tobacco smoke), 223
euphoria, 284*f*
evacuation plans, 378
exercise, 68–73. *See also* **fitness**
  active rest, 86
  aerobic and anaerobic, 72–73
  clothing for, 86
  FIT, 70

  fitness tests, 69, 69*t*
  frequency of, 85
  with friends, 87
  heart rate monitoring, 71
  importance of, 68, 127
  injuries, 80–87
  machines, 77
  overexercising, 121
  overtraining, 81, 83
  Physical Activity Pyramid, 411, 411*f*
  recovery time, 71
  to release anger, 212
  safety equipment, 87
  weight training, 76–79, 78–79*f*
extended families, 180
eye contact, 41, 138, 178
eye, of a hurricane, 389*f*
eyes, 340–341, 340*f*

facial expressions, 203. *See also* **body language**
fad diets, 120
fallopian tube, 354, 354*f*, 355*f*. *See also* **female reproductive system**
families, 180–183
  conflicts within, 199
  different roles in, 180
  drug abuse and, 280
  forms of, 180
  help for emotional problems, 149
  help for serious problems, 183
  influences on body image, 119
  influences on decisions, 28
  influences on self-esteem, 52
  nurturing in, 181
  problems in, 182–183

Index   **445**

families (continued)
  respect within, 181
  working toward goals with, 35
FAS (fetal alcohol syndrome), 255
fast-food meals, 108. *See also* **diet**
fat, dietary, 99
fatigue, from stress, 162–163
fear, 137*t*, 147
FEMA (Federal Emergency Management Agency), 405
female reproductive system
  menstrual cycle, 354–355, 355*f*
  problems of reproductive system, 356, 356*t*
  reproductive system, 354–357, 354*f*
  self care, 357
fetal alcohol syndrome (FAS), 255
fetus, 360, 361*f*
fight-or-flight response, 162
fire extinguishers, 379
fire safety, 374, **378–379**
first aid, 392–401
  bleeding, 398
  burns, 399, 399*t*
  choking, 394–395, 394*f*, 395*f*
  definition, 392
  dislocations, 400
  first-aid kits, 414
  fractures, 400
  head, neck, and back injuries, 401
  poisoning, 399
  rescue breathing, 396–397, 396*f*, 397*f*
  RICE, 82
first-aid kits, 414
FIT, 70

fitness, 66–89. *See also* **exercise**
  body composition, 67
  endurance, 66
  exercise and, 68–73
  FIT, 70
  flexibility, 67
  goals for, 70
  heart rate monitoring, 71
  Physical Activity Pyramid, 411, 411*f*
  strength, 66
  tests of, 69, 69*t*
  weight training, 76–79
fitness zones, 69, 69*t*
flashbacks, 288
flash floods, 390
Fleming, Alexander, 305, 305*f*
flexibility, 67, 69
floods, 390
flu (influenza), 307, 307*t*
food, 94–109. *See also* **nutrition**
  Calorie and nutrient contents, 408–409*t*
  choices, 96
  Dietary Guidelines for Americans, 102, 102*t*
  digestion of, 95
  eating at home, 109
  eating disorders, 120–123
  eating out, 108
  essential nutrients, 98–100
  feelings and, 97, 126
  healthy breakfasts, 106
  healthy snacks, 107, 107*f*
  Nutrition Facts label, 104, 104*f*
  reasons for eating, 126
  safety, 410
  serving sizes and portions, 105
Food Guide Pyramid, 103
  alternative, 407, 407*f*
  description of, 103, 103*f*, 406, 406*f*
  servings sizes in, 105

fractures, 82–83, 400. *See also* **injuries**
Freud, Sigmund, 141
friends, 176–193. *See also* **relationships**
  abstinence, 190–191, 191*t*
  affection between, 188, 188*t*
  conflicts with, 200
  drug abuse and, 280, 290
  healthy friendships, 186
  help with emotional problems, 149
  influences on body image, 119
  positive peer pressure, 187
  support for not drinking alcohol, 262
  unhealthy relationships, 189
frostbite, 384

G

gangs, 375
generic and brand-name products, 13
genes, 348, 351*f*
genital herpes, 311*t*. *See also* **sexually transmitted diseases**
gestures, 203
girls
  menstrual cycle, 354–355, 355*f*
  problems of reproductive system, 356, 356*t*
  reproductive system, 354–357, 354*f*
  self care, 357
glands, 332, 332*t*
glasses, 341
glaucoma, 341
glucose, 72
gluten, 335
glycogen, 72

goals, 32–39
  changing your plans, 39
  definition, 32
  fitness, 70
  importance of, 32
  learning from mistakes, 37
  measuring progress toward, 38
  self-esteem and, 58
  short-term and long-term, 34
  steps in reaching, 36
  values and interests and, 33, 33*t*
  working with others toward, 35, 187
gonorrhea, 311*t*. *See also* **sexually transmitted diseases**
good sport, being a, 74
grief, 367
group pressure, for violence, 209
growth and development, 360–367
  adolescence, 364–365
  adulthood, 365
  aging, 366
  death, 367
  infancy and early childhood, 362
  late childhood, 363
  middle childhood, 362
  pregnancy, 360, 361*f*
growth hormone, 359*t*
Guillain-Barré syndrome, 331*t*. *See also* **diseases**
gun safety, 376

H

hairy cell leukemia, 327*f*
hallucinations, 146. *See also* **mental illness**
hallucinogens, 288. *See also* **drugs**
hamstring curl, 79*f*
head injuries, 331, 381, 401
health, 4–17
  definition, 4
  effect of environment on, 9
  emotional, 5
  heredity and inherited traits, 8
  lifestyle choices and, 10, 15
  mental, 5
  nine life skills for, 12–15, 13*t*
  nutrition and, 94
  personal responsibility for, 11
  physical health, 4
  relationships and, 176
  social, 6
  wellness and, 7
health assessments, 7, 14
healthcare, preventive, 11
healthy weight range, 124. *See also* **weight**
heart, 324–325, 325*f*
heart attacks, 325
heart disease
  congenital, 325
  drug abuse and, 282*f*
  fighting, 325
  inherited traits and, 8
  overview, 325
  from smoking, 225
heart failure, 325
heart rate monitoring, 71
heat exhaustion, 385
heatstroke, 385
Heimlich maneuver, 394–395, 394*f*, 395*f*
helmets, safety, 381
helping, self-esteem and, 59
heredity
  alcoholism and, 258
  definition, 348
  diseases, 322*t*
  genes, 348
  inherited traits, 8
hernias, 352*t*
herpes, 311*t*. *See also* **diseases**
high blood pressure
  drug abuse and, 282*f*
  hypertension, 326, 326*f*
  kidney disease and, 337
hiking safety, 386, 386*f*
HIV (human immunodeficiency virus), 271, 282, **312–313**
hobbies, 262
home alone, 413
hormones, 358–359
  effects on emotions, 134
  endocrine system and, 332, 359*t*
  functions of, 358–359, 359*t*
  during puberty, 364
  as response to stress, 162
hot weather safety, 385
HPV (human papillomavirus), 311*t*
human growth hormone, 359*t*
human immunodeficiency virus (HIV), 271, 282, **312–313**
human papillomavirus (HPV), 311*t*
humor, 59, 141, 168
hurricanes, 389, 389*f*
hygiene, 4
hypertension, 326, 326*f*, 337
hyperthyroidism, 333
hypodermic needles, 271, 271*f*
hypothermia, 384

I

IBD (inflammatory bowel disease), 335. *See also* **diseases**

INDEX

immune system, smoking and, 227
infants
  development of, 362
  first aid for choking, 394, 394*f*
infectious diseases, 300–317. See also *specific diseases*
  antibiotics for, 305
  bacterial infections, 302–305
  definition, 300
  sexually transmitted diseases, 310–313
  spread of, 301, 314–315
  viral infections, 306–309
inflammatory bowel disease (IBD), 335. See also **diseases**
influenza, 307, 307*t*
inguinal hernias, 352*t*
inhalants, 289
inhalers, 272, 272*f*
inherited diseases, 8
injuries, 80–87. See also **first aid**
  accidents at home, 374, 374*f*
  acute, 82
  avoiding, 84–87
  chronic, 83
  first aid for, 398–401
  head, neck, and back, 331, 381, 401
  of the nervous system, 331
  overtraining, 81
  safety equipment, 87
  warning signs of, 80
insulin, 333
integrity, 56
interests, 33, 33*t*, 58
Internet safety, 415
intestines, 334, 334*f*
intoxication, 249, 249*f*, 250*f*
IQ, stress and, 163

"I" statements, 119

jock itch, 352*t*
journal writing, 38

kidney disease, 337. See also **diseases**
kidneys, 336–337, 336*f*
knowing yourself, 57

laughter, importance of, 59, 141, 168
leukemia, 327, 327*f*, 341. See also **cancer**
life expectancy, 367
life jackets, 412
life skills for health, 12–15, 13*t*
lifestyles, healthy, 10, 15
ligaments, 82
liking yourself, 57
listening skills
  active listening, 138
  body language, 41
  during conflicts, 204
  in relationships, 178
liver, 334
long-term goals, 34
LSD, 288
lung cancer, 9, 226. See also **cancer**
lunge exercise, 79*f*
lungs, 226*f*, 282*f*, 328
lymph nodes, 308

M

male reproductive system
  problems of the reproductive system, 352, 352*t*
  reproductive system, 350–353, 350*f*
  self care, 353
  sperm, 351, 351*f*
mania, 146
marijuana, 272, 286–287
maximum heart rate (MHR), 71
MD (muscular dystrophy), 339
media
  alcohol use shown in, 260–261
  influences on body image, 118
  influences on decisions, 30–31
  influences on self-esteem, 53
  smoking shown in, 31, 233
mediation, 207
mediators, 207
medicines, 274–277
  abuse of, 277
  antibiotics, 305
  antiviral, 308
  definition, 274
  inhalers, 272, 272*f*
  misuse of, 276
  over-the-counter, 275, 275*f*
  prescription, 274, 274*f*
  taken by injection, 272
  taken by transdermal patch, 273
  taken orally, 272
Mediterranean diets, 407, 407*f*
meningitis, 341
menstrual cycle, 354–355, 355*f*. See also **female reproductive system**
menstruation, 355–356, 355*f*
mental health, definition of, 5

mental illness, 144–151
  anxiety disorders, 147
  bipolar mood disorder, 146
  definition, 144
  depression, 145
  getting help for, 148–151
  helping others with, 151
  professional help for, 150
  schizophrenia, 146
  signs that help is needed, 148
mentors, 59
metabolism, 95, 332–333
methamphetamine, 284t. *See also* **drugs**
MHR (maximum heart rate), 71
microorganisms, 300
minerals, 100
misdirection, 136
mononucleosis, 308
mood disorders, 145
mountain biking safety, 387f
mouth cancer, 226. *See also* **cancer**
muscles, 338, 419, 419f
muscle soreness, 80
muscular dystrophy (MD), 339
mushrooms, magic, 288. *See also* **drugs**
mycobacteria, 304

natural disasters, 388–391
  earthquakes, 388
  emergency kits, 391, 414
  FEMA, 405
  floods, 390
  preparation for, 391
  tornadoes and hurricanes, 389, 389f
neck injuries, 401. *See also* **injuries**
negative peer pressure, 29

negative thinking, 140
neglect, 182–183
negotiation, 204
nephrons, 336–337
nervous system, 330–331
  anatomy, 330, 330f, 418
  diseases of, 331, 331t
  drug abuse and, 282f
nicotine, 230–231
  addiction to, 230–231
  effects and dangers of, 221, 284t
  quitting smoking and, 235, 273
  in tobacco smoke, 272
Nicotine Replacement Therapy (NRT), 235, 273. *See also* **smoking**
noninfectious diseases, 322–342. *See also specific diseases*
  aging and, 366
  blood diseases, 327
  bone diseases, 339
  causes of, 322t
  definition, 322
  digestive system, 335, 335f
  endocrine system, 333
  of the eyes and ears, 341
  food-related, 410
  heart disease, 325
  muscle diseases, 339
  nervous system, 330f, 331t
  respiratory system, 329
  skin diseases, 339
  urinary system, 337
NRT (Nicotine Replacement Therapy), 235, 273. *See also* **smoking**
nurturing, 181
nutrients. *See also* **diet; nutrition**
  definition, 95
  essential, 98–100
  table of, 408–409t

  vitamins and minerals, 100
  water, 101
nutrition, 94–111. *See also* **diet; nutrients**
  ABCs of, 102, 102t
  carbohydrates, 99
  definition, 94
  Dietary Guidelines for Americans, 102, 102t
  digestion and metabolism, 95
  eating at home, 109
  eating healthfully, 126
  eating out, 108
  essential nutrients, 98–100
  fats, 99
  feelings and, 97, 126
  food choices, 96
  Food Guide Pyramid, 103, 103f
  health and, 94
  Nutrition Facts label, 104–105, 104f
  proteins, 99
  serving sizes and portions, 105
  snacks, 107, 107f
  vitamins and minerals, 100
Nutrition Facts label, 104–105, 104f

obesity, 123. *See also* **diet; weight**
obsessions, 147. *See also* **mental illness**
obsessive-compulsive disorder (OCD), 147. *See also* **mental illness**
open-ended questions, 41
options, 25. *See also* **decisions**

oral cancer, 226. *See also* **cancer**
organs, 322, 323*f*
osteoporosis, 338*f*, 339. *See also* **diet; nutrition**
outdoor safety, 386, 386*f*
ovarian cancer, 356*t*. *See also* **cancer**
ovaries. *See also* **female reproductive system**
  anatomy of, 354, 354*f*
  hormones from, 332*t*, 358*f*, 359*t*
  in menstrual cycle, 355*f*
overexercising, 121. *See also* **exercise**
over-the-counter medicines, 275, 275*f*
overtraining, 81
ovulation, 355, 355*f*. *See also* **female reproductive system**

pain, 80
pancreas, 334, 358*f*
panic attacks, 147. *See also* **mental illness**
panic disorders, 147. *See also* **mental illness**
Pap tests, 357. *See also* **female reproductive system**
parathyroid gland, 332*t*, 358*f*
Parkinson's disease, 331*t*. *See also* **diseases**
peer pressure
  influences on decisions, 29
  positive, 29, 187
  to start smoking, 232
  to use alcohol, 246, 260
  violence and, 209
peers, definition of, 29, 200

pelvic examinations, 357. *See also* **female reproductive system**
penicillin, 305, 305*f*. *See also* **medicines**
penis, 350*f*. *See also* **male reproductive system**
periods (menstrual), 355–356, 355*f*. *See also* **female reproductive system**
peripheral nervous system (PNS), 330
persistence, 37
personal responsibility, 177
phobias, 147. *See also* **mental illness**
phone calls, emergency, 393, 393*f*
phosphorous, 100
physical abuse, 182*t*
physical activity, 127. *See also* **exercise**
Physical Activity Pyramid, 411, 411*f*
physical dependence, 258, 279. *See also* **drugs**
physical fitness, 66–89. *See also* **exercise**
  body composition, 67
  endurance, 66
  exercise and, 68–73
  FIT, 70
  flexibility, 67
  goals for, 70
  heart rate monitoring, 71
  Physical Activity Pyramid, 411, 411*f*
  strength, 66
  tests of, 69, 69*t*
  weight training, 76–79
physical health, 4
physical self-concept, 55
pipe tobacco, 222. *See also* **tobacco**

pituitary gland, 332*t*, 358*f*, 359*t*
PKD (polycystic kidney disease), 337. *See also* **diseases**
placenta, 360
plasma, blood, 326
platelets, 326–327
PNS (peripheral nervous system), 330
poisoning, 374, 399
polycystic kidney disease (PKD), 337. *See also* **diseases**
portions, 105
positive peer pressure, 29, 187
positive self-talk, 58, 58*t*, 140
positive stress, 159. *See also* **stress**
posture, during conflict, 203
potassium, 100
pregnancy, 360–361
  alcohol use during, 255
  fetal development, 360–361
  HIV infection during, 312
  smoking during, 227
prejudice, 136
prescription medicines, 274, 274*f*
preventive healthcare, 11
problems, identifying, 24. *See also* **decisions**
progesterone, 359*t*
projection, as defense mechanism, 165*t*
prostate gland, 350*f*, 351
proteins, 99
psychiatrists, 150
psychological dependence, 279. *See also* **drugs**
psychological fatigue, 163
puberty, changes during, 364

rape, 251, 267
rationalization, 165t
reaction time, alcohol use and, 249f, 250, 256
receptors, nicotine, 230, 230f
recovery, from alcoholism, 259
recovery time, 71
red blood cells, 326
redirection, 167
reframing, 167
refusal skills
  abstinence, 191
  dealing with peer pressure, 42
  drugs, 292, 293t
  using, 43
regression, as defense mechanism, 165t
relationships, 176–193. See also **friends**
  abstinence in, 190–191, 191t
  affection in, 188, 188t
  assertiveness in, 179
  in communities, 184–185
  definition, 176
  drug abuse and, 290
  goals and, 35
  healthy, 176, 186
  positive peer pressure, 187
  teamwork and personal responsibility in, 177
  tolerance in, 184
  unhealthy, 189
relaxation, 167, 236
repetitions, in weight training, 76
repression, as defense mechanism, 165, 165t
reproductive systems, 350–357
  care of, 353
  female, 354–357, 354f
  male, 350–353, 350f
  problems of, 352, 352t, 356, 356t
rescue breathing, 396–397, 396f, 397f
respect, 56, 181, 190
respiratory system, 328–329, 328f
resting heart rate (RHR), 71
retina, 340
rheumatic fever, 303
RICE, 82
rickets, 339
risks, 26, 191
role models, 59

SAD (seasonal affective disorder), 9
sadness, 135
safety, 374–403
  accidents at home, 374
  alcohol and, 252–254
  automobile, 382, 382f
  baby sitter, 416–417
  bicycle, 381, 387f
  in class, 375
  in cold weather, 384
  fire, 378–379
  food, 410
  gun, 376
  home safety tips, 374f
  in hot weather, 385
  Internet, 415
  natural disasters, 388–391
  outdoor adventures, 386, 386–387f
  preparation, 391
  school bus, 383
  staying home alone, 413
  swimming, 386f
  violence at school, 375
  water, 386, 386f, 412
  ways to protect yourself, 377
  in weight training, 77
  while walking, 380
safety equipment
  boating, 412
  helmets, 381
  seat belts, 382
  sports, 87
schizophrenia, 146. See also **mental illness**
school
  conflicts at, 201
  problems from drug abuse, 281, 281f
  safety in class, 375
school bus safety, 383
scrotum, 350f. See also **male reproductive system**
seasonal affective disorder (SAD), 9
seat belts, 382, 382f
self-concept, 54–55
self-esteem, 50–59
  definition, 32, 50
  high and low, 51
  influences on, 52
  keys to, 56
  media and, 53
  from meeting goals, 32
  self-concept and, 54–55
  ways to develop, 57–59
self-talk, 58, 58t, 140
semen, 351
serving sizes, 105
setbacks, 37
sets, in weight training, 76
sex cells, 348
sexual abstinence, 190–191, 191t, 310
sexual abuse, 182t
sexual activity, 190, 191, 253
sexual assaults, 251, 267

sexually transmitted diseases (STDs), 310–313. See also **diseases**
  common, 311, 311*t*
  definition, 310
  in females, 356*t*
  HIV and AIDS, 312–313, 313*f*
  in males, 352*t*
  symptoms, 310
short-term goals, 34
sickle cell anemia, 327
sinus infections, 303, 307*t*
sinusitis, 303
skeletal system, 338–339, 338*f*, 419
skiing safety, 387*f*
skin, 338
skin cancer, 339. See also **cancer**
sleep, stress and, 168
small children, rescue breathing for, 397, 397*f*
smoke detectors, 378
smokeless tobacco, 222, 226, 272
smoking. See also **tobacco**
  addiction to, 230, 230*f*
  advertising, 233
  breaking rules, 228
  cancer from, 226
  cardiovascular disease from, 225
  early effects of, 221
  environmental tobacco smoke, 223
  harmful effects of, 227, 329
  media influences on, 31
  Nicotine Replacement Therapy, 235
  quitting, 234–239
  reasons for, 232–233, 232*t*
  reasons not to start, 239
  relaxation without, 236
  respiratory problems, 224
  social strain, 229
  tolerance, dependence, and withdrawal, 231, 234
snacks, healthy, 107, 107*f*
sneezing, 301, 315, 315*f*
snowboarding safety, 387*f*
social health, 6
social self-concept, 55
social strain, 229
sodium, 100
somatic nervous system, 330
sperm, 351, 351*f*. See also **male reproductive system**
spinal cord, 330
spinal cord injuries, 331
sports
  aerobic and anaerobic energy in, 72–73
  competition, 74
  getting started in, 75
  injuries, 80–87
  overtraining, 81
  sportsmanship, 74
  winning, 75
sportsmanship, 74
sports physicals, 70
spotters, 77
sprains, 82
STDs (sexually transmitted diseases), 310–313. See also **diseases**
  common, 311, 311*t*
  definition, 310
  in females, 356*t*
  HIV and AIDS, 312–313, 313*f*
  in males, 352*t*
  symptoms, 310
stimulants, 284, 284*t*. See also **drugs**
stomach cancer, 335, 335*f*. See also **cancer**
storms, 389–390, 389*f*
strains, 82
strains, of influenza, 207
strength, 66, 69, 76–79
strep throat, 303
stress, 158–171
  avoiding distress, 168–169, 168*f*
  common causes of, 160–161*f*
  coping with, 141
  defense mechanisms, 164–165, 165*t*
  definition, 158
  distress and positive stress, 159
  emotional and mental effects of, 163, 163*t*
  management of, 141, 167
  as part of life, 158
  personal stress inventory, 161
  physical effects of, 162
  violent behavior and, 209
  warning signs, 166, 166*t*
stress fractures, 83, 85
stress management, 141, 167
stressors, 158, 160*f*
stress response, 162
stretching, 67, 84
stroke, 225, 225*f*
suicide, 145
sunscreen, 86, 386
support groups, 235
swimming safety, 386*f*, 412
syphilis, 311*t*. See also **sexually transmitted diseases**

tablets, 271
tar, 220, 272
targeted marketing, 233
target heart rate zone, 71
teachers, conflicts with, 201
teasing, 200, 210
television, body image and, 118. See also **media**
temperature, body, 101
tendinitis, 83, 85
tendons, 82–83
testes (singular, *testis*). See also **male reproductive system**
  anatomy of, 350*f*
  hormones from, 332*t*, 358*f*, 359*t*
  problems of, 352*t*
testicular cancer, 352*t*. See also **cancer**
testicular torsion, 352*t*
testosterone, 359*t*
THC, 286
therapists, 150
therapy, 144
threats, 210
throat cultures, 303
thymus gland, 358*f*
thyroid gland, 332*t*, 358*f*, 359*t*
thyroid hormones, 359*t*
tissues, 322
tobacco, 220–240
  addiction to, 230, 230*f*
  advertising, 233
  breaking rules, 228
  cancer from, 226
  cardiovascular disease from, 225
  chemicals in, 220, 272
  early effects of, 221
  environmental tobacco smoke, 223
  harmful effects of, 227, 329
  Nicotine Replacement Therapy, 235
  quitting, 234–239
  reasons for using, 232–233, 232*t*
  reasons not to start, 239
  relaxation without, 236
  respiratory problems, 224
  smokeless products, 222, 226, 272
  social strain, 229
  tolerance, dependence, and withdrawal, 231, 234
tolerance, in communities, 184–185
tolerance, to tobacco, 231
tornadoes, 389
toxic shock syndrome, 356*t*
transdermal patch, 273
trauma, 352*t*
trichomoniasis, 311*t*
triggers for emotion, 142
trimesters, in pregnancy, 360
tuberculosis, 304, 304*f*
type 1 diabetes, 333
type 2 diabetes, 333
typhoons, 389

ulcerative colitis, 335
ultrasound imagery, 360*f*
umbilical cords, 360
unhealthy eating behaviors, 120. See also **eating disorders**
ureters, 336
urethra, 336, 351
urinary system, 336–337, 336*f*, 420
urinary tract infections (UTIs), 352*t*, 356*t*
urination, 336
urine, 336
uterine cancer, 356*t*. See also **cancer**
uterus, 354*f*, 355*f*. See also **female reproductive system**

vaccines, 307, 309
vagina, 354*f*, 355*f*. See also **female reproductive system**
vaginitis, 356*t*
Valium, 285. See also **medicines**
values
  conflict over, 199
  decisions and, 25
  family influences on, 28
  goals and, 33, 33*t*
vas deferens, 350*f*, 351. See also **male reproductive system**
vegetarian diets, 407, 407*f*
veins, 325, 325*f*
ventricles, 324, 325*f*
verbal communication, 138. See also **communication**
villi, 334*f*
violence, 208–213. See also **conflicts**
  aggression and, 210
  alcohol use and, 254, 267
  conflicts turning into, 209
  definition, 208
  gun safety, 376
  preventing, 212–213

violence *(continued)*
 protecting yourself, 213
 reporting threats, 211
 at school, 375
 signs of, 209
 threats of, 210–211
 walking away, 209, 213
viral infections, 306–309. *See also* **diseases**
 colds, 307, 307*t*
 fighting, 308
 influenza, 307, 307*t*
 mononucleosis, 308
 sinus infections, 307*t*
 spreading of, 306
 symptoms of, 307, 307*t*
 vaccines, 307, 309
viral sinus infections, 307*t*
viruses, 306. *See also* **viral infections**
vitamin A, 100, 104. *See also* **nutrition**
vitamin C, 100, 104. *See also* **nutrition**
vitamins, 100. *See also* **nutrition**
volunteering, 59

walking safety, 380
warm-ups, 84
washing hands, 314
water, importance of, 101, 386, 414
water safety, 386, 386*f*, 412
weather alerts, 389
weight, 115–129. *See also* **diet; fitness; nutrition**
 binge eating disorder and, 123
 drug abuse and, 282*f*
 factors affecting, 125
 fitness and, 67
 keeping a healthy weight, 124, 125
 obesity, 123
 overexercising to control, 121
weight training, 76–79, 78–79*f*, 85. *See also* **exercise**
wellness, 7. *See also* **health**
white blood cells, 326
withdrawal
 from alcohol, 259
 from drugs, 278, 278*f*
 from tobacco, 231, 234

Xanax, 285

Acknowledgments continued from page iv.

Academic Reviewers
(continued)

Marianne Suarez, Ph.D.
Postdoctoral Psychology Fellow
Center on Child Abuse and Neglect
The University of Oklahoma
   Health Sciences Center
Oklahoma City, Oklahoma

Nathan R. Sullivan, M.S.W.
Associate Professor
College of Social Work
The University of Kentucky
Lexington, Kentucky

Josey Templeton, Ed.D.
Associate Professor
Department of Health, Exercise,
   and Sports Medicine
The Citadel, The Military College
   of South Carolina
Charleston, South Carolina

Martin Van Dyke, Ph.D.
Professor of Chemistry Emeritus
Front Range Community College
Westminster, Colorado

Graham Watts, Ph.D.
*Assistant Professor
   of Health and Safety*
The University of Indiana
Bloomington, Indiana

Teacher Reviewers

Dan Aude
Magnet Programs Coordinator
Montgomery Public Schools
Montgomery, Alabama

Judy Blanchard
District Health Coordinator
Newtown Public Schools
Newtown, Connecticut

David Blinn
Secondary Sciences Teacher
Wrenshall School District
Wrenshall, Minnesota

Johanna Chase
School Health Educator
Los Angeles County Office
   of Education
Downey, California

JeNean Erickson
*Sports Coach, Physical Education
   and Health Teacher*
New Prague Middle School
New Prague, Montana

Stacy Feinberg, L.M.H.C.
Family Counselor for Autism
Broward County School System
Coral Gables, Florida

Arthur Goldsmith
Secondary Sciences Teacher
Hallendale High School
Hallendale, Florida

Jacqueline Horowitz-Olstfeld
Exceptional Student Educator
Broward County School District
Fort Lauderdale, Florida

Kathy LaRoe
Teacher
St. Paul School District
St. Paul, Nebraska

Regina Logan
*Sports Coach, Physical Education
   and Health Teacher*
Dade County Middle School
Trenton, Georgia

Alyson Mike
*Sports Coach, Science
   and Health Teacher*
East Valley Middle School
East Helena, Montana

Elizabeth Rustad
*Sports Coach, Life Science
   and Health Teacher*
Centennial Middle School
Yuma, Arizona

Rodney Sandefur
Principal
Nucla Middle School
Nucla, Colorado

Helen Schiller
Science and Health Teacher
Northwood Middle School
Taylor, South Carolina

Gayle Seymour
Health Teacher
Newton Middle School
Newtown, Connecticut

Bert Sherwood
Science and Health Specialist
Socorro Independent School
   District
El Paso, Texas

Beth Truax, R.N.
Science Teacher
Lewiston-Porter Central School
Lewiston, New York

Dan Utley
Sports Coach and Health Teacher
Hilton Head School District
Hilton Head Island, South
   Carolina

Jenny Wallace
Science Teacher
Whitehouse Middle School
Whitehouse, Texas

Kim Walls
Alternative Education Teacher
Lockhart Independent School
   District
Lockhart, Texas

Alexis Wright
Principal, Middle School
Rye Country Day School
Rye, New York

Joe Zelmanski
Curriculum Coordinator
Rochester Adams High School
Rochester Hills, Michigan

Teen Advisory Board

Teachers

Melissa Landrum
Physical Education Teacher
Hopewell Middle School
Round Rock, Texas

Stephanie Scott
Physical Education Teacher
Hopewell Middle School
Round Rock, Texas

Krista Robinson
Physical Education Teacher
Hopewell Middle School
Round Rock, Texas

Teen Advisory Board
(continued)

Hopewell Middle School Students

Efrain Nicolas Avila
Darius T. Bell
Micki Bevka
Kalthoom A. Bouderdaben
La Joya M. Brown
Jennafer Chew
Seth Cowan
Mariana Diaz
Marcus Duran
Timothy Galvan
Megan Ann Giessregen
Shane Harkins
Ryan Landrum
Maria Elizabeth Ortiz Lopez
Travis Wilmer

Staff Credits

Editorial

Robert Todd, *Associate Director, Secondary Science*
Debbie Starr, *Managing Editor*

Senior Editors

Leigh Ann García
Kelly Rizk
Laura Zapanta

Editorial Development Team

Karin Akre
Shari Husain
Kristen McCardel
Laura Prescott
Betsy Roll
Kenneth Shepardson
Ann Welch
David Westerberg

Copyeditors

Dawn Marie Spinozza, *Copyediting Manager*
Anne-Marie De Witt
Jane A. Kirschman
Kira J. Watkins

Editorial Support Staff

Jeanne Graham
Mary Helbling
Shannon Oehler
Stephanie S. Sanchez
Tanu'e White

Editorial Interns

Kristina Bigelow
Erica Garza
Sarah Ray
Kenneth G. Raymond
Kyle Stock
Audra Teinert

Online Products

Bob Tucek, *Executive Editor*
Wesley M. Bain
Catherine Gallagher
Douglas P. Rutley

Production

Eddie Dawson, *Production Manager*
Sherry Sprague, *Senior Production Coordinator*
Mary T. King, *Administrative Assistant*

Design

Book Design

Bruce Bond, *Design Director*
Mary Wages, *Senior Designer*
Cristina Bowerman, *Design Associate*
Ruth Limon, *Design Associate*
Alicia Sullivan, *Designer, Teacher Edition*
Sally Bess, *Designer, Teacher Edition*
Charlie Taliaferro, *Design Associate, Teacher Edition*

Image Acquisitions

Curtis Riker, *Director*
Jeannie Taylor, *Photo Research Supervisor*
Stephanie Morris, *Photo Researcher*
Sarah Hudgens, *Photo Researcher*
Elaine Tate, *Art Buyer Supervisor*
Angela Parisi, *Art Buyer*

Design New Media

Ed Blake, *Design Director*
Kimberly Cammerata, *Design Manager*

Media Design

Richard Metzger, *Director*
Chris Smith, *Senior Designer*

Graphic Services

Kristen Darby, *Director*
Jeff Robinson, *Senior Ancillary Designer*

Cover Design

Bruce Bond, *Design Director*

Design Implementation and Page Production

Preface, Inc., Schaumburg, Illinois

Electronic Publishing

EP Manager

Robert Franklin

EP Team Leaders

Juan Baquera
Sally Dewhirst
Christopher Lucas
Nanda Patel
JoAnn Stringer

Senior Production Artists

Katrina Gnader
Lana Kaupp
Kim Orne

Production Artists

Sara Buller
Ellen Kennedy
Patty Zepeda

Quality Control

Barry Bishop
Becky Golden-Harrell
Angela Priddy
Ellen Rees

New Media

Armin Gutzmer, *Director of Development*
Melanie Baccus, *New Media Coordinator*
Lydia Doty, *Senior Project Manager*
Cathy Kuhles, *Technical Assistant*
Marsh Flournoy, *Quality Assurance Project Manager*
Tara F. Ross, *Senior Project Manager*

Ancillary Development and Production

General Learning Communications, Northbrook, Illinois

Illustration and Photography Credits

Abbreviations used: (t) top, (c) center, (b) bottom, (l) left, (r) right, (bkgd) background

Illustrations

All work, unless otherwise noted, contributed by Holt, Rinehart & Winston.

Chapter One: Chapter One: L1: Page 7 (tr), Leslie Kell; REV: 17 (tr), Leslie Kell.

Chapter Two: L1: Page 22 (b), Marty Roper/Planet Rep; L2: 24 (b), Rita Lascaro; L3: 30 (t), Laura Bailie; L4: 34 (t), Argosy; REV: 45 (tr), Leslie Kell.

Chapter Three: L1: Page 51 (r), Marty Roper/Planet Rep; 52-53 (t), Rita Lascaro; REV: 61 (tr), Leslie Kell; FEA: 62 Laura Bailie.

Chapter Four: L2: Page 68 (b), Marty Roper/Planet Rep; 70 (tl), Argosy; L6: 81 (t), Argosy; L8: 85 (b), Mark Heine.

Chapter Five: L3: Page 104 (c), Argosy; L4: 108 (tr), Argosy; FEA: 112 Argosy.

Chapter Six: L2: Page 118 (bl), (bc), (br), Rick Herman; L4: 125 (b), Argosy; REV: 129 (tr), Leslie Kell.

Chapter Seven: L1: Page 135 (b), Marty Roper/Planet Rep; L5: 150 (tr), Leslie Kell; FEA: 155 Rita Lascaro.

Chapter Eight: L4: Page 168-169 (t), Argosy; FEA: 173 Argosy.

Chapter Nine: L4: Page 187 (tl), Marty Roper/Planet Rep; FEA: 195 Laura Bailie.

Chapter Ten: L1: Page 200 (t), Marty Roper/Planet Rep; L2: 202 (b), Rita Lascaro; 204 (tr), Marty Roper/Planet Rep; L4: 209 (t), Stephen Durke/Washington Artists.

Chapter Eleven: L1: Page 220 (b), Rick Herman; L2: 225 (tl), Christy Krames; L4: 230 (b), Stephen Durke/Washington Artists; L6: 234 (br), Leslie Kell; L7: 238 (b), Leslie Kell.

Chapter Twelve: L2: Page 249 (b), Leslie Kell; 250 (b), Mark Heine; 251 (tr), Mark Heine; L4: 257 (tl), Leslie Kell; L5: 258 (bl), Mark Heine; REV: 265 (tr), Marty Roper/Planet Rep.

Chapter Thirteen: L2: Page 274 (br), Leslie Kell; 275 (t), Leslie Kell; L4: 278 (bl), Leslie Kell; L5: 281 (t), Stephen Durke/Washington Artists; 282 (b), Christy Krames; L7: 287 (t), Mark Heine.

Chapter Fourteen: L1: Page 300 (b), Argosy; L2: 302 (b), Stephen Durke/Washington Artists; L4: 313 (t), Argosy; REV: 317 (tr), Leslie Kell.

Chapter Fifteen: L2: Page 324 (bl), (br), Christy Krames; 326 (br), Leslie Kell; L3: 328 (bl), Christy Krames; L4: 330 (bl), Christy Krames; L5: 332 (bl), Christy Krames; L6: 334 (bl), Christy Krames; L7: 336 (bl), Christy Krames; L8: 338 (bl), Christy Krames; L9: 340 (bl), (br), Christy Krames; REV: 343 (tr), Leslie Kell.

Chapter Sixteen: L2: Page 350 (b), Christy Krames; L3: 354 (b), Christy Krames; 355 (t), Christy Krames; L4: 358 (b), Christy Krames; REV: 369 (tr), Leslie Kell; FEA: 371 Laura Bailie.

Chapter Seventeen: L2: Page 378 (b), Argosy; 379 (tl), (tr), Mark Heine; L3: 382 (t), Leslie Kell; L4: 386 (tl), (tr), Stephen Durke/Washington Artists; 387 (tl), (tr), Stephen Durke/Washington Artists; L6: 393 (cl), Argosy; L7: 396 (b), Marcia Hartsock/The Medical Art Company; 397 (t), Marcia Hartsock/The Medical Art Company; REV: 403 (tr), Leslie Kell.

Appendix: 406 (c), Argosy; 407 (cl), (bl), (cr), Rick Herman; 411 (c), Rick Herman; 413 (br), Argosy; 418 (tl), (tr), Christy Krames; 419 (tl), (br), Christy Krames; 420 (tl), (tr), Christy Krames; 421 (tl), (tr), Christy Krames.

Photography

Cover: Gary Russ/HRW.

Table of Contents: v, Index Stock Imagery; vi (t), Peter Van Steen/HRW; (b), Victoria Smith/HRW; vii (t), Sam Dudgeon/HRW; (b), Jim Cummins/Getty Images/FPG International; viii (t), Bill Bachmann/The Image Works; (b), Sam Dudgeon/HRW; ix (tl), David Young-Wolff/PhotoEdit; (bl), Thom DeSanto Photography, Inc./StockFood; (br), John Kelly/Getty Images/Stone; x (tl,tr), Sam Dudgeon/HRW; (bl), Image Copyright 2004 PhotoDisc, Inc.; xi (t), Dennis Curran/Index Stock; (c), David Young-Wolff/PhotoEdit; (b), Catrina Genovese/Index Stock; xii (t), Image Copyright 2004 PhotoDisc, Inc.; (b), Michael Newman/PhotoEdit; xiii (t), David Young-Wolff/PhotoEdit; (b), Myrleen Ferguson Cate/PhotoEdit; xiv (t), Mary Kate Denny/PhotoEdit; (b), Image Copyright 2004 PhotoDisc, Inc.; xv (t), Yoav Levy/Phototake; (b), Kwame Zikomo/Superstock; xvi (t), Index Stock/Steve Stroud; (bl), E. Dygas/Getty Images/FPG International; (br), Mark Reinstein/Index Stock; xvii (t), Image Copyright 2004 PhotoDisc, Inc.; (b), Damien Lovegrove/SPL/Photo Researchers, Inc.; xviii (t), Peter Van Steen/HRW; (b), A. Davidhazy/Custom Medical Stock Photo; xix (t), Paul Windsor/Getty Images/FPG International; (bl), Gavin Wickham; Eye Ubiquitous/Corbis; (br), Microworks/Phototake; xx (t,bl), David Young-Wolff/PhotoEdit; (br), Duomo/Corbis; xxi (t), Sam Dudgeon/HRW; (bl), Bob Daemmrich/The Image Works; xxii (t), Victoria Smith/HRW; (c), Sam Dudgeon/HRW; (b), PhotoSpin, Inc.; xxiii, Network Productions/Index Stock; xv, Victoria Smith/HRW.

Chapter One: 2-3, SW Productions/Index Stock Imagery, Inc.; L1: 4, Sean Cayton/The Image Works; 5, Dana White/PhotoEdit; 6, Paul A. Souders/Corbis; 7, Victoria Smith/HRW; L2: 8, Dick Luria/Getty Images/FPG International; 9, AP Photo/Steve Frischling; L3: 10, Victoria Smith/HRW; 11, David Young-Wolff/PhotoEdit; L4: 12 (all), Peter Van Steen/HRW; 14,

Photography (continued)

Rachel Epstein/PhotoEdit; 15, Jennie Woodcock; Reflections Photolibrary/Corbis; FEA: 18, Gibson Photography; 19, Jose Luis Pelaez, Inc./Corbis.

Chapter Two: 20-21, Denis Felix/Getty Images/FPG International; L1: 23, Bob Mitchell/Corbis; L2: 25, Sam Dudgeon/HRW; 26, Sam Dudgeon/HRW; 27, David Young-Wolff; L3: 28, Jonathan Nourok/PhotoEdit; 29, Ghislain & Marie David de Lossy/Getty Images/The Image Bank; 31, Amy E. Conn/AP/Wide World Photos; L4: 32, Jim Cummins/Getty Images/FPG International; 33, Image Copyright 2004 PhotoDisc, Inc.; 35, Mary Kate Denny/PhotoEdit; L5: 36, Mug Shots/Corbis Stock Market; 37 (l), Mark Humphrey, AP Staff; (r), Mark J. Terrill, AP Staff; L6: 38, David Madison/Getty Images/Stone; 39 (all), Peter Van Steen/HRW; L7: 40, Cleve Bryant/PhotoEdit; 41, David Young-Wolff/PhotoEdit; FEA: 46, LWA-Dann Tardif/Corbis; 47, Armen Kachaturian/Comstock.

Chapter Three: 48-49, Maria Taglienti/Getty Images/The Image Bank; L1: 50, Corbis Images/PictureQuest; L2: 54, Index Stock/Table Mesa Prod.; 55 (all), Victoria Smith/HRW; L3: 56, Tom Stewart/Corbis Stock Market; 57, Tom Stewart/Corbis; 59, Bill Bachmann/The Image Works; FEA: 63, David Young-Wolff/PhotoEdit.

Chapter Four: 64-65, Richard Hutchings/Corbis; L1: 66, Terje Rakke/Getty Images/The Image Bank; 67, A. Ramey/PhotoEdit; L2: 69, Image Stock/Omni Photo Communications Inc.; 71, Tom Prettyman/PhotoEdit; L3: 72 (l), Dennis MacDonald/PhotoEdit; (r), Sylvain Grandadam/Getty Images/Stone; 73, Index Stock/Ellen Skye; L4: 74, David Young-Wolff/PhotoEdit; 75, John Langford/HRW; L5: 76, Steve Smith/Getty Images/FPG International; 77, Bob Rowan; Progressive Image/Corbis; 78 (all), Sam Dudgeon/HRW; 79 (all), Sam Dudgeon/HRW; L6: 80, Shelby Thorner/David Madison; L7: 82, Mark E. Gibson/Gibson Stock Photography; 83, Dana White/PhotoEdit; 84, Spencer Grant/PhotoEdit; 86, David Young-Wolff/PhotoEdit; 87, Steve Bly/Getty Images/Stone; FEA: 90, Victoria Smith/HRW; 91, Tony Freeman/PhotoEdit.

Chapter Five: 92-93, Getty Images/The Image Bank; L1: 94 (all), Peter Van Steen/HRW; 95 (b), Corbis Images/HRW; (c), Image Copyright 2004 PhotoDisc, Inc./HRW; (bl), Image Copyright 2004 PhotoDisc, Inc.; (tr,tl), Sam Dudgeon/HRW; 96, Index Stock/Lonnie Duka; 97, David Young-Wolff/PhotoEdit; L2: 98, Don Couch/HRW; 99 (t), Thom DeSanto Photography, Inc./StockFood; (c), Steven Mark Needham/FoodPix; (b), Brian Hagiwara/Getty Images/FoodPix; 100 (c), PhotoSpin, Inc.; (br,tl,cl,cr,t), Image Copyright (c)2004 PhotoDisc, Inc./HRW; (bl,cl), Corbis Images/HRW; Richard Hutchings; L3: 103, John Kelly/Getty Images/Stone; 105, Victoria Smith/HRW; L4: 106 (tr), Index Stock/Roberto Santos; (tl), Thomas Eckerle/Getty Images/FoodPix; (bc), Eisenhut & Mayer/Getty Images/FoodPix; 108 (all), Peter Van Steen/HRW; 109 (l), John Langford/HRW; (r), Victoria Smith/HRW; FEA: 113, Myrleen Ferguson Cate/PhotoEdit.

Chapter Six: 114-15, James Muldowney/Getty Images/Stone; L1: 116,117, Image Copyright 2004 PhotoDisc, Inc.; L2: 118 (l), Camille/Getty Images/FPG International; (c), Anne-Marie Weber/Getty Images/FPG International; (r), Lawrence Manning/Getty Images; L3: 120, Peter Van Steen/HRW; 123, Mary Kate Denny/PhotoEdit; L4: 124, Sam Dudgeon/HRW; 126 (all), Sam Dugeon/HRW; 127, Robert Brenner/PhotoEdit; FEA: 130 (t,b), Burke/Triolo Productions/FoodPix; (c), Brian Hagiwara/FoodPix; 131, Chuck Savage/Corbis.

Chapter Seven: 132-33, E. Dygas/Getty Images/FPG International; L1: 134, Mary Kate Denny/PhotoEdit; 136, Davis Barber/PhotoEdit; L2: 138, Jack Hollingsworth/Corbis; 139, Burstein Collection/Corbis; L3: 140, Sam Dudgeon/HRW; 141, Index Stock/Dennis Curran; 142, Index Stock/Catrina Genovese; 143, David Young-Wolff/PhotoEdit; L4: 144, Bruce Ayres/Getty Images/Stone; 145, David Kelly Crow/PhotoEdit; 146, Hulton Archive/Getty Images; 147, Image Copyright 2004 PhotoDisc, Inc.; L5: 148, Image Copyright 2004 PhotoDisc, Inc.; 149, Image 100/Royalty-Free/Corbis; 150, Tom Stewart/Corbis Stock Market; 151, Dennis MacDonald/PhotoEdit; FEA: 154, David Young-Wolff/PhotoEdit.

Chapter Eight: 156-57 Kelly/Corbis; L1: 158 (l), Mary Kate Denny/PhotoEdit; (r), Will Hart/PhotoEdit; 159 (l), Michael Newman/PhotoEdit; (r), Tony Freeman/PhotoEdit; 160, PhotoDisc, Inc.; L2: 162, Russell Dian/HRW; L3: 164, David Young-Wolff/PhotoEdit; L4: 167 (c), David Young-Wolff/PhotoEdit; (t), Jonathan Nourok/PhotoEdit; (b), David Young-Wolff/PhotoEdit; FEA: 173, Ian Shaw/Getty Images/Stone.

Chapter Nine: 174-75, David M. Grossman/Photo Researchers, Inc.; L1: 176, JILL SABELLA/Getty Images/FPG International; 177, Mark Gibson; 178 (l), Victoria Smith/HRW; (r), Sam Dudgeon/HRW; 179, David Young-Wolff/PhotoEdit; L2: 180, Bob Daemmrich/Bob Daemmrich Photo, Inc.; 181, Myrleen Ferguson Cate/PhotoEdit; 183, Mary Kate Denny/PhotoEdit; L3: 184, Index Stock/Jeff Greenberg; 185, Syracuse Newspapers/The Image Works; L4: 186, David Young-Wolff/PhotoEdit; 188, Zigy Kaluzny/Getty Images/Stone; 189, Index Stock/SW Production; L5: 190, David Young-Wolff/PhotoEdit; FEA: 194, Kwame Zikomo/SuperStock.

Chapter Ten: 196-97, SW Productions/Index Stock Imagery, Inc.; L1: 198, Index Stock/SW Production; 199, Image Copyright 2004 PhotoDisc, Inc.; 201, Mug Shots/CorbisStock Market; L2: 203 (all), Sam Dudgeon/HRW; 205 (all), Peter Van Steen/HRW; L3: 207, Mary Kate Denny/PhotoEdit; L4: 208, Sam Dudgeon/HRW; 210, Mary Kate Denny/PhotoEdit; 211, Michael Newman/PhotoEdit; L5: 212, David Young-Wolff/PhotoEdit; 213, Image Copyright 2004 PhotoDisc, Inc.; FEA: 216, Mark Richards/PhotoEdit; 217, Mary Kate Denny/PhotoEdit.

Chapter Eleven: 218-19, Joe McBride/Getty Images/Stone; L1: 221, Bill Aron/PhotoEdit; 222, Peter Van Steen/HRW; 223, Index Stock/Doug Mazell; L2: 224, Spencer Grant/PhotoEdit; 225, Moredun Scientific/Photo

Researchers; 226 (b), AP Photo/Eric Paul Erickson; (tl), Siebert/Custom Medical Stock Photo; (tr), SIU BioMed/Custom Medical Stock Photo; 227, Yoav Levy/Phototake; L3: 228, Index Stock/Brian Drake; 229, Ron Chapple/Getty Images/FPG International; L4: 231, Victoria Smith/HRW; L5: 233, Corbis Stock Market; L6: 235, Victoria Smith/HRW; 236, Bob Child/AP/Wide World Photos; 237, David Young-Wolff/PhotoEdit; L7: 239, Kwame Zikomo/Superstock; FEA: 242, Peter Van Steen/HRW; 243, Image Copyright 2004 PhotoDisc, Inc.

Chapter Twelve: 244-45, Corbis Images/HRW; L1: 246, Tony Arruza/Corbis; 247, E. Dygas/Getty Images/FPG International; L2: 248, Index Stock/David Davis; L3: 52, David Young-Wolff/PhotoEdit; 253, Image Copyright 2004 PhotoDisc, Inc.; 254, Rachel Epstein/PhotoEdit; 255, George Steinmetz; L4: 256, Index Stock/Mark Reinstein; L5: 259, Spencer Grant/PhotoEdit; L6: 260, Index Stock/SW Production; 261, Chuck Savage/Corbis; L7: 262, Myrleen Ferguson Cate/PhotoEdit; 263, Index Stock/Steve Stroud; FEA: 266, Victoria Smith/HRW; 267, EyeWire.

Chapter Thirteen: 268-69, David Young-Wolff/PhotoEdit; L1: 270, Victoria Smith/HRW; 271 (t), Jonathan Nourok/PhotoEdit; (b), Image Copyright 2004 PhotoDisc, Inc./HRW; 272, Damien Lovegrove/SPL/Photo Researchers, Inc.; 273, Victoria Smith/HRW; L3: 276, Walter Hodges/Getty Images/Stone; 277, Michael P. Gadomski/Photo Researchers; L4: 278, Mike Siluk/The Image Works; 279, Jeff Greenberg/PhotoEdit; L5: 280, Image Copyright 2004 PhotoDisc, Inc.; 282, Victoria Smith/HRW; 283, Paul Conklin/PhotoEdit; L6: 285, Peter Van Steen/HRW; L7: 286, Henry Diltz/Corbis; L8: 288, H. Schleichkorn/Custom Medical Stock Photo; 289, Tom Stewart/Corbis; L9: 290, Network Productions/Index Stock; 291, Skjold Photographs; 294, Index Stock/Dave Ryan; FEA: 296, PUSH/Index Stock; 297, Eric Horan/Index Stock.

Chapter Fourteen: 298-99, Bob Daemmrich/Stock Boston; L1: 301, Ghislain & Marie David de Lossy/Getty Images/The Image Bank; L2: 303 (l), DR Marazzi Science Photo Library; (r), Barts Medical Library/Phototake; 304 (l), Sam Dudgeon/HRW; (r), Barts Medical Library/Phototake; 305 (l), Corbis; (r), Bettmann/Corbis; L3: 306 (l), CDC/Photo Researchers, Inc.; (r), Kwangshin Kim/Photo Researchers, Inc.; 308, Peter Van Steen/HRW; 309, Michael Newman/PhotoEdit; L4: 310, Victoria Smith/HRW; 312, AP Photo/Amy Sancetta; L5: 314, T.Bannor/Custom Medical Stock Photo; 315, A. Davidhazy/Custom Medical Stock Photo; FEA: 318 (t), Image Copyright 2004 PhotoDisc, Inc.; (b), EyeWire; 319, Will Hart/PhotoEdit.

Chapter Fifteen: 320-21, Kindra Clineff/Index Stock Imagery, Inc.; L2: 324, Sam Dudgeon/HRW; 325, Lester V. Bergman/Corbis; 326 (all), Custom Medical Stock Photo; 327 (tr), Microworks/Phototake; (tl), Sam Dudgeon/HRW; (l), Microworks/Phototake; L3: 328 (l), Sam Dudgeon/HRW; (c), Clark Overton/Phototake; (r), Custom Medical Stock Photo; 329, Mary Steinbacher/PhotoEdit; L4: 330 (r), Collection CNRI/Phototake; (l), Sam Dudgeon/HRW; L5: 332, Sam Dudgeon/HRW; 333, Paul Windsor/Getty Images/FPG International; L6: 334 (l), Sam Dudgeon/HRW; (r), Eye Of Science/Photo Researchers; 335, Salisbury District Hospital/Photo Researchers; L7: 336 (l), Sam Dudgeon/HRW; (c), Lester V. Bergman/Corbis; (r), Siebert/Custom Medical Stock Photo; 337, Jay Daniel/Photo 20-20/PictureQuest; L8: 338 (l), Sam Dudgeon/HRW; 338 (c,r), P. Motta/Photo Researchers; L9: 341, Gavin Wickham/Eye Ubiquitous/Corbis; FEA: 344, Gabriela Medina/SuperStock; 345, Mary Kate Denny/PhotoEdit.

Chapter Sixteen: 346-47, Richard Hutching/Photo Researchers; L1: 348 (br, bl), Michael Newman/PhotoEdit; (bc), Skjold Photographs; 349, Courtesy Mary Wages; L2: 351, C.N.R.I./Phototake; 353, Duomo/Corbis; L3: 357, Will Hart/PhotoEdit; L4: 358, Sam Dudgeon/HRW; L5: 360, EURELIOS/Phototake; 361 (t), Lennart Nilsson; (c), Claude Edelmann/Photo Reseachers; (b), Lennart Nilsson/Albert Bonniers Forlag AB, A CHILD IS BORN; 362 (tl), Courtesy Leigh Ann Garcia; (tr), David Young-Wolff/PhotoEdit; 363 (tl), Painet Inc./Cleo Freelance Photography; (tr), Tom Stewart/Corbis; L6: 364, 365, 366, 367, David Young-Wolff/PhotoEdit; FEA: 370, Image Copyright 2004 PhotoDisc, Inc.; 371, Victoria Smith/HRW.

Chapter Seventeen: 372-73, Stephen Simpson/Getty Images/FPG International; L1: 375, Sam Dudgeon/HRW; 376, West Stock; 377, Spencer Ainsley/The Image Works; L3: 380, Dana White/PhotoEdit; 381, Index Stock/Don Romero; 383, Tom Stewart/Corbis Stock Market; L4: 384, Richard Hutchings/PhotoEdit; 385, Bob Daemmrich/The Image Works; L5: 388, Roger Ressmeyer/Corbis; 390, Chris Todd/Getty Images; 391, Peter Van Steen/HRW; L6: 392, Peter Van Steen/HRW; L7: 394, Watson/Custom Medical Stock Photo; 395 (all), Peter Van Steen/HRW; L8: 398, Peter Van Steen/HRW; 400, SPL/Photo Researchers, Inc.; 401, G. Brad Lewis/Getty Images/Stone; FEA: 404, Victoria Smith/HRW; 405, Lonnie Duka/Index Stock.

Appendix: 410, Victoria Smith/HRW; 411 (tr), Nathan Bilow/Getty Images; (cr), David Young-Wolff/PhotoEdit; (br), Davis Barber/PhotoEdit; (tl), Mark Gibson Photography; 412, Terje Rakke/Getty Images/The Image Bank; 414, Peter Van Steen/HRW; 415, 416, Mary Kate Denny/PhotoEdit; 417, Victoria Smith/HRW.